ENDOSCOPIC
SURGERY

Frederick L. Greene, M.D.
Professor of Surgery
Director of Surgical Oncology and Surgical Endoscopy
University of South Carolina School of Medicine
Columbia, South Carolina

Jeffrey L. Ponsky, M.D.
Professor of Surgery
Case Western Reserve University School of Medicine
Director, Department of Surgery
Mount Sinai Medical Center
Cleveland, Ohio

W.B. SAUNDERS COMPANY
A Division of Harcourt Brace & Company
Philadelphia   London   Toronto   Montreal   Sydney   Tokyo

W.B. SAUNDERS COMPANY
A Division of
Harcourt Brace & Company

The Curtis Center
Independence Square West
Philadelphia, Pennsylvania 19106

Library of Congress Cataloging-in-Publication Data

Endoscopic surgery / [edited by] Frederick L. Greene,
Jeffrey L. Ponsky.

    p.   cm.

ISBN 0–7216–4504–6

1. Endoscopic surgery.   2. Endoscopy.   I. Greene, Frederick L.
  II. Ponsky, Jeffrey L.

[DNLM: 1. Endoscopy—methods.   2. Surgery, Operative—methods. WO
500 E5652 1994]

RD33.53.E533 1994

617′.05—dc20

DNLM/DLC   93–4600

ENDOSCOPIC SURGERY   ISBN 0–7216–4504–6

Printed in the United States of America

Last digit is the print number: 9   8   7   6   5   4   3   2   1

Contributors

Frederick W. Ackroyd, M.D.
Associate Professor of Surgery,
Harvard Medical School; Visiting
Surgeon, Massachusetts General
Hospital, Boston, Massachusetts.
Complications of Flexible Endoscopy

David B. Adams, M.D.
Associate Professor of Surgery and
Head, Section of General and
Gastrointestinal Surgery, Medical
University of South Carolina,
Charleston, South Carolina.
*Endoscopic Management of
Esophageal Stricture*

Mohan C. Airan, M.D.
Clinical Professor of Surgery,
Chicago Medical School; Associate
Chairman, Department of Surgery,
Mount Sinai Hospital Medical
Center, Chicago, Illinois.
Laparoscopic Cholangiography

Riccardo G. Annibali, M.D.
Research Fellow, Creighton
University School of Medicine,
Omaha, Nebraska.
Laparoscopic Inguinal Hernia Repair

George Berci, M.D.
Clinical Professor of Surgery, UCLA
School of Medicine; Senior
Consultant, Department of Surgery,

Cedars-Sinai Medical Center, Los
Angeles, California.
*History of Endoscopic Surgery;
Intraoperative Biliary Endoscopy*

Kenneth F. Binmoeller, M.D.
Lecturer, University of Hamburg
School of Medicine; Senior
Consultant, Department of
Endoscopic Surgery, University
Hospital Eppendorf, Hamburg,
Germany.
*Endoscopic Management of
Malignant Biliary Obstruction*

Joe W. R. Bolton, M.D.
Staff Cardiothoracic Surgeon,
Wilford Hall, USAF Medical Center,
Lackland Air Force Base, Texas;
Clinical Assistant Professor,
University of Texas Health Science
Center, Division of Cardiothoracic
Surgery, San Antonio, Texas.
Bronchoscopy and Mediastinoscopy

Brock M. Bordelon, M.D.
Resident, University of Utah
Hospital, Salt Lake City, Utah.
Endoscopic Technology

Talmadge A. Bowden, Jr., M.D.
Professor of Surgery, Medical
College of Georgia; Consultant in
Surgery, Veterans Administration
Hospital; Consultant in Surgery,

University Hospital, Augusta, Georgia.
Small Bowel Enteroscopy and Intraoperative Endoscopy

Gerhard Buess, M.D.

Professor of Minimally Invasive Surgery, Klinikum Schnarrenberg, Eberhard-Karls-Universität, Tübingen, Germany.
Transanal Microsurgical Techniques

Denis Collet, M.D., Ph.D.

Associate Professor of Surgery, University of Bordeaux; Surgeon, Surgical Unit, Laparoscopic Center, Bordeaux, France.
Laparoscopic Cholecystectomy

Alfred Cuschieri, M.D.

Professor and Chairman, Department of Surgery, Ninewells Hospital and Medical School, Dundee, Scotland.
Minimal Access Approaches for the Treatment of Peptic Ulcer Disease

Thomas L. Dent, M.D.

Professor of Surgery, Temple University School of Medicine, Philadelphia, Pennsylvania; Chairman, Department of Surgery, Abington Memorial Hospital, Abington, Pennsylvania.
Credentialing and Privileging for Endoscopic and Laparoscopic Surgery

Philip E. Donahue, M.D.

Professor of Surgery, University of Illinois at Chicago; Chairman, General Surgery, Cook County Hospital; Attending Surgeon, University of Illinois Hospital; Senior Attending Surgeon, Rush-Presbyterian-St. Luke's Medical Center; Attending Surgeon, West Side Veterans Administration Hospital, Chicago, Illinois.
Endoscopic Evaluation of the Postoperative Stomach

Marc L. Eckhauser, M.D.

Associate Professor of Surgery and Director, Surgical Endoscopy, Metro Health Medical Center, Case Western Reserve University, Cleveland, Ohio.
Endoscopic Transintestinal Ultrasonography

Michael Edye, M.D.

Assistant Professor, Division of Laparoscopic Surgery, Department of Surgery, Mount Sinai School of Medicine, New York, New York.
Laparoscopic Cholecystectomy

Francis D. Ferdinand, M.D.

Chief Resident in Thoracic Surgery, University of Chicago, Pritzker School of Medicine, Chicago, Illinois; Formerly, Chief Resident in General Surgery, The Medical College of Pennsylvania, Philadelphia, Pennsylvania.
Bronchoscopy and Mediastinoscopy

Charles J. Filipi, M.D., F.A.C.S.

Assistant Professor, Creighton University School of Medicine, Omaha, Nebraska; Attending Physician, St. Joseph Hospital, Omaha, Nebraska; Consultant, Memorial Community Hospital, Blair, Nebraska.
Laparoscopic Inguinal Hernia Repair

Robert J. Fitzgibbons, Jr., M.D.

Professor, Chief of Division of General Surgery, Creighton University and St. Joseph Hospital, Omaha, Nebraska.
Laparoscopic Inguinal Hernia Repair

Kenneth A. Forde, M.D.

Professor of Clinical Surgery, College of Physicians and Surgeons, Columbia University; Attending Surgeon, Presbyterian Hospital, New York, New York.
Technique of Diagnostic Colonoscopy

Vito Forte, M.D.

Assistant Professor of Otolaryngology, Faculty of Medicine,

University of Toronto; Staff
Otolaryngologist, Hospital for Sick
Children, Toronto, Ontario, Canada.
Endoscopic Surgery in Children

Ali Ghazi, M.D.
Associate Professor of Clinical
Surgery, Mount Sinai School of
Medicine; Attending Surgeon, Beth
Israel Medical Center, New York,
New York.
*Endoscopic Techniques of
Sphincterotomy*

Frederick L. Greene, M.D.
Professor of Surgery, Director of
Surgical Oncology and Surgical
Endoscopy, University of South
Carolina School of Medicine,
Columbia, South Carolina.
*Esophagogastroduodenoscopy:
Indications, Technique, and
Interpretation; Endoscopic Screening
and Surveillance for Gastrointestinal
Malignancy; Endoscopic
Management of Gastrointestinal
Tract Foreign Bodies*

Timothy R. S. Harward, M.D.
Assistant Professor of Surgery,
University of Florida College of
Medicine; Attending Physician,
Shands Hospital; Staff Surgeon,
Veterans Administration Hospital,
Gainesville, Florida.
*Angioscopy in Peripheral Vascular
Disease*

Harry S. Himal, M.D.
Associate Professor, Department of
Surgery, University of Toronto,
Toronto, Ontario, Canada.
*Endoscopic Techniques of
Sphincterotomy*

John G. Hunter, M.D.
Associate Professor of Surgery,
Emory University School of
Medicine; Chief of Gastrointestinal
Surgery, Emory University Hospital,
Atlanta, Georgia.
Endoscopic Technology

Anthony L. Joseph, M.D.
Resident Physician in Surgery,
Wayne State University Affiliated
Hospitals, Detroit, Michigan.
*Management of Nonvariceal Upper
Gastrointestinal Bleeding*

Sung-Tao Ko, M.D.
Clinical Professor of Surgery,
Chicago Medical School; Chief,
Department of Surgical Endoscopy,
Mount Sinai Hospital Medical Center
of Chicago, Chicago, Illinois.
Laparoscopic Cholangiography

Howard L. Levine, M.D.
Adjunct Member, Department of
Otolaryngology and Communication
Disorders, Cleveland Clinic
Foundation; Chief, Section of Nasal-
Sinus Surgery, Division of
Otolaryngology, Department of
Surgery, Mount Sinai Medical
Center, Cleveland, Ohio.
*Nasopharyngeal and Laryngeal
Endoscopy*

Bradley S. Litke, M.D.
General Surgical Resident, and
Laparoendoscopic Surgical Fellow,
Creighton University, Omaha,
Nebraska.
Laparoscopic Inguinal Hernia Repair

Thom E Lobe, M.D.
Chairman, Section of Pediatric
Surgery, University of Tennessee
Medical School, LeBonheur
Children's Medical Center, St. Jude
Children's Research Hospital,
Memphis, Tennessee.
Endoscopic Surgery in Children

Bruce V. MacFadyen, Jr., M.D.
Professor, Department of Surgery,
The University of Texas Medical
School; Attending Physician,
Hermann Hospital and M. D.
Anderson Hospital and Tumor
Institute, Houston, Texas.
*Endoscopic Placement of Enteral
Feeding Tubes*

Gerald Marks, M.D.
Professor, Jefferson Medical College
of Thomas Jefferson University;
Director, Division of Colorectal
Surgery, Thomas Jefferson University
Hospital, Philadelphia, Pennsylvania.
*Anoscopy and Flexible Fiberoptic
Sigmoidoscopy: Evaluation of the
Distal 50 Cm of Colorectum*

John Marks, M.D.
Chief Surgical Resident, Department
of Surgery, Thomas Jefferson
University Hospital, Philadelphia,
Pennsylvania.
*Anoscopy and Flexible Fiberoptic
Sigmoidoscopy: Evaluation of the
Distal 50 Cm of Colorectum*

Daniel T. Martin, M.D.
Assistant Professor of Surgery,
Division of Surgical Endoscopy and
Laparoscopy, Department of Surgery,
University of New Mexico School of
Medicine; Attending Surgeon,
University of New Mexico Hospital
and Albuquerque Veterans
Administration Medical Center,
Albuquerque, New Mexico.
*Laparoscopic Surgery of the
Gastrointestinal Tract*

J. Barry McKernan, M.D., Ph.D.
Clinical Professor, The Medical
College of Georgia, Augusta,
Georgia; Attending Physician at
Metropolitan Hospital and HCA West
Paces Ferry Hospital, Atlanta,
Georgia; Attending Physician,
Kennestone Hospital, Marietta,
Georgia.
Laparoscopic Appendectomy

Anna D. Miller, R.N.
Head Nurse, Department of Surgery,
University of Virginia Health
Sciences Center, Charlottesville,
Virginia.
*Cleaning and Disinfecting
Endoscopic Equipment*

Jacques Périssat, M.D.
Professor of Surgery, University of
Bordeaux; Head of Surgical Unit,
Head of Laparoscopic Center,
Bordeaux, France.
Laparoscopic Cholecystectomy

Edward H. Phillips, M.D.
Clinical Associate Professor of
Surgery, University of Southern
California and Los Angeles County
Hospital; Attending Surgeon, Cedars-
Sinai Medical Center and Century
City Hospital, Los Angeles,
California.
*Laparoscopic Approaches to the
Common Bile Duct*

Jeffrey L. Ponsky, M.D.
Professor of Surgery, Case Western
Reserve University School of
Medicine; Director, Department of
Surgery, Mount Sinai Medical
Center, Cleveland, Ohio.
*Percutaneous Endoscopic
Gastrostomy and Jejunostomy;
Endoscopic Retrograde
Cholangiopancreatography;
Endoscopic Retrograde
Cholangiopancreatography and the
Management of Common Bile Duct
Stones*

Carolyn E. Reed, M.D.
Associate Professor of Surgery,
Division of Cardiothoracic Surgery,
Medical University of South
Carolina, Charleston, South Carolina.
*Diagnostic and Therapeutic
Thoracoscopy*

William P. Reed, M.D.
Professor of Surgery, Tufts
University School of Medicine,
Boston, Massachusetts; Director of
Surgical Oncology, Baystate Medical
Center, Springfield, Massachusetts.
*Endoscopic Screening and
Surveillance for Gastrointestinal
Malignancy*

Jonathan M. Sackier, M.B.
Associate Professor of Surgery,
University of California, San Diego
School of Medicine, San Diego,
California.
Emergent Laparoscopy

Samir Said, M.D.
Department of Surgery, University of
Cologne, Köln, Germany
Transanal Microsurgical Techniques

Giovanni M. Salerno, M.D.
Laparoscopic Research Fellow,
Creighton University and St. Joseph
Hospital, Omaha, Nebraska.
Laparoscopic Inguinal Hernia Repair

Richard M. Satava, M.D.
Special Assistant to the Director,
Biomedical Technology for
Advanced Research Projects Agency
(ARPA), Arlington, Maryland;
Associate Professor, Department of
Surgery, Uniformed Services
University of Health Science,
Bethesda, Maryland.
*Endoscopic Training for the General
Surgeon*

Bruce D. Schirmer, M.D.
Associate Professor of Surgery,
University of Virginia Health
Sciences Center, Charlottesville,
Virginia.
Complications of Laparoscopy

Robert E. Schmieg, Jr., M.D.
Resident in General Surgery,
University of Virginia, University of
Virginia Health Sciences Center,
Charlottesville, Virginia.
*Cleaning and Disinfecting
Endoscopic Equipment*

Theodore R. Schrock, M.D.
Professor of Surgery, University of
California, San Francisco School of
Medicine, San Francisco, California.
*Colonoscopy in the Diagnosis and
Treatment of Colorectal Malignancy*

James M. Seeger, M.D.
Professor and Chief, Section of
Vascular Surgery, Department of
Surgery, University of Florida
College of Medicine; Attending
Physician, Shands Hospital; Staff
Surgeon, Veterans Administration
Hospital, Gainesville, Florida.
*Angioscopy in Peripheral Vascular
Disease*

Hiromi Shinya, M.D.
Clinical Professor of Surgery, Mount
Sinai School of Medicine; Chief of
Surgical Endoscopy Unit, Beth Israel
Medical Center, New York, New
York.
*Therapeutic Colonoscopy:
Polypectomy, Management of
Bleeding, and Decompressive
Techniques*

Irwin B. Simon, M.D.
Director of Surgical Endoscopy, Silas
B. Hays Army Hospital, Fort Ord,
California.
*Endoscopic Training for the General
Surgeon*

Nib Soehendra, M.D.
Professor of Surgery, University of
Hamburg Medical School; Head,
Department of Endoscopic Surgery,
University Hospital Eppendorf,
Hamburg, Germany.
*Endoscopic Management of
Malignant Biliary Obstruction*

Thomas A. Stellato, M.D.
Professor of Surgery, Case Western
Reserve University School of
Medicine; Chief, Division of General
Surgery, University Hospitals of
Cleveland, Cleveland, Ohio.
*Diagnostic Laparoscopy for Benign
and Malignant Disease*

Greg V. Stiegmann, M.D.
Associate Professor of Surgery,
University of Colorado School of
Medicine, University of Colorado at
Denver; Chief, Endoscopic Surgery,

Veterans Affairs Hospital, Denver, Colorado.
Endoscopic Management of Esophageal Varices

Choichi Sugawa, M.D.
Professor of Surgery and Director of Surgical Endoscopy, Wayne State University School of Medicine; Attending Physician at Detroit Receiving Hospital, Harper Hospital, and Grace Hospital, Detroit, Michigan.
Management of Nonvariceal Upper Gastrointestinal Bleeding

Sanford Timen, M.D.
Assistant Clinical Professor of Otolaryngology, Case Western Reserve University School of Medicine; Chief, Division of Otolaryngology, Department of Surgery, Mount Sinai Medical Center, Cleveland, Ohio.
Nasopharyngeal and Laryngeal Endoscopy

Michael R. Treat, M.D.
Associate Professor of Clinical Surgery, Columbia University College of Physicians and Surgeons; Attending Surgeon, Columbia-Presbyterian Medical Center, New York, New York.
New Technologies and Future Developments for Endoscopic Surgery

Darryl S. Weiman, M.D.
Associate Professor of Surgery, Division of Cardiothoracic Surgery, University of Tennessee Medical School, Memphis, Tennessee.
Bronchoscopy and Mediastinoscopy

David E. Wesson, M.D.
Associate Professor of Surgery, Faculty of Medicine, University of Toronto; Head, Division of General Surgery, Hospital for Sick Children, Toronto, Ontario, Canada.
Endoscopic Surgery in Children

Glenn J. R. Whitman, M.D.
Associate Professor and Chief, Cardiothoracic Surgery, The Medical College of Pennsylvania; Consultant, Veterans Administration Hospital, Philadelphia, Pennsylvania.
Bronchoscopy and Mediastinoscopy

William I. Wolff, M.D.
Attending Surgeon and Former Director of Surgery, Beth Israel Medical Center; Attending, New York Infirmary-Beekman Downtown Hospital, New York, New York.
Therapeutic Colonoscopy: Polypectomy, Management of Bleeding, and Decompressive Techniques

Karl A. Zucker, M.D.
Professor of Surgery and Chief, Division of Surgical Endoscopy, University of New Mexico School of Medicine; Staff Surgeon, Albuquerque Veterans Hospital, Albuquerque, New Mexico.
Laparoscopic Surgery of the Gastrointestinal Tract

Foreword

Within the last century, the field of surgery has witnessed a number of essential innovations, ranging from daring laparotomies and safer general anesthetics to the development of adjunctive measures, such as blood transfusions and sophisticated parenteral fluid therapy. Some of the most profound advances within the recent past have been technical advances related to highly focused specialty undertakings such as cardiopulmonary bypass and transplantation techniques and immunosuppression. It has been only within the past 5 years that such technical advances have focused primarily on the field of general surgery. It was the introduction of the fiberoptic endoscope and the logical extension of laparoscopy into the field of surgery that substantially changed the course of current medical practice and revitalized the fundamental discipline of general surgery.

The two editors of *Endoscopic Surgery,* Professors Greene and Ponsky, have been at the forefront of endoscopy and laparoscopy, leading the way through their organizational, personal, and scientific contributions to these fields. The editors have provided many of their own contributions to this book. They have also made a valid effort to convey the clinical historical aspects of endoscopy, as well as some of the latest technical advances that have made less-invasive surgical procedures the standard for medical practice in much of the Western Hemisphere. As a matter of fact, many of the procedures discussed in this book have already become the standard against which other procedures are compared; inevitably, many of the other procedures will establish the groundwork for future standards. It is by testing the limits of progress that virtually all advances of this surgical century have been made, and within the pages of this book are many of those groundbreaking suggestions.

Endoscopic Surgery contains some of the finest illustrations and color reproductions of laparoscopic and endoscopic images that I have seen.

It is clear that the surgeon and the medical practitioner of the next century will have to master all of these techniques and must be able to offer their patients the choice of the less-invasive forms of both diagnostic and therapeutic procedures. One can envision the clinician of the next era providing a full range of traditional open versus closed operative choices, using whichever is best suited to the specific pathologic state or the overall well-being of a given patient.

Endoscopic Surgery brings the discipline of surgery to the brink of the 21st century, and I think that it will be a widely used and consistent resource throughout the current era. I find it as stimulating to imagine how this compendium will influence the next generation of surgical innovations as it is to see what current concepts and prototypical ideas Professors Greene and Ponsky directly convey in this well-organized book.

HIRAM C. POLK, JR., M.D.

Preface

"Diseases that harm call for treatments that harm less."
William Osler

The melding of the terms "endoscopic" and "surgery," while a natural phenomenon, has evolved only in the last decade as general, thoracic, and pediatric surgeons have realized not only that their patients benefited from well-done endoscopic studies, but also that these endoscopic studies should ideally be performed by the specialist, who might use the information directly to effect a surgical cure. Only recently have surgical training programs embraced the concept of endoscopic training as an integral part of a well-structured didactic and practical general surgical education. The American Board of Surgery has supported the need for specific training in endoscopic procedures and has entrusted Program Directors to ensure that all surgical trainees are exposed to these principles.

The need for a textbook that covers the principles of flexible endoscopy as well as the exciting new concepts of diagnostic and therapeutic laparoscopy had been obvious to us during the last several years. The result of experience in resident teaching and in directing courses in postgraduate education in surgical endoscopy, this textbook has evolved from course syllabi, course contents, discussions with faculty and colleagues, and lengthy discussions of the future needs of the well-trained general surgeon.

The concepts of endoscopic surgery now transcend both general surgical education and the principles of gastrointestinal surgery. Modern technological advances have allowed us to look into orifices and hollow organs that could not have been approached a decade ago. The excitement generated by these advances has rejuvenated general surgery as a discipline and has created strong bonding with disciplines dedicated to treatment of the peripheral vascular and respiratory systems.

We dedicate this textbook to the surgical and technological pioneers who have helped to forge the rebirth of surgical endoscopy and to create an atmosphere in which future advances are limitless. We especially dedicate this effort to all surgical residents who may benefit by this work during their training and beyond.

FREDERICK L. GREENE, M.D.
JEFFREY L. PONSKY, M.D.

Acknowledgments

A textbook planned to be a comprehensive treatment of the topic of surgical endoscopy cannot be developed without the input and dedication of many leaders in the field. We appreciate and acknowledge the many long hours generously devoted by our authors in developing what we believe are outstanding contributions to the literature in the areas of endoscopic surgery. We recognized that many times we pressured and cajoled them in order to meet deadlines and to develop a textbook worthy of our readership. We appreciate very much our authors' understanding of our tyrannical approach, and if we offended, we apologize!

We also wish to express our sincere gratitude to the very professional editorial staff at the W.B. Saunders Company, especially to Melissa McGrath, our Developmental Editor, and Carolyn Naylor, our Production Manager. It is obvious that this textbook could not have been produced without the excellent leadership of these individuals. We further acknowledge all of the other professionals at Saunders who made it possible to produce first-rate artwork, which is so important in the field of laparoscopic and endoscopic surgery. We are indebted to Mr. Edward Wickland, formerly of Saunders, who gave us guidance in the initial preparation phase, and Lisette Bralow, Vice President and Editor-in-Chief, for her faith and support.

Finally, we acknowledge our wonderful families, who for many years have allowed us to develop our interests in endoscopic surgery and who were willing, despite the sacrifices, to give us the time and the freedom to steal energies from them in the development of this labor of love.

FREDERICK L. GREENE, M.D.
JEFFREY L. PONSKY, M.D.

Contents

1

History of Endoscopic Surgery

George Berci

The first reports about endoscopic procedures attest to the ingenuity of the pioneers who conceived the idea, the motivation behind it, and the circumstances under which theoretic concepts were transformed into functioning units. Around the turn of the century, the investigators and their assistants were able to complete a sophisticated design of an operating tool without the consultation of engineering specialists and without access to data, compiling libraries, and computers. It was obvious that there were internal organs with external orifices that would be worthwhile to explore if access to these deeply located cavities could be achieved without harming the patient.

Bozzini, an Italian physician living and practicing medicine in Germany (Fig. 1–1), built a system in which the illumination consisted of the reflected light of a candle directed to deeply situated organs by a metal tube shaped according to the size and configuration of the organ.[1] Desormeaux, who used as a light source a mixture of alcohol and turpentine, was the first to condense the beam to a narrower area to achieve a brighter spot.[2] Bevan extracted foreign bodies from the esophagus.[3]

The open tube system underwent revolutionary changes with the introduction of a telescope. In 1879, the first optical system was invented by Nitze, a general practitioner, who with an optician and an instrument maker made a cystoscope to examine the inside of the urinary bladder. A platinum wire was heated to create light, and the system was cooled by a separate water circulation. After the discovery of Edison's filament globe, the first gastroscope employed a miniature electric globe.[4] It was first used by a surgeon, Mikulicz, in 1881 (Fig. 1–

2).[5] The examinations at that time were performed using topical cocaine or morphine anesthesia. Many details and refinements were included by the pioneers of gastroscopy and cystoscopy and by the instrument makers of that time.

Before the turn of the century, Lange and Meltzing developed the first flexible gastro-

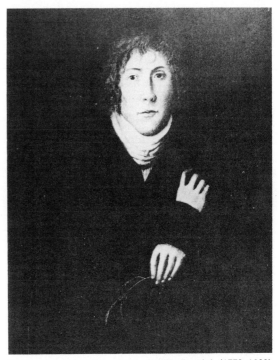

Figure 1–1. Portrait of Dr. Phillip Bozzini (1773–1809). (From Reuter HJ, Reuter MA. Phillip Bozzini und Die Endoskopie des 19. Copyright 1988 by Max-Nitze-Museum, Stuttgart, Germany.)

1

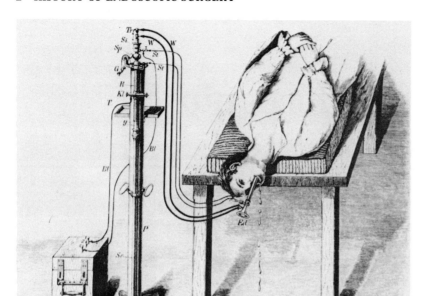

Figure 1–2. The first documentation of a gastroscopy by Dr. Johann Von Mikulicz (Vienna, 1881). The system used the Nitze telescope with miniature electric globes. (From Reuter HJ, Reuter MA. Phillip Bozzini und Die Endoskopie des 19. Copyright 1988 by Max-Nitze-Museum, Stuttgart, Germany.)

camera and published the results of treating 15 patients.[6] Exposure time was 0.5 to 1 second. A small film roll was placed at the distal end of the scope and was pulled after each exposure. The image was 4 mm in diameter, and the rigid head was only 66 mm long. The mechanism was divided into three compartments: the film magazine, the camera head, and the electric globe. Fifty exposures were made per examination. The rest of the camera consisted of a rubber tube with electric wires, air insufflation, and the pulling mechanism of the film transport. Sixty-two years later, the modern version of the gastrocamera was developed.

There were two milestone inventions that advanced the evolution of endoscopy. One was a flexible image transmitting system, invented by Heel and Hopkins in 1954.[7, 8] A few years later, the first clinical tool, the flexible gastroscope, was introduced by Hirschowitz.[9] In the rigid endoscopy field, the introduction of a new optical transmitting system, the rod lenses by Hopkins and its clinical applications by Berci broadened the possibilities for endoscopic examinations.[10, 11]

DOCUMENTATION

The need for a permanent record was recognized since the invention of the endoscope and the introduction of visual examinations. Nitze developed the first photocystoscope in 1893 and published the first atlas of pathology of the urinary bladder a few years later.[12] In 1938, Henning and Keilhack produced the first color pictures from the stomach using a semirigid Schindler-type gastroscope with an overburned filament (Figs. 1–3 and 1–4).[13]

TELEVISION

The first use of studio television cameras with endoscopes was reported from France in the field of bronchology in 1956.[14] My colleagues and I produced the first black and white miniature television camera for endoscopy in 1962 and at a later stage, substituted larger, color devices and miniature chip cameras.[15, 16] The first videotapes were made in the field of laparoscopic gynecology.[17]

LAPAROSCOPY

In 1901, Kelling, a German surgeon, lectured at the meeting of the Society of German Doctors in Hamburg about the endoscopic visualization of the esophagus and stomach.[18] At the end of his lecture, he mentioned that he also was experimenting with "coelioscopy" by using room air for creation of pneumoperitoneum and a trocar, developed by Fiedler, through which

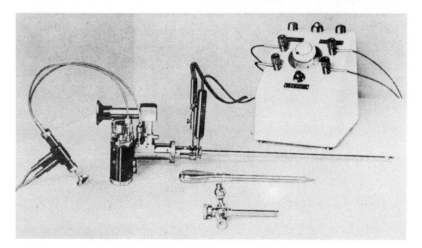

Figure 1–3. A photolaparoscope developed by Sass and Wolf in 1957. In its double-filament globe, one filament was overburned to create a flash. (From Reuter HJ, Reuter MA. Phillip Bozzini und Die Endoskopie des 19. Copyright 1988 by Max-Nitze-Museum, Stuttgart, Germany.)

a cystoscope was advanced. These first reports did not find any response in the medical community. In 1910, Jacobaeus, who was not informed about Kelling's pioneer work, produced the first 109 cases in Sweden within 1.5 years (Fig. 1–5).[19] He originated the idea of systematic endoscopic inspection of the abdominal cavity. Sporadic reports came from Brazil, Denmark, Finland, France, Italy, Hungary, and other locations throughout Europe. In 1911, Bernheim, at Johns Hopkins Hospital, took a 12-mm-diameter proctoscope and introduced it through a

small incision into the epigastrium. With the help of an ENT mirror, he examined parts of the anterior surface of the stomach, liver, and diaphragm.[20] Kalk, a gastroenterologist from Germany, was the real father and promoter of diagnostic laparoscopy. He developed a Foroblique optic system and the dual trocar approach, and he designed biopsy instruments. A decade later, he published a monograph of 2000 liver biopsies performed using local anesthesia without mortality.[21]

Ruddock, an American internist, recom-

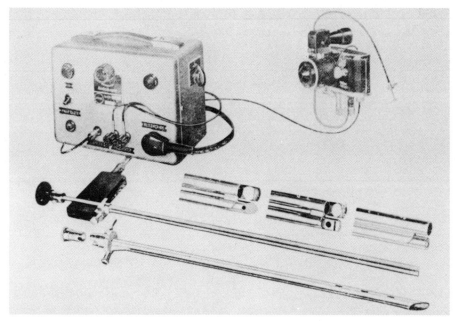

Figure 1–4. The first electroflash discharge telescopic system for the bronchoscope and laparoscope was used for documentation. Below the eyepiece and along the shaft, a flat flash globe was interposed outside the patient, and the discharge was transmitted into the body cavity by a quartz rod. A reflex 35-mm camera could be attached. This was developed by Karl Storz in 1959. (Courtesy of Karl Storz, Tuttlingen, Germany.)

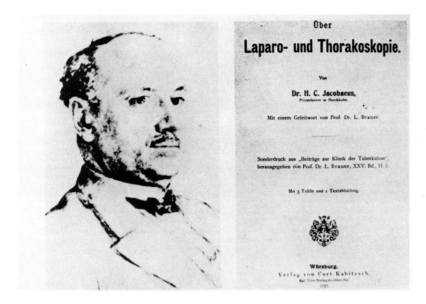

Figure 1–5. Dr. Jacobaeus published his first series of *Laparoscopy in Humans* in 1912. (Courtesy of N. Henning, Laparoskopie. Stuttgart, Germany: Georg Thieme Verlag, 1985.)

mended this important examination in 1937 based on 500 successful cases, but he did not find followers.[22] Benedict, a pioneer of American endoscopy, tried to promote laparoscopy in 1938 with a minimum of success.[23] Segal made the first laparoscopic movies of liver diseases in 1959 (Fig. 1–6). I started using laparoscopy in oncology cases in 1960 and published the first results in 1962.[24] Most surgeons preferred to explore surgically the questionable or advanced

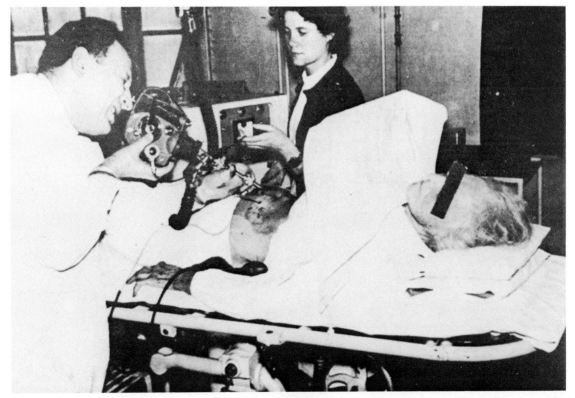

Figure 1–6. Filming laparoscopy was first performed by Dr. H. Segal in France in 1959. A projector globe is attached outside the endoscope, and the beam is reflected through a condenser lens into the abdominal cavity by a quartz rod. With this excellent illumination, movie records could be obtained. The operator in this picture was a gastroenterologist. (Courtesy of Photo Cinema Publication, Paul Montel, Paris, 1960.)

cases of abdominal malignancy rather than first obtain a tissue diagnosis through the laparoscope and assess the operability or stage of disease. The instrumentation was vastly improved by the introduction of a new image transmitting system (*i.e.,* Hopkins rod-lens system). My colleagues and I tried to popularize laparoscopy for a variety of indications but found few followers. The gynecologists were much more progressive and adopted laparoscopy earlier for diagnostic and therapeutic procedures. Today, in our institution, one third of all gynecologic operations are diagnostic or therapeutic laparoscopies. We publicized this examination procedure for 20 years before finding some resonance after the first laparoscopic cholecystectomy was reported in 1986 in Germany by Muhe, followed by Dubois and Perissat in France and Reddick and Olsen and by Phillips, Berci, and colleagues in the United States.[24–27] After this, the picture changed drastically. Program directors recognized the need to insert surgical endoscopy in the curricula. General surgeons participated in training courses to become acquainted with laparoscopic surgery.

The progress of instrumentation and image transmission is far from complete. New developments in various areas will allow us to replace open surgery with endoscopic or minimal access procedures, resulting in less discomfort, shorter hospitalization, and faster rehabilitation for the patient. We do hope that in a few years' time there will be enough data to prove the effectiveness and safety of this new era of endoscopic or laparoscopic surgery.

References

1. Bozzini PH. Lichtleiter, eine Erfindung zur Anschauung innerer Teile und Krankheiten. J Prak Heilk 24:107, 1806.
2. Desormeaux AJ. Endoscope and its application to the diagnosis and treatment of affections of the genitourinary passages. Chicago Med J, 1867.
3. Bevan L. The esophagoscope. Lancet 1:470, 1868.
4. Nitze M. Beobachtungs und Untersuchungsmethode fur Harnrohre Harnblase und Rectum. Wien Med Wochenschr 24:651, 1879.
5. Mikulicz J. Uber Gastroskopie und Osophagoskopie. Wien Med Presse 45:1405, 1881.
6. Lange F, Meltzing. Die photography des Mageninnern. Munch Med Wochenschr 50:1585, 1898.
7. Heel ACS. A new method of transporting optical images without aberrations. Nature 173:39, 1954.
8. Hopkins HH, Kapany NS. A flexible fiberscope. Nature 173:39, 1954.
9. Hirschowitz BI, Curtis LE, Peters CW, et al. The fiberscope. Gastroenterology 35:50, 1958.
10. Hopkins HH. Optical principles of the endoscope. In: Berci G, ed. Endoscopy. New York: Appleton-Century-Crofts, 1976:3–27.
11. Berci G, Kont LA. A new optical system in endoscopy with special reference to cystoscopy. Br J Urol 41:564, 1969.
12. Nitze M. Zur Photographie der menschlichen Harnblase. Med Wochenschr 2:744, 1893.
13. Henning N, Keilhack H. Farbenphotography der Magenhohle. Dtsch Med Wochenschr 64:1328, 1938.
14. Soulas A. Televised bronchoscopy. Presse Med 64:97, 1956.
15. Berci G, Davids J. Endoscopy and television. Br Med J 1:1610, 1962.
16. Berci G, Schulman AG, Morgenstern L, Paz-Partlow M, Cuschieri A, Wood RA. Television choledochoscopy. Surg Gynecol Obstet 160:176, 1985.
17. Berci G, Brooks PG, Paz-Partlow M. TV laparoscopy—a new dimension in visualization and documentation of pelvic pathology. J Reprod Med 31:585, 1986.
18. Kelling G. Endoscopie fur Speiserohre und Magen. Munch Med Wochenschr 34:934, 1897.
19. Jacobeus HC. Uber die Moglichkeit die Zystoskopie bei Untersuchungen, seroser Hohlungen anzuwenden. Munch Med Wochenschr 57:2090, 1910.
20. Berheim BM. Organoscopy. Ann Surg 53:764, 1911.
21. Kalk H, Bruhl W. Leitfaden der Laparoskopie und Gastroskopie. Stuttgart: Thieme, 1951.
22. Ruddock JC. Peritoneoscopy. Surg Gynecol Obstet 65:623, 1937.
23. Benedict EB. Peritoneoscopy. New Engl J Med 218:713, 1938.
24. Muhe E. Die erste Cholecystectomy durch das Laparoskope. Langenbecks Arch Chir 369:804, 1986.
25. Dubois F, Berthelots G, Levard H. Cholecystectomy par Coelioscopie. Presse Med 18:980, 1989.
26. Perissat J, Belliard R, Collet DC, Bikandou G. Cholecystectomy par Laparoscopie. J Chir (Paris) 127:347, 1990.
27. Phillips E, Berci G, Carroll B, et al. The importance of intraoperative cholangiography during laparoscopic cholecystectomy. Am J Surg 56:792, 1990.

2

Endoscopic Technology

Brock M. Bordelon and John G. Hunter

Surgical endoscopy has developed as a discipline within general surgery as a result of surgical imagination and engineering progress. Technologic development has freed creative surgeons from the stagnation of older surgical approaches. Although it is not absolutely necessary to know how a photon of light becomes an electronic signal to be a creative and competent endoscopic surgeon, such knowledge helps the surgeon participate in purchasing and maintaining the most appropriate equipment for his or her needs.

This chapter introduces basic and "cutting edge" endoscopic equipment, including video cameras, endoscopes, light sources, electrosurgery, laser, and ultrasound. Although it is impossible to discuss every available device for endoscopic surgery, the reader should be able to take away sufficient technical information to enhance his or her knowledge about the equipment used daily.

OPTICS

Video Imaging

High-resolution, color-accurate video imaging has played a vital role in facilitating quality diagnostic and therapeutic endoscopy. Transferring the endoscopic image through a video camera to a high-resolution video monitor has several advantages over direct monocular visualization (i.e., looking through the scope), including the ability to operate with upright posture, reduce eye strain, free both hands for operating, and share the video image with the first assistant and others in the room. The shared image allows participation of the entire operating team in complicated procedures and facilitates the teaching of operative technique to

residents and detailed anatomy to medical students. The video image can be recorded for documentation, quality assurance, and subsequent demonstration.

To be useful in diagnostic and therapeutic procedures, the endoscopic video camera must be small, lightweight, and sterile and incorporate excellent light sensitivity and color resolution. The first endoscopic video camera was introduced in 1962, but it was bulky and had poor imaging characteristics.[1] Several engineering developments in the 1970s and 1980s improved video technology to the extent that the size and quality of the image became acceptable to surgeons.[2]

The basis of modern endoscopic video imaging systems is the silicon charge-couple device (CCD) or "chip" camera. The CCD camera incorporates a dense grid of photocell receptors in a single silicon chip. Each photocell receptor passes an electronic signal to an image processor, which generates a single pixel of the video image. The pixel represents the smallest unit of the video image, with an outer diameter of 17 $\times$ 13 μm. The image resolution depends on the number of pixels packed onto the chip; the current generation of CCD cameras contain 150,000 to 300,000 pixels. The organized compilation of individual pixels is displayed on the video monitor as the final image.

A one-chip camera contains a single black and white chip. There are two methods used for adding color. In most laparoscopy systems with separate camera and light source, the camera "box" translates the black and white image into color by using gray scale approximations of the visible spectrum. This reconstituted color is least accurate at the longer wavelengths (red, purple) but provides adequate resolution for most laparoscopic procedures.

In flexible endoscopic systems in which red-purple accuracy is important for diagnosis, a color wheel that runs through the color sequence at a rate faster than the flicker frequency of the visual cortex is placed in front of the light source. The reflected light, received by the black and white chip, will vary with the color of the incident (light source) light. Very close approximations of true color can be achieved with this system. Current generation one-chip CCD cameras achieve a picture resolution of 400 lines or greater, some have built-in zoom capabilities, and most have freeze-frame imaging for detailed evaluation or photographic documentation of the image. An automatic iris is incoporated in most video cameras to reduce glare from reflective tissue surfaces.

A variety of manufacturers have developed endoscopic video systems incorporating three CCD chips. The three-chip camera contains a CCD chip for each of three colors: red, green, and blue (RGB). The signal from each chip is reintegrated at the level of a high-resolution RGB monitor, offering the most accurate color representation. Excellent horizontal resolution, greater than 700 lines, and a superior dynamic range in the red spectrum combine to make this state-of-the-art technology. An almost identical RGB CCD chip system is used in network television cameras. This is an expensive system, but it may become the standard for many applications.

The CCD sensor may be attached to the eyepiece of the endoscope, as is the fashion with video laparoscopy, or it may be placed at the tip of the instrument to fashion a true video endoscope. Positioning the video sensor at the tip of the instrument bypasses the relatively inferior light transmission of flexible fiberoptic systems. Although commonly used in flexible endoscopy, the video endoscope has not yet achieved much popularity in laparoscopy because light and color losses are not as severe in the short, large, solid quartz rods of the laparoscope as they are in long, flexible fiberoptic endoscopes. Current flexible video laparoscopes are afflicted with image distortion and diminished illumination compared with a three-chip camera attached to a quartz rod-lens system and a 300 W xenon light source.

Optical Principles of the Rigid Endoscope

The first endoscope incorporating a lens system and illumination was developed by Nitze in 1879 for examination of the urinary bladder.[3]

The Nitze cytoscope used small lenses with large intervening air spaces. A glowing platinum wire was originally used for illumination but later replaced with a small, low-voltage electric light bulb.[4] This simple system remained essentially unchanged for decades and, with the addition of a high-intensity light source, was quite adequate for diagnosis and photography. However, the image quality of the conventional endoscope suffered from a narrow viewing angle, poor color resolution, poor illumination, and inefficient light transmission.

A major innovation in rigid endoscopy was the development of the Hopkins rod-lens system.[5] Instead of relying on image relay through many lenses separated by air, the rod-lens system transmits the image through a series of quartz rods with small air interspaces (Fig. 2–1). Light transmission is many times better than with air-filled scopes, yielding a brighter, clearer image with better color resolution. The Hopkins rod-lens system also incorporates a larger viewing angle, providing a larger field of visualization.

Despite these advantages, rigid endoscopic systems have their shortcomings. The image quality, although superior to fiberoptic systems, is mildly distorted. Light transmission remains quite inefficient, with only 3% to 7% of the light energy produced by the light source reaching the target.[6] Seventy percent to 80% of losses occur in the fiberoptic cable, and a smaller percentage is lost through the optics of the telescope. Fiber mismatch at the cable-telescope interface results in further reduction of light transmission.

The standard Hopkins rod-lens telescope, familiar to most laparoscopists, is a forward-viewing (0°) telescope, which provides visualization of objects directly in line with the telescope. Rotation of the telescope does not change the view obtained. A forward-oblique telescope (30° or 45°) has many advantages over the 0° instrument. A more complete inspection of the body cavity can be attained. As the angled telescope is rotated, a different perspective is gained, which provides more information for diagnosis and therapy. This is an extremely important advantage, permitting the performance of advanced endoscopic procedures without frequent camera position changes. More light is lost with an angled telescope than with a 0° telescope, providing a slightly darker image and necessitating a 300 W light source for therapeutic procedures.

Before the advent of video laparoscopy, 10-mm operating telescopes were commonly used (Fig. 2–2). This type of telescope is unsatisfactory for

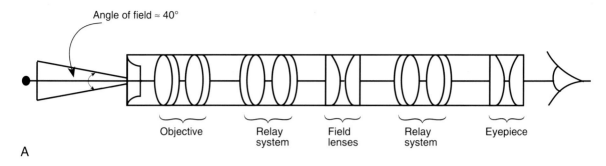

A

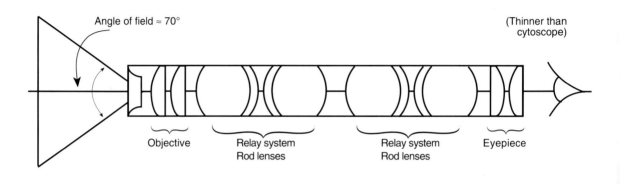

B

Figure 2–1. **(A)** The optics of a traditional cystoscope in which several lenses in a relay system were placed in a hollow tube. **(B)** The Hopkins rod-lens system contains four solid quartz rods with little intervening air.

most applications, requiring alignment of the operating instrument and telescope in a coaxial fashion such that the tip of the instrument is poorly visualized. The quartz rods are of a reduced diameter to allow room for the operating channel, which reduces light transmission. These operating telescopes are quite dangerous when monopolar electrosurgical instruments are passed through the operating channel, especially if nonconductive trocars are used. If current leaks into the telescope by one of several mechanisms (*e.g.,* insulation failure, capacitive coupling), the telescope may act as a large electrode, passing current to the intestine out of the visual field of the telescopic image. Operating telescopes were never popular among general surgeons because of these difficulties and because it became clear that little morbidity or discomfort was associated with the use of secondary trocars.

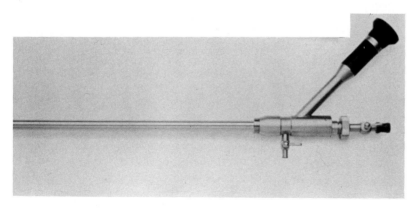

Figure 2–2. The single-puncture operating laparoscope has the inherent disadvantage of a smaller quartz rod and coaxial visualization.

Optical Principles of the Flexible Endoscope

A light beam entering one end of a glass rod passes through the rod in a zigzag pattern, reflecting on the walls of the rod until it exits the opposite end (Fig. 2–3). This phenomenon is mathematically explained by the physics of ray optics, in which light waves originating from a light source travel along rays that are refracted or reflected at any optically clear surface they meet. Total internal reflection occurs in a glass rod if the angle of refraction exceeds the incident angle (*i.e.,* the angle at which the light ray is encountering the wall of the rod). Because the ray cannot escape the cylinder, there is 100% transmission of light energy through the rod without loss of light during a multitude of reflections. This characteristic of light transmission applies to flexible glass fibers as small as 8 μm in diameter, which allowed the development of multifiber, small caliber, fiberoptic endoscopes.[7]

The principles of ray optics do not apply to glass fibers less than approximately 8 μm in diameter, in which case the fiber diameter is less than several times the wavelength of visible light. This state is mathematically defined by wave optics, in which light is propagated in waves. A fiber with a diameter less than several times the wavelength of the light in question is unable to capture and transmit all of the modes of the light wave, and certain modes are lost through the fiber walls as diffraction losses.[8] Increases in fiber diameter are quickly matched by increases in wave mode transmission, such that fibers 10 μm or greater in diameter transmit any wave form without significant light loss over extended lengths. Most flexible fiberoptic en-

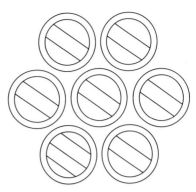

Figure 2–4. The mesh-like appearance of fiberoptic endoscopes is a result of the cladding around each fiber and the gaps created by arranging round fibers in parallel.

doscopes use fibers with approximately 10-μm diameters.

Fiberoptic cables are composed of numerous bundles, each of which incorporates thousands of individual glass fibers. To ensure a 100% reflection coefficient (*i.e.,* total internal reflection), each fiber is optically fused to a glass sheath that has a lower optical density than the core fiber. This cladding does not transmit light and constitutes the packing fraction, which is responsible for the mesh-like appearance of fiberoptic images (Fig. 2–4). Despite the high quality of currently available fiberoptic instruments, they can never achieve the image quality of rigid endoscopes.

Accurate image transmission through a fiberoptic bundle can only be achieved by bundle construction with identical fiber orientation at both ends. This type of coherent bundle usually contains fibers 10 μm in diameter and is expensive to manufacture (Fig. 2–5). Light transmission for illumination does not require exact fiber orientation, and the fibers in a bundle may be randomly arranged. These incoherent bundles are typically constructed of 25-μm-diameter fibers.

Stereo Optics

Minimally invasive, video-assisted surgical techniques suffer from an inherent disadvantage: a lack of normal depth perception. This shortcoming requires that the surgeon develop strategies to obtain three-dimensional clues from the two-dimensional representation of the peritoneal or chest cavity. The information necessary for the brain to recreate a three-dimensional image can be gained by comparing the

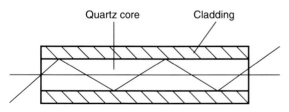

Figure 2–3. In a quartz fiber, light is refracted as it enters the fiber, but it cannot escape (*i.e.,* because of total internal reflection) until it reaches the end of the fiber, where it is again refracted to recreate the true image.

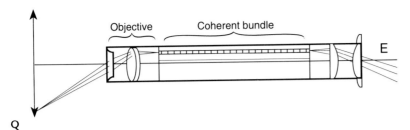

Figure 2–5. With a coherent bundle of fibers, light from a particular point Q is focused on a single fiber. The image is recreated with a second lens at the viewing end of the endoscope *(E)*. Accurate image representation depends on the fiber bundle's being absolutely coherent.

apparent size of structures to the memory of the actual size (perspective) and by moving the telescope, tissues, and instruments to obtain different perspectives. Creating three-dimensional space from the two-dimensional information is mentally tiring. Three-dimensional stereoscopic visualization, providing "natural" depth perception, would be a tremendous advantage over current two-dimensional video technology.

The technology for three-dimensional, video-assisted surgery is still in its infancy, but affordable, reliable systems should become available in the next few years. Stereoscopic endoscopy can be achieved by using a telescope with parallel but separate rod-lens systems and placing a CCD camera on the end of each optical system. The individual images are processed and polarized by a computer, which sends the two image signals to the video monitor in a rapidly alternating fashion (120 cycles/sec). Polarized filters on the monitor and in the eyewear deliver only the image from the ipsilateral quartz rod to each eye, 60 images/sec, which restores stereo vision. Although simple in concept, three-dimensional video is a difficult and costly engineering task.

DOCUMENTATION

The earliest photographic documentation of an endoscopic image was performed by Nitze with his photocystoscope.[9] These initial efforts were followed by Ruddock in 1935 and Holinger in 1940, who published an endoscopic color atlas of the tracheobronchial tree.[10] The advent of intracorporeal flash photography in the 1960s was a major advance for photographic documentation. With subsequent improvements in light source technology, the same light source was able to be used for diagnostic and photographic purposes.[11] Despite the diligent efforts of many investigators, endoscopic cinematography failed to achieve much success and was abandoned in favor of endoscopic video imaging using television.[12]

The move toward video imaging was an im-portant step, permitting accurate documentation with standard video cassette recorders. Advancements in technology have allowed freeze-frame capability with still photography and the incorporation of patient data with the video images. The next stage in documentation will probably be digital video image processing and storage. Currently available technology permits digital compact disc image recording with data input. A 1-gigabyte compact disc has enough space for 10,000 video images, which can be stored, rearranged, removed, or integrated with database information.

LIGHT SOURCES AND CABLES

Before the 1950s, endoscopic illumination was provided by a small tungsten filament lamp positioned at the tip of the viewing instrument. This arrangement was usually less than satisfactory, furnishing poor illumination and significant color distortion. These light sources suffered from excess heat production, causing tissue damage. This system was modified by placing the tungsten lamp in a steel housing at the proximal end of the telescope, with light transmitted directly down the quartz rod.[13]

The advent of fiberoptic systems allowed light transmission through a flexible cable from a remote high-intensity light source. Quartz, mercury, xenon, and halide light sources provide continuous, high-intensity light that is bright enough for endoscopic illumination despite the inefficiencies alluded to previously. Although flexible endoscopy is performed using lower-intensity light sources, laparoscopy requires exceedingly bright light to adequately illuminate the more cavernous abdominal cavity. Xenon light sources provide up to 300 W of continuous illumination, and some units have stroboscopic flash capabilities for still photography.

An alternative to fiberoptic light cables is the fluid cable, capable of transmitting 30% more light than a standard 1.8-m (6-ft) glass fiber cable. The improvement in light transmission is gained by eliminating the packing fraction losses of standard fiberoptic cables. This benefit is small, however, compared with the increased bulk and decreased flexibility of fluid cables.

ENERGY SOURCES

The ability to look into bodily cavities inevitably led surgeons to seek the means to treat the abnormalities encountered so that therapeutic procedures could accompany diagnostic endoscopy. In addition to stents, baskets, scissors, and balloons, most therapeutic endoscopy requires the application of thermal energy to control bleeding.

Laser and electrosurgical energy, despite their vastly different physical characteristics, affect tissue by the production of heat at the tissue level. An adequate understanding of laser and electrosurgical principles is requisite to the safe performance of therapeutic endoscopic procedures.

Principles of Monopolar Electrosurgery

Monopolar electrosurgical generators produce electrical current at a frequency of 500,000 to 750,000 cycles per second. These frequencies are characteristic of radio waves, and electrosurgical energy is known as radiofrequency (RF) electricity. With monopolar electrosurgical circuits, current passes from the active electrode ("Bovie" tip) through tissue and back to the indifferent electrode (ground plate). The rapidly alternating current catapults ionized species in tissue to and fro, generating kinetic energy. Coagulating, cutting, and blended electrosurgical waveforms use this principle to create different types of thermal tissue injury.

Electrosurgical tissue heating depends on the square of the current (I) flowing through a particular cross-sectional area of tissue: $T = k(I/cm^2)^2$. Current density is directly proportional to applied power (voltage [V]) and inversely proportional to tissue resistance (impedance [R]): $I = V/R$.

Initial application of a constant-voltage RF current to tissue results in low current flow, because undisturbed tissue resistance is fairly high. Continued current application raises tissue temperature sufficiently to create highly conductive ionized species. As resistance falls, current flow and tissue temperature increase. An increase in tissue temperature leads to water evaporation, and the tissue desiccation increases tissue resistance, decreases current, and slows the heating process.

An example of this phenomenon is the frequent observation by the surgeon that the electrosurgery electrode sparks furiously, abruptly ceases sparking, and then sticks to a carbonized eschar that does not melt away no matter how high the power is adjusted or how long the electrode is activated. Bipolar coagulating forceps use this principle of desiccation to the surgeon's advantage. When the current flow between two activated electrodes falls to zero, it signifies that the conductor in that tissue (primarily water) has been eliminated. It is then safe to cut across the tissue without the risk of bleeding.

Effective tissue coagulation requires deep and even heat distribution. Monopolar coagulating current is characterized by a rapid discharge of short bursts of high-voltage energy, which drives electrons across a high-resistance, non-ionized air gap between tissue and the electrode. These short bursts are interrupted by longer pauses that slow the heating of tissue, permitting coagulation rather than vaporization. When used in a noncontact fashion, effective surface coagulation (i.e., fulguration) is achieved.

Electrosurgical cutting is obtained with a continuous, high-frequency (500 kHz), low-voltage sine wave discharge without intervening pauses, yielding rapid tissue heating. This leads to tissue vaporization, producing a gap of steam between electrode and tissue. The steam facilitates conduction of energy across the gap. Electrosurgical cutting current rapidly vaporizes tissue without tissue contact, giving the surgeon the sensation of floating through tissue. This results in limited lateral thermal injury but inadequate thermocoagulation.

When the electrode is placed firmly against tissue with a high water content and a cutting or coagulation current is applied, the slowest and deepest tissue desiccation (for maximal large vessel coagulation) is achievable. The slow application of energy allows the surgeon to remove the electrode before carbonization and electrode sticking occurs.

The major shortcoming of monopolar electrosurgery is related to the path taken by electrical current as it passes from the active electrode to the ground plate. Current pathways may originate in unsuspected locations, causing unsuspected tissue injury remote from the surgical field. Current division may be a consequence of inadequately insulated instruments, damaged insulation, or capacitively coupled current.

Current division originating from uninsulated portions of instruments or through defective electrode insulation is an obvious and preventable mechanism of accidental tissue injury. Judicious inspection of monopolar electrodes is an important step in preparing for any endoscopic procedure. The surgeon should be acutely aware that electrical injury may occur from any bare metal outside his or her field of view, and this serious injury may be unseen or manifested only by tissue blanching.

Capacitive coupling occurs when electrical charge on a monopolar electrode not being drained by an electron sink (*e.g.*, tissue) induces a charge on a coaxial cylinder of metal (*e.g.*, trocar, operating telescope), and this capacitor is not allowed to drain electrons into the abdominal wall because of insulation (*e.g.*, plastic screw anchor) between the metal of the capacitor and the abdominal wall. This phenomenon was classically associated with the use of an operating telescope, through which an insulated monopolar electrode was passed. As much as 80% of available power in the activated but ungrounded electrode is capacitively coupled to the operating telescope if the circuit is incomplete. If a metal trocar is used, capacitively coupled current is returned to the ground plate through the abdominal wall and back to the ground plate, with low power density at all points. If the operating telescope is passed through a plastic trocar, capacitively coupled current may return to the ground pad through a loop of intestine adjacent to the telescope, because the current cannot penetrate the plastic trocar to return to the ground pad through the abdominal wall.

Another dangerous situation exists when undesirable points of high current density are created by narrow-diameter return circuits. Examples of these dangerous conditions are poor ground pad application (alleviated with tandem test circuits in modern electrosurgical generators), an adhesion with a single small contact point to the intestine undergoing electrothermal division, or a waist in a structure being transected, such as the tightly ligated base of the appendix (Fig. 2–6).

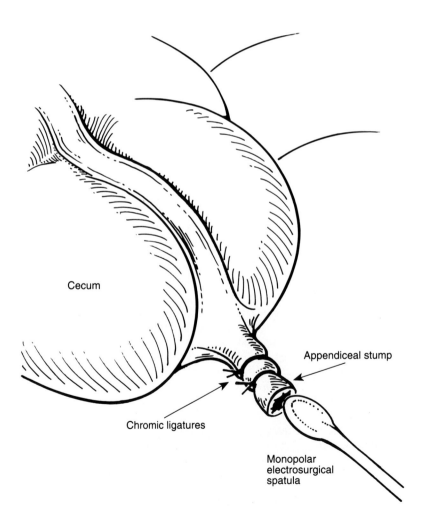

Cecum

Appendiceal stump

Chromic ligatures

Monopolar
electrosurgical
spatula

Figure 2–6. If a monopolar electrosurgical probe is used to coagulate the mucosa after ligature appendectomy, the current return through the appendiceal stump may cause areas of extremely high current density at the point of the ligatures. The high current density may cause coagulation necrosis of the tissue in this area and lead to stump "blowout."

Principles of Bipolar Electrosurgery

The fundamental difference between monopolar and bipolar electrosurgery is the path taken by the electrical current. Monopolar current flows from the active electrode, through tissue, and back to the ground plate. Bipolar electrosurgical instruments place the active and indifferent electrodes in proximity, and current flows only through tissue contiguous with both electrodes. This safe alternative to monopolar electrosurgery has been successfully applied in all disciplines of surgery. Although bipolar use in laparoscopy was previously limited to coagulating forceps, a host of new instruments using bipolar technology are being evaluated. Despite the advantages of bipolar electrosurgery, it is unlikely that laparoscopic monopolar electrosurgery will be replaced by this burgeoning technology.

Principles of Lasers

A medical laser (*l*ight *a*mplification by *s*timulated *e*mission of *r*adiation) is a device capable of converting electrical energy to photon energy. Electrical current is passed to a bright lamp (*i.e.*, flashlamp), which emits photons directed at the lasing medium. When a photon strikes an electron within the lasing medium, the electron absorbs the photon energy and is excited to a higher energy state. Return of the electron to its resting state is accompanied by release of the absorbed energy as another photon, whose wavelength is characteristic of the lasing medium (*i.e.*, spontaneous emission). Stimulated emission occurs when this photon strikes an electron already excited to a higher energy state, and return to the resting state stimulates release of an identical photon. These photons are of the same wavelength and have synchronized wavefronts (*i.e.*, in phase) with each other. This process multiplies exponentially as the photons are amplified between a pair of mirrors.

This process generates monochromatic (*i.e.*, single wavelength), coherent light (*i.e.*, all photons in phase with each other across time and space). The wavelength produced depends on the lasing medium. Millions of coherent photons with the same wavelength act as wavefronts, falling on one another and generating the power of the laser.

Laser light interaction with tissue produces heat, and the extent of tissue heating and damage depends on the laser wavelength, its power density, and the concentration of tissue pigments (*i.e.*, chromophores). Water, melanin, and hemoglobin are the most common tissue chromophores, and each selectively absorbs light of different wavelengths. Laser light penetration and absorption depend on the concentration and content of the various tissue chromophores. This also means that the tissue effect of a given laser and its surgical applications depend on its wavelength.

Four lasers are commonly used in endoscopic surgical procedures: the CO_2, Nd:YAG, KTP, and argon lasers. The carbon dioxide laser (λ = 10.6 μm) produces light in the far-infrared portion of the electromagnetic spectrum and is highly absorbed by water. The neodymium-doped yttrium-aluminum-garnet laser (Nd:YAG, λ = 1064 nm) generates light in the near-infrared portion of the spectrum and is poorly absorbed by oxyhemoglobin or water, penetrating deeply into tissue. The potassium-titanyl-phosphate laser (KTP, λ = 532 nm) is a frequency-doubled (wavelength-halved) Nd:YAG laser that produces green light, poorly absorbed by water but well absorbed by melanin and oxyhemoglobin. The argon laser (λ = 488–514 nm) emits blue light and has an absorption spectrum similar to the KTP laser. These latter two wavelengths are useful for superficial coagulation (*e.g.*, arteriovenous malformations of the colon) or tissue cutting.

Laser energy is most commonly delivered through quartz glass fibers with high internal reflectance. When the light reaches the end of the fiber, it diverges if a lens or thermal coupler is not placed at the end of the fiber. When it is allowed to diverge, the laser beam is used in a noncontact mode. The power density of the laser beam depends on the distance the fiber tip is held from tissue. Commonly used thermal couplers are metal (*e.g.*, laser angioplasty) or crystal. Sapphire has been used for contact laser surgery because of its high melting point, but it appears that the tip of the quartz laser fiber may be sculpted to provide a fine cutting tip or a broad coagulating contact tip at a fraction of the cost of sapphire tips.

Laser or Electrosurgery?

Rigid Endoscopic Surgery

There is a diversity of opinion regarding the superiority of laser or electrosurgical use in rigid endoscopic surgical procedures. This debate raged for many years in gynecologic circles, with laser taking the upper hand because of monopolar intestinal injury occurring in pelviscopic tubal ligation at a rate of 0.1% to 1.0%.[14, 15] The advent of laparoscopic cholecystectomy resurrected this controversy.[16–18] Despite the emotional tone of this argument, the only prospective, randomized study that has been performed to evaluate the two energy sources in laparoscopic cholecystectomy found electrosurgical dissection to be faster and provide superior bleeding control than laser dissection.[19] There was no difference in surgical complications related to the use of monopolar electrosurgery in this or any other study of laparoscopic cholecystectomy.

Flexible Endoscopic Surgery

Although most procedures in laparoscopic surgery can be performed using a combination of monopolar and bipolar electrosurgery, the laser has some unique features that prove advantageous in the realm of flexible endoscopic surgery. The first of these advantages is color selectivity. Argon, KTP, and flashlamp pumped dye lasers with green and yellow dyes are highly absorbed by hemoglobin compounds and poorly absorbed by water. Selective ablation of red-pigmented lesions, such as arteriovenous malformations of the colon, can be performed using these lasers. Electrosurgery is moisture selective but not color selective, and it is therefore less safe than the aforementioned lasers.

The major drawback to using monopolar electrosurgery through flexible telescopes in the gastrointestinal (GI) tract is that the injury this instrument creates is erratic and frequently of full thickness.[19] An additional danger inherent in monopolar surgery is that insufflation of the GI tract causes a thinning of the bowel wall, making it more susceptible to perforation. The probe placed against the bleeding point puts added pressure on the GI tract wall, resulting in further thinning. The electrical current follows the perforating vessels that supply mucosal blood flow, heating the entire bowel wall and risking full-thickness bowel injury.

Although the bipolar probes have been effective in arresting GI hemorrhage without the risks of monopolar technology, there are limitations to this device as a means of recanalizing an obstructed viscus. It is poorly able to vaporize a large volume of tissue at a single setting. If the surgeon is endoscopically attempting to palliate a large, bulky neoplasm of the GI tract, the best instrument appears to be an Nd:YAG laser, because it has a predictable, deep penetration in tissue.

The optimal manner in which to use lasers in endoscopic procedures is to exercise their unique tissue interaction properties. Because each laser has characteristic tissue absorption, it is reasonable to employ lasers in situations that maximize the advantages of those attributes. Examples of resourceful laser use include argon laser photoablation of endometriosis deposits in the pelvis and Nd:YAG laser palliation of obstructing rectal carcinoma. Although more applications for lasers will undoubtedly become apparent during the next few years, monopolar electrosurgery will probably remain the workhorse of therapeutic endoscopic procedures.

ENDOSCOPIC ULTRASOUND

Physics

Ultrasound is an acoustic wave with alternating regions of high and low pressure. These waves travel through the body like sound waves through water. Although sound waves have very low frequency oscillation (i.e., hundreds of cycles per second), ultrasound waves oscillate at frequencies from 1 to 30 million cycles per second (MHz). Higher ultrasound frequencies penetrate tissue to a lesser depth than lower frequencies, but they offer a better spatial resolution of superficial structures. To calculate the penetration depth of a particular ultrasound probe, 40 divided by the frequency of the probe equals the depth of penetration in centimeters. For example, a 20 MHz probe penetrates approximately 2 cm in tissue.

The ultrasound probe is a transducer that transmits and receives the ultrasound energy. The ultrasound image is generated by reflection of the sound waves at various tissue interfaces. In a homogeneous medium such as water (e.g., the bladder), no interfaces are encountered, and no echoes are generated. In a heterogenous mixture of gas, fluid, and solid tissue such as the intestinal tract, much of the ultrasound wave is reflected. When a solid substance with little water content is encountered, propagation is arrested, and a bright shadow is reflected back to the transducer. Beyond this area of reflection, no further reflections are seen. This area is known as the acoustic shadow. Examples of substances creating acoustic shadows are bones and renal or biliary stones.

If ultrasound waves were only able to differentiate water, bone, and soft tissue, their value for diagnosis would be limited. However, the heterogeneity of soft tissue causes different degrees of ultrasound attenuation and a different appearance of the reflected signal. A good example of this phenomenon is seen during endoluminal ultrasound of the intestinal wall, which demonstrates five distinct layers of alternating hyperechogenicity and hypoechogenicity. The hyperechoic areas are the mucosa, submucosa, and serosa. Despite almost identical water content, the homogeneity of the muscularis mucosa and muscularis propria produces hypoechoic bands.

The ultrasound wave is produced by a piezoelectric disc, in which electrical energy is converted into acoustic energy by slight changes in the disc thickness. A reverse coupling occurs when the sound wave is received by the disc. When the signal returns to the transducer, the sound wave alters the configuration of the disc, generating an electrical signal that is transmitted to a digital processor. With B-mode probes, the rapidity of signal generation (15–30/second) allows viewing of anatomy in real time as the transducer is moved across the abdominal wall.

Several ultrasound transducers available for medical application. The most elementary type of scanner is the sector scanner, in which a single element is oscillated, producing a pie-shaped image that views a small array of elements close to the scanner and a wide array of elements more distant from the scanner. To avoid the pie-shaped image, a rectangular image may be obtained by mounting multiple transducers along a path. These are known as linear array transducers. A final type is the phased array transducer, which is similar to the linear array transducer except that slight time delays in the transducer activation (phase differences) may allow control of the imaging direction.

Clinical Application

Flexible endoscopic ultrasound may be performed using small, high-frequency transducers (20 MHz) that can be passed through the operating channel of the endoscope. These transducers produce a limited amount of information because of the shallow depth of ultrasound penetration and the small sector of tissue that can be examined.

Most flexible endoscopic imaging employs a dedicated endoscope fitted with a fluid coupler (i.e., water-filled balloon) that is mounted over the transducer at the end of the scope. All three types of transducers (i.e., linear array, phased array, and sector scanners) have been attached to endoscopes, and some units have the unique capability of being tunable to frequencies between 7 and 12 MHz.

The primary clinical use of endoscopic ultrasound in the GI tract has been to stage esophageal, gastric, and rectal carcinomas. In one series of esophageal carcinoma staged using endoscopic ultrasound, 89% accuracy was obtained, with an equal distribution of overstaging and understaging.[20] The size of lymph nodes adjacent to the gut wall can be accurately determined with endoscopic ultrasound. However, despite the development of criteria for predicting the benign or malignant nature of these nodes, the accuracy has been less than ideal.

For preoperative staging of colorectal malignancies, endoscopic ultrasound has been used extensively to determine the appropriateness of local therapy or radical extirpation.[21, 22] In these series, it has been easier to determine the depth of primary tumor invasion than to predict whether enlarged lymph nodes contain cancer.

LAPAROSCOPIC ULTRASOUND

The disadvantage of transcutaneous ultrasound for fine detail of small anatomic structures is that the low-frequency units necessary to penetrate deeply into the abdomen do not provide the resolution necessary to make the diagnosis of small pathologic lesions, such as small bile duct stones or carcinomas. Laparoscopic ultrasound using high-frequency, high-resolution probes can be a tremendous advantage. Studies have looked at the ability of laparoscopic ultrasound probes to visualize the anatomy of deep-seated hepatic metastases that might change an operative approach or guide ablative surgery.[23] Laparoscopic ultrasound may replace cholangiography as a more accurate method of looking at the extrahepatic biliary system without using ionizing radiation or potentially toxic contrast mediums (Fig. 2–7). In previous studies of open cholecystectomy, the accuracy of ultrasonographic imaging of the biliary system was superior to cholangiography for detecting choledocholithiasis.[24, 25]

CONCLUSION

Endoscopic technology is rapidly expanding. Ultrasonic aspirating devices are entering the field of therapeutic endoscopy, and harmonic scalpels have been created for mechanical or

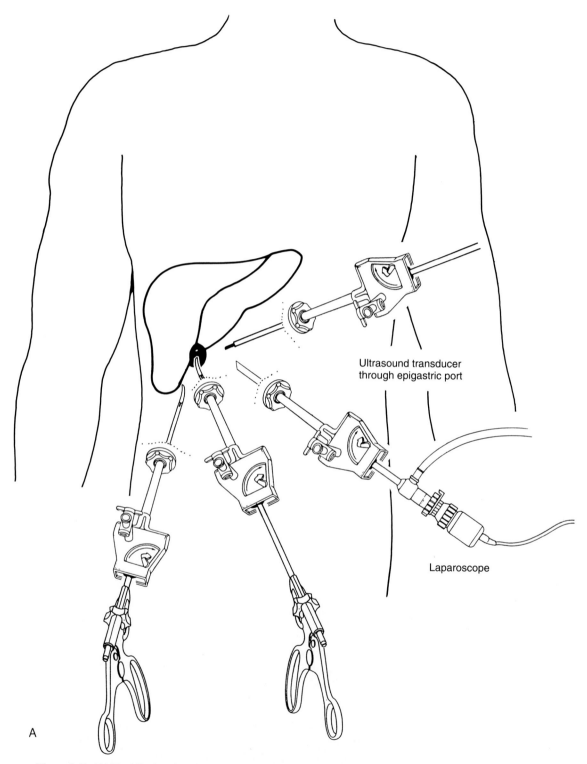

Ultrasound transducer
through epigastric port

Laparoscope

A

Figure 2–7. (A) For bile duct imaging, a sector scanner is introduced through a 10-mm port in the epigastrium.

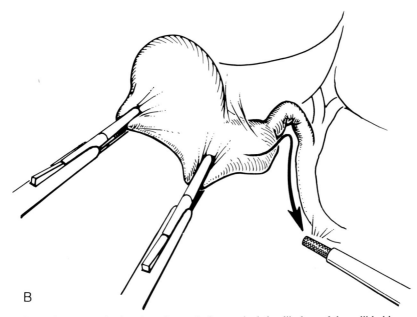

B

Figure 2–7 *Continued* **(B)** The scanner is placed on the cystic duct at the infundibulum of the gallbladder, and swept medially and inferiorly to scan the cystic, common hepatic, and common bile ducts.

thermal dissection. Rotary mechanical bits have been developed for gallstone fragmentation and tissue morcellation.

Although the surgeon is frequently tempted or pressured to buy every new piece of endoscopic technology that comes along, it is his or her duty to evaluate each of these new technologies for equipment safety, expense to the patient, and cost to society. Only if patient outcome will be better and cost can be curtailed should the physician heartily embrace a new bit of endoscopic technology.

References

1. Berci G, Davids J. Endoscopy and television. Br Med J 1:1610, 1962.
2. Berci G, Urban JC. Miniature black and white TV camera for endoscopy and other medical applications. Biomed Eng 7:116, 1972.
3. Nitze M. Biobachtungs und Untersuchungsmethode für Harnrohre Harnblase und Rectum. Wein Med Wochenschr 24:651, 1879.
4. Gunning JE. The history of laparoscopy. J Reprod Med 12:222, 1974.
5. Hopkins HH. Optical principles of the endoscope. In: Berci G, ed. Endoscopy. New York: Appleton-Century-Crofts, 1976:3.
6. Olsen V. Light sources. In: Berci G, ed. Endoscopy. New York: Appleton-Century-Crofts, 1976:64.
7. Hopkins HH. Physics of the fiberoptic endoscope. In: Berci G, ed. Endoscopy. New York: Appleton-Century-Crofts, 1976:27.
8. Hopkins HH. Physics of the fiberoptic endoscope. In: Berci G, ed. Endoscopy. New York: Appleton-Century-Crofts, 1976:27.
9. Nitze M. Zur Photography der meinschlichen Harnrohe. Berl Med Wochenschr 31:744, 1893.
10. Paz-Partlow M. Documentation for laparoscopy. In: Berci G, Cuschieri A, eds. Practical laparoscopy. London: Balliere Tindall, 1986:19.
11. Paz-Partlow M. Documentation for laparoscopy. In: Berci G, Cuschieri A, eds. Practical laparoscopy. London: Balliere Tindall, 1986:19.
12. Berci G. Techniques for improving illumination and recording in endoscopy. Optics Laser Technol 2:31, 1976.
13. Fourestier M, Bladu A, Vulmière J. Perfectionnement de l'endoscopie medicale. Presse Med 60:1292, 1952.
14. Phillips JM. Survey of gynecologic laparoscopy for 1974. J Reprod Med 15:45, 1975.
15. Thompson BH, Wheeless CR. Gastrointestinal complications of laparoscopy sterilization. Obstet Gynecol 41:669, 1973.
16. Voyles CR, Petro AB, Meena AL, et al. A practical approach to laparoscopic cholecystectomy. Am J Surg 161:365, 1991.
17. Corbitt JD. Laparoscopic cholecystectomy: laser versus electrosurgery. Surg Lap Endosc 1:85, 1991.
18. Hunter JG. Laser or electrocautery for laparoscopic cholecystectomy? Am J Surg 161:345, 1991.
19. Bordelon BM, Hobday KA, Hunter JG. Laser versus electrosurgery in laparoscopic cholecystectomy: a prospective, randomized trial. Arch Surg 128:233, 1993.
20. Tio TL, Coene PPLO, Luiken GJHN, Tytgat GNJ. Endosonography in the clinical staging of esophagogastric carcinoma. Gastrointest Endosc 36:S2, 1990.
21. Beynon J, Mortensen NJ, Foy DMA, et al. Pre-operative assessment of local invasion in rectal cancer: digital examination, endoluminal sonography, or computed tomography. Br J Surg 73:1015, 1986.

22. Buess G, Mentges B, Manncke K, Starlinger M, Becker HD. Technique and results of transanal endoscopic microsurgery in early rectal cancer. Am J Surg 163:63, 1992.
23. Boenhof JA, Linhart P, Bettendorf U, et al. Liver biopsy guided by laparoscopic sonography. Endoscopy 16:237, 1984.
24. Jakimowicz JJ, Rutten H, Jurgens PJ, Carol EJ. Comparison of operative ultrasonography and radiology in screening of the common bile duct for calculi. World J Surg 11:628, 1987.
25. Sigel B, Machi J, Beitler JC, et al. Comparative accuracy of operative ultrasonography and cholangiography in detecting common bile duct calculi. Surgery 94:715, 1983.

3

Nasopharyngeal and Laryngeal Endoscopy

Howard L. Levine and Sanford Timen

Physicians performing endoscopy of the upper gastrointestinal and respiratory tracts pass their endoscopes through the nasal cavity or mouth, through the hypopharynx, and into the trachea or the esophagus. For these endoscopists, it is important to understand the techniques involved in endoscopy of the upper airway and the pathologic conditions encountered in this region.

NASAL ENDOSCOPY

Nasal endoscopy provides an efficient and thorough method of diagnosis and management of nasal and sinus disorders. Many patients with nasal symptoms who have normal traditional nasal examinations have treatable abnormalities found on nasal endoscopy.[1]

Equipment

Nasal endoscopy can be performed with rigid or flexible endoscopes. Rigid endoscopes permit one hand to hold the endoscope while the other is free to manipulate any instrument that is inserted into the nasal cavity. These endoscopes are available in different lens configurations to allow a straightforward view (0°) or angled view (30° or 70°) (Fig. 3–1). Some endoscopes provide a wide-angle view of the field.

Flexible endoscopes require two hands to manipulate the instrument. Typically, one hand holds the endoscope near the body orifice while the other holds the observer ocular portion and manipulates the endoscope tip. Some of these endoscopes have suction and biopsy channels that are useful only for minimal secretions and small biopsies. These scopes are available in different outer diameters for use in pediatric and adult patients. Although not allowing the freedom of a second hand for instrumentation that the rigid endoscopes provide, the flexible endoscopes often permit a more thorough view into the orifices of the nasal and sinus cavities because the tip of the endoscope can be manipulated.

Several light sources are available for endoscopy, depending on the needs and goals of the examiner. Hand-held light sources can be carried from one examining room to another or to the patient's bedside. Although convenient, they provide enough illumination for only a general overview of the region. Larger, portable light sources employ a slide projector bulb and

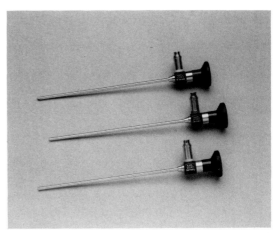

Figure 3–1. Nasal endoscopes with 0° forward viewing, 30°, and 70° lenses.

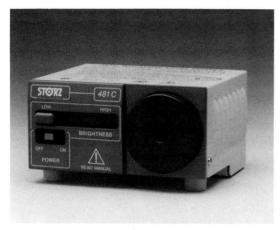

Figure 3–2. Portable office or bedside light source.

Table 3–1. BOYETTE'S SOLUTION

4% xylocaine HCl monohydrate, 8 g
1% phenylephrine HCl, 2 g
0.9% sodium chloride granules, 1.8 g
Q. suff. to 200 mL with distilled H_2O
Add 1 drop of peppermint oil
Add 5 drops of zephrine chloride concentrate to preserve
  solution

can be used for both office or bedside examinations (Fig. 3–2). For photographic or video
documentation, halogen or xenon light sources
are best (Fig. 3–3).

Technique

The nasal cavity is topically anesthetized and
decongested using Boyette's nasal spray (Table
3–1). If there is moderate or marked nasal
congestion, the nose is sprayed again. After 5
to 10 minutes, the nose is examined.

For most of the examination, the 0° 4-mm
endoscope is used. This permits an overview of
the nasal cavity (Fig. 3–4). The relationship
between the nasal turbinates and the nasal septum is observed, looking for septal deviations,
septal spurs, and contact points between the
nasal septum and lateral nasal wall that may be
a source of nasal airway or sinus obstruction

(Fig. 3–5). Sometimes, systemic pathology manifests within the nose (Figs. 3–6 and 3–7). The
nasal endoscope is passed along the floor of the
nose into the nasopharynx to visualize the eustachian tube orifice, looking for neoplasms,
adenoid hypertrophy, or infection (Figs. 3–8
and 3–9).

The endoscope is withdrawn into the nose
and angled upward to examine the sphenoethmoid recess, the area between the middle and
superior nasal turbinates, where the sphenoid
and posterior ethmoid sinuses drain into the
nose (Fig. 3–10). The recess is often narrow
because the superior turbinate is in proximity
to the nasal septum. In these cases, a 30° 2.7-
mm endoscope may be needed. The angled
endoscope allows better visualization into the
superior meatus. Infection or nasal polyps may
be found here, and they may be the source of
nasal drainage or facial pain and pressure.

As the endoscope is withdrawn in the nose,
the area of the middle meatus is examined
carefully. This region is named the ostiomeatal
complex (*i.e.*, the ostia of the frontal, maxillary,
and anterior ethmoid sinuses and the middle
meatus of the nose). This area is the origin of

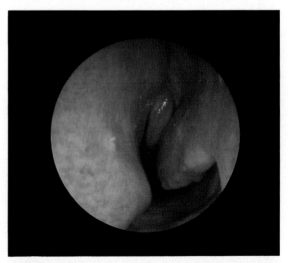

Figure 3–4. Endoscopic overview of the right side of the
nasal cavity demonstrates the nasal septum to the left and
the inferior and middle turbinates to the right.

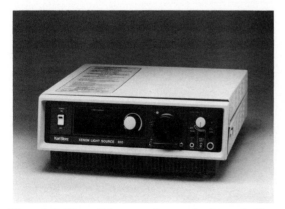

Figure 3–3. Xenon light source for examination and still or
video documentation.

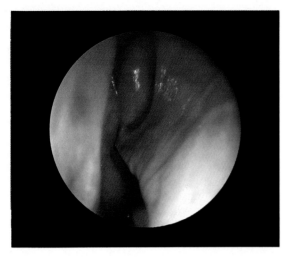

Figure 3–5. Right side of the nose with deviated nasal septum with contact point between the septum and the lateral nasal wall.

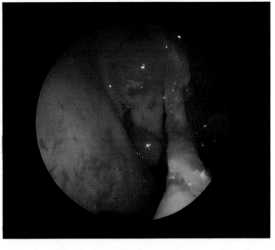

Figure 3–7. Total nasal septal perforation in hereditary hemorrhagic telangiectasia of the nasal cavity.

most nasal and sinus pathology. It is best examined by beginning posteriorly in the middle meatus and rotating the endoscope upward and laterally beneath the middle turbinate. Much like the sphenoethmoid recess, this region may be narrow and necessitate the use of the 30° 2.7-mm endoscope. The ostiomeatal complex is the frequent site of polyps and infection (Figs. 3–11 and 3–12).

Surgical Nasal Endoscopy

Nasal endoscopy provides a superb method for diagnosing nasal disorders, and it offers a surgical approach to the sinuses.[2-4] Endoscopic sinus surgery can be performed on an outpatient basis under attended local or general anesthesia. The 0° 4-mm endoscope is usually employed with a xenon or halogen light source. Most surgeons operate looking through the endoscope, but more are beginning to use a video camera and monitor. Use of a video camera and monitor provides a magnified and illuminated image that aids surgery.

Many operations can be performed with the nasal endoscopes, depending on the extent and nature of the pathology. If the disease is extensive and there have been multiple previous operations (*e.g.,* sinus and nasal polyposis), an endoscopic marsupialization procedure is per-

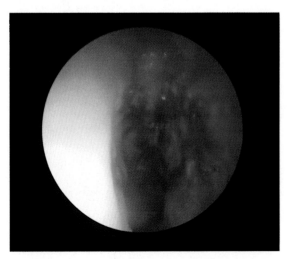

Figure 3–6. Crohn's disease with nasal ulceration.

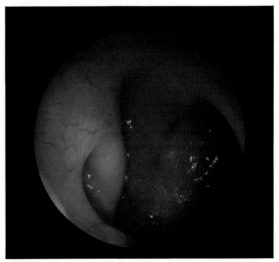

Figure 3–8. Normal nasopharynx, posterior pharyngeal wall, and right eustachian tube orifice.

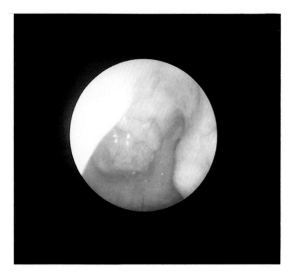

Figure 3–9. Adenoid hypertrophy on the roof of the nasopharynx.

anterior cranial fossa, and the lamina papyracea, the lateral wall of the ethmoid sinus that separates it from the orbit, can be identified and preserved.

If disease is limited and there has been minimal or no previous sinus surgery, a true functional endoscopic sinus surgical (FESS) procedure can be performed. Normal structures such as the middle turbinate can be preserved with much of the sinus mucosa, which minimizes crusting in the nose. The results of FESS are more physiologic because the procedure restores more normal nasal airflow and ciliary clearance of the sinus cavity. The natural ostia of the sinuses can be refashioned to permit efficient and natural sinus drainage.

LARYNGEAL ENDOSCOPY

Endoscopy of the larynx was first described by a singing teacher, Garcia, in 1854, when he examined his own vocal cords using a candle and mirror. Since that time, indirect laryngoscopy (using a mirror to reflect the image) has been the standard method for examining the larynx.

The technique of indirect laryngoscopy is

formed. This is similar to the traditional intranasal ethmoidectomy, except it is done with endoscopes. The use of the endoscopes allows more thorough removal of the pathologic tissue. At the same time, the fovea ethmoidalis, the roof of the ethmoid sinus and floor of the

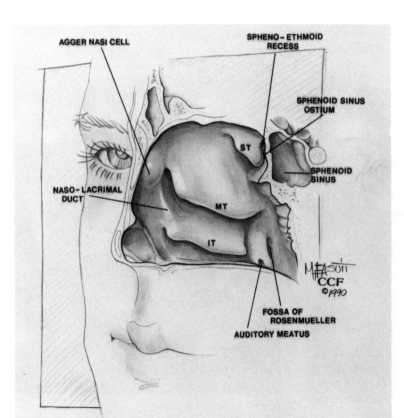

Figure 3–10. Lateral nasal wall and the sphenoethmoid recess.

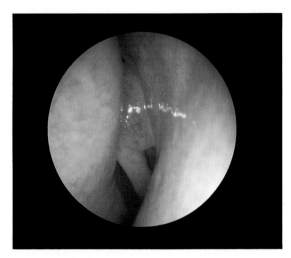

Figure 3–11. Mucosal edema of the left nasal cavity. The left middle turbinate with early polyp formation is beginning to obstruct the ostiomeatal complex.

rapid, inexpensive, transportable, and noninvasive. For generations, experienced general surgeons and otolaryngologists have relied on indirect mirror laryngoscopy to provide accurate diagnosis of laryngeal pathology. Disadvantages of the mirror examination include the need for patient cooperation and participation. This requirement often precludes examining small children, some adults, and bedridden or unconscious patients. Documentation of the examination with an indirect mirror is limited to the examiner verbally describing or sketching findings. There are some laryngeal disorders, such as neuromuscular and subtle functional problems, that are not easily detected with the mirror, but the

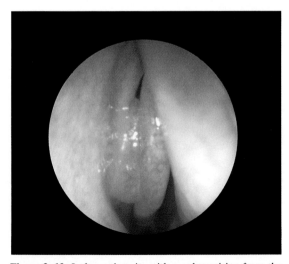

Figure 3–12. Left nasal cavity with a polyp arising from the anterior ethmoid sinus that obstructs the ostiomeatal complex.

mirror remains an excellent method for surveying laryngeal pathology.

Flexible fiberoptic laryngoscopy (FFL) has become an excellent method for examination of the larynx. The major advantage over mirror examination is the ease with which the flexible laryngoscope may be passed into the larynx in patients with an excessive gag reflex. Patients with depressed states of consciousness and recumbent patients can be examined without their active cooperation. A small child may often be encouraged to permit passage of a narrow-diameter laryngoscope. Another valuable use of the FFL is retrograde passage through a tracheostomy to examine the underside of the vocal cords. Disadvantages of FFL are few. Compared with the indirect mirror laryngoscopy, FFL is expensive, and unless used frequently for laryngeal or nasal examinations, having a flexible laryngoscope may not be cost effective.

Direct or operative laryngoscopy has its greatest use in examination of the larynx for referable signs, evaluation and biopsy of laryngeal neoplasia, part of complete endoscopic examination for known squamous cell carcinoma of the aerodigestive tract looking for a second primary lesion, evaluation of a patient with an occult metastatic carcinoma to the neck, evaluation of a trauma, and removal of a foreign body.[5]

Technique

Indirect laryngoscopy requires experience and patience to master. Using a No. 4 or No. 6 laryngeal mirror, the examiner positions the patient's head to a level slightly higher than his own. The patient is positioned straight backed with the head and neck extended as if he were sniffing a flower. The examiner's thumb is placed on the dorsum of the tongue, the second finger opposes the thumb on the ventral surface, and the index finger lifts the patient's upper lip. The patient is asked to breathe gently through the mouth, often imitating a soft panting sound. The mirror is introduced into the mouth. Deliberately touching the corner of the upper lip with the handle of the mirror reduces the patient's tendency to gag. The mirror is used to displace and elevate the uvula. Care is taken to touch neither the lateral pharyngeal wall nor the base of the tongue, which might trigger the gag reflex.

Having the patient phonate "ahhh . . ." or "heee . . ." raises and tilts the larynx, bringing it into the examiner's view and adducting the vocal cords. The hypopharynx is examined during quiet breathing and phonation. The physician examines each portion of the hypopharynx:

base of tongue, lingual tonsil, lingual surface and free margin of the epiglottis, arytenoid and aryepiglottic folds, false vocal folds, laryngeal ventricle and true vocal folds, subglottis and trachea, piriform sinus, esophageal introitus, and walls of the hypopharynx. Vocal cord mobility is determined by having the patient alternate inspiration with phonation of "heee." Patients with a sensitive gag reflex benefit from placement of topical anesthesia on the middle one third of the tongue and soft palate.

Flexible fiberoptic laryngoscopy requires patient preparation. The patient's nasal cavity is anesthetized with 4% xylocaine and 1% phenylephrine to vasoconstrict the mucosa and provide comfort. While the patient breathes through his nose, the examiner views through the laryngoscope as it is advanced along the floor of the nose. On reaching the nasopharynx, as the tip of the laryngoscope passes the free margin of the soft palate, the patient often finds mouth breathing more comfortable. The larynx and hypopharynx are easily examined and the various structures systematically viewed as with the mirror. With the FFL, the piriform sinuses can be seen particularly well. The patient is instructed to inhale against the closed glottis, mimicking a bilateral vocal cord paralysis (i.e., vocal cords adducted). This causes the piriform fossae to expand with air, and exposes each mucosal wall.

Operative laryngoscopy techniques require close cooperation between the endoscopist and the anesthesiologist. It is important that both examine the patient before the procedure, especially if a potential airway problem might occur. The choice of anesthesia technique is also a consideration that requires cooperation and communication between surgeon and anesthetist. General anesthesia is most commonly used. Preoperative apprehension is less if patients are sure they will be comfortably asleep, and the endoscopist is less pressured with the patient under general anesthesia. General anesthesia permits the surgeon to proceed with a detailed examination of all the hypopharyngeal structures and teach or photograph as desired. The disadvantages of general anesthesia are the inability to determine active vocal cord mobility and the interference of the endotracheal tube in viewing some parts of the larynx. Special care is required for a large tumor. It may be necessary to perform a tracheostomy before anesthesia is safely given.

Operative direct laryngoscopy is performed with oral-endotracheal intubation using a 5.5- to 6.0-mm cuffed endotracheal tube. The endotracheal tube occasionally interferes with examination of the posterior larynx between the arytenoid aryteroid cartilages.

Apneic anesthetic techniques eliminate the problems of the endotracheal tube obscuring structures. Ventilation proceeds with a face mask. While asleep, the patient is hyperventilated with oxygen. The oxygen saturation is monitored by pulse oximetry. When deemed appropriate by the anesthesiologist, ventilation is discontinued while the surgeon carries out 1 or 2 minutes of unencumbered inspection of the larynx. The technique is of great value if there is a marginal airway and the surgeon thinks that minimal trauma to the larynx may trigger frank airway obstruction.

Percutaneous jet ventilation originally used a needle placed into the trachea and pressurized oxygen to fill the lungs. Difficulties with complications, such as trauma to the tracheal mucosa, subcutaneous emphysema, pneumomediastinum, pneumothorax, and hematoma, make this method undesirable for most situations. Safe and convenient jet ventilation is accomplished using a 3.5-mm endotracheal tube and ventilating with 15 to 20 psi of oxygen at 10 to 16 respirations per minute.

After the anesthesia method has been decided, a laryngoscope must be chosen. The largest laryngoscope that can fit without causing injury to the oral and pharyngeal mucosa should be used. The Holinger anterior commissure laryngoscope and the Dedo-Pilling modified anterior commissure laryngoscope are instruments that have been relied on for years.

The patient is positioned with a shoulder roll under the lower neck to extend the neck if anatomy permits. Hyperextension is not absolutely necessary and should be avoided in patients with substantial cervical arthritis. After the patient is asleep and positioned, the evaluation proceeds. The blade tip is inserted superior and posterior to the tongue while the teeth are protected by a gauze sponge or rubber teeth protector. The epiglottis is examined first, with care taken to view the vallecula and lingual and laryngeal surfaces of the epiglottis. The laryngoscope is directed anteriorly, carefully avoiding the use of the teeth as a fulcrum. The remainder of the supraglottic, glottic, and hypopharyngeal structures are subsequently examined.

Pathologic Conditions Requiring Endoscopy

The pathologic conditions that may require endoscopic examination of the larynx are evaluation of a neck mass or tumor, impairment of respiration, dysfunction of deglutition, and problems of phonation.

Appropriate evaluation of a neck mass in an adult requires endoscopic examination of the upper aerodigestive tract.[6] In a patient older than 50 years of age, a neck mass has a chance of being a metastasis from the upper air or food passageway approaching 85%. Many of the areas can easily be seen with a headlight, tongue depressor, and mirror on FFL. Failure to identify a primary site should be followed by fine-needle aspiration of the neck mass. Operative endoscopic examination should be considered next to confirm, biopsy, or search for an undiscovered second primary. Open biopsy of a lymph node in the neck should be employed selectively, and preparation should be in place for neck dissection if a frozen section proves positive for squamous cell carcinoma.

Impaired respiration from laryngeal compromise occurs in conditions such as neoplasia, a neurogenic abnormality, or trauma. A common neurologic problem encountered in surgery is whether the recurrent laryngeal nerve is intact after thyroidectomy or parathyroidectomy. All patients having thyroid or parathyroid surgery should have their larynges examined preoperatively. This simple, but often overlooked examination determines whether recurrent laryngeal nerves are intact and functioning. Failure to recognize a vocal cord paralysis preoperatively may cause the patient unnecessary morbidity. Although unusual, asymptomatic or minimally symptomatic unilateral vocal cord paralysis that had not been previously diagnosed occurs often enough to be of concern.

Extubation of the patient after total thyroidectomy causes occasional consternation about the airway. Some surgeons are in the habit of asking the anesthesiologist whether the vocal cords move adequately. Most anesthesiologists agree that this practice has little validity. The extraneous movements that occur when the patient is being extubated include frequent coughing and occasional laryngospasm. Under these conditions, vocal cord mobility cannot be observed reliably. Any patient whose airway is significantly impaired needs to be reintubated and awakened. A controlled endoscopic examination can be carried out with mirror or FFL.

Bilateral vocal cord paralysis may cause respiratory distress while a normal voice is retained. Injury to the recurrent laryngeal nerve(s) results in loss of the posterior cricoarytenoid muscle function, the only abductor of the glottis. Variation in the neurology of the larynx probably accounts for the inability to always predict correctly the position of the vocal

cords in an acute injury. The posterior ramus of the recurrent laryngeal nerve usually innervates the posterior cricoarytenoid muscle and injury results in the vocal cords assuming a paramedian position. Occasionally, the anterior ramus may carry the posterior cricoarytenoid fibers. This branch may become entrapped between the cricoarytenoid joint and the thyroid cartilage during endotracheal intubation, with recurrent nerve dysfunction occurring without the nerve being sectioned. Frank airway obstruction with bilateral vocal cord paralysis does not always occur immediately. As the muscle tone of the denervated muscle decreases and the vocal cord falls passively toward the midline, progressive dyspnea and stridor develop.

Injury to the superior laryngeal nerve can occur in thyroid surgery. This nerve carries sensory and motor fibers by its internal and external branches to the supraglottic mucosal surfaces and to the cricothyroid muscle. Damage to the nerve results in loss of ability to reach the upper end of the pitch register when singing and the sensation of a foreign body irritating the pharynx. Endoscopy of the larynx reveals the larynx to be rotated on a vertical axis with the anterior commissure directed away from the injured nerve and the posterior commissure pointed to the damaged side.

Hoarseness frequently occurs as a complication of intubation. Direct pressure from a stiff endotracheal tube can easily erode the mucosa of the posterior glottis. This condition does not take long to develop and has been seen in patients who were intubated only for several hours. After extubation, the patients complain of hoarseness and have sore throat, dysphagia, and odynophagia. Prolonged intubation of several days increases the frequency of the irritation. Endoscopic examination may reveal granuloma formation or ulceration of the vocal process of the arytenoid process or on the anteromedial surface of the arytenoid cartilages. Patients with gastroesophageal reflux are prone to this problem. The extreme extent of such difficulties may be seen in patients who have been intubated and require nasogastric tubes with stiff, large lumens. After extubation, pain, hoarseness, and aspiration may indicate the presence of a postcricoid ulcer that would only be visualized by direct operative laryngoscopy.

Unilateral vocal cord paralysis is often the cause of hoarseness.[6] The recurrent laryngeal nerve is placed at risk during thyroid, parathyroid, and carotid artery surgery. Carotid endarterectomy has been associated with postoperative cranial neuropathy of the glossopharyngeal, vagus, accessory, and hypoglossal nerves. When one recurrent laryngeal nerve is nonfunctional, the vocal cord often is positioned just off the midline. During adduction, the contralateral vocal cord may fail to compensate by moving across the midline. Air escape during phonation results in a breathy voice, and ineffective coaptation of the vocal cords during swallowing causes aspiration.

The surgeon may be required to evaluate laryngeal function in the trauma patient. Most cases involve blunt trauma, but the principles of management are the same for penetrating injuries. If emergent tracheostomy is not needed, a complete history of the traumatic event is usually useful. An estimate of the extent of force transmitted to the neck provides the examiner with the sense of the severity of the injury. Symptoms of hoarseness, pain, and dysphagia are indicators of mild injury. Hemoptysis and stridor indicate a more serious injury. Physical examination may reveal anterior neck discoloration and swelling. Palpation can determine subcutaneous emphysema, pain over the hyoid bone, thyroid cartilage, or cricoid cartilages or displacement of the cartilages.

FFL is preferred to mirror laryngoscopy in these patients because of improved patient compliance and superior visualization. Examination should include observation of the patency of the airway, should establish the status of vocal cord mobility, and should determine the extent of hematoma and laceration of the laryngeal mucosa. Although beyond the scope of this chapter to discuss the treatment of laryngeal trauma, it is important to realize that some of these injuries are best treated by tracheotomy, and others require open exploration within 24 hours to preserve the voice and protect function of the larynx.

References

1. Levine HL. The office diagnosis of nasal and sinus disorders using rigid nasal endoscopy. Otolaryngol Head Neck Surg 102:370, 1990.
2. Kennedy DW, Zinnreich SJ, Rosenbaum AE, et al. Functional endoscopic sinus surgery: theory and diagnostic evaluation. Arch Otolaryngol 111:576–582, 1985.
3. Stammberger H. Endoscopic sinus surgery–new concepts and treatment of recurring rhinosinusitis. I. Anatomic and pathophysiologic considerations. II. Surgical technique. Otolaryngol Head Neck Surg 94:143–156, 1986.
4. Messerklinger W. Endoscopy of the nose. Baltimore: Urban & Schwartzenberg, 1978.
5. Johnson J, Myers, EN. Recent advances in operative endoscopy. Otolaryngol Clin North Am 17:35, 1984.
6. Tucker HM. Vocal cord paralysis; etiology and management. Laryngoscope 90:585, 1980.

4

Esophagogastroduodenoscopy
Indications, Technique, and Interpretation

Frederick L. Greene

Disease is very old and nothing about it has changed. It is we who change as we understand what was formerly imperceptible.

CHARCOT

The approach to upper gastrointestinal (GI) tract disease depends on a clear understanding of symptoms and signs. The evaluation should take into consideration patient safety, cost issues, the ability to make histologic interpretation, and record keeping, including retrievable data to allow for review of interpretation. Although contrast studies continue to have a role in the assessment of upper GI disease, our ability to assess the esophagus, stomach, and duodenum endoscopically has enabled increased accuracy and earlier histologic determination of mucosal lesions.

For surgeons performing curative and palliative procedures for GI tract malignancies, the need to be directly involved in endoscopic assessment of the upper GI tract has taken on greater importance in recent years. Although less aggressive surgical approaches to benign GI tract disease, such as those related to acid peptic processes and reflux, have evolved because of efficient and potent medical therapies, the surgeon's role will continue to be important in the management of complications of these illnesses. The surgeon must become proficient in the performance of gastrointestinal endoscopy for upper GI tract disease.

INDICATIONS

The primary reasons to perform esophago-gastroduodenoscopy (EGD) are to provide early evidence of esophageal or gastric malignancy, to assess sites of bleeding from the proximal GI tract, to identify active lesions attributable to acid peptic disease or reflux, or to assess the likelihood of congenital processes in adults and children. Symptoms of dysphagia or odynophagia should be evaluated initially by EGD because of the likelihood of finding esophageal malignancy. Most patients seeking treatment for dysphagia tend to present after symptoms have existed for weeks to months, and the earliest endoscopic evaluation and histologic assessment are mandatory. Many patients continue to undergo contrast studies of the esophagus, which may display anatomic abnormalities that require endoscopic assessment before definitive treatment.

A second frequent indication for EGD is substernal or epigastric pain or burning associated with "waterbrash" or the report of a sour or acid taste by the patient. The symptoms are indicative of acid reflux and require a complete EGD evaluation. Symptoms of vague abdominal or back pain may be associated with symptoms of reflux and may indicate associated peptic ulcer disease in the stomach or duodenum.

Signs or symptoms of acute or chronic bleeding from the upper GI tract should prompt early EGD evaluation. Melanic stool, usually indicating active upper GI bleeding, may be assessed endoscopically with the additional benefit of applying therapeutic modalities through endoscopic means if needed. The need for emergent endoscopic evaluation in the patient with acute upper GI bleeding has been debated in terms of the effect on overall outcome after early endoscopic visualization of the bleeding site.[1] Although a clear benefit of early EGD has not been universally established, early recognition and localization of a proximal GI bleeding site often leads to directed treatment planning and specific surgical therapy.

If radiographic contrast studies have been obtained to evaluate the possibility of proximal GI disease, a clear indication for EGD is the elucidation of an abnormal or indeterminate radiographic study. A careful review of contrast studies is mandatory to plan for full endoscopic evaluation and to direct the surgical endoscopist. Evaluation of the contrast studies provides valuable information about potential hazardous areas such as Zenker's or duodenal diverticula, paraesophageal hernia, or other acquired or congenital upper GI tract abnormalities.

Many patients who have had previous upper GI tract resection, reconstruction, or other procedures continue to have symptoms requiring early endoscopic evaluation.[2] The surgical endoscopist is best suited to evaluate these patients, to interpret postoperative anatomic changes, to identify new lesions, and determine the need and extent of operative reconstruction.

ENDOSCOPIC EQUIPMENT AND PATIENT PREPARATION

The availability and safety of upper GI endoscopy are directly related to the major advances in technology ushered in during the modern age of fiberoptic technology, beginning in the early 1960s. Before the era of flexible scopes, rigid endoscopic techniques were dangerous and difficult for patient and endoscopist. The historic development of adequate light sources, optic design, directional control, and adaptation to photographic and modern data recording techniques are examples of successful physician-technology interaction.[3]

The surgical endoscopist has a wide choice of available endoscopic equipment. Instrument diameter, suction, instrument channel size, still photographic or video recording capability, and additional endoscopic characteristics may enhance diagnostic and therapeutic capability. Because most EGD procedures are performed in a hospital-based or free-standing endoscopic suite, a variety of endoscopes should be available to manage adult and pediatric problems. Improved endoscopic technology, using the chip camera and television display, has created new opportunities for the endoscopist and for those taking part in the interpretation of findings.

Most upper GI endoscopic studies are performed in the outpatient setting. Patients should be instructed to take nothing orally for at least 6 to 8 hours before the examination and to avoid the ingestion of antacids or other medicinals that interfere with interpretation of mucosal lesions. Because sedation is used for most upper endoscopic techniques, the patient should be accompanied to the hospital and driven home after the procedure.

A full explanation of the plans for the endoscopic procedure is mandatory and should be followed by appropriate completion of an informed consent document by the patient. Printed material, including a diagram of the planned procedure, is helpful and should be distributed to the patient during the initial office or clinic appointments. It is important to assess the competency and cooperation of each patient undergoing an endoscopic procedure. Uncooperative patients pose a threat to themselves, the endoscopic team, and the instrumentation, and they should be managed using general anesthetic techniques. Appropriate informed consent must be obtained from the patient's family or guardian if competency is questioned.

Patient preparation using oropharyngeal topical anesthesia, intravenous sedation, or both returns dividends if performed adequately by the surgeon-endoscopist. Several minutes should be taken to spray the pharynx with an appropriate topical agent. Taking a full history to uncover possible allergy to xylocaine or other agents is mandatory before administering any agent. The gag response of each patient has to be assessed to achieve optimal pharyngeal sedation. Supplementation with intravenous sedation is necessary for most patients. An intravenous catheter should be placed in the right forearm or hand before the procedure to allow titration of intravenous sedation during the procedure. Because the patient is placed in the left lateral recumbent position, placement of the catheter in the right upper extremity avoids the possibility of venous obstruction secondary to positioning.

Traditionally, intravenous narcotics or benzodiazepines have been used to achieve sedation for upper and lower gastrointestinal endoscopy. Midazolam (Versed) has become popular because of the reduction in respiratory depression and thrombophlebitis associated with this drug. Small doses of midazolam can achieve significant sedation and amnesia, and it should be used in doses ranging from 1 to 3 mg, especially in elderly patients. Benzodiazepine receptor antagonists are effective in reversal of drug effects. One such drug is flumazenil (Mazicon), which is recommended to be given intravenously in a dose of 0.2 mg over 15 seconds with follow-up doses of 0.2 mg every 60 seconds until a maximal dose of 1 mg is reached. These antagonists and traditional narcotic antagonists should be available in the endoscopy suite. If intravenous opiates are used, naloxone (Narcan) may be given in a dose ranging from 0.2 to 0.4 mg. The short-lived effect of the intravenous drug supports the administration of an equal and simultaneous intramuscular dose. The use of atropine to reduce oral secretions, although popular in past years, is rare today during upper GI endoscopic examination.

Before beginning the endoscopic procedure, evaluation of instrumentation by the gastrointestinal assistant and surgeon-endoscopist is mandatory to ensure that mechanical problems do not create hazardous situations or interfere with optimal assessment and interpretation. A checklist to ensure proper functioning of air and water channels, suction capability, and optics is important (Table 4–1). If biopsy, cytology, or photographic capability is anticipated, the availability of these accessories should be determined before the endoscope is introduced.

For most upper endoscopic examinations, the patient is placed in the left lateral recumbent position. Routine monitoring of oxygen saturation, pulse rate, and blood pressure is mandatory, especially if intravenous sedation is employed.[4–7] Oral suction capability should be readily available and located for easy access to the patient and endoscopic assistant. Full assessment of the intraoral area should be made, and dentures should be removed.

ENDOSCOPIC TECHNIQUE

After optimal topical or intravenous sedation has been achieved, the tip of the endoscope is placed into the posterior pharynx. A bite block, previously placed over the scope, is inserted gradually and gently into the patient's mouth with instructions to the patient to bite gently on the plastic device. The patient is encouraged to

Table 4–1. CHECKLIST BEFORE ESOPHAGOGASTRODUODENOSCOPY

Functioning of air and water channels
Availability of suction
Monitoring equipment (*e.g.,* pulse oximeter, EKG, blood pressure cuff)
Nasal oxygen if needed
Accessories (*e.g.,* biopsy forceps, snare, electrocautery)
Intravenous access
Proper informed consent
Photographic or video recording capability

swallow as the posterior pharynx is visualized through the endoscope or on the television monitor if video endoscopy is used. Because swallowing may be difficult with a bite block in place, in the cooperative patient swallowing of the endoscope may be facilitated by removing the bite block until the endoscope is advanced into the upper esophagus. The bite block is then replaced for the remainder of the examination. Flexion of the neck may facilitate passage of the endoscope into the upper esophagus.

The most important principles in performing safe gastrointestinal endoscopy are the visualization of the lumen of the bowel at all times and advancing the endoscope only when the lumen is clearly evident. Although full evaluation of the upper GI tract is usually achieved during withdrawal of the instrument, careful assessment of the esophagus, stomach, and duodenum during intubation may identify abnormalities that should be reevaluated during scope withdrawal.

The scope is advanced using the endoscopist's right hand while the left hand controls the directional dials and regulates air, water, and suction. Much of the examination may be performed using torquing techniques with the shaft of the instrument, employing tip deflection during intubation of the duodenum and retroflexion for assessment of the gastric cardia and gastroesophageal junction. The endoscope should be advanced initially to the level of the pylorus and advanced through the pyloric channel during sphincter relaxation (Fig. 4–1). A minimal amount of air insufflation allows patient comfort. After the duodenum is entered, the concentric rings of mucosal folds become evident (Fig. 4–2) and allow the duodenal lumen to be followed to at least the third portion, where the ampulla of Vater may be visualized. Identification of the ampulla may be difficult using the conventional end-viewing instrument.

A careful evaluation of the duodenum is performed during withdrawal. The duodenal bulb is best visualized during withdrawal and is characterized by a flattening of the mucosa with loss of the characteristic duodenal folds. Before withdrawing the endoscope into the pyloric channel, suctioning air from within the duodenum enhances patient comfort.

The pylorus and gastric antrum are visualized fully as the endoscope is withdrawn proximally into the stomach. Optimal use of insufflation allows flattening of the gastric rugal folds to fully assess the gastric mucosa. Full use of tip deflection and shaft rotation is necessary to survey the gastric body and fundus (Fig. 4–3). While the tip of the endoscope is positioned in

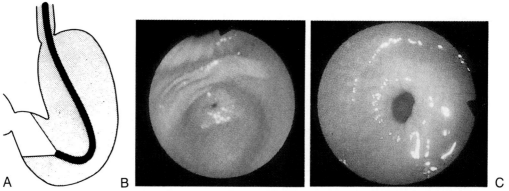

Figure 4–1. (A) View of the body and antrum of the stomach. **(B)** Prepyloric area before intubation of the pyloric channel. **(C)** Pyloric channel.

the central portion of the body of the stomach, the instrument is retroflexed 180° to allow complete evaluation of the gastric cardia and gastroesophageal (GE) junction. This maneuver is facilitated by a full deflection of the tip of the endoscope and simultaneous clockwise torque of the shaft of the instrument. This combination of maneuvers should position the tip of the instrument for visualization of the incisura angularis along the lesser gastric curve and a view of the GE junction in the distance (Fig. 4–4). By maintaining the tip deflection, gentle withdrawal of the instrument brings the cardia and GE junction into close view, allowing a complete evaluation of the cardia by rotating the instrument in a clockwise and counterclockwise manner (Fig. 4–5). Localization of the GE junction may be confirmed by asking the patient to

sniff or cough, causing the diaphragm to contract at the level of the esophageal hiatus.

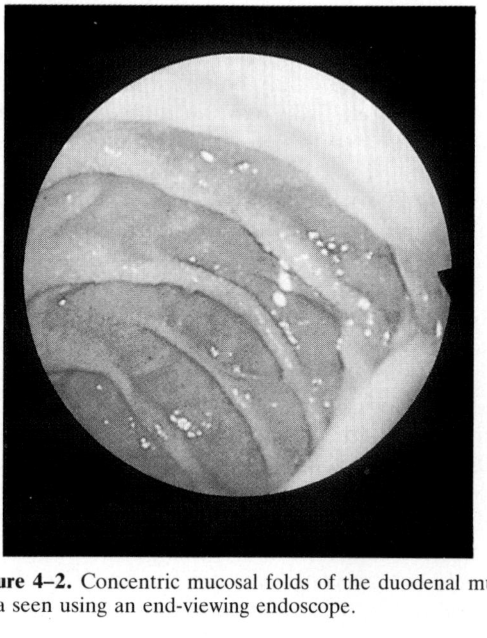

After the examination using retroflexion is complete, the tip of the scope is straightened, which allows a global view of the gastric fundus and antrum. Insufflated air should be suctioned before withdrawal of the scope into the esophagus. After the instrument is withdrawn to the level of the GE junction, the "Z" line, representing the squamocolumnar junction, should be identified, and the distance in centimeters of this landmark from the upper incisors should be recorded (Fig. 4–6). In the adult patient, the normal position of the GE junction is 40 cm from the upper incisors. This distance may be less if there is a hiatal hernia. During continued withdrawal of the instrument, the entire esophagus is carefully visualized (Fig. 4–7). Before complete withdrawal, the larynx is usually identified, and the status of the cords can be assessed easily in most patients (Fig. 4–8).

BIOPSY TECHNIQUES

EGD in the evaluation of upper GI symptoms and disease allows definitive histologic assessment. Biopsy or cytologic sampling should be anticipated whenever this endoscopic procedure is undertaken, and proper informed consent for a biopsy should be obtained from the patient. The surgeon-endoscopist must assume that proper instrumentation is available to allow adequate and efficient biopsy, and he or she must supervise the handling of all tissue for histologic or cytologic interpretation.

The decision to biopsy lesions seen during upper endoscopic evaluation is based initially on the accessibility and the microscopic determination, which indicates whether biopsy is the proper course of action. Knowledge of the gross

Figure 4–2. Concentric mucosal folds of the duodenal mucosa seen using an end-viewing endoscope.

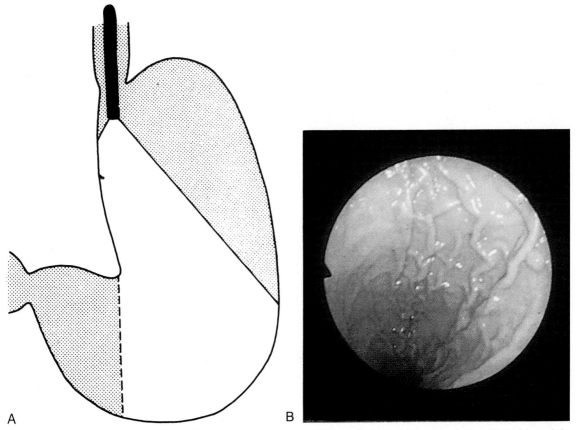

Figure 4–3. (A) Retroflexion of the endoscope allowing for full examination of the proximal stomach. **(B)** Position of the endoscope allowing for full examination of the gastric body.

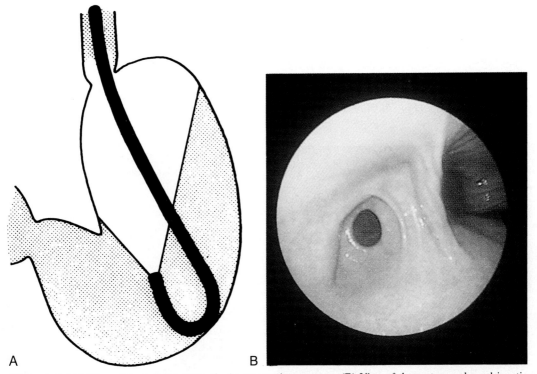

Figure 4–4. (A) View of the incisura along the lesser gastric curvature. **(B)** View of the gastroesophageal junction.

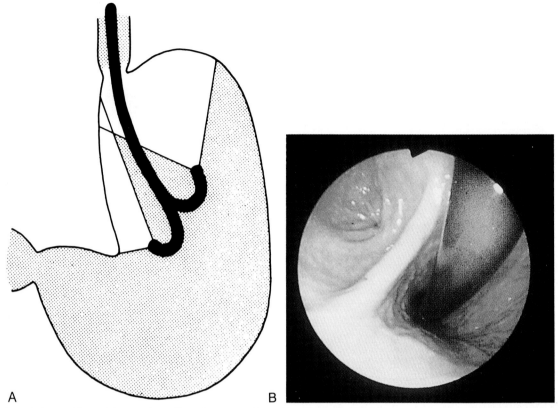

A   B

Figure 4–5. (A) View of the gastric cardia and gastroesophageal junction. **(B)** Complete examination of the gastroesophageal junction using rotation of the endoscope while it is retroflexed.

appearance of certain lesions is mandatory to interdict biopsy decisions. The gross appearance of esophageal or gastric varices can immediately determine the proper decision to avoid biopsy of this type of lesion (Fig. 4–9). Evaluation of an esophageal submucosal lesion should indicate that biopsy should be avoided if a subsequent transthoracic, submucosal removal of the lesion is planned. Although a diagnosis of an esophageal leiomyoma (Fig. 4–10) may be obtained

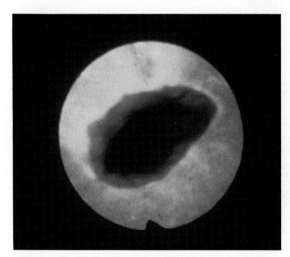

Figure 4–6. Squamocolumnar junction represented by the "Z-line" occurring approximately 40 cm from the upper incisors in the adult.

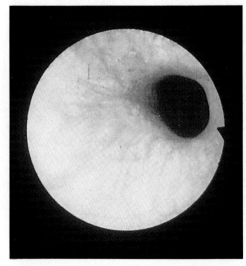

Figure 4–7. View of the distal esophagus.

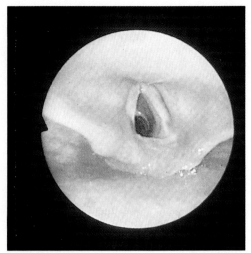

Figure 4–8. Visualization of the larynx during withdrawal of the endoscope.

during endoscopic biopsy, the violation of the mucosa of the esophagus renders the eventual transthoracic procedure more difficult, with the greater likelihood of creating an esophageal-pleural fistula postoperatively.

Interpretation and microscopic identification of other lesions such as erosions, ulcers, or exophytic masses mandate biopsies. Multiple biopsies of these lesions may be necessary to allow the pathologist to interpret the biopsy specimen, especially if a neoplasm may exist. Although the surgeon-endoscopist may have a high level of expectation that a gross, exophytic lesion of the gastric cardia may be an adenocarcinoma, the small size of the biopsy forceps may give an unrepresentative portion of tissue from

the surface of the lesion. Frequently, this biopsy material is interpreted as "inflammation only—no tumor seen." This pitfall may be avoided by taking multiple samples from the periphery and central portion of the lesion, with deeper penetration of the biopsy forceps after superficial biopsy has been completed. This approach should be used when ulcerating lesions are biopsied, because necrotic debris in the center of the ulcer crater may not be representative of malignancy. Several biopsy specimens should be taken from the inside "rim" of the ulcer crater to achieve optimal histologic interpretation (Fig. 4–11).

Interpretation of some pathologic processes may dictate identification of bacterial or fungal pathogens. During esophageal inspection, the finding of multiple, white patches on the esophageal mucosa indicates the possibility of *Candida* esophagitis (Fig. 4–12). Biopsy or cytologic brushing for fungal culture or traditional potassium hydroxide preparation of the specimen can support the microscopic interpretation and lead to proper therapy. For a gastric ulcer or diffuse gastritis, the recent association of *Helicobacter pylori* with these processes (Fig. 4–13) compels the surgeon-endoscopist to obtain representative biopsies to perform the "CLO" enzymatic test (Tri-Med Specialties, Overland Park, KS) or traditional culture and microbiologic identification of the organism.

Biopsy may be important even though gross mucosal lesions are not evident. In these circumstances, histologic assessment of "normal" mucosa may identify microscopic evidence of malignant or dysplastic tissue and determine therapy. If a grossly ulcerating lesion of the

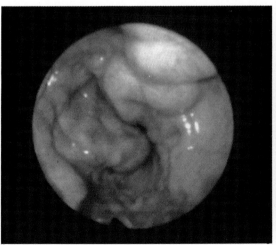

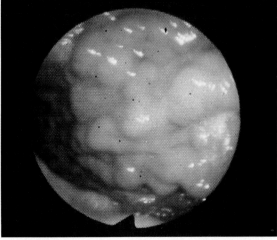

A B

Figure 4–9. (A, B) Esophageal and gastric varices.

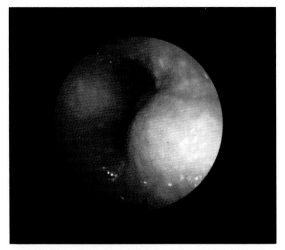

Figure 4–10. Submucosal lesion of esophagus representing a leiomyoma.

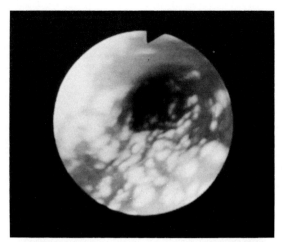

Figure 4–12. Classic appearance of *Candida* esophagitis.

middle third of the esophagus is seen, additional mucosal biopsies should be obtained from the proximal and distal esophagus for a distance of at least 5 cm. The propensity of esophageal carcinoma to spread along the mucosa and submucosa demands sampling of tissue at various distances from the gross lesion. Similarly, in the endoscopic evaluation of the remaining stomach after a recent partial gastrectomy and reconstruction, representative samples of tissue should be obtained from the gastric remnant and anastomotic areas, even though these mucosal sites are microscopically pristine. Dysplastic tissue or early invasive carcinoma may be identified, mandating resection of the remaining gastric remnant.[9]

INTERPRETATION OF FINDINGS

Although there are a multitude of lesions that can be identified during endoscopic evaluation of the upper GI tract, realization of normal mucosal anatomy is the most important goal because the greatest amount of surface area of the upper GI tract evaluated is normal. Overestimation of disease and the misreading of normal variations ultimately leads to overdiagnosis, which increases the incorrect usage of drugs, surgical intervention, and other manipulation. Misinterpretation also affects a patient's ability to become insured, resulting in an economic burden created because of the use of inappropriate therapeutic maneuvers.

Only experience with upper endoscopy can

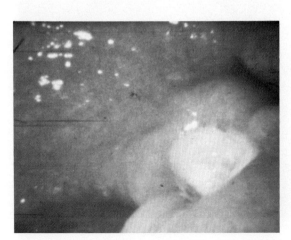

Figure 4–11. Ulcerating gastric lesion, showing the typical rim of an ulcer crater and the necrotic central debris.

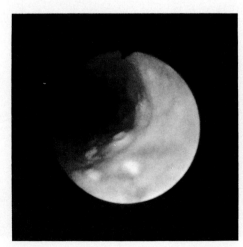

Figure 4–13. Endoscopic appearance of diffuse gastritis. The patient was *H. pylori* positive on traditional culture and CLO enzymatic test.

ensure that the surgeon-endoscopist becomes facile enough with common and uncommon lesions to make the appropriate interpretive call. The greatest challenge for any endoscopist is to make the appropriate differentiation between benign and malignant processes, which depends on the frequent use of biopsy and cytologic techniques for gross lesions. Any ulcerating or exophytic lesion should be biopsied to detect an early esophageal or gastric carcinoma. The use of still photography and video allow corroboration of the interpretation by other physicians.[10]

Many lesions observed in the esophagus, stomach, and duodenum represent various forms of inflammation resulting from peptic disease or opportunistic infection, which is seen more frequently in the immunocompromised host (see Fig. 4–13). The association of GI lesions in patients with infection due to human immunodeficiency virus has become more common and represents a genre of diseases that should be familiar to the surgeon-endoscopist.[11] For surgeons who treat inflammatory bowel disease, especially Crohn's disease, it should be remembered that this transmural process may involve the entire GI tract and should be appropriately documented during upper gastrointestinal evaluation. Although these changes may be subtle, appropriate biopsy can help in the interpretation of inflammatory bowel disease and lead to appropriate medical management.

The diagnostic use of EGD has given way to exciting therapeutic modalities that can be used in conjunction with traditional endoscopic surgical methods.[12] The foundation for the safe implementation of these therapeutic modalities, such as laser therapy, stent placement, endoscopic sclerotherapy (Chapter 5), or ligation of esophageal varices (Chapter 10), depends on meticulous use of the technology and polished interpretive skills.[13–15]

References

1. Schuman BM, Sugawa C. Diagnostic endoscopy of upper gastrointestinal bleeding. In: Sugawa C, Schuman BM, Lucas CE, eds. Gastrointestinal bleeding. New York: Igaku-Shoin, 1992:222–229.
2. Strodel WE, Johnson SF. Endoscopic examination in the evaluation of the postoperative stomach and duodenum. Probl Gen Surg 7:141, 1990.
3. Edmonson JM. History of the instruments for gastrointestinal endoscopy. Gastrointest Endosc 37(Suppl):27, 1991.
4. Fleischer D. Monitoring the patient receiving conscious sedation for gastrointestinal endoscopy: issues and guidelines. Gastrointest Endosc 35:262, 1989.
5. Bell GD, Mccloy RF, Charlton JE, et al. Recommendations for standards of sedation and patient monitoring during gastrointestinal endoscopy. Gut 32:823, 1991.
6. Andrus CH, Dean PA, Ponsky JL. Evaluation of safe, effective intravenous sedation for utilization in endoscopic procedures. Surg Endosc 4:179, 1990.
7. Steffes CP, Sugawa C, Wilson RF, et al. Oxygen saturation monitoring during endoscopy. Surg Endosc 4:175, 1990.
8. Schubert T, Schubert A, Ma CK. Symptoms, gastritis, and *Helicobacter pylori* in patients referred for endoscopy. Gastrointest Endosc 38:357, 1992.
9. Greene FL. Neoplastic changes in the post-gastrectomy stomach. Probl Gen Surg 7:55, 1990.
10. Paz-Partlow M. The importance of permanent documentation of endoscopic findings. Probl Gen Surg 8:487, 1991.
11. Wheeler RR, Peacock JE Jr, Cruz JM, et al. Esophagitis in the immunocompromised host: role of esophagoscopy in diagnosis. Rev Infect Dis 9:88, 1987.
12. Hunter JG. Endoscopic methods for palliation of malignant tumors of the gastrointestinal tract. Probl Gen Surg 7:103, 1990.
13. Brown SC, Hawes R, Matthewson K, et al. Endoscopic laser palliation for advanced malignant dysphagia. Gut 28:799, 1987.
14. Tytgat CMJ, den Hartog Jager FCA, Bartelsman J. Endoscopic prosthesis for advanced esophageal cancer. Endoscopy 18:32, 1986.
15. Stiegmann GV, Goff JS, Michael-Onody PA, et al. Endoscopic sclerotherapy as compared with endoscopic ligation for bleeding esophageal varices. N Engl J Med 326:1527, 1992.

5

Endoscopic Management of Esophageal Stricture

David B. Adams

Stricture formation is a common complication of many diseases of the esophagus. Easily accessible to the narrow diameter endoscope, esophageal strictures are readily visualized for endoscopic diagnosis and treatment. The underlying cause of a stricture is suggested by its endoscopic appearance, which can be confirmed by endoscopic biopsy or cytologic brushings. Clinical history, physical examination, radiologic evaluation, and esophageal manometry all have their place in the diagnosis and treatment of esophageal strictures. Rushing the patient with an esophageal stricture to the endoscopy suite is rarely indicated, and an organized approach with a gathering of history, physical examination, and laboratory findings should not be neglected.

Therapeutic endoscopy has a major role in the management of benign and malignant esophageal strictures. Direct dilation with mercury-weighted bougies is the simplest technique available for treating benign esophageal strictures. Blind bougienage has been supplemented by several techniques that incorporate endoscopic and fluoroscopic visualization. New choices with graduated dilators and balloon dilators offer promises of improved safety and efficacy. The 1980s witnessed the maturation of techniques using flexible fiber lasers and endoscopic intubation with plastic stents, which dramatically diminished the morbidity and mortality in managing malignant esophageal strictures.

The plan of this chapter is to review the following aspects of esophageal stricture disease:

1. Early history of nonoperative treatment
2. Pathogenesis and classification
3. Clinical history
4. Physical examination
5. Radiologic evaluation

This will be followed by a discussion of the endoscopic diagnosis and treatment of disorders associated with esophageal strictures listed in Table 5–1. A review of the complications of treatment of esophageal strictures concludes the chapter.

HISTORY

The principle of dilating an esophageal stricture with a bougie was introduced in the 16th century, when Fabricius ab Acquapendente used a wax taper in blind bougienage of a

Table 5–1. CAUSES OF STRICTURES OF THE ESOPHAGUS

Peptic strictures
Associated with reflux esophagitis
Associated with scleroderma
Associated with Barrett's esophagus
Schatzki's ring
Congenital web
Traumatic strictures
Corrosive
Sclerotherapy
Foreign body
Postoperative
Inflammatory strictures
Radiation
Crohn's disease
Eosinophilic gastroenteritis
Cutaneous bullous disease
Achalasia
Malignant strictures

36

stricture. The word bougie is derived from the Arabic name of Boujiyah, Algeria, a medieval center for the wax candle trade. Willis was the first to dilate the distal esophagus for achalasia using a whalebone probe with a sponge on the end.[1] The current principles of endoscopic treatment of esophageal strictures were introduced more than 100 years ago. The English physician J.C. Russell introduced a balloon dilator in 1887 that was similar to those used today.[2] Russell described this device as "an instrument consisting of a tube, or a hollow bougie. This was passed through the stricture in a collapsed state, and blown up with air in a syringe when in position." Samuel Mixter of Boston developed a technique for passing a bougie over a guiding string.[3] In 1909, Mixter described a technique of allowing the patient to swallow a string. After it was beyond the stomach and anchored in the small intestine, the string served as a guidewire over which the dilating bougie was passed. H.S. Plummer of the Mayo Clinic was responsible for major advances in the treatment of esophageal narrowing associated with achalasia.[4, 5] The Plummer dilator was constructed with a rubber balloon, cemented to the end of a rubber tube so that the tube passed through the balloon. Diathermy incision of a congenital stricture was described in 1900 by Frazier. Sir Arthur Hurst introduced the mercury-filled flexible bougie in 1915.[1]

The flexible endoscope, introduced in 1957, revolutionized the diagnosis and management of esophageal stricture. Although the eponyms of esophageal bougie and balloon dilators change, there are limited ways to mechanically enlarge a luminal narrowing, and the principles remain the same.

PATHOGENESIS AND CLASSIFICATION

Esophageal stricture is defined as a narrowing or stenosis of the tubular esophagus, which usually consists of contracting scar or deposition of abnormal tissue.[6] There are many causes of esophageal stricture, which are related to three general factors: epithelial injury, motility disorders, and malignant tumor growth.[7] Strictures are not rare and most commonly are associated with epithelial injury due to peptic esophagitis. Most strictures are located in the distal esophagus. Middle and proximal esophageal strictures are associated with malignancy, Barrett's esophagus, Crohn's disease, radiation injury, congenital webs, eosinophilic gastroenteritis, bullous disorders of the skin, and medication ingestion.

Epithelial Injury

Epithelial injury of the esophagus may be produced by gastroesophageal reflux of acid, duodenogastroesophageal reflux of bile, accidental ingestion of alkaline (e.g., lye) or acid liquid, trauma by foreign bodies (e.g., tubes, pills, bones), and external-beam irradiation. Injury and destruction of the epithelial mucosa leads to repair with inflammation and fibrosis. As wound healing progresses, connective tissue proliferates, leaving a ring of scar tissue that may narrow or obstruct the lumen. The cicatricial ring usually develops in the submucosa, unprotected by the injured epithelium. If the injury is superficial and minimal, the shallow, short, soft stricture can be easily dilated. If the underlying disorder is arrested, repair may occur with reepithelization and absence of scar contraction.

Wound healing is synonymous with inflammation, and there is a narrow margin between healing with an intact, epithelialized open lumen and healing with luminal stenosis due to recurrent fibrosis and scar contracture. The destruction and necrosis associated with lye ingestion, for example, produces deep and long cicatrization. This noncompliant, rigid scar may not yield to bougie dilation. The anastomotic stricture associated with early postoperative edema and inflammation may respond readily to simple dilation. However, the late postoperative stricture may produce a dense fibrotic scar that does not dilate but cracks or tears with attempts at balloon or bougie dilation. Collagen deposited in strictures is constantly remodeling, with concomitant collagen synthesis and lysis. Although a fresh scar may be readily dilated, it may mature into a rigid, undilatable stricture. Chronic, dense strictures may not be dilatable. Fixed strictures "crack" and may be torn by the dilating instrument, initiating a cycle of injury and repair with dense recurrent scar formation.

The benefits of dilation may be brief, frequently requiring another approach to provide longer-lasting success. Patients who have persistent dysphagia after dilation of peptic strictures have developed transmucosal fibrosis of the distal esophagus with fibrotic tissue infiltration extending through the full thickness of the wall of the esophagus.[8]

Motility Disorders

Esophageal motility dysfunction is associated with many connective tissue, endocrine, and neuromuscular disorders. The connective tissue disease most commonly associated with peptic stricture formation is scleroderma. In scleroderma, motor abnormalities in the distal esophagus are associated with low-amplitude contractions in the body. Loss of the lower esophageal high-pressure zone results in acid reflux and frequent stricture formation due to mucosal acid injury. In achalasia, another cause of luminal narrowing of the distal esophagus, the lower esophageal high-pressure zone is hypertensive with failure of receptive relaxation. The distal esophageal narrowing of achalasia is related entirely to a disorder of esophageal motor function. In patients with benign peptic strictures, low-amplitude pressure waves may be encountered in the distal esophagus.[1] Whether this is a cause or effect of acid injury to the esophagus is uncertain. Studies have indicated that reflux-induced esophageal stricture is associated with a major disorder of the distal high-pressure zone that leads to increased acid exposure of the distal esophagus.[8, 9]

Malignancy

There are several ways that malignant tumors cause esophageal strictures. The most common cause is infiltrating squamous cell carcinoma, which infiltrates the submucosa with occasional disruption of the mucosa.[7] Infiltrating adenocarcinoma arises most commonly from the cardia of the stomach and leads to obstruction of the distal esophagus. Less frequently, adenocarcinoma arises in Barrett's epithelium. In both types of adenocarcinoma, the typical stricture presents a nodular appearance with asymmetric narrowing. Esophageal stricture caused by extrinsic compression may result from breast, pancreas, or lung cancer metastatic to the mediastinum. Usually located in the midesophagus or cardia, strictures due to extrinsic tumor compression are rare. The appearance of the esophagus is similar to a benign stricture with intact mucosa and concentric narrowing in the midesophagus or distal esophagus.

CLINICAL HISTORY

Symptoms associated with esophageal stricture include dysphagia, odynophagia, regurgitation, and bleeding (*i.e.,* hematemesis, melena). Dysphagia, which is difficulty with swallowing, may be related to a disorder of physiology or anatomy. True dysphagia is never psychogenic and must always be investigated to determine an underlying cause.[10] Patients with luminal narrowing caused by strictures usually complain of solid food dysphagia. Liquid and solid dysphagia, particularly if associated with hot and cold temperatures, is usually related to motility disorders. It is not unusual, however, for patients with benign or malignant nonobstructing strictures to complain of dysphagia. Patients may point to their throat or lower chest to pinpoint the location of dysphagia, which may indicate an approximate location of the stricture site. In 293 patients with benign disease evaluated for dysphagia, strictures were identified in 84%. The most common cause was peptic stricture (65%). Less frequent causes were postoperative stricture (18 patients), cervical web (14 patients), Schatzki's ring (11 patients), achalasia (10 patients), and caustic stricture (1 patient).[11]

Odynophagia, which is pain with swallowing, is frequently associated with motility disorders. Impaction of a food bolus may progress from dysphagia to odynophagia. Odynophagia varies in severity from a mild discomfort to an intense pressure radiating to the back and arms. Patients with strictures due to Crohn's disease, radiation esophagitis, and malignancy may complain of odynophagia. Regurgitation of a solid bolus of food suggests unusual narrowing due to stricture, particularly if unable to pass food by repeated swallowing.

Heartburn, a unique esophageal symptom, may also radiate into the neck, back, and arm.[10] The disappearance of long-standing heartburn may herald the onset of distal esophageal stricture formation, with luminal narrowing preventing acid reflux. Major gastrointestinal bleeding is rarely related to benign strictures, but strictures related to Crohn's disease or radiation esophagitis may be associated with hemorrhage. Malignant strictures are less commonly associated with bleeding than with obstruction. Cervical webs associated with Plummer-Vinson syndrome are usually not associated with hemorrhage but are accompanied by a sideropenic anemia of unknown cause.

PHYSICAL EXAMINATION

The diagnosis of esophageal stricture disease may be made for most patients by history alone.[10] Physical examination is less specific in diagnosing esophageal stricture. Evidence of previous abdominal surgery on abdominal examination should confirm the clinical history. Scleroderma presents initially in many cases with esophageal manifestation. However, skin changes typical of scleroderma should be sought, and these include telangiectasia, cutaneous fibrosis, and subcutaneous calcification. The arms and hands are chiefly involved and may be associated with Raynaud's phenomenon of digital ulceration and shortening.[12] Most patients with malignant strictures demonstrate muscle wasting and other evidence of weight loss on examination.

RADIOLOGIC EVALUATION

The standard barium swallow examination is complementary to endoscopic examination in evaluating patients with esophageal stricture. It is important to identify a high cervical stricture before endoscopy to diminish the risk of instrument perforation (Fig. 5–1).[13] Zenker's diverticulum, a cause of cervical dysphagia, may be an unexpected hazard if not identified before endoscopy. In the past, barium swallow had been considered mandatory before endoscopy for dysphagia. Currently, endoscopy can be safely performed without a barium study if endoscopic intubation is done gently and carefully; if the patient is unable to swallow the endoscope or if there is any impediment to advancement of the endoscope, particularly at the level of the cervical esophagus, endoscopy should be delayed until the completion of a barium swallow. The safest practice is to use the barium swallow as the initial step in the workup of the patient with dysphagia. Uncooperative patients, elderly patients, and patients with cervical arthritis are at increased risk for perforation and are a group of patients who benefit in particular from preendoscopy barium swallow.

Strictures that block passage of the endoscope should be evaluated with a barium swallow to identify the location and extent of the lesion. Most strictures are due to esophagitis or carcinoma, and radiologic differentiation of the two may be difficult. Mucosal irregularity from esophagitis is difficult to differentiate from malignant changes in many cases.[14] Typical radiologic features of a benign peptic stricture are gradual, smooth, symmetric narrowing of the distal esophagus. Malignant strictures may present more proximally with asymmetric narrowing, gross mucosal irregularity, and shouldering at the proximal and distal stricture. Radiologic examination is more likely to confuse a benign stricture for a malignant one than vice versa. If a radiologic diagnosis of malignancy is not confirmed endoscopically, endoscopic biopsy should be repeated. Squamous cell carcinoma typically infiltrates the submucosa, and evidence of malignancy may be absent on the initial biopsy. An infiltrating squamous cell carcinoma occa-

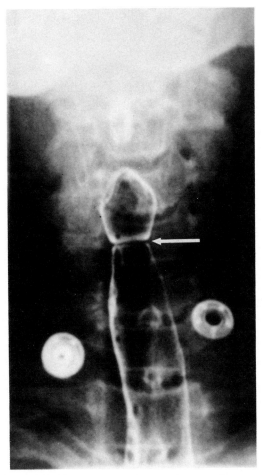

Figure 5–1. Air contrast esophagram demonstrating a cervical web *(white arrow)*, which may be difficult to identify by endoscopy.

sionally produces a benign appearing stricture, mimicking the radiologic appearance of achalasia with a smooth distal stricture and proximal dilation. Manometric and endoscopic studies can clarify the diagnosis.[14]

The roles of endoscopy and radiology in the diagnosis of esophageal strictures have been controversial, resolved favorably on the side of endoscopy. In a retrospective review of 52 patients with significant strictures identified with endoscopy, the frequency of radiographic diagnosis of the stricture ranged from 34% to 40%, varying inversely with the preceding time interval (1–8 months).[15] The routine use of endoscopy to evaluate dysphagia was recommended. For all patients evaluated with dysphagia using endoscopy, 23% have normal studies.[16] When those with negative esophagrams are studied endoscopically, strictures are identified in only 2% of patients.[17] Cancer is rarely missed on radiologic diagnosis; nevertheless, the consensus is that endoscopy is indicated for patients with dysphagia who have undergone a barium swallow that is normal.

ENDOSCOPIC DIAGNOSIS AND TREATMENT

Benign Peptic Stricture

Diagnosis

Strictures complicate reflux esophagitis in approximately 10% of cases. Most commonly located in the distal esophagus, benign peptic strictures may occur without the symptoms of reflux esophagitis. The typical endoscopic appearance of a peptic stricture is concentric narrowing of the tubular lumen with a symmetric opening and loss of the normal appearance of the mucosal columns.[7] In endoscopic grading of the degree of esophagitis, stricture formation represents severe or grade IV esophagitis.[18] Evidence of esophagitis may appear adjacent to the stricture with erythema, touch bleeding, erosions, ulceration, or exudates in about half of the patients.[19] The adjacent esophageal mucosa may appear normal. An endoscopic biopsy should be taken of esophageal strictures, and the examiner should have a high index of suspicion of malignancy for strictures with asymmetric narrowing and strictures located in the middle and proximal esophagus. Biopsies should be taken from all quadrants. Brushings for cytology may be valuable if pinch biopsies are negative. If microscopic examination does not confirm an endoscopic impression of malignancy, biopsies and cytologic brushings should be repeated.

Stricture dilation is often necessary before obtaining adequate biopsies of the distal margin. Biopsies taken proximal to a stricture may show microscopic evidence of esophagitis even if the endoscopic appearance of the esophageal mucosa is normal. The size of a stricture can be estimated by comparison to the jaws of the open biopsy forceps. Strictures are graded as three degrees of severity:[8]

Grade I (mild): Diameter greater than or equal to 12 mm; a No. 36 French (12 mm) endoscope passes easily

Grade II (moderate): Diameter greater than 10 but less than 12 mm; a No. 36 French endoscope passes with difficulty

Grade III (severe): Diameter less than 10 mm; a No. 36 French does not pass. A minimal area of stenosis may prevent passage of the endoscope.

Although length varies from 1 to 8 cm, most strictures are short and may be associated with marked luminal narrowing.[20] Length of the stricture frequently is not assessed until after dilation. Long strictures or strictures that are not clearly defined at endoscopy should be evaluated by barium esophagram to define anatomy before undertaking dilation. A microscopic diagnosis should be sought before dilation, because the cause of the stricture influences the choice of therapy. At endoscopy, stricture diameter and length, distance from incisors, mucosal appearance, and associated hiatal hernia and Barrett's epithelium should be observed. If possible, an examination of the upper gastrointestinal tract should be completed after dilation to determine the presence of associated foregut disorders.[13]

Technique

Mercury-Filled Bougie Dilation. Most benign peptic strictures of the esophagus should initially be treated by dilation techniques (Fig. 5–2). The technique depends on the anatomy and pathology of the stricture. Although a clear anatomic and pathologic diagnosis cannot always be defined at initial endoscopy, for 90% of patients the diagnosis of benign strictures can be made at endoscopy. Dilation can usually be performed at the time of endoscopic evaluation.[13]

Short, soft strictures larger than 1.5 cm in diameter can safely be dilated with mercury-filled rubber dilators. The round-tipped Hurst dilator and the taper-tipped Maloney dilator are most commonly used. They are available in sizes of No. 12 to No. 60 French (4–20 mm). The Maloney dilator is easier to use than the Hurst dilator because the tapered tip of the Maloney dilator seems to find the ostium of the stricture more readily.[21] Treatment is performed on an outpatient basis using topical pharyngeal anesthesia without intravenous sedation in most cases. An awake, unsedated patient is an asset in avoiding complications, because pain may be an early indication that excessive force is being used and suggests that an alternative method is necessary. With the patient in a sitting position, gravity can be enlisted to assist in carrying the dilator past the stricture as the patient swallows, gradually stretching the fibrotic stricture (Fig. 5–3).

The procedure is initiated by selecting a dilator smaller than the stricture and increasing dilator size by 4 French units (1.3 mm) with each passage. A stricture should never be forcibly stretched. The force of dilation may be

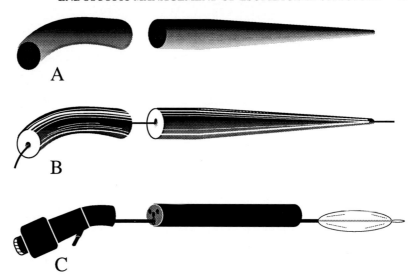

Figure 5–2. Most esophageal stricture dilation is done with these three instruments. **(A)** Mercury-filled red rubber Maloney bougie. **(B)** Taper-tipped polyvinyl chloride Savary dilator with a hollow core for introduction of a guidewire. **(C)** Through-the-scope (TTS) balloon dilator, which passes through the endoscope biopsy channel and is inflated under endoscopic visualization.

limited by gripping the dilator with two fingers, using a right-handed colonoscopy grip and not a "ski-pole" grip.[1, 21] Dilators are increased to a size 50 (16.5 mm) if possible or until extreme

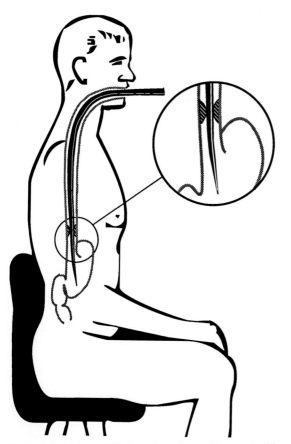

Figure 5–3. Maloney dilation of a stricture illustrated with the patient in sitting position. The dilator is lubricated and advanced with gentle rotation. Resistance to dilation determines the number of dilators that may be passed.

pain or resistance is encountered. If resistance or uncertainty are encountered, the procedure may be repeated at another session with a similar or alternate technique. Safety is enhanced by proceeding slowly. The size of the first and last dilator passed and the size of the largest dilator that can be easily passed should be recorded.[1]

Savary Dilation. The olive-tipped metallic Eder-Puestow dilator passed over a guidewire was the preferred technique for dilating complicated strictures for many years. In the 1980s, the Savary dilator replaced the Eder-Puestow system and, in many situations, mercury-weighted bougienage. The Savary dilator is a semiflexible polyvinyl chloride bougie with a graduated tip, similar in shape to the Maloney dilator.[22] A standard set is composed of dilators of 5, 7, 9, 11, 12.8, 14, and 15 mm. (To convert millimeters to French units, multiply millimeters by pi, 3.14.) Available in 70- and 100-cm lengths, the 70-cm Savary dilators are satisfactory for esophageal work. The Savary dilator has a central hollow core that allows the dilator to be placed over a guidewire. Although the guidewire may be passed across the stricture under endoscopic visualization, fluoroscopy diminishes complication risks by confirming the presence of the guidewire tip within the stomach. Frequent dislodgement and repositioning of the guidewire occurs during the exchange of dilators, and it is not a simple matter to ensure that the guidewire is out of harm's way. Tortuous strictures, diverticula, and proximal strictures are situations in which the risk of perforation is increased, and a guidewire could perforate the esophagus or the stomach. Fluoroscopy adds to the safety of Savary dilation and, except for selected patients who have been taught self-dilation, is considered mandatory for all esophageal dilation by many endoscopists.[23]

In dilation using the Savary dilator, the patient is placed in the left lateral decubitus position (Fig. 5–4). The Savary dilator is passed over the guidewire and manually directed through the hypopharynx into the upper esophagus. An assistant holds the wire steady as the dilator is gently advanced with a two-handed motion past the stricture. The stricture type determines how much dilation can be achieved at one sitting. In general, no more than three sizes above the initial size of dilation should be used at the first session.[24]

It has been suggested that the Savary system has several advantages over the Eder-Puestow system of bougienage. The long, smooth shaft of constant diameter allows the Savary dilation to be passed over a long stenosis. The Savary guidewire is designed so that it will not bend at acute angles, which diminishes risk of perforation. The tapered end of the flexible tip may allow progressive entry and reduces the risk of perforation compared with the rigid and short, metallic olive tips of Eder-Puestow system.[25] In a comparison between Savary and through-the-scope (TTS) balloon dilation of benign esophageal strictures, both methods were without major morbidity or mortality. Savary dilators were judged to be more effective and simpler to use than balloons.[26] The TTS balloon dilators were preferred for long and tortuous strictures in multiple, closely place strictures in the cervical esophagus.

Through-the-Scope and Over-the-Wire Dilation. Alternative treatment for tight, long, or asymmetric strictures includes TTS and over-the-wire (OTW) balloon dilators. Both techniques are used in dilating simple strictures. The TTS dilator is a hydrostatic balloon dilator 8 cm long. The balloon is made of an inelastic polymer and has an inflated outer diameter of No. 18 to No. 54 French (6–18 mm), which can pass through a 2.8-mm biopsy channel. The catheters have a 180-cm usable length and are reusable, although fragile and prone to breakage. The TTS balloons can be passed across the stricture under direct endoscopic vision. The TTS balloon dilators may be difficult to pass through the narrow-diameter gastroscope and may pass more readily through a 3.5-mm working channel, available with therapeutic gastroscopes or a narrow-diameter sigmoidoscope. A variation on this technique involves the use of OTW dilators. A guidewire is positioned endoscopically or fluoroscopically and special OTW balloon catheters are positioned. Radiopaque markers assist in effective fluoroscopic placement. Controlled dilation is provided by visualizing the disappearance of the balloon waist by fluoroscopy. OTW dilators as large as No. 60 French (20 mm) are available.

A major advantage of the TTS dilator is avoiding the use of a guidewire and fluoroscopy. Using TTS balloon dilator, the endoscope is

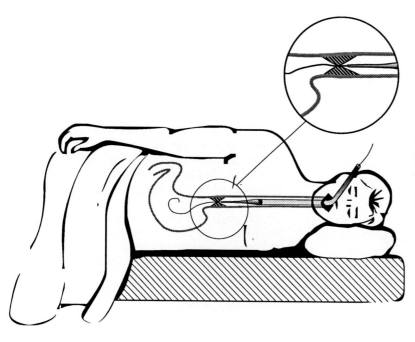

Figure 5–4. Savary dilation is done with the patient sedated and placed in the lateral decubitus position. The guidewire is positioned with fluoroscopic visualization. The dilator is loaded over the guidewire, which is placed on traction as the dilator is advanced.

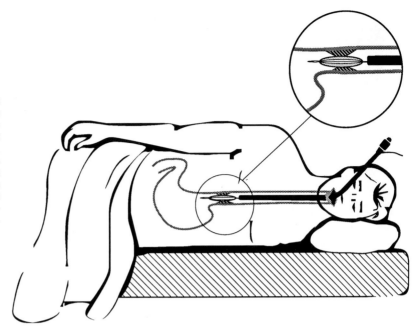

Figure 5–5. Through-the-scope (TTS) balloon dilation is done with the patient in the lateral decubitus position. The endoscope is placed proximal to the stricture. The balloon is passed through the biopsy channel of the endoscope and into the stricture under direct visualization. The balloon is slowly inflated and held for 1 minute. Fluoroscopy is not used routinely.

positioned above the stricture under direct vision (Fig. 5–5). The deflated TTS balloon is placed within the stricture, and the balloon is inflated with water, using a hand-held pressure gauge that is helpful in preventing balloon rupture due to overinflation. The TTS balloon is constructed of a noncompliant plastic, and after the maximal balloon volume is instilled, further pressure leads to a rapid rise in internal balloon pressure, causing the balloon to become fixed and rigid. Further pressure leads to balloon rupture. A controlled pressure and volume syringe that delivers a fixed pressure is available and may be simpler to use than the hand-held pressure gauge. Balloons remain distended for 1 minute and are released several times. Larger balloons are introduced to achieve the desired dilation.[27] To relieve dysphagia, it is necessary to increase the lumen size to at least 40 French (13 mm).[13] The final result of TTS and OTW balloon dilation may be gauged by passing a Hurst or Maloney dilator. For example, after a 15-mm balloon dilation, the No. 44 French Maloney dilator should pass without resistance.[27]

The effects of a bougie dilator on esophageal stricture size have been studied.[28] The postdilation stricture diameter was always less than the maximal bougie passed. The difference ranged from 1 to 11 mm and depended on the stricture "rigidity." An inelastic, rigid stricture was more difficult to dilate but showed less rebound after dilation.

After dilation, the stricture can be examined,

biopsy of the distal margin of the stricture can be taken, and the stomach and duodenum can be examined, if possible. Advantages suggested for balloon dilation include increased patient comfort, diminished mucosal injury, decreased risk of perforation, and avoidance of guidewires and fluoroscopy. It is not certain that TTS balloon dilation will replace the mercury-filled bougie dilators or reduce the need for Savary dilators. In some patients with complicated strictures, a combination of techniques is needed. Narrow, tortuous strictures may be successfully dilated with TTS balloon dilators followed by Savary dilation.[26] Complicated strictures may be dilated with balloon dilators to achieve a 47 French (15 mm) lumen. Subsequent dilation to 50 or 60 French may be accomplished with direct bougienage. Balloon dilation may be safer than Savary or Maloney dilators because the radial force delivered to the stricture waist by the balloon is more evenly distributed circumferentially and a gradually controlled dilation is less traumatic than the shearing axial force of the graduated bougie dilators.[27] Whether this advantage is other than theoretic has not been demonstrated (Fig. 5–6).

Results of Peptic Stricture Dilation

The long-term results of dilation of benign esophageal strictures are difficult to quantify. It has been estimated that a successful outcome is achieved in 80% to 90% of patients.[28, 29] About half of patients have long-term success after a

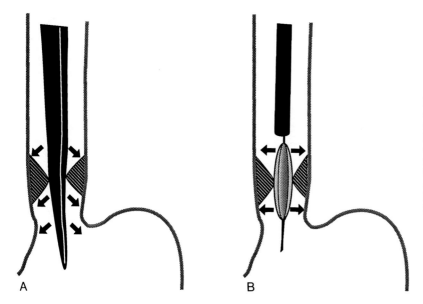

Figure 5–6. Axial shearing forces of **(A)** a taper-tipped dilator are thought to increase the risk of laceration and perforation of the esophagus compared with **(B)** the radial forces of balloon dilation. Gradual stretching of a stricture done by a Maloney or Savary dilator may be less traumatic than the sudden dilation of a balloon.

single dilation, and approximately 40% to 60% of patients require repeat dilations.[30] A few patients with recurrent peptic strictures learn self-dilation techniques, which they do at home.[31]

Good results with dilation of peptic strictures and medical management is achieved in 65% to 88% of patients.[32–35] Success with dilation may be related to technique. An 88% overall success rate was ascribed to routinely dilating to an 18- to 20-mm diameter.[35] A lower success rate of 70% was achieved with dilations up to 12 mm.[36] Success in 79% of patients was achieved if dilations were carried up to 15 mm. However, the question of optimal diameter of dilation has not been definitively answered. Bigger may not always be better because of scar formation after tearing injury. Earlam advises: "Do not attempt to achieve perfection by dilating to 60 F if the patient is satisfied with a smaller diameter. Each stricture has its own individual property and must be treated as a separate entity."[1]

The frequency of dilation is a clinical decision with no rigid guidelines; dilation should be done as frequently as necessary to achieve adequate relief of dysphagia. Which patients will require further dilation is not always predictable.[1] If one is unable to dilate a stricture sufficiently to relieve dysphagia or if the procedure needs to be done too frequently, an operative solution should be considered.

Preoperative and Postoperative Stricture Dilation

Stricture formation represents an end stage of gastroesophageal reflux disease and esopha-

gitis, and it has been called an indication for antireflux surgery.[37] Others recommend that surgical treatment of benign esophageal strictures is indicated only in selected cases. The young patient with a severe stricture that does not respond to dilation is an appropriate candidate for operation.[35] Although some physicians have reported that results of operation for reflux-induced strictures are equal to results for antireflux surgery for uncomplicated disease, others have had a lower success rate with stricture disease.[8] Extensive periesophagitis and defective esophageal propulsion are factors that may limit the success of operative and nonoperative treatments.

Endoscopy is important in the preoperative evaluation of patients with peptic stricture disease. Preoperative stricture dilation is usually safe, but with severe strictures, intraoperative dilation may be more prudent.[38] Preoperative dilation is helpful as a means of selecting patients for surgery. A course of medical therapy is beneficial in arresting further damage in the preoperative period, and as the local edema and inflammation resolve, esophageal compliance may improve and allow increasing dilation of the fibrotic scar tissue.[37] Many patients who undergo antireflux surgery for peptic strictures require postoperative dilation. In one series, 48% of patients with severe strictures and 26% with mild or moderate strictures needed postoperative dilation.[38]

Scleroderma

Esophageal involvement is common in scleroderma. Esophageal motor disturbances may be the initial manifestation of the disease and may occur without skin changes. Progressive atrophy of the smooth muscle in the distal two thirds of the esophagus leads to reduced amplitude of contraction. Submucosal sclerosis develops, and eventually there is loss of function in the lower esophageal sphincter. Acid reflux occurs after the loss of the protective high-pressure zone, and esophagitis and stricture formation are common. The typical patient with scleroderma develops increasing symptoms of heartburn, which progress to dysphagia as stricture formation occurs.[39] The endoscopic appearance of scleroderma is that of severe reflux esophagitis with ulceration, exudate, and a narrow, rigid stricture. Early in the disease, the esophageal mucosa may appear normal, with no evidence of narrowing in proximity to the gastroesophageal junction. The distal two thirds of the esophagus is aperistaltic.

Endoscopy is indicated as an adjunct to diagnosis and in managing complications. Strictures are managed as previously discussed for benign peptic strictures. The outcome is less favorable, because the underlying disorder is poorly managed with standard medical therapy for gastroesophageal reflux. These patients present difficult problems in management with antireflux operative procedures because of the underlying motility disorder. Scleroderma predicts an adverse outcome of operative management of esophageal stricture. Postoperative dilation is needed in 45% of patients after antireflux operations for strictures associated with scleroderma.[38] Dilation and medical therapy are warranted for initial and recurrent stricture management.

Strictures Associated with Barrett's Esophagus

Barrett's esophagus is a condition in which columnar epithelium replaces the squamous epithelium that normally lines the distal esophagus and extends over a distance of 3 cm into the tubular esophagus.[40] The endoscopic diagnosis of Barrett's esophagus and the issue of adenocarcinoma in patients with Barrett's esophagus are discussed in Chapter 7. Dysphagia and benign strictures occur in approximately 50% of patients with Barrett's esophagus and are usually associated with a hiatal hernia.[41, 42] Most strictures associated with Barrett's esophagus are short, located at or below the squamocolumnar junction. Stricture distance from the incisors ranges from 20 to 35 cm. The concept that benign strictures can be differented from malignant strictures on the basis of location has been discounted.[43] Strictures in Barrett's esophagus are associated with an increased prevalence of a mechanically defective lower esophageal sphincter. In patients with uncomplicated reflux esophagitis, the prevalence of defective sphincter function is 50%; this increases to 84% in patients with strictures and 92% in patients with Barrett's epithelium.[8] The combination of Barrett's epithelium and a stricture has an almost 100% prevalence of sphincter dysfunction.

Schatzki's Ring

Schatzki's ring is circumferential narrowing of the lower esophagus related to submucosal fibrotic thickening. Clinically associated with dysphagia and food impaction, the ring is located at the squamocolumnar junction and is usually associated with hiatal hernia. The cause of Schatzki's ring is unclear. A congenital variant, chemical injury, and acid reflux have all been suggested as possible causes.[44] The reported prevalence ranges from 0.2% to 14% in the general population.

Histologically, the core of the ring consists of areolar tissue with bundles of smooth muscle fibers belonging to the muscularis mucosa. Muscularis propria is not involved, nor is there histologic evidence of inflammation.[45] Rings are classified on the basis of internal diameter: mild, >12 mm; moderate, 9 to 12 mm; severe, ≤8 mm.[46] Patients with severe rings have repeated dysphagia, and about half of those with moderate rings have dysphagia. Endoscopy detects mild rings in 25% of patients and is better at detecting moderate (54%) or severe rings (82%).[47]

Diagnosis of a Schatzki's ring is best made by barium swallow, because mild or moderate rings are frequently missed at endoscopy (Fig. 5–7). Rings were confirmed at endoscopy in 59% of patients with radiologically determined rings.[44]

A variety of techniques to dilate rings associated with esophageal symptoms has been employed. Dilation with a single No. 60 French (20 mm) bougie is thought to produce good long-term results, because disruption of the ring is more likely to occur than with gradual dilation.[48] After dilation, endoscopy may be performed to confirm ring disruption, evident by some bleeding and tearing of the mucosa and submucosa. Patients who failed mercury-weighted bougie dilation have been successfully treated with pneumatic dilation.[49] Operative interruption of the ring is rarely indicated but has

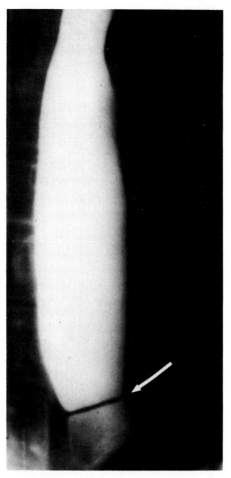

Figure 5–7. Esophagram showing Schatzki's ring *(white arrow)* located in the distal esophagus.

been used successfully in combination with an antireflux procedure.[50] Patients who have no gastroesophageal reflux associated with the ring usually respond to a single dilation. Most patients with proven reflux require repeat dilations.[44] Patients who do not have reflux are likely to have a history of ingestion of mucosa-damaging drugs, supporting the theory that Schatzki's ring is probably an acquired chemical- or acid-induced injury.

An innovative technique using endoscopic electrosurgical incision of the ring has been introduced.[52, 53] By cutting the distal part of a standard papillotomy sphincterotome, a straight, retractable sphincterotome was constructed. Introduced through a forward-viewing scope, electrocautery radial incisions are made in each quadrant of the ring. A successful long-term outcome (26–74 months) was obtained in 82% of patients without major complications.[53] This technique has not been widely adopted because Maloney dilation has an acceptable success rate.

Esophageal Webs

Esophageal webs are thin, ring-like strictures usually located in the cervical esophagus. Cervical webs were present in 7.5% of 1334 patients examined by cineradiography for dysphagia.[54] Their proximal location may lead to difficulties in endoscopic visualization; webs should be suspected if there is difficulty in passing the endoscope into the midesophagus, and diagnosis may require a barium swallow and cineradiography.

If associated with dysphagia and iron-deficiency anemia, esophageal webs are part of the Plummer-Vinson or Patterson-Kelly syndromes, seen most frequently in premenopausal, edentulous females in the fourth or fifth decades of life. On endoscopy, the web arises from the posterior esophageal wall several centimeters below the cricopharyngeus. The lumen of the web has an eccentric location surrounded by a thin membrane that becomes thicker as it approaches the esophageal wall. The treatment of a web associated with dysphagia is dilation.[55] Webs may be characterized as soft or fibrous. Fibrous webs frequently require multiple dilations to relieve dysphagia. Dilation with a No. 50 French (16.5 mm) bougie or balloon dilation is adequate treatment for most webs, but it is not without complications. Perforation and subsequent mortality has been reported after dilation of a cervical web.[13] Transendoscopic scissor incision and electrocautery incision have also been used to treat cervical webs.[55, 56] Endoscopic biopsy should be undertaken if abnormal mucosal lesions are found, because cervical webs can be associated with carcinoma.

Traumatic Strictures

A variety of physical and chemical agents causes injury to the esophageal mucosa and leads to the development of strictures. Traumatic strictures include those due to caustic injury, sclerotherapy, nasogastric tubes, medications, and postoperative strictures. Strictures due to lye ingestion and postoperative anastomotic strictures pose challenging management problems and are frequently difficult to dilate.

Caustic Injury

Severe, intraluminal, long, or multiple strictures develop in 4% to 33% of patients who swallow a corrosive agent.[57] Endoscopic evaluation of injury caused by caustic ingestion is controversial. With the narrow-diameter scopes, early evaluation is safe and helpful in developing management plans. If mucosal injury is found, steps can be taken to prevent stricture complications. Other physicians claim that early endoscopy is of limited value because only 24% of cases suspected of corrosive injury show evidence of mucosal injury at endoscopy. Endoscopic examination affords no evidence of the depth of the burn nor the prognosis in terms of stricture formation.[58]

In patients with severe mucosal injury, therapy usually consists of steroids, antibiotics, and serial endoscopy. Dilation is indicated if there is evidence of stricture formation.[57] However, early dilation of caustic strictures may be dangerous and ineffective for severe burns.[59] Steroids are routinely used but are of unproven benefit. In children, it is claimed that intensive steroid therapy and hydrostatic balloon dilation under fluoroscopic control prevents all but localized areas of stricture.[60] Stricture formation becomes apparent clinically 3 weeks after injury, when dysphagia appears. Endoscopy provides information on the extent of injury, the severity of the stricture, and expected response to treatment, which can best be determined after attempts at dilation. Patients may be categorized into three groups: the easily dilatable, the intermediate, and the nondilatable. Patients in the first two categories are initially managed with dilation. Nondilatable strictures require operative treatment.[58]

The coagulation necrosis of acid injury leads to deep penetration of the esophageal wall and severe fibrotic strictures. Acid ingestion has a higher incidence of stricture formation than lye ingestion. In acid injury, dilation of strictures must be repeated many times and frequently proves to be unsuccessful.[61]

An innovative approach to severe caustic injury features the use of plastic stents.[62] Four patients with severe, nontransmucosal injury were treated with esophageal stents with good results and no strictures during a 20-month follow-up period.

Foreign Bodies

Foreign bodies are rare causes of esophageal strictures. Strictures have been associated with long-term indwelling nasogastric tubes, complicating tube placement in less than 0.1% of cases.[7, 63, 64] Distal esophageal strictures have been associated with ingestion of medications, particularly potassium supplements and tetracycline. Nighttime medication ingestion, minimal fluid intake with ingestion, and the supine position have been associated with the development of medication strictures. Motility disorders and esophageal narrowing have also been associated with medication strictures.[7, 65] Medications that become impacted in the esophagus slowly dissolve and release their contents in high concentration. The resultant mucosal injury may lead to stricture formation, dysphagia, and odynophagia. In a review of 142 patients with drug-induced esophagitis, 17 medications were cited and 3 agents accounted for 83% of the cases: emepronium bromide (an anticholinergic available in Europe), tetracycline, and potassium chloride. Fourteen patients (1%) developed strictures. These strictures responded to dilation and avoiding the foreign body.[66]

Sclerosant Injury

Endoscopic injection sclerotherapy of esophageal varices is associated with stricture formation in 0% to 50% of patients, with most researchers reporting rates of 10% to 25%.[67-69] Sclerosant injury causes fibrosis and may induce a disorder of motility, predisposing the distal esophagus to acid injury. Strictures are usually solitary and located in the distal esophagus. Although stricture formation has been attributed to the amount of sclerosant used, others have identified no predisposing factors except patient gender and persistent ulceration.[68, 69] The mean interval from sclerotherapy to stricture development ranges from 55 to 131 days, with patients presenting with variable dysphagia.[67, 68] Most strictures respond to dilation and interrupting the sclerotherapy. Strictures can be dilated over two to four sessions, with an expected success rate of 85%. Mercury-weighted bougie dilation is routine, with balloon and Savary dilation used for complex structures.[69]

Postoperative Strictures

Strictures develop after many procedures involving the esophagus. Vagotomy and Nissen fundoplication may be complicated by dysphagia associated with anatomic and physiologic disorders of the distal esophagus. If stenosis is evident at endoscopy, a single dilation usually eliminates the dysphagia. Strictures that develop after esophageal resection and anastomosis are more problematic, because the underlying cause is frequently related to ischemia and a difficult anastomosis. Mucosal injury may be evident at the stricture site, suggesting acid reflux as a contributing factor. After construction of an esophagogastric anastomosis with a circular stapling device, anastomotic strictures develop in 10% to 20% of patients.[70] A relation between the size of the stapler head and the development of stricture formation has been suggested. There does not appear to be an increased stricture rate when stapled anastomoses are compared with hand-sewn anastomoses.[71] The development of anastomotic stricture after resection for benign stricture is reported to be as high as 39% and typically requires multiple dilations.[72] Anastomoses for benign disease are more difficult to dilate than those associated with malignant disease. Most postoperative anastomotic strictures develop within the first 6 months after surgery and respond to one or two dilations. After ileocolic transposition for caustic strictures of the hypopharynx and esophagus, endoscopy was undertaken in the early postoperative period. If strictures were found, they were dilated weekly for 1 month and then every 2 or 3 weeks, with a successful outcome for most patients.[73]

Inflammatory Strictures

Unusual causes of strictures include strictures due to external-beam irradiation, Crohn's disease, eosinophilic gastroenteritis, and cutaneous bullous disorders. Irradiation for lymphoma, breast cancer, and lung cancer at doses from 30 to 60 Gy has led to the development of cervical or midesophageal strictures.[7, 74] Concomitant chemotherapy appears to potentiate radiation-induced esophageal injury.[75] The appearance of a radiation stricture is usually characterized by normal-appearing mucosa proximal to the narrow, smooth stricture.[76] Successful dilation of a radiation-induced stricture under guidewire control with subsequent Maloney dilation was reported with minimal radiographic narrowing of the esophagus on radiographic follow-up at 1 year.[74]

Crohn's disease may mimic esophageal cancer, with an endoscopic picture showing an irregular, friable mucosa in the stricture region (Fig. 5–8). Patients with strictures associated with Crohn's disease present with a brief history of dysphagia and weight loss. Giant cell lesions that are pathognomic of Crohn's disease may be absent, and the diagnosis can be elusive. Edema and chronic inflammation with an intact epithelium suggest Crohn's disease. The treatment of choice is dilation with medical therapy.[77] Repetitive dilation over a prolonged period may be required.[74]

Bullous pemphigoid and epidermolysis bullosa are rarely associated with pharyngeal ex-

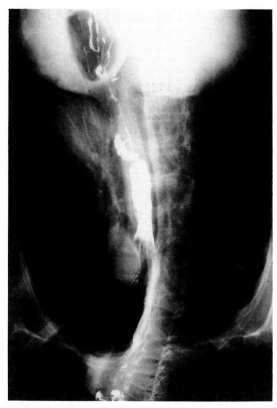

Figure 5–8. Esophagram of patient with stricture caused by Crohn's disease. The radiographic picture of Crohn's disease may mimic carcinoma, and endoscopic diagnosis may be difficult.

tension into the proximal esophagus and the development of a severe stricture but may occur in the absence of cutaneous disease.[78] Eosinophilic gastroenteritis is another unusual disorder rarely complicated by stricture formation in the proximal esophagus.[79]

Achalasia

Achalasia is a disorder of esophageal motility associated with abnormal esophageal peristalsis and obstruction of the distal esophagus due to failure of relaxation of the distal esophageal sphincter. Achalasia is clinically characterized by progressive dysphagia and regurgitation, anatomically by the absence of an organic lesion, and endoscopically by the absence of esophageal peristalsis.[80] A dilated "megaesophagus" appears late in the disease. Esophageal mucosa is normal, with symmetric narrowing at the cardia.

Forceful dilation of the gastroesophageal junction, directed at diminishing the resisting pressures of the lower esophageal sphincter through pneumatic dilation, is one mode of therapy. Indications for operative therapy include unsuccessful dilation, perforation with dilation, massive esophageal dilation, inability to exclude cancer, and achalasia in children.[80] Operative therapy with transthoracic long esophagomyotomy has an excellent success rate and is selected as initial therapy for many patients.[81, 82]

Dilators are available in multiple sizes and styles for use in pneumatic balloon dilation in achalasia. In the past, latex and nylon balloons were used, but polyethylene OTW balloons are now used by most centers.[83] Available in balloon diameters of 30, 35, and 40 mm, the actual size for dilation depends on patient size and comfort. Fluoroscopic control is required to direct guidewire placement and to identify the waist of the balloon in relation to the area of stenosis. A success rate of 70% was achieved using a mean distention pressure of 7 psi, 1 to 2 psi greater than that necessary for waist obliteration, which is maintained for 30 seconds.[84] Success in 85% of patients was achieved using a single dilation with a 30-mm balloon under endoscopic control for 1 minute of maximal pressure time.[85]

Although pneumatic dilation is the preferred dilation treatment of achalasia, mercury bougienage has not been abandoned. Mercury bougienage to a diameter of 56 French (18.5 mm) had a 50% success rate in one study and was recommended because of its simplicity and safety.[86] There was an acceptable success rate with subsequent pneumatic dilation in those who failed mercury bougienage. Success rates for pneumatic dilation in achalasia range from 48% to

100%, with an average of 71% in a collected review of 899 patients.[87] Perforation rates ranged from 0% to 12% (mean, 1.4%). There is concern that the rigidity of the polyethylene balloon dilator may lead to an increased bleeding and perforation rate.[88] After dilation, patients have pain that may persist, making the diagnosis of perforation difficult. Patients should be evaluated with an esophagram after dilation, although some researchers think that clinical observation is sufficient. Pneumatic balloon dilation on an outpatient basis has been practiced and found to be safe and effective.[89]

Malignant Strictures

Ninety percent of malignant strictures can be identified during endoscopic inspection; however, the diagnosis of cancer may be elusive and should be suspected in strictures that require repeated dilation.[13] Most tumors in patients who present with dysphagia due to malignant strictures are unresectable and require palliation with a combination of radiation, Nd:YAG laser therapy, and plastic stents (Fig. 5–9). Relief of dysphagia can be obtained by tumor destruction by heat energy supplied with electrocautery or the Nd:YAG laser. Laser therapy is safe and provides relief of dysphagia, but it must be repeated at frequent intervals to prevent recurrent dysphagia.[90, 91] Intubation therapy with plastic stents provides longer-lasting relief of dysphagia and is instituted as initial therapy for

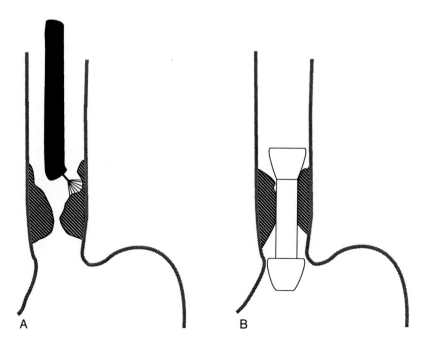

Figure 5–9. Palliation of inoperable malignant strictures is usually achieved with **(A)** Nd:YAG tumor ablation after dilation or **(B)** plastic tube endoscopic intubation after dilation and guidewire placement.

tumors that are extrinsic, submucosal, or associated with fistulas.

Most malignant strictures can be dilated with Savary dilators to achieve temporary relief of dysphagia. Success rates greater than 90 percent and low mortality rates has been reported.[92] There does not seem to be an increased risk of perforation of malignant strictures compared with benign strictures. Because dilation provides only transient relief of dysphagia, measured in days to weeks, longer-lasting palliation can be achieved by peroral intubation with plastic stents.

In 1977, Atkinson described a technique of palliative intubation for inoperable malignant strictures using an endoscopic technique.[93] After stricture dilation, a Celestin tube mounted on an introducer was passed over a guidewire that had been endoscopically inserted. The early experience with this technique, reported from Nottingham in 1982, described successful relief of dysphagia in 94.9% of 118 patients.[94] The perforation rate was 12.7% and the mortality rate was 11.0%. Approximately 25% of patients survived for 6 months, and 8.5% survived for 1 year. Endoscopic palliation had markedly lower morbidity and mortality rates and improved survival time than that reported for operative palliation, and it was judged to be the treatment of choice for palliation of malignant strictures.

This viewpoint was echoed in a study of 409 patients reported 10 years later.[95] Intubation could not be accomplished in 8% of the 409 patients. Mortality was 3.4%, and major complications included bleeding (2%), perforation (4.9%), dislodgement (12.7%), and obstruction (4.4%). Early semisolid feeding was achieved in 80% of patients discharged from the hospital. The 1-year survival rate was 7.7% with a median survival of 3.9 months. Others have equalled these results with relief of dysphagia in 80% of patients, but with complication rates as high as 20%.[96]

The results appear to be directly related to patient selection and operator expertise. Principles of dilation of malignant strictures include patience, gentleness, and control.[97] Progressive dilation over several sessions may be needed. Passing no more than three dilators per sitting if moderate resistance is encountered is recommended. Fluoroscopy is essential to control the guidewire and dilator tip position.[97] Most failures occur in tight, angular strictures in the gastroesophageal junction region.[95]

Endoscopic intubation is a successful treatment for patients with inoperable esophageal cancer with long, infiltrating, circumferential cancer of the thoracic esophagus. In patients with fistulas, it may be the only treatment option.

Nd:YAG laser therapy has a major role in the palliation of malignant strictures and is the initial treatment in many centers. Stricture dilation is required before laser therapy. Laser ablation is more safely applied from the distal to the proximal stricture, which diminishes perforation complications. Usually three to five sessions are required to relieve dysphagia. Success rates are about 75% with a 5% perforation rate.[97]

The outcome of 28 patients treated with Nd:YAG therapy was compared with 116 patients treated with intubation.[98] The laser had a higher success rate (100% vs. 95%) and lower morbidity (3.6% vs. 13.8%) and mortality rates (0% vs. 4.3%) than intubation. Intubation was recommended for fistulas and extensive, long, stenotic lesions. Intubation was compared with laser therapy in a three-armed prospective study incorporating radiation therapy in patients with squamous cell carcinoma and strictures of the middle or distal esophagus.[99] Laser and radiation therapy were thought to be the treatment of choice based on a significantly lower complication rate and prolonged palliation compared with patients treated with intubation with and without radiation therapy. Tumor ablation using the bipolar coagulation probe has been used in the treatment of malignant strictures with success.[100] With this technique, dilation is followed by passing an olive-tipped electrocautery probe over a wire with endoscopic and fluoroscopic control. Acceptable complications rates have been reported, but this technique has not been widely adopted.

Metallic self-expanding stents were introduced in an attempt to overcome complications of tumor ingrowth and tube displacement associated with plastic stents. These metallic stents are compressible and can be delivered through narrow strictures, exerting an outward force after placement. Problems with aspiration and tissue overgrowth have been reported, although long-term patency (≤ 6 months) has been good.[101] Silicone-coated self-expanding metallic stents have produced good results in relieving dysphagia relief, but stent migration, silicone disruption with tumor ingrowth, food impaction, and perforation have been reported.[102] Although the self-expanding stent has several theoretic advantages, it has not yet been shown to be an improvement over plastic stents and Nd:YAG laser palliation of malignant strictures.

COMPLICATIONS

Diagnostic endoscopy of esophageal strictures is associated with a low complication rate. Although transient bacteremia is common after esophageal manipulation, symptomatic bacteremia is rare. Serious bleeding complications are extremely rare, and the perforation rate is less than 0.01%.[103]

In diagnostic endoscopy, the most common site of perforation is the cricopharyngeal region of the cervical esophagus. The next most common site is the distal esophagus near the aortic arch.[104] Old age, cervical arthritis, and Zenker's diverticulum are factors known to increase the risk of perforation. Instrumentation is the most common cause of esophageal perforation, acounting for approximately half of all cases.[104, 105] In the 1974 American Society for Gastrointestinal Endoscopy survey, the perforation rate for diagnostic endoscopy was 0.03%, which increased to 0.25% with dilation procedures.[106] In a collected series of 511 endoscopic instrumental perforations of the esophagus, 40% of patients had no underlying esophageal disease. Benign strictures existed in 27%, anatomic lesions in 17%, tumors in 10%, and achalasia in 6%. The causes of instrumental perforation were diagnostic esophagoscopy in 35% of patients, pneumatic dilation in 25%, bougienage in 20%, and other causes in 20%.[107] Esophageal perforation rates were reported in 1831 endoscopic procedures, and no increases in perforation rates with diagnostic and mercury bougie dilation procedures were described.[108] There was a tenfold increase in perforations with complex strictures treated with the Celestin tube, Eder-Puestow dilator, and pneumatic dilation.

The underlying disorder influences the perforation rate. Achalasia and caustic stricture dilation have an increased perforation rate compared with benign peptic strictures. An increased rate of perforation of malignant strictures after dilation has not been shown. Pneumatic dilation for achalasia appears to have the greatest risk of perforation, and it has been recommended that an esophagram be done after all dilations for achalasia. Eder-Puestow dilators have a higher risk of perforation than the Maloney dilators.

Instrumental perforation of the esophagus is a true emergency. Mortality increases directly as the length of time from injury to treatment increases. The prudent endoscopist must always consider the possibility of perforation after stricture dilation.[13] A high index of suspicion and prompt contrast radiography will lead to early, lifesaving treatment. The diagnosis of esophageal perforation may be subtle. With perforation, there is an early chemical mediastinitis for approximately 6 to 8 hours, which is followed by bacterial invasion and sepsis. Mediastinitis may be followed by pleuritis, pyopneumothorax, and empyema. Early signs and symptoms of esophageal perforation include subcutaneous emphysema in the neck and thorax and persistent pain. Late symptoms are fever, dysphagia, neck pain, vocal changes, retrosternal pain, pleuritic pain, and odynophagia.[103] If perforation is a possibility, the patient should be given nothing orally, and neck and chest radiographs should be obtained. Noncontrasted radiography is normal in 12% to 33% of patients and should not delay a contrast esophagram if perforation remains a possibility.[104] Water-soluble contrast media is preferred in the initial study to avoid instilling barium into the mediastinum. However, if a patient is at risk for aspiration, high osmotic contrast medicine should be avoided, and a low osmotic solution, such as metrizamide, may be employed. If the water-soluble contrast study is normal, a study with dilute barium should be obtained. The false-negative rate using barium is less than that with water-soluble contrast, which may miss 8% of perforations.[109] Overall, esophagrams have a 10% false-negative rate, and if there remains a suspicion of perforation after a normal barium study, repeat endoscopy and a computed tomography scan may be indicated.

Instrumental perforations of the esophagus differ from spontaneous perforations, for which early recognition and an empty esophagus are uncommon. If recognition is delayed, the outcome is similar to noninstrumental perforation. Nonoperative management is selected for most small perforations after dilation of a peptic stricture or achalasia. Criteria for nonoperative management of esophageal perforation include the presence of a recent or walled-off perforation, containment in the mediastinum, drainage back into the esophagus, absence of tumor or obstruction, and minimal physiologic derangement.[110] Most instrumental perforations meet these criteria and can be successfully managed with nothing administered orally, total parenteral nutrition, and nasogastric suction for 10 days, intravenous broad-spectrum antibiotics for 7 to 14 days, and closed chest tube thoracostomy if pleural effusion develops. If there is no improvement with this treatment, a computed tomography scan should be done to seek undrained collections. Perforation of a malignant stricture is an indication for operative therapy.[111, 112]

References

1. Earlam R. Benign oesophageal strictures: historical and technical aspects of dilation. Br J Surg 68:829, 1981.
2. Russell JC. Diagnosis and treatment of spasmodic stricture of the oesophagus. Br Med J 1450, 1898.
3. Mixter SJ. Symposium on the surgery of the esophagus from the standpoint of the general surgeon. Trans Am Laryngol Assoc 31:342, 1909.
4. Plummer HS. Cardiospasm with a report of forty cases. JAMA 51:549, 1908.
5. Meade RH. Thoracic surgery. In: An introduction to the history of general surgery. Philadelphia: WB Saunders, 1968:173–196.
6. Basmajian JV, Burke MD, Burnett GW, et al, eds. Stedman's medical dictionary. Baltimore: Williams & Wilkins, 1982:1351.
7. Blackstone MO. Esophageal strictures. In: Endoscopic interpretation: normal and pathologic appearances of the gastrointestinal tract. New York: Raven Press, 1984:34–42.
8. Zaninotto G, DeMeester TR, Bremmer CG, Smyrk TC, Cheng SC. Esophageal function in patients with reflux-induced strictures and its relevance to surgical treatment. Ann Thorac Surg 47:362, 1989.
9. Liberman DA. Medical therapy for chronic reflux esophagitis. Long-term follow-up. Arch Intern Med 147:1717, 1987.
10. Pope CE II. Heartburn, dysphagia, and other esophageal symptoms. In: Sleisenger M, Fordtran JS, eds. Gastrointestinal disease: pathophysiology, diagnosis, and management. Philadelphia: WB Saunders, 1989: 200–203.
11. Webb WA, McDaniel L, Jones L. Endoscopic evaluation of dysphagia in two hundred and ninety-three patients with benign disease. Surg Gynecol Obstet 158:152, 1984.
12. Harris ED Jr. Scleroderma. In: Wyngaarden JB, Smith LH Jr, eds. Cecil textbook of medicine. Philadelphia: WB Saunders, 1982:1857–1860.
13. Webb WA, McDaniel L, Jones L. The use of endoscopy in assessment and treatment of peptic strictures of the esophagus. Am Surg 50:476, 1984.
14. Bartram CI, Kumar P. Oesophagus. In: Clinical radiology in gastroenterology. Boston: Blackwell Scientific Publications, 1981:50–72.
15. Hiatt GA. The roles of esophagoscopy vs. radiography in diagnosing benign peptic esophageal strictures. Gastrointest Endosc 23:194, 1977.
16. Halpert RD, Feczko PJ, Spickler EM, Ackerman LV. Radiological assessment of dysphagia with endoscopic correlation. Radiology 157:599, 1985.
17. DiPalma JA, Prechter CC, Brady CE III. X-ray negative dysphagia: Is endoscopy necessary? J Clin Gastroenterol 6:409, 1984.
18. Little AG, DeMeester TR, Kirchner PT, et al. Pathogenesis of esophagitis in patients with gastroesophageal reflux. Surgery 88:101, 1980.
19. Buchin PJ, Spiro HM. Therapy of esophageal stricture. A review of 84 patients. J Clin Gastroenterol 3:121, 1981.
20. Mukhopadhyay AK. Idiopathic lower esophageal sphincter incompetence and esophageal stricture. Arch Intern Med 140:1493, 1980.
21. Webb WA. Esophageal dilation: personal experience with current instruments and techniques. Am J Gastroenterol 83:471, 1988.
22. Monnier PH, Hsiek V, Savary M. Endoscopic treatment of esophageal stenosis using Savary-Gilliard bougies: technical innovations. Acta Endoscopica 15:119, 1985.
23. McClure SA, Wright RA, Brady PG. Prospective randomized study of Maloney esophageal dilation—blinded versus fluoroscopic guidance. Gastrointest Endosc 36:272, 1990.
24. Chung RS. Dilation of strictures. In: Therapeutic endoscopy in gastrointestinal surgery. New York: Churchill-Livingstone, 1987:181–208.
25. Fuentes P, Giudicelli P, Riera P, Dumon JF, Dupin B, Rebond E. Treatment of esophageal peptic strictures. In: DeMeester TR, Skinner DB, eds. Esophageal disorders: pathophysiology and therapy. New York: Raven Press, 1985:253–256.
26. Shemesh E, Czerniak A. Comparison between Savary-Gilliard and balloon dilatation of benign esophageal strictures. World J Surg 14:518, 1990.
27. Graham DY, Tabibian N, Schwartz JT, Smith JL. Evaluation of the effectiveness of through-the-scope balloons as dilators of benign and malignant gastrointestinal strictures. Gastrointest Endosc 33:432, 1987.
28. Bennett JR, Sutton DR, Price JF, Dyet JF. Effects of bougie dilation on esophageal stricture size. In: DeMeester TR, Skinner DB, eds. Esophageal disorders: pathophysiology and therapy. New York: Raven Press, 1985:221–224.
29. Patterson DJ, Graham DY, Smith JL, et al. Natural history of benign esophageal stricture treated by dilatation. Gastroenterology 85:346, 1983.
30. Anderson PE, Cook A, Amery AH. A review of the practice of fibreoptic endoscopic dilation of oesophageal stricture. Ann R Coll Surg Engl 71:124, 1989.
31. Grobe JL, Kozarek RA, Sanowski RI. Self-bougienage in the treatment of benign esophageal strictures. J Clin Gastroenterol 6:109, 1984.
32. Burkhart KL, Sullivan BH. Course and treatment of benign esophageal strictures. Am J Gastroenterol 58:531, 1972.
33. Lanza FL, Graham DY. Bougienage is effective therapy for most benign esophageal strictures. JAMA 240:844, 1978.
34. Watson A. The role of antireflux surgery combined with fiberoptic endoscopic dilation in peptic esophageal stricture. Am J Surg 148:346, 1984.
35. Wesdorp ICE, Tytgat GN. Results of conservative treatment of benign esophageal strictures in 100 patients. In: DeMeester TR, Skinner DB, eds. Esophageal disorders: pathophysiology and therapy. New York: Raven Press, 1985:247–252.
36. Benedict EB. Peptic stenosis of the esophagus—a study of 233 patients treated with bougienage, surgery or both. Am J Dig Dis 11:761, 1966.
37. Little AG, Naunheim KS, Ferguson MK, Skinner DB. Surgical management of esophageal stricture. Ann Thorac Surg 45:144, 1988.
38. Henderson RD, Henderson RF, Marryatt GV. Surgical management of 100 consecutive esophageal strictures. J Thorac Cardiovasc Surg 99:1, 1990.
39. Sack TL, Sleisenger MH. Effects of systemic extraintestinal disease on the gut. In: Sleisenger MH, Fordtran JS, eds. Gastrointestinal disease: pathophysiology, diagnosis, management. Philadelphia: WB Saunders, 1989:488–517.
40. Spechler SJ, Goyal RK. Barrett's esophagus. N Engl J Med 315:362, 1986.
41. Iascone C, DeMeester TR, Little A, Skinner DB. Barrett's esophagus. Arch Surg 118:543, 1983.
42. Sjogren RW, Johnson LF. Barrett's esophagus: a review. Am J Med 74:313, 1983.
43. Lackey C, Rankin RA, Welsh JD. Stricture location

in Barrett's esophagus. Gastrointest Endosc 30:331, 1984.

44. Jamieson J, Hinder RA, DeMeester TR, Litchfield D, Barlow A, Bailey RT. Analysis of thirty-two patients with Schatzki's ring. Am J Surg 158:563, 1989.

45. Schatzki R, Gary JE. Dysphagia due to a diaphragm-like localized narrowing in the lower esophagus ("lower esophageal ring"). AJR 60:911, 1953.

46. Groskreutz JL, Kim CH. Schatzki's ring. Long-term results following dilation. Gastrointest Endosc 36:479, 1990.

47. Ott DJ, Gelfand DW, Wu WC, Castell DO. Review: esophagogastric region and its rings. AJR 142:281, 1984.

48. Goyal RK, Glancy JJ, Spiro HM. Lower esophageal ring (part two). N Engl J Med 282:1355, 1970.

49. Sanowski RA, Riegel N. Pneumatic dilatation of lower esophageal ring. Am J Dig Dis 15:407, 1970.

50. Eastridge CE, Pate JW, Mann JA. Lower esophageal ring: experiences in treatment of 88 patients. Ann Thorac Surg 37:103, 1984.

51. Raskin JB, Manten H, Harary A, Redlhammer DE, Rogers AL. Transendoscopic electrosurgical incision of lower esophageal (Schatzki) rings: a new treatment modality. Gastrointest Endosc 31:391, 1985.

52. Auchzermeyer A, Burdeljki M, Hruby M. Endoscopic therapy of a congenital oesophageal stricture. Endoscopy 11:259, 1979.

53. Guelrud M, Villasmil L, Mendez R. Late results in patients with Schatzki ring treated by endoscopic electrosurgical incision of the ring. Gastrointest Endosc 33:96, 1987.

54. Ekbery O, Malmquist J, Lindren S. Pharyngo-oesophageal webs in dysphageal patients—a radiologic and clinical investigation in 1134 patients. Fortschr Rontgenstr 145:75, 1986.

55. Acosta JC. Congenital stenosis of the esophagus. Gastrointest Endosc 27:197, 1981.

56. Mares AJ, BarZiv, Liberman A, et al. Congenital esophageal stenosis—transendoscopic web incision. J Clin Gastroenterol 8:555, 1986.

57. Tucker JA, Yarington CT Jr. The treatment of caustic ingestion. Otolaryngol Clin North Am 12:343, 1979.

58. Belsey RHR. Corrosive strictures of the esophagus. In: DeMeester TR, Skinner DB, eds. Esophageal disorders: pathophysiology and therapy. New York: Raven Press, 1985:261–270.

59. Oakes DD, Sherck JP, Mark JBD. Lye ingestion: clinical patterns and therapeutic options. J Thorac Cardiovasc Surg 83:194, 1982.

60. Othersen HB Jr, Parker EF, Smith CD. The surgical management of esophageal stricture in children. Ann Surg 207:590, 1988.

61. Gerzic ZB, Knezevic JB, Milicevic MN, Jovanovic BK. Esophagocoloplasty in the management of post-corrosive strictures of the esophagus. Ann Surg 211:329, 1990.

62. Mills LJ, Estrera AS, Platt MR. Avoidance of esophageal stricture following severe caustic burns by the use of an intraluminal stent. Ann Thorac Surg 28:60, 1979.

63. Nagler K, Spiro HM. Persistant gastroesophageal reflux induced during prolonged gastric intubation. N Engl J Med 269:495, 1963.

64. Hussain R. Oesophageal stricture following use of an indwelling Ryle's tube. Br J Surg 51:525, 1964.

65. Kikendall JW, Friedman OC, Oyewole MA, Fleischer D, Johnson LF. Pill-induced esophageal injury: Case reports and review of the medical literature. Dig Dis Sci 28:174, 1983.

66. Oakes DD, Sherck JP. Drug-induced esophagitis. In:

DeMeester TR, Skinner DB, eds. Esophageal disorders: pathophysiology and therapy. New York: Raven Press, 1985:241–246.

67. Haynes WC, Sanowski RA, Foutch PG, Bellapravalu S. Esophageal strictures following endoscopic variceal sclerotherapy: clinical course and response to dilation therapy. Gastrointest Endosc 32:202, 1986.

68. Guynn TP, Eckhauser FE, Knol JA, et al. Injection sclerotherapy-induced esophageal strictures. Risk factors and prognosis. Am J Surg 57:567, 1991.

69. Kochhar R, Goenka MK, Mehta SK. Esophageal strictures following endoscopic variceal sclerotherapy. Antecedents, clinical profile, and management. Dig Dis Sci 37:347, 1992.

70. Muehrcke DD, Kaplan DK, Donnelly RJ. Anastomotic narrowing after esophagogastrectomy with the EEA stapling device. J Thorac Cardiovasc Surg 97:434, 1989.

71. Hopkins RA, Alexander JC, Postlethwait RW. Stapled esophagogastric anastomosis. Am J Surg 147:283, 1984.

72. Bender EM, Walbaun PR. Esophagogastrectomy for benign esophageal stricture. Ann Surg 205:385, 1987.

73. Tran Ba Huy P, Celerier M. Management of severe caustic stenosis of the hypopharynx and esophagus by ileocolic transposition via suprahyoid or transepiglottic approach. Ann Surg 207:439, 1988.

74. Little AG, DeMeester TR, Skinner BD. Strictures of the proximal esophagus. In: DeMeester TR, Skinner DB, eds. Esophageal disorders: pathophysiology and therapy. New York: Raven Press, 1985:277–284.

75. Nelson RS, Hernandez AJ, Goldstein HM, Saca A. Treatment of irradiation esophagitis. Am J Gastroenterol 71:17, 1979.

76. Silverstein FE, Tytgat GNJ. Esophagus. III: Motor dysfunction, vascular abnormalities, and trauma. In: Atlas of gastrointestinal endoscopy. Philadelphia: WB Saunders, 1987:3.1–3.18.

77. Iascone C, Morald A, Zerillim J, et al. Unusual benign stenosis of the esophagus: four case reports. In: DeMeester TR, Skinner DB, eds. Esophageal disorders: pathophysiology and therapy. New York: Raven Press, 1985:285–291.

78. Sharon P, Greene ML, Rachmilewitz D. Esophageal involvement in bullous pemphigoid. Gastrointest Endosc 24:122–123, 1978.

79. Dobbins JW, Sheahan DG, Behar J. Eosinophilic gastroenteritis with esophageal involvement. Gastroenterology 72:1312, 1978.

80. Castell DO. Achalasia and diffuse esophageal spasm. Arch Intern Med 136:571, 1976.

81. Ellis FH, Crozier RE, Watkins E. Operation for esophageal achalasia: results of esophagomyotomy without an antireflux operation. J Thorac Cardiovasc Surg 88:344, 1984.

82. Sauer L, Pellegrini CA, Way LW. The treatment of achalasia: a current perspective. Arch Surg 124:929, 1989.

83. Richter JE, Stark GA, Wu WC, et al. Randomized comparison of Browne-McHardy and Microvasive Rigiflex dilators in the treatment of achalasia. Am J Gastroenterol 83:1024, 1988.

84. Gelfand MD, Kozarek RA. An experience with polyethylene balloons for pneumatic dilation in achalasia. Am J Gastroenterol 84:924, 1989.

85. Levine ML, Moskowitz GW, Doy BS, Bank R. Pneumatic dilation in patients with achalasia with a modified Gruntzig dilator (Levine) under direct endoscopic control: results after 5 years. Am J Gastroenterol 86:1581, 1991.

86. McJunkin B, McMillan WO, Duncan HE, Harman

KM, White JJ, McJunkin JE. Assessment of dilation methods in achalasia: large diameter mercury bougienage followed by pneumatic dilation as needed. Gastrointest Endosc 37:18, 1991.

87. Ferguson MK. Achalasia: current evaluation and therapy. Ann Thorac Surg 52:336, 1991.

88. Fried RL, Rosenberg S, Goyal R. Perforation rate in achalasia with polyethylene balloon dilators. [letter] Gastrointest Endosc 37:405, 1991.

89. Barkin JS, Guelrud M, Reiner DK, Goldbery RI, Phillips RS. Forceful balloon dilation: an outpatient procedure for achalasia. Gastrointest Endosc 36:123, 1990.

90. Fleischer D, Kessler F, Haye O. Endoscopic Nd:YAG laser therapy for carcinoma of the esophagus: a new palliative approach. Am J Surg 143:280, 1982.

91. Lightdale CJ, Zimbalist E, Winawer SJ. Outpatient management of esophageal cancer with endoscopic Nd:YAG laser. Am J Gastroenterol 82:46, 1987.

92. Heit HA, Johnson LF, Siegel SR, Boyce HW Jr. Palliative dilation for dysphagia in esophageal carcinoma. Ann Intern Med 89:629, 1978.

93. Atkinson M, Ferguson R. Fibreoptic endoscopic palliative intubation of inoperable oesophagogastric neoplasms. Br Med J 1:266, 1977.

94. Ogilivie AL, Dronfield MW, Ferguson R, Atkinson M. Palliative intubation of oesophagogastric neoplasms at fibreoptic endoscopy. Gut 23:1060, 1982.

95. Cusumano A, Ruol A, Segalin A, et al. Push-through intubation: effective palliation in 409 patients with cancer of the esophagus. Ann Thorac Surg 53:1010, 1992.

96. Chavy AL, Rougier PM, Pieddeloup C, et al. Esophageal prosthesis for neoplastic stenosis. Cancer 57:1426, 1986.

97. Boyce HW. Palliation of advanced esophageal cancer. Semin Oncol 9:186, 195, 1984.

98. Buset M, des Marez B, Baize M, et al. Palliative endoscopic management of obstructive esophagogastric cancer: Laser or prosthesis? Gastrointest Endosc 33:357, 1987.

99. Reed CE, Marsh WH, Carlson LS, Seymore CH, Kratz JM. Prospective, randomized trial of palliative treatment for unresectable cancer of the esophagus. Ann Thorac Surg 51:552, 1991.

100. Johnston J, Fleischer D, Petrini J, Nord J. Palliative bicap therapy of obstructing esophageal cancer. Gastrointest Endosc 32:141, 1986.

101. Kozarek RA, Bull TJ, Patterson DJ. Metallic self-expanding stent application in the upper gastrointestinal tract: caveats and concerns. Gastrointest Endosc 38:1, 1992.

102. Schaer J, Katon RM, Ivancev K, Uchida B, Rosch J, Binmoeller K. Treatment of malignant esophageal obstruction with silicone-coated metallic self-expanding stents. Gastrointest Endosc 38:7, 1992.

103. Wesdorp ICE, Bartelsman JFWM, Huibregtse K, Den Hartog Jager FCA, Tytgat GN. Treatment of instrumental oesophageal perforation. Gut 25:398, 1984.

104. Jones WG II, Ginsberg RJ. Esophageal perforation: a continuing challenge. Ann Thorac Surg 53:534, 1992.

105. Ancona E, Gayet B. Esophageal perforations. I: Etiology, diagnostic localization and symptoms. A GEEMO questionaire. In: Stewart JR, Holsher AH, eds. Diseases of the esophagus. New York: Springer-Verlag, 1988:1327–1330.

106. Silvis SE, Nebel O, Rogers G, Sugawa C, Mandelstam P. Endoscopic complications: results of the 1974 American Society of Gastrointestinal Endoscopy survey. JAMA 235:928, 1976.

107. Jones JD, Bozymski EM. Instrument esophageal perforation. Dig Dis Sci 24:319, 1979.

108. Nashef SAM, Pagliero KM. Instrumental perforation of the esophagus in benign disease. Ann Thorac Surg 44:360, 1987.

109. Attar S, Hankins JR, Suter CM, Coughlin TR, Sequeira A, McLaughlin JS. Esophageal perforation: a therapeutic challenge. Ann Thorac Surg 50:45, 1990.

110. Cameron JL, Kieffer RF, Hendrix TR, Mehigan DG, Baker RR. Selective nonoperative management of contained intrathoracic esophageal disruptions. Ann Thorac Surg 27:404, 1979.

111. Yeo CJ, Lillemore KD, Klein AS, Zinner MJ. Treatment of instrumental perforation of esophageal malignancy by transhiatal esophagectomy. Arch Surg 123:1016, 1988.

112. Orringer MD, Stirling MC. Esophagectomy for esophageal disruption. Ann Thorac Surg 49:35, 1990.

6

Endoscopic Management of Malignant Biliary Obstruction

Kenneth F. Binmoeller and Nib Soehendra

Malignant biliary obstruction is commonly caused by carcinoma of the pancreas, bile duct, and gallbladder and by extrinsic compression from metastatic lymph nodes. The treatment of malignant jaundice was primarily surgical bypass, but during the past 20 years, the introduction of endoscopic and percutaneous biliary drainage has made a dramatic impact on management.

The importance of nonoperative treatment is primarily related to the poor resectability of most cancers that cause biliary obstruction at the time of their presentation. These cancers are usually diagnosed late in their course, after contiguous or metastatic spread has already occurred. For most patients, treatment is palliative. Nonoperative palliation is attractive because it is less invasive than surgery and rarely requires general anaesthesia. Malignant biliary obstruction tends to occur in elderly patients who usually have other comorbid diseases, which increase the morbidity and mortality from surgery.

Whether biliary drainage is performed by the endoscopic or percutaneous approach depends largely on the local expertise. The endoscopic method has steadily gained popularity over the percutaneous approach because it is regarded as less invasive and can be combined with diagnostic endoscopic retrograde cholangiopancreatography (ERCP). However, individual cases may be better suited for the one or the other approach, and ideally both modalities should be available. In this chapter, we primar-ily describe endoscopic management of obstructive jaundice due to malignancy.

CONFIRMATION OF MALIGNANCY

Diagnostic imaging studies, including sonography (transabdominal and endoscopic), computed tomography, and findings on ERCP, usually suggest the diagnosis of malignancy. However, this should be confirmed by histologic or cytologic tissue examination before committing the patient to endoscopic treatment. Biopsies and cytology can be obtained endoscopically with forceps and brushes that can be passed into the bile duct.[1, 2] It is possible to pass ultrathin endoscopes through the working channel of duodenoscopes to evaluate the macroscopic appearance of the bile duct and to obtain biopsies under direct vision.[3, 4] Lesions seen on ultrasound or computed tomography can be biopsied under imaging guidance.

GOALS OF PALLIATION

The main objective of palliative management is the relief of symptomatic jaundice while maximizing the quality of life. The decision to perform biliary drainage depends on several factors, including the severity of the patient's symptoms, laboratory data, psychosocial factors, and the patient's wishes. The clinician should not always feel compelled to treat; supportive treatment may be the best option for the terminally ill patient with a short life expectancy.

Jaundice alone may not warrant a drainage procedure. However, mechanical biliary obstruction is often associated with other deleterious effects on the liver and other organs. Byproducts of bilirubin metabolism and toxic bile salts impair hepatic, renal, and immunologic functions.[5] Jaundice may decrease appetite and lead to a deterioration of the patient's overall sense of well-being. It is important to recognize that the terminal appearance of the jaundiced patient—commonly attributed to the underlying malignancy—may have a reversible component.

Jaundice in the patient with metastatic liver disease is generally attributed to hepatic parenchymal disease. Biliary drainage is not thought to be indicated. However, it is our experience that approximately 67% of patients with metastatic liver disease have concomitant extrahepatic obstruction. We have found that biliary decompression can relieve jaundice in most of these patients. ERCP should be considered for patients with metastatic liver disease to assess concomitant extrahepatic obstruction.

SITE OF BILIARY OBSTRUCTION

Tumors can cause obstruction at all levels of the biliary tract, from the papilla to the intrahepatic branches. Analysis of our patient collective revealed the distal common bile duct to be the most common site of obstruction (47%), followed by the hilar (23%), middle common bile duct (19%), and ampullary (11%) regions. Endoscopic management and success rates of treatment vary according to the level of involvement.

Ampulla of Vater

Tumors at the ampulla of Vater deserve special mention. In contrast to most other malignancies involving the biliary tract, tumors involving the ampulla may have a high rate of surgical resectability. The 5-year survival rate of ampullary tumors after radical surgery has been as high as 50%.[6-8] Surgery should be the treatment of choice, and endoscopic treatment should be reserved for patients who are poor surgical candidates. Endoscopic methods of palliation include stenting, snare papillectomy, and laser tumor ablation.[9, 10]

Distal Common Bile Duct

The most frequent cause of malignant distal common bile duct obstruction is pancreatic head carcinoma, followed by cholangiocarcinoma. Differentiation may be difficult based on the cholangiogram alone. Filling of the pancreatic duct usually demonstrates a double-duct sign (Fig. 6–1), indicating a tumor in the head of the pancreas.[11] Endoscopic stenting of distal common duct obstruction is usually easy after cannulation has been achieved. Success rates of 90% or higher have been reported.[12, 13]

Middle Common Bile Duct

Obstruction involving the middle third of the bile duct is primarily due to cholangiocarcinoma or carcinoma of the gallbladder. In gallbladder cancer, the gallbladder usually fails to opacify or incompletely fills. Tumor invasion of the bile duct typically laterally displaces the bile duct, causing an eccentric stricture (Fig. 6–2). Cholangiocarcinoma tends to cause concentric narrowing (Fig. 6–3). Differentiation of the two is

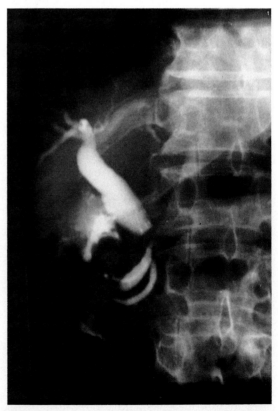

Figure 6–1. Endoscopic retrograde cholangiopancreatogram showing obstruction of the distal bile and pancreatic ducts (*i.e.,* double duct sign).

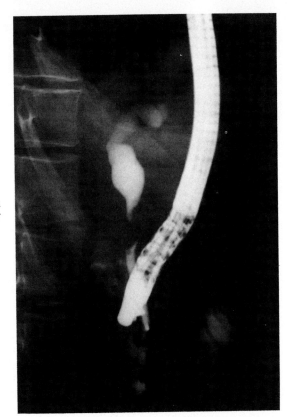

Figure 6–2. Endoscopic retrograde cholangiogram showing a middle common bile duct stricture secondary to gallbladder carcinoma.

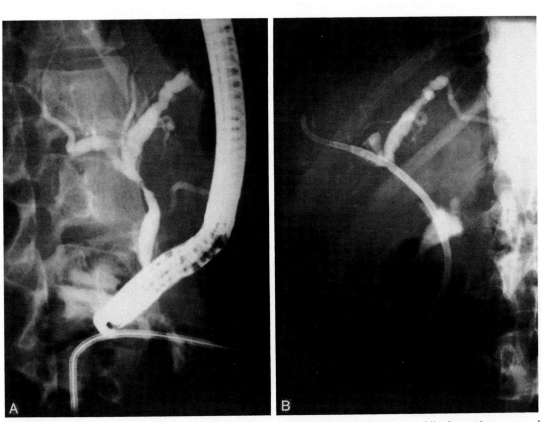

Figure 6–3. (A) Endoscopic retrograde cholangiogram showing a concentric middle common bile duct stricture secondary to cholangiocarcinoma. **(B)** After placement of a pigtail stent across the stricture into the right hepatic duct.

perhaps academic, because both cancers are burdened with equally dismal prognoses. These tumors may extend up to bifurcation, and it is important to carefully define the proximal extent of tumor growth. Some surgeons have advocated placement of bilateral endoprosthesis before the bifurcation becomes involved, but we have found single stent placement to be sufficient in most cases (see Fig. 6–3B).[14]

Hilar Strictures

Malignant obstruction involving the bifurcation and hepatic branches may be due to cholangiocarcinoma, gallbladder carcinoma, or metastases. This location is diagnostically and therapeutically difficult. An optimal cholangiogram may be difficult to obtain because of backflow of the contrast media. In such cases, it is helpful to inject contrast media under pressure, using the occlusion balloon catheter. This maneuver may "open" a seemingly complete obstruction (Fig. 6–4).

The management of hilar strictures depends on the extent of hepatic duct involvement. Strictures limited to the common hepatic duct (type I, Fig. 6–5) are relatively easy to stent. A single stent is placed across the obstruction into the right or left intrahepatic duct. Jaundice is relieved in more than 90% of patients.[12, 15] Strictures involving both hepatic ducts (type II, Fig. 6–6A) or their branches (type III, Fig. 6–7) are considerably more difficult to stent, and success rates of bilateral drainage have been as low as 25%.[12] There is some controversy about whether type II and III strictures require bilateral (Fig. 6–6B) or even multiple stents to completely drain obstructed segments. We recommend complete drainage whenever this is technically feasible. Cremer and colleagues reported a significantly higher incidence of early cholangitis and mortality from sepsis when endoscopic drainage was complete (bilateral) compared with incomplete (unilateral) in type II and III hilar strictures.[16] Complete drainage is mandatory if contrast medium fails to drain after ductal filling, because retained contrast may induce cholangitis. If endoscopic drainage fails, percutaneous drainage should be attempted.

ENDOSCOPIC TECHNIQUE

Before embarking on the therapeutic procedure, a diagnostic ERCP is performed, and the

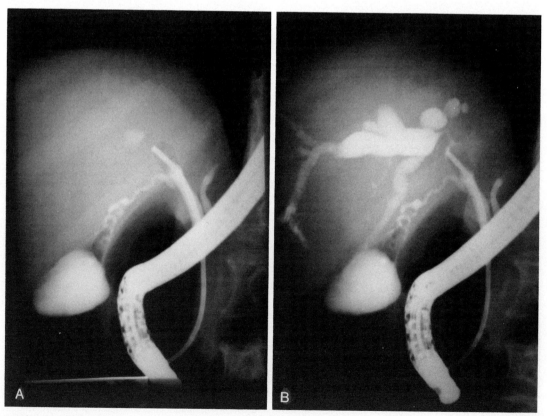

Figure 6–4. (A) Endoscopic retrograde cholangiogram showing an abrupt cutoff at the bifurcation. The balloon catheter has been inserted into the common hepatic duct and inflated to occlude the duct. **(B)** Complete cholangiogram after injection of contrast medium under pressure shows dilated hepatic branches.

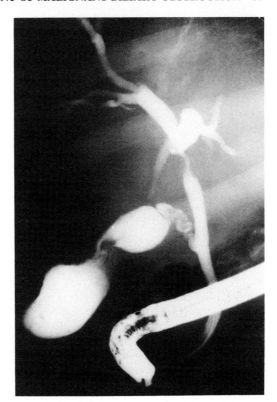

Figure 6–5. Endoscopic retrograde cholangiogram showing a carcinomatous stricture limited to the common hepatic duct (type I).

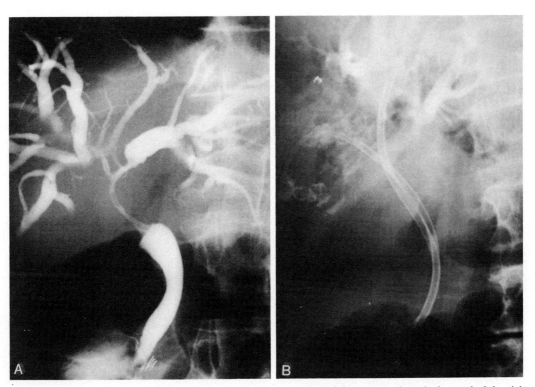

Figure 6–6. (A) Endoscopic retrograde cholangiogram showing narrowing of the common hepatic duct and of the right and left hepatic ducts owing to cholangiocarcinoma (type II). **(B)** After bilateral placement of pigtail stents into the right and left hepatic ducts.

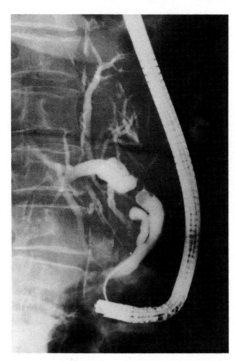

Figure 6–7. Endoscopic retrograde cholangiogram showing diffuse tumor spread to the hepatic ducts and branches (type III).

anatomic details of the malignant stricture are assessed. The procedure is performed under sedation with intravenous benzodiazepam, which can be supplemented with an opiate if necessary. Buscopan (*N*-butylscopolammonium bromide) or glucagon is administered to counter peristaltic bowel activity.

Standard duodenoscopes with a 3.2-mm channel only accommodate stents up to a No. 8 French (2.6 mm) in diameter. A large-channel duodenoscope (3.7 or 4.2 mm) is required for placement of No. 10 and No. 11.5 French stents. We generally perform the initial diagnostic ERCP, papillotomy, and stent placement with the large-channel instrument. However, larger endoscopes are more difficult to manipulate than standard duodenoscopes. Some endoscopists prefer to perform the cholangiogram and papillotomy with the standard duodenoscope, and exchange this for the large-channel instrument for stent placement.

We perform a small papillotomy to facilitate stent placement. The orifice of the papilla is cannulated with a curved, tapered-tip catheter (Universal catheter [distal end, 4.5 French; proximal end, No. 6 French], Wilson-Cook Inc, Winston-Salem, NC). A flexible guidewire is passed through the catheter and extended slightly beyond the catheter tip. With the catheter resting below the stricture, the guidewire is maneuvered through the stricture under fluoroscopic monitoring (Fig. 6–8*A,B*).

An assortment of flexible guidewires is commercially available for passing strictures. The conventional 0.035-in (0.8 mm) stainless steel guidewire has a 3-cm flexible tip but is fairly rigid and difficult to steer. Forceful probing of tight or angulated strictures risks perforation. In these difficult cases, hydrophilic guidewires (Terumo Glidewire, Tokyo, Japan; Tracer wire, Wilson-Cook Inc, Winston-Salem, NC) should be used. A special polymer coating of this wire

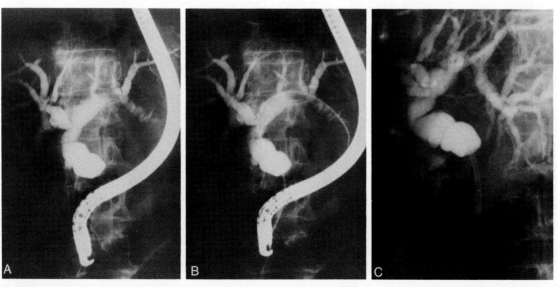

Figure 6–8. Endoscopic insertion of a straight plastic stent. **(A)** Initial endoscopic retrograde cholangiogram showing an obstruction of the distal common bile duct with prestenotic dilation. **(B)** A conventional guidewire has been inserted through the stricture into the left hepatic duct. **(C)** Prosthesis in place across the tumor.

gives it a lower coefficient of friction, which allows it to pass through strictures more easily. The wire tip is steerable because of effective transmission of torque. The stricture is negotiated by combining torque with backward and forward movements. Adjusting the position of the catheter tip can improve the angle of access to the stricture.

After the guidewire is passed through the stricture, the catheter follows the guidewire. Contrast medium is injected at this point to more completely opacify the biliary tree above the stricture. A Y-adapter can be connected to the proximal end of the catheter to enable instillation of contrast media without having to remove the guidewire.

Stent placement is performed over an indwelling 400-mm guidewire using the Seldinger technique (Fig. 6–8C). Hydrophilic wires are generally too floppy for stent insertion and should be exchanged for a conventional guidewire. An exception is the Tracer wire, which uniquely combines properties of a hydrophilic and conventional guidewire. The hydrophilic coating is limited to the distal 60 cm, making this wire suitable for passing difficult strictures and for stent placement. Depending on the type of plastic stent used, one of the two variations of stent insertion technique is used. Pigtail stents (Fig. 6–9A) gradually taper toward the tip and can be threaded directly over the guidewire. Straight stents (Fig. 6–9B) are not tapered and must be inserted coaxially over an inner catheter to reduce step-off between the stent and wire (*i.e.,* two-layer technique). The stent is advanced over the guidewire or inner catheter with a pusher tube.

Hilar strictures are often technically difficult to stent. These strictures tend to be tight, tortuous, and firm. They are also farther away from the endoscope. We prefer pigtail stents for these strictures, which are easier to insert because of the tapered tip. If bilateral placement of stents into the right and left hepatic ducts is indicated, difficulties often arise in placing the second stent. It is advisable to initially place smaller-caliber (7 French, 2.3 mm) stents. The stents can be exchanged for larger-diameter stents 1 to 2 weeks later. It is helpful to exchange stents over a guidewire using the Soehendra retriever (Wilson-Cook Inc, Winston-Salem, NC) to avoid having to recannulate the strictures (see later section on Stent Replacement).

STENTS

The most commonly used stents are made of plastic material. Two basic designs are available: pigtail and straight stents (see Fig. 6–9A,B). Pigtail stents are straightened over a guidewire for insertion and resume their pigtail shape after withdrawal of the guidewire. The pigtail provides anchorage in the bile duct and is tapered to minimize step-off between the guidewire and stent. Multiple side holes at the proximal end provide for drainage. Straight stents have side flaps to prevent dislodgement and side holes for drainage. In one model, the side holes are formed where the side flaps are cut out of the wall of the stent. The advantage of pigtail stents is that they are easier to place through tight strictures. However, in vitro studies have shown that straight stents have better flow rates than pigtail stents.[17, 18]

Stent Clogging

The major complication of all plastic stents is their tendency to clog over time, leading to recurrent jaundice and cholangitis. Occlusion rates have been 30% at 3 months and 70% at 6 months, and the mean duration of patency was 5 months.[12, 19] This problem has been the subject of considerable research over the past years and continues to remain unsolved.

Mechanism of Clogging

The major contributors to stent clogging are thought to be the adherence of bacteria to the inner wall of the stent and the reflux of chyme

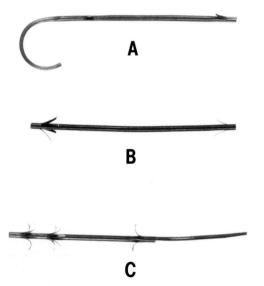

Figure 6–9. Plastic stent designs. **(A)** Single pigtail stent. **(B)** Straight stent without side holes. **(C)** Straight stent with tail-like appendage (*i.e.,* gutter stent).

from the duodenum. Light and electron microscopic analysis of occluded stents has demonstrated bacterial contamination (mostly *Escherichia coli*), encrusted plant fibers, and deposits of amorphous material.[20–22] A bacterial biofilm forms on the surface of the plastic prosthesis that is composed of a matrix of bacterial cells and fibrillar anionic extracellular products.[22] It is thought that bacteria form biofilms by polysaccharide production, which cements bacterial cells to the surface and mediates further adhesion of bacteria. Bacterial enzymatic activity leads to the deposition of crystals of calcium bilirubinate, calcium palmitate, and cholesterol, which contribute to sludge formation.[23]

Antibacterial Coating of Stents

Antibacterial coating of stents has been proposed to reduce bacterial contamination, which may trigger biofilm formation. An in vitro study demonstrated that impregnation of stents with silver or chlorhexidine significantly reduced *E. coli* growth.[24] However, this has not translated to prolonged stent patency in in vivo studies. The patency of stents coated with silver or antibiotics such as cephalosporin was no better than that of conventional stents.[25, 26] Systemic antibiotics and aspirin affect the content of stent sludge, but their effect on stent patency is still unclear.[27]

Stent Material

Plastic prostheses may be constructed from different polymers including Teflon, polyurethane, polyethylene, polyvinyl chloride, and silicone. In vitro studies suggest that the encrustation rates depend on the material for stent construction. In one study comparing various polymers perfused with human bile over a 2-week period, the frictional coefficient of the polymer correlated with the amount of encrusted material.[28] Teflon had the lowest frictional coefficient and accrued the least amount of encrusted sludge. However, in another study, Teflon had the highest (and polyurethane the lowest) encrustation rates.[29] Clinical studies are needed to clarify the role of plastic stent material on clogging rates. It has been our experience that Teflon stents have lower occlusion rates than the commercially available polyethylene stents.

Stent Design

We analyzed the sites of stent occlusion and found these to be especially prominent around

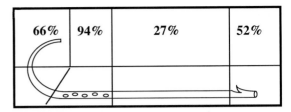

Figure 6–10. Diagram of pigtail stent showing frequency of occlusion according to site.

the side holes and side flaps (Fig. 6–10). This can be explained by turbulent flow at the site of side holes and the rough-cut edges that promote bacteria and sludge adherence. Stents without side holes form significantly less sludge than stents with side holes. In a clinical trial, patients treated with polyethylene stents with side holes accrued significantly more sludge than patients with polyethylene stents without side holes.[28] Whether side holes really improve biliary drainage is not clear; it has been suggested that side holes may actually decrease bile flow due to flow turbulence.[17]

We compared the patency rates of 60 straight stents without side holes and 60 pigtail stents. Stents were uniformly manufactured from Teflon. Side flaps of straight stents were cut out of the wall without opening the lumen of the stent. The straight Teflon stents had significantly longer median patency rates compared with pigtail stents (175 vs. 99 days), and stent exchanges were required more frequently in patients with pigtail stents ($p<0.01$). The median patency of straight stents without side holes was longer than that reported in the literature for straight stents with side holes.[12]

Using conventional technique, stents are left protruding into the lumen of the duodenum to allow for easy retrieval in the event of clogging. Duodenal contents (*e.g.,* bacteria, chyme) can reflux into the lumen of the stent, which promotes clogging. To minimize duodenal reflux, we modified plastic stents by adding a tail-like "gutter" appendage to the distal end of the stent (Fig. 6–9*C*). The stent was positioned above the papilla, and the gutter portion was left extending into the duodenum for the purpose of stent removal (Fig. 6–11). This prosthesis was placed in the usual manner and was not difficult to insert. Stents can be removed with a snare or forceps or can be exchanged over a guidewire using the Soehendra stent retriever. In a prospective clinical study, gutter pigtail stents had a trend toward longer patency than conventional pigtail stents.[26]

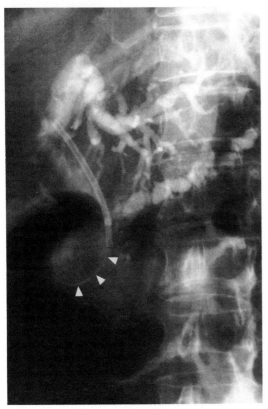

Figure 6–11. Endoscopic retrograde cholangiogram after placement of a gutter stent with a tail-like appendage *(arrowheads)* extending into the duodenum.

Expandable Metal Stents

Several studies have shown that increasing the stent diameter increases the duration of patency. In a comparison of No. 7 or No. 8 French stents with No. 10 French stents, the larger stents had longer periods of patency.[30] Although bigger appears to be better, the maximal outside diameter of plastic stents is limited by the instrument channel of the duodenoscope. This is an a No. 11.5 French (3.8-mm) stent for the larger-channel (4.2-mm) duodenoscope. To overcome this, expandable metal stents have been used in the biliary tract. These stents can be inserted through the duodenoscope in a compressed state and expand passively or actively after deployment in the bile duct (Fig. 6–12).

Three expandable stents are undergoing evaluation for use in the bile duct. These include the Gianturco "Z" stent (Cook, Bloomington, IN), the Wallstent (Medivent SA, Lausanne, Switzerland), and the Strecker Stent (Meditech, Boston Scientific Corp., Watertown, MA). A comparison of these stents is provided in Table 6–1. The Gianturco and Wallstent stents are self-expanding, and the Strecker stent requires balloon inflation for expansion.

Preliminary results suggest that expandable metal stents clog less often than plastic prostheses.[31–36] With the exception of one study, which reported sludge clogging in 15% of cases, clogging was rarely observed.[36] However, recurrent jaundice still occurred in 13% to 42% of patients over various follow-up periods. In most cases, this was due to tumor ingrowth through the wire struts or overgrowth proximal or distal to the stent. Occlusion has also been secondary to mucosal hyperplasia induced by the metal wires. This was most prominent at the proximal and distal edges of the stents and may decrease luminal diameter by as much as 60%.[29, 32, 37]

The role of expandable stents in the management of malignant biliary obstruction remains to be defined. The preliminary results of a prospective randomized trial comparing patency rates of the Wallstent and straight polyethylene stents failed to show a statistical difference after a mean follow-up of 147 days.[38] Coating of expandable stents has been proposed to inhibit tumor ingrowth, but tumor overgrowth and mucosal hyperplasia may still cause recurrent obstruction. The high commercial cost of these stents discourages their widespread use. The potential advantages must be weighed against the limited life expectancy associated with malignant biliary obstruction; in one study of 17 patients who underwent Wallstent placement, 9 patients died within 4 months, and 2 of 5 patients followed for more than 4 months developed stent obstruction due to tumor ingrowth.[39]

A disadvantage of these expandable stents is the inability to move or remove them after they are implanted. We are investigating the use of a prototype expandable stent made of a shape-memory alloy (nitinol), which can be easily removed after placement. The stent is coil-shaped and has the unique property of resuming a predefined shape when heated (Fig. 6–13). The prototype being investigated can be delivered over a No. 7 French catheter and expands to a lumen diameter of No. 14 to No. 16 French when irrigated with warm water (55°C). The stent is highly flexible. With warming, the length of the stent shrinks by approximately 40%. There are practically no open spaces through which tumor can grow. The stent is removed by pulling on the proximal end, which uncoils the stent. We have found the stent technically easy to deploy. Studies of long-term tolerance and patency rates are pending.

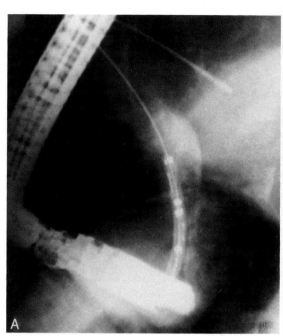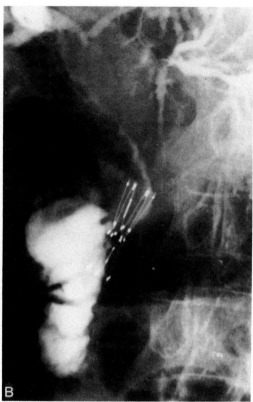

Figure 6–12. Endoscopic retrograde cholangiogram showing deployment of a self-expandable stent (Gianturco stent, Cook, Bloomington, IN) across a distal common bile duct stricture. **(A)** Coaxial insertion of the compressed stent over a guidewire. **(B)** Expanded stent after release from the delivery catheter.

Results and Complications of Biliary Stenting

Endoscopic transpapillary stent placement is a standardized technique. Success rates exceed 90% for the drainage of distal strictures. Failure is primarily due to inaccessibility of the papilla. Common causes are duodenal tumor stenosis and prior gastroduodenal surgery (*e.g.,* Billroth II gastrectomy, Roux-en-Y anastomosis). Inability to cannulate the papilla, particularly if the papilla is infiltrated by tumor, may also cause failure.

The overall procedure-related complication rate requiring interventional therapy is 1.5% to 2%, and the mortality rate is less than 1%. Early complications are mainly related to papillotomy and include hemorrhage, pancreatitis, and retroduodenal perforation. We perform a small papillotomy, which reduces these complications. Rarely, guidewire insertion may perforate the bile duct. Incomplete drainage of contrast media after injection may lead to cholangitis. If transpapillary drainage is not successful after injection of contrast media, endoscopic drainage should be reattempted or per-

Table 6–1. COMPARISON OF EXPANDABLE METALLIC STENTS

Characteristics	Stent Type			
	Wallstent	*Gianturco*	*Strecker*	*Nitinol*
Manufacturer	Medivent	Cook	Meditech	Olympus
Metal used	Stainless steel	Stainless steel	Tantulum	Titanium-nickel alloy
Mechanism	Self-expandable	Self-expandable	Balloon expandable	Heat expandable
Diameter compressed	2.3–3 mm	4 mm	3 mm	3.3 mm
Diameter expanded	8–10 mm	12 mm	8 mm	5–6 mm
Removable	No	No	No	Yes

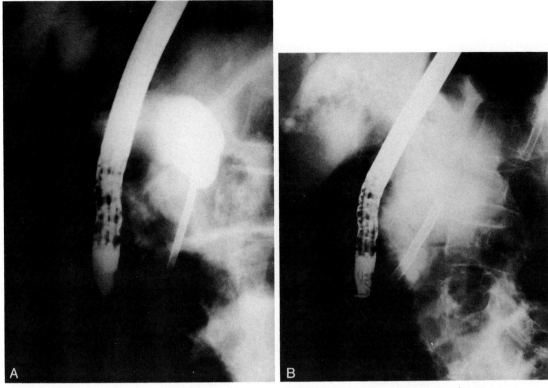

Figure 6–13. Endoscopic retrograde cholangiogram showing deployment of a nitinol expandable stent for a distal common bile duct stricture. **(A)** Stent with native diameter after insertion across the tumor. **(B)** Expanded stent after instillation of warm water.

cutaneous drainage performed no later than the next day. The incidence of cholangitis was found to increase from 2.7% to 22% if drainage required two or more attempts.[40]

Late complications of stent placement are primarily related to stent clogging. The clinical presentation may range from mild flu-like symptoms to septic cholangitis and is usually accompanied by recurrent jaundice.[12, 19] Stents may also migrate. Distal migration may impact the duodenal wall and cause ulceration with complications such as bleeding and perforation. Acute cholecystitis due to obstruction of the cystic duct has been reported as a late complication.[12, 19]

Stent Replacement

Stent replacement can be performed by removing the clogged stent with a snare or forceps and inserting a new stent or by exchanging the stent over a guidewire using the Soehendra stent retriever (Fig. 6–14). Using the latter technique, a conventional guidewire is inserted through the stent and serves as a guide for stent exchange. The stent retriever is used to remove the stent through the instrumentation channel of the duodenoscope. The advantage of this method is that stent replacement can be performed without losing access to the stricture. This is particularly helpful if bilateral stent replacement is indicated.

STENTING VERSUS SURGERY

Randomized trials comparing the results of surgery and endoscopic stenting for the palliation of low bile duct and pancreatic head cancer have demonstrated both methods to be equally effective in relieving jaundice.[41–43] Overall survival in both groups was similar. Endoscopic stenting had the advantage of a significantly shorter initial hospital stay, lower procedural complications, and lower 30-day mortality rate (Table 6–2). However, recurrent jaundice occurred more often in the stented patients. Despite hospital readmissions for stent exchanges, the overall time spent in the hospital until death was significantly less for patients treated endoscopically.[41]

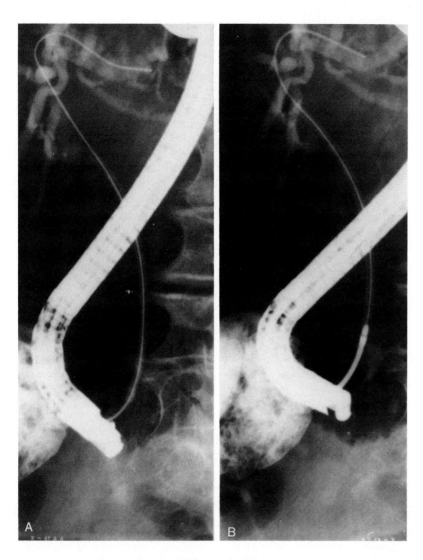

Figure 6–14. Over-the-guidewire stent replacement using the Soehendra retriever. **(A)** Endoscopic retrograde cholangiogram showing insertion of a Teflon-coated guidewire through the stent. **(B)** The retriever is passed over the guidewire and screws into the distal end of the prosthesis. The stent is removed through the duodenoscope instrumentation channel, leaving the guidewire in place for insertion of a new stent.

Table 6–2. RANDOMIZED TRIALS COMPARING BYPASS SURGERY WITH ENDOSCOPIC STENT PLACEMENT

Characteristics	Shepherd, 1988[41]		Andersen, 1989[42]		Dowsett, 1989[43]	
	Stent	*Surgery*	*Stent*	*Surgery*	*Stent*	*Surgery*
No. of patients	23	25	30	19	65	62
Jaundice relieved (%)	91	92	96	76	94	94
Complications (%)	22	40	36	20	11	5
30-day mortality (%)	9	20	17	32	6	15
Recurrent jaundice (%)	43	0	28	16	17	3
Duodenal stenosis (%)	9	4	0	0	14	3
Survival (weeks)	22	18	12	15	22	16

In our experience, most stent exchanges can be performed on an outpatient basis if there are no signs of cholangitis. Cost analysis of surgical drainage and endoscopic treatment until death revealed significant savings (average of $8000 per patient) for the endoscopic group.[44] These results and the intuitively less invasive nature of endoscopic treatment argue in favor of the endoscopic approach.

Duodenal obstruction due to progressive tumor growth may develop in patients with low bile duct or pancreatic head tumors, eventually necessitating duodenal bypass surgery. In surgical series, duodenal obstruction requiring reoperation was reported in as many as 50% of patients who underwent biliary bypass.[45] This has been an argument in favor of a prophylactic gastroenterostomy at the initial presentation of patients with malignant distal bile duct obstruction. However, follow-up studies after endoscopic drainage have shown that the incidence of duodenal obstruction was much lower than that reported in surgical series (7.5% and 6.0%) in two large series from Amsterdam and the Middlesex Hospitals.[43, 46] This is probably explained by the fact that endoscopic drainage preselects patients with minimal or no duodenal tumor involvement. In the face of a shortened life expectancy, duodenal obstruction is not likely to become a clinically relevant problem in patients undergoing endoscopic drainage.

In contrast to distal common bile duct obstruction, the results of endoscopic stenting of tumors involving the bifurcation are often unsatisfactory. Speer and colleagues reported relief of jaundice in only 56% of patients with type III hilar strictures.[15] Failure to adequately drain obstructed segments may result in cholangitis. Even when drainage is initially successful, the results are often short-lived due to progressive intraductal tumor extension. It has increasingly been our policy to refer patients with type III strictures for percutaneous drainage. There are no randomized trials comparing results of surgery and endoscopy as palliative treatments for obstructing bifurcation tumors.

PREOPERATIVE DECOMPRESSION

The value of preoperative biliary drainage by the endoscopic or percutaneous route is still a subject of debate. Theoretically, reducing the level of hyperbilirubinemia should reduce the operative morbidity and mortality.[5, 47] Retrospective studies have suggested that preopera-

tive percutaneous drainage could reduce the risk of surgery.[48, 49] However, of two prospective studies comparing preoperative percutaneous drainage with no preoperative drainage, one study did not show a difference in surgical mortality, and another showed an increased mortality after preoperative drainage.[50, 51] Complications of percutaneous drainage may offset the potential advantages. Preoperative endoscopic drainage has not been adequately studied. One small study of 39 patients showed preoperative endoscopic drainage to result in significantly fewer early complications than no preoperative drainage.[52]

ENDOSCOPIC VERSUS PERCUTANEOUS MANAGEMENT

The endoscopic approach is generally preferable to the percutaneous approach, because it avoids liver puncture. A prospective study by Speer and colleagues showed better success rates of endoscopic stent placement for relief of jaundice (81% vs. 61%) and a significantly lower 30-day mortality rate (15% vs. 33%).[53] The complication rates of endoscopic and percutaneous drainage were 19% and 67%, respectively. Most complications (i.e., hemorrhage, bile leaks) in the percutaneous group were due to liver puncture.

For biliary drainage procedures that cannot be accomplished by endoscopy, a combined endoscopic and percutaneous method approach ("rendezvous" procedure) can be used.[54–57] A guidewire is passed transhepatically into the duodenum to lead the endoscopic placement of a prosthesis. The advantage of this combined approach is that a large-diameter prosthesis can be implanted with a lower risk than by percutaneous placement alone. Self-expandable metallic stents have also reduced the risk of liver trauma associated with percutaneous stent placement.[33, 34]

References

1. Foutch PG, Kerr DM, Harlan JR, Manne RK, Kummet TD, Sanowski RA. Endoscopic retrograde wire-guided cytology for diagnosis of patients with malignant obstruction of the bile duct. Am J Gastroenterol 85:891, 1990.
2. Venu RP, Geenen JE, Kini M, Hogan WJ, Payne M, Johnson GK, Schmalz MJ. Endoscopic retrograde brush cytology. A new technique. Gastroenterology 99:1475, 1990.

3. Ponchon T, Chavaillon A, Ayela P. Retrograde biliary ultrathin endoscopy enhances biopsy of stenoses and lithotripsy. Gastrointest Endosc 35:292, 1989.
4. Rustgi AK, Kelsey PB, Guelrud M, et al. Malignant tumors of the bile ducts: diagnosis by biopsy during endoscopic cannulation. Gastrointest Endosc 35:248, 1989.
5. O'Connor, MJ. Mechanical biliary obstruction. A review of the multisystemic consequences of obstructive jaundice and their impact on perioperative morbidity and mortality. Am Surg 5:245, 1985.
6. Warren KW, Choe DS, Plaza J, Relihan M. Results of radical resection for periampullary cancer. Ann Surg 181:534, 1975.
7. Cohen JR, Kuchta N, Geller N, Shires GT, Dineen P. Pancreaticoduodenectomy. A 30 year experience. Ann Surg 195:608, 1982.
8. Kellum JM, Clark J, Miller HH. Pancreaticoduodenectomy for resectable malignant periampullary tumors. Surg Gynecol Obstet 157:362, 1983.
9. Lambert R, Ponchon T, Chavaillon A, Berger F. Laser treatment of tumors of the papilla of Vater. Endoscopy 20:227, 1988.
10. Huibregtse K, Tytgat GNJ. Carcinoma of the ampulla of Vater: the endoscopic approach. Endoscopy 20:223, 1988.
11. Freeny PC, Bilbvao MK, Katon RM. "Blind" evaluation of endoscopic retrograde cholangiopancreatography (ERCP) in the diagnosis of pancreatic carcinoma: the "double duct" and other signs. Radiology 119:271, 1976.
12. Huibregtse K, Katon RM, Coene PPL, Tytgat GNJ. Endoscopic palliative treatment in pancreatic cancer. Gastrointest Endosc 32:334, 1986.
13. Soehendra N, Grimm H, Berger B, Nam VC. Malignant jaundice: results of diagnostic and therapeutic endoscopy. World J Surg 13:171, 1989.
14. Huibregtse K, Tytgat GN. Endoscopic biliary drainage. In: Lygidakis NJ, Tytgat GNJ, eds. Hepatobiliary and pancreatic malignancies: diagnosis, medical, and surgical treatment. Stuttgart: Georg Thieme Verlag, 1989:426–438.
15. Speer AG, Cotton PB. Endoscopic stents for biliary obstruction due to malignancy. In: Jacobson IM, ed. ERCP: diagnostic and therapeutic applications. New York: Elsevier, 1989:203–224.
16. Deviere J, Baize M, de Toeuf J, Cremer M. Long-term follow-up of patients with hilar malignant stricture treated by endoscopic internal biliary drainage. Gastrointest Endosc 34:95, 1988.
17. Rey JF, Maupetit P, Greff M. Experimental study of biliary endoprosthesis efficiency. Endoscopy 17:145, 1985.
18. Leung JWC, Del Favero G, Cotton PB. Endoscopic biliary prosthesis: a comparison of materials. Gastrointest Endosc 31:93, 1985.
19. Siegel JH, Snady H. The significance of endoscopically placed prostheses in the management of biliary obstruction due to carcinoma of the pancreas: results of nonoperative decompression in 277 patients. Am J Gastroenterol 81:634, 1986.
20. Leung JWC, Ling TKW, Kung JLS, Vallance-Owen J. The role of bacteria in the blockage of biliary stents. Gastrointest Endosc 34:19–22, 1988.
21. Groen AK, Huibregtse K, Delzenne B, Hoek FJ, Tytgat GNJ. Characterization of the content of occluded biliary endoprostheses. Endoscopy 19:57, 1987.
22. Speer AG, Cotton PB, Rode J, Seddon AM, Neal CR, Holton J, Costerton JW. Biliary stent blockage with bacterial biofilm. Ann Intern Med 108:546, 1988.
23. Leung JWC, Banez VP. Clogging of biliary stents: mechanisms and possible solution. Dig Endosc 2:97, 1990.
24. Haulk A, Danilewitz M. Prevention of bacterial growth and colonization with antimicrobial impregnated stents—an in vitro study. [Abstract] Gastrointest Endosc 35:163, 1989.
25. Browne S, Schmalz M, Geenen J, Venu R, Johnson GK. A comparison of biliary and pancreatic stent occlusion in antibiotic-coated vs. conventional stents. [Abstract] Gastrointest Endosc 36:206, 1990.
26. Brückner M, Seitz U, Mack D, Grimm H, Eckman B, Soehendra N. Vergleichende Untersuchung über Rinnen- und Silberprothesen bei der Drainage maligner Gallengangsstenosen. In: Henning N, Soehendra N, eds. Fortschritte der gastroenterologischen Endoskopie. Gräfelfing: Demeter Verlag, 1990:17–21.
27. Smit JM, Out MMJ, Groen AK, Huibregste K, Jansen PLM, van Marle J, Tytgat GNJ. A placebo-controlled study on the efficacy of aspirin and doxycycline in preventing clogging of biliary endoprostheses. Gastrointest Endosc 35:485, 1989.
28. Coene PPLO, Groen AK, Cheng J, Out MMJ, Tytgat GNJ, Huibregtse K. Clogging of biliary endoprostheses: a new perspective. Gut 31:913, 1990.
29. Lammer J. Biliary endoprostheses. Plastic versus metal stents. Radiol Clin North Am 28:1211, 1990.
30. Speer AG, Cotton PB, MacRae KD. Endoscopic management of malignant biliary obstruction: stents of 10 French gauge are preferable to stents of 8 French gauge. Gastrointest Endosc 35:412, 1988.
31. Irving JD, Adam A, Dick R, Dondelinger RF, Lunderquist A, Roche A. Gianturco expandable metallic stents: result of a European clinical trial. Radiology 172:321, 1989.
32. Yoshioka T, Sakaguchi H, Yoshimura H, Tamada T, Ohishi H, Uchica H, Wallace S. Expandable metallic biliary endoprostheses: preliminary clinical evaluation. Radiology 177:253, 1990.
33. Lammer J, Klein GE, Kleinert R, Hausegger K, Einspieler R. Obstructive jaundice: use of expandable metal endoprosthesis for biliary drainage. Work in progress. Radiology 177:789, 1990.
34. Adam A, Chetty N, Roddie M, Yeung E, Benjamin IS. Self-expandable stainless steel endoprostheses for treatment of malignant bile duct obstruction. Am J Roentgenol 156:321, 1991.
35. Neuhaus H, Hagenmüller F, Griebel M, Classen M. Percutaneous cholangioscopic or transpapillary insertion in self-expanding biliary stents. Gastrointest Endosc 37:31, 1991.
36. Gillams A, Dick R, Dooley JS, Wallsten H, Eldin A. Self-expandable stainless steel braided endoprosthesis for biliary strictures. Radiology 174:137, 1990.
37. Alvarado R, Palmaz JC, Garcia OJ, Tio FO, Rees CR. Evaluation of polymer-coated balloon-expandable stents in bile ducts. Radiology 170:975, 1988.
38. Davids PHP, Fockens P, Groen AK, Tytgat GNJ, Huibregtse K. Prospective randomized trial of self expanding metal stents vs polyethylene stents for malignant biliary obstruction: preliminary results. [Abstract] Gastrointest Endosc 38:249, 1992.
39. Cremer M, Deviere J, Sugai B, Baize M. Expandable biliary metal stents for malignancies: endoscopic insertion and diathermic cleaning for tumor ingrowth. Gastrointest Endosc 36:451, 1990.
40. Huibregtse K, Katon RM, Coene PP, Tytgat GNJ. Endoscopic palliative treatment in pancreatic cancer. Gastrointest Endosc 32:334, 1986.
41. Shepherd HA, Royle G, Ross APR, Diba A, Arthur

M, Colin-Jones D. Endoscopic biliary endosprothesis in the palliation of malignant obstruction of the distal common bile duct: a randomized trial. Br J Surg 75:1166, 1988.

42. Andersen JR, Sorensen SM, Kruse A, Rokkjaer M, Matzen P. Randomised trial of endoscopic versus operative bypass in malignant obstructive jaundice. Gut 30:1132, 1989.

43. Dowsett JF, Russell RCG, Hatfield ARW, et al. Malignant obstructive jaundice: prospective randomized trial of by-pass surgery versus endoscopic stenting. Gastroenterology 96:A128, 1989.

44. Brandabur JJ, Kozarek RA, Ball TJ, et al. Nonoperative versus operative treatment of obstructive jaundice in pancreatic cancer: cost and survival analysis. Am J Gastroenterol 83:1132, 1988.

45. Saar MG, Cameron JL. Surgical palliation of unresectable carcinoma of the pancreas. World J Surg 8:906, 1984.

46. Huibregtse K. Endoscopic palliation in malignant bile duct strictures: the Amsterdam experience. Dig Endosc 2:203, 1990.

47. Braasch JW, Gray BN. Considerations that lower pancreaticoduodenectomy mortality. Am J Surg 133:480, 1977.

48. Denning DA, Ellison EC, Carey L. Preoperative percutaneous transhepatic biliary decompression lowers operative morbidity in patients with obstructive jaundice. Am J Surg 141:61, 1981.

49. Nakayama T, Ikeda A, Okuda K. Percutaneous trans-hepatic drainage of the biliary tract. Technique and results in 104 cases. Gastroenterology 74:554, 1978.

50. Hatfield ARW, Tobias R, Terblanche J, et al. Preoperative percutaneous biliary drainage in obstructive jaundice: a prospective controlled trial. Br J Surg 71:371, 1984.

51. McPherson GAD, Benjhamin IS, Hodgson HJF, et al. Preoperative percutaneous biliary drainage: the results of a controlled trial. Br J Surg 71:371, 1984.

52. Lygidakis NJ, van der Heyde MN, Lubbers MJ. Evaluation of preoperative biliary drainage in the surgical management of pancreatic head carcinoma. Acta Chir Scand 153:665, 1987.

53. Speer AG, Cotton PB, Russell RCG, et al. Randomised trial of endoscopic versus percutaneous stent insertion in malignant obstructive jaundice. Lancet 2:57, 1987.

54. Dowsett JF, Vaira D, Hatfield ARW, et al. Endoscopic biliary therapy using the combined percutaneous and endoscopic technique. Gastroenterology 96:1180, 1989.

55. Hall RI, Denyer ME, Chapman AH. Percutaneous-endoscopic placement of endoprostheses for relief of jaundice caused by inoperable bile duct strictures. Surgery 107:224, 1990.

56. Kerlan RK, Ring EJ, Pogancy AC, Jeffrey RB. Biliary endoprosthesis insertion using a combined peroral method. Radiology 150:828, 1984.

57. Robertson DAF, Hacking CN, Birch S, Ayres R, Shepherd H, Wright R. Experience with a combined percutaneous and endoscopic approach to stent insertion in malignant obstructive jaundice. Lancet 2:1449, 1987.

7

Endoscopic Screening and Surveillance for Gastrointestinal Malignancy

William P. Reed and Frederick L. Greene

Each year, almost 250,000 people in the United States are diagnosed as having cancer of the digestive organs. Almost half will die of their disease, accounting for approximately 25% of all cancer deaths.[1] Because more than 80% of these tumors arise from mucosal surfaces that are within the optical range of modern endoscopic equipment, it is natural to ask whether periodic endoscopic evaluation of asymptomatic persons can promote earlier detection and treatment and improve long-term survival.

Supporting widespread screening are the demonstrated accuracy and therapeutic potential of endoscopy. Endoscopy has greater sensitivity in the detection of small mucosal lesions than barium contrast radiography or fecal occult blood testing.[2, 3] Endoscopic screening permits immediate biopsy or complete removal of suspicious-appearing lesions, unlike radiologic examination, which requires additional intervention for histologic confirmation.

Despite its advantages, endoscopy does not satisfy the criteria for a cost-effective screening test that can be applied to a target population, most of whose members are expected to be healthy. Because the equipment must be manipulated by a skilled physician, endoscopy is costly. The procedure produces significant discomfort and is associated with too high a rate of morbidity to be used routinely on healthy people.[4] If mass screening of asymptomatic groups or targeted surveillance of high-risk groups is to be justified, physicians must identify groups whose risk of disease warrants the expense and morbidity of endoscopy (Table 7–1).[5]

UPPER GASTROINTESTINAL TRACT

Risk and Dectection of Malignancies

Twenty-four thousand cases of gastric cancer and fewer than 12,000 cases of esophageal cancer are expected in the United States in 1993.[1]

Table 7–1. PREMALIGNANT CONDITIONS OF THE STOMACH, COLON, AND RECTUM USED AS THE BASES OF SCREENING PROGRAMS

Premalignant Conditions	Percent of Patients
Stomach	
Severe atrophic gastritis	5–10 (?)
Pernicious anemia	2
Gastric adenomas	0.5
Gastric stump	1–3
Hereditary carcinoma (diffuse type)	1–2
Total	10–15
Colon and rectum	
Previous colorectal carcinoma treated	5
Previous colorectal adenoma(s) treated	2–5
Cancer family syndrome	5–10
Familial adenomatous polyposis	0.5
Ulcerative colitis	1–2
Juvenile polyposis	0.1
Peutz-Jeghers syndrome	0.1
Ureterosigmoidostomy	0.1
Total	10–20

(From Jarvinen HJ. Premalignant conditions of the gastrointestinal tract: a basis for selective screening programs. Ann Med 21:285–286, 1989.)

There will be only 3400 cancers involving the small bowel. Although current methods of detection allow early resection and cure of relatively few patients, the overall number of Americans who die of these diseases each year is small. Increments in survival attributed to improved methods of early detection are also likely to be small and difficult to document.

Mass Screening of Asymptomatic Patients

The cumulative lifetime risk of developing cancer in the upper gastrointestinal tract is less than 1% for Americans.[6] For more than 99% of the population, there is no benefit to offset the risk, discomfort, and cost of periodic endoscopic inspection of the upper gastrointestinal mucosa. The most common malignancies of this region, those of the esophagus and stomach, do not usually develop from defined premalignant lesions that can be removed endoscopically, as is the case with many colorectal cancers. The growth rate of these tumors, which is rapid compared with that of other gastrointestinal cancers, makes it more likely that these lesions will appear in the interval between examinations.[7] For these reasons, mass endoscopic screening of asymptomatic people for early detection of cancers of the upper gastrointestinal tract is not warranted in the United States.

Surveillance of High-Risk Groups

Groups with premalignant conditions of the gastrointestinal mucosa and those at high risk for developing cancer in this region offer favorable targets for screening endoscopy. These patients are identified because of symptoms that draw attention to the upper gastrointestinal tract. The discomfort and cost of endoscopy become more acceptable, because the complaints lend themselves to endoscopic evaluation and possible treatment, even if malignancy is not found. Unfortunately, identifying a risk factor does not provide a clear indication for further treatment. Most tumors of the esophagus and stomach do not develop from polyps, which can be removed; they develop in areas of dysplasia that may regress or progress. If esophagectomy or gastrectomy is needed to remove the abnormal mucosa, most surgeons require assurance that the changes are progressing in the direction of malignancy before proceeding. Certainty necessitates repeated examinations over many months or years, always with the risk that a given lesion could progress beyond the limits of curative resection in the interval between examinations.

Most data on the value of endoscopic surveillance for high-risk conditions of the stomach and esophagus come from small, retrospective reports rather than from long-term, population-based, prospective studies. The applicability of these data to clinical practice is open to question, especially because different studies give conflicting results. To clarify matters, the American Society for Gastrointestinal Endoscopy (ASGE) developed guidelines in 1986 for endoscopic surveillance in the more commonly encountered premalignant conditions of the upper gastrointestinal tract, recommending surveillance for achalasia and columnar epithelium-lined esophagus (i.e., Barrett's esophagus) but not for pernicious anemia or for patients with prior gastric resection for benign disease.[8] Although based on the best available data, these recommendations may need modification as the results of other studies become published.

Esophageal Conditions

Achalasia. Achalasia is a disease brought on by a disturbance in esophageal motility. Absent peristalsis in the body of the esophagus and failure of the lower sphincter to relax in response to swallowing leads to progressive stasis of food within the organ and dilation. Squamous cancer develops in 1.7% to 8.2% of patients with untreated achalasia after an average of 17 to 28 years from the onset of symptoms.[6, 8–10] This represents a risk that is approximately seven times that of the general population.

Treatment of achalasia is directed toward relieving the distal obstruction through balloon dilation of the sphincter or esophagomyotomy. Effective early treatment appears to restore the risk of esophageal cancer in these patients to that of the general population.[10] The ASGE consensus group recommends endoscopic surveillance after successful treatment of achalasia only for patients whose treatment came late in the course of the disease, usually after 15 years of symptoms.[8]

Because the treatment for achalasia disrupts the lower esophageal sphincter, gastric contents may reflux after successful myotomy, leading to another premalignant lesion of the esophagus, Barrett's esophagus, in which columnar epithelium replaces the normal squamous mucosa.[11, 12] The true incidence of this complication is unknown but was reported as 4.3% for a series of 70 patients with achalasia who were treated with esophagomyotomy and concomitant antireflux procedure.[12] One of the patients in this series also had carcinoma in situ, and invasive adenocarcinoma has been reported in this setting in at least one patient.[13] Fortunately, the patients with these esophageal changes had symptoms of heartburn to aid the identification. Until more data are available, we recommend yearly surveillance of any patient remaining symptomatic or developing symptoms of reflux after effective treatment of achalasia.

Barrett's Esophagus. Barrett's esophagus (*i.e.,* columnar epithelium-lined esophagus) is an acquired condition that results from chronic injury to the lining mucosa of the esophagus through exposure to gastric acid (Fig. 7–1). The stratified squamous epithelium normally present above the gastroesophageal junction is replaced in various degrees by columnar epithelium. That these changes are secondary to reflux esophagitis is supported by the observation that metaplasia is only observed in the presence of gastroesophageal reflux.[14] The severity of esophagitis producing Barrett's metaplasia may be caused by the reflux of bile and pancreatic enzymes in addition to gastric acid, as has been demonstrated in a significantly higher proportion of these patients by esophageal and gastric pH monitoring and by hepatobiliary scan.[15, 16] Barrett's mucosa can also develop after surgical procedures that disrupt the integrity of the gastroesophageal sphincter. Retrospective studies indicate that metaplastic mucosa occurs in 10% to 12% of patients with chronic gastroesophageal reflux, but the prevalence of this disorder is increasing as more experience is gained with endoscopic diagnosis, indicating that earlier estimates could be low.[6, 9, 17]

Columnar epithelium within the esophagus does not produce symptoms, although symptoms of the inciting reflux affect most patients.

The major clinical significance of the condition is the predisposition of this epithelium to develop into adenocarcinomas in 8% to 10% of patients.[8, 17, 18] Correction of the gastroesophageal reflux seldom causes the columnar epithelium to regress, nor does it reduce the risk of cancer.[8, 19] The mechanism of cancer induction is not completely understood, but it may be related to the suppression of interleukin-2 production with subsequent T- and B-lymphocyte dysfunction that is demonstrated in these patients.[20] Bile acids modulate lymphocyte function in the colon and may contribute to tumor induction in that site.[21] It is possible that similar effects occur when bile repeatedly contacts the distal esophageal mucosa. Squamous carcinoma associated with Barrett's esophagus is unusual, but it can occur, most often in patients with concomitant risk factors, such as tobacco and alcohol abuse.[22]

There is evidence that progression to adenocarcinoma occurs in areas of columnar epithelium that have first developed dysplasia.[23–26] This provides a rationale for employing endoscopic evaluation and biopsy for routine surveillance in patients with Barrett's esophagus. Long-term survival rates of resected patients whose carcinomas were detected by endoscopic surveillance of Barrett's mucosa were twice as high as those of patients who developed adenocarcinoma without Barrett's esophagus or surveillance in one small series.[27] More experience is needed to confirm these results.

There is agreement that patients with adenocarcinoma within the region lined by columnar epithelium should undergo esophagectomy. Whether esophagectomy should be offered to patients with dysplasia alone and, if so, at what degree of dysplasia is controversial.[27, 28] Esophagogastrectomy is associated with such high morbidity and mortality rates that it is inappropriate as prophylaxis for a condition that could regress after further follow-up.[29, 30] However, there is considerable sampling error involved in detecting malignant change by biopsy. Depending on the extent of Barrett's change, four-quadrant biopsies are made every 1 cm from 0 to 6 cm above the gastroesophageal junction and then every 2 cm to the squamocolumnar junction. This technique leaves large areas of the surface mucosa untouched. Brush cytology allows surface sampling of a wider area of abnormal mucosa, but without visible changes to identify early carcinoma, cancers next to areas of dysplasia can be missed.[31] There is no vital dye that can outline areas of dysplasia within Barrett's mucosa the way Lugol's solution can for squamous cancers of the esophagus.[32] In

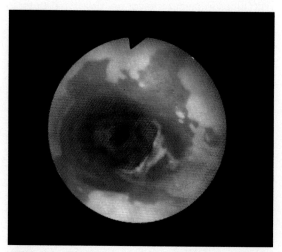

Figure 7–1. Endoscopic appearance of Barrett's changes in the distal esophagus. The biopsy demonstrated adenocarcinoma.

the future, flow cytometric analysis of the DNA content of esophageal biopsies may be able to identify tissue likely to progress to dysplasia and carcinoma. Dysplasia can be found in 44% of patients with aneuploidy.[33]

Although most investigators agree with the recommendations of the ASGE for periodic endoscopic surveillance of patients with Barrett's mucosa, the frequency of examination recommended varies from twice yearly to once every 2 years.[8, 34] Because men account for a disporportionate number of esophageal adenocarcinomas and as many as 94% of the adenocarcinomas that develop in Barrett's mucosa, we recommend annual surveillance for men and biennial surveillance for women.[35, 36] If there is evidence of dysplasia, the interval between examinations should be shortened to 6 months. If severe dysplasia (i.e., carcinoma in situ) is detected, resection of the segment of esophagus containing the abnormal mucosa should be strongly considered if the patient can tolerate the procedure.

Celiac Disease. Celiac disease (i.e., nontropical sprue, gluten-sensitive enteropathy) is a malabsorptive disorder brought on by exposure to gluten-containing foods. Histologically, it is characterized by flattenning of the intestinal mucosa and infiltration by chronic inflammatory cells, particularly in the jejunum. These changes and the malabsorption can be reversed by gluten withdrawal. The condition may be familial, with as many as 10% of first-degree relatives affected.[9]

Malignancies occur in as many as 14% of patients with celiac disease.[37] Half of these malignancies are lymphomas of the gastrointestinal tract, most commonly of the jejunum. Lymphomas develop with equal frequency in patients who have shown complete resolution of the celiac disease after treatment and in those who have not.

Gastric cancers are no more frequent than expected in celiac disease, but adenocarcinomas of the small intestine and squamous carcinoma of the esophagus are seen at 32 and 5 times their expected rates, respectively.[38] It is thought that nutritional deficiency may play a role in the development of esophageal carcinoma, but the precise mechanism for development of these tumors is poorly understood, as is the relation of risk to gluten ingestion.

No specific recommendations for endoscopic surveillance can be made, because many of the malignancies associated with celiac disease are not in endoscopic viewing range. Any patient with symptoms suggesting malignancy should promptly undergo appropriate evaluation.

Index Cancers of the Upper Aerodigestive Tract. Cancers of the upper aerodigestive tract are usually associated with alcohol and tobacco abuse. Because these agents affect multiple sites in the head and neck region, it is not surprising that 8% to 16% of patients with squamous cell cancer of the head or neck have synchronous second primary tumors of the upper aerodigestive tract.[39] Most of these develop in another head or neck site, but 0.6% to 5.1% are in the esophagus.[33, 39–43] This has prompted the recommendation that routine esophagoscopy be included in the evaluation of patients with head and neck cancers, although there are no prospective trials showing a survival benefit from this approach.[40, 41, 43]

Some researchers question the need for esophagoscopy in the absence of an abnormal barium swallow.[39, 42, 44] The yield under these circumstances is low, and the chance that patients identified with synchronous esophageal cancers can survive resection appears to be negligible. However, an interesting study using Lugol's solution to enhance the endoscopic detection of early esophageal cancers yielded nine (5.1%) asymptomatic esophageal cancers in 198 patients with head and neck cancers.[33] Seven (78%) of these cancers had early-stage disease that was amenable to resection. If confirmed by others, these results could add weight to the argument in favor of routine esophagoscopy in this group of patients.

For patients with previous resection of an esophageal cancer, the value of periodic surveillance endoscopy is not established.[6] A patient with esophageal recurrence after resection for esophageal cancer is unlikely to benefit from further therapy. Nevertheless, patients with early esophageal squamous cell cancers whose anticipated prognosis is good should be monitored for other primary tumors of the aerodigestive tract by periodic chest radiographs and head and neck examinations to preclude shortening their survival by overlooking metachronous lesions in these sites.

Lye Corrosion. Squamous cell carcinoma of the esophagus can develop in areas of stricture produced by lye corrosion. This usually develops years after the injury; the shortest interval reported was 13 years.[45] The most common site is at the level of the tracheal bifurcation, where the injury and subsequent stricture are most severe.[45, 46] The incidence ranges from 0.8% to 5.5%.[9, 47] Because these tumors may have a high rate of resectability and survival (i.e., 83% and 33%, respectively, at 5 years in one large study), periodic surveillance seems justified, although probably not until 15 to 20 years after the injury.[45]

Scleroderma. There is no evidence that patients with scleroderma are at increased risk for esophageal carcinoma.[48] Scleroderma does produce smooth muscle atrophy and esophageal fibrosis, which may lead to gastroesophageal reflux with secondary Barrett's esophagus.[49, 50] Esophageal carcinoma has been reported in patients with chronic reflux esophagitis complicating scleroderma, probably as a consequence of the mucosal metaplasia.[50] Routine endoscopic surveillance is not justified for patients with uncomplicated scleroderma but should be strongly considered after reflux develops. Any patient with scleroderma who develops dysphagia or symptoms of reflux should undergo prompt endoscopic examination to determine if Barrett's mucosa, dysplasia, or neoplasia has occurred.

Tylosis. Family clusters of esophageal cancer may occur in areas of the world where this tumor is endemic. This probably represents a commonly shared dietary deficiency rather than a genetic predisposition.[51] Similar deficiencies (*e.g.*, Plummer-Vinson syndrome) may have played a role in the development of the esophageal cancers in Scandinavian women seen earlier in this century.[9, 52, 53]

Other than celiac disease, the only recognized familial cause of esophageal cancer in the United States is the rare autosomal dominant dyskeratosis called tylosis.[51, 52] Tylosis is characterized by keratosis of the palms and soles and an increased risk of esophageal cancer that may reach as high as 95%.[9] Any patient identified with this disorder should have yearly endoscopic surveillance.

Gastric Conditions

Chronic Atrophic Gastritis. Chronic atrophic gastritis was classified as two types by Strickland and Mackay.[54] Type A atrophic gastritis, which may be autoimmune in origin, shows diffuse gastric involvement with antral sparing, impairment of acid secretion, and antibodies to parietal cells (PCA).[55] Pernicious anemia is associated with this type of atrophic gastritis, but carcinoma is unusual.[56] Type B atrophic gastritis, which is more common than type A and may be related to environmental factors, is associated with antral involvement and focal changes within the gastric body. The test for PCA is negative, and there is only moderate impairment of gastric function.

Intestinal metaplasia occurring with type B atrophic gastritis may progress through dysplasia to carcinoma in 5% to 10% of patients.[57, 58] *Helicobacter pylori* infection may promote this form of gastritis and subsequent cancer.[59–62] Yearly endoscopic surveillance seems reasonable for patients with this type of gastritis, with shortened intervals between examinations after dysplasia develops. Unfortunately, type B atrophic gastritis is often an asymptomatic finding that is unlikely to be detected without mass screening. *Helicobacter pylori* infection, which has been proposed by some as an indication for endoscopic surveillance, progresses to carcinoma in few patients.[62, 63]

Patients with type A gastritis or pernicious anemia probably do not need surveillance in accordance with the guidelines established by ASGE, because carcinoma develops in no more than 2% of patients during 5 years.[8, 64]

Familial Polyposis. Familial polyposis coli and Gardner's syndrome are associated with gastric and duodenal polyps and the premalignant adenomatous polyps of the lower gastrointestinal tract.[65] Gastric polyps can be adenomatous or hyperplastic and occur in 39% to 100% of patients with these conditions.[66, 67] Nevertheless, very few gastric cancers develop in these patients (*e.g.*, approximately 0.5% in one series of 1255 patients).[68] Duodenal polyps, which occur in 46% to 93% of patients with these disorders, are usually adenomatous and more frequently lead to carcinoma (*i.e.*, 4.0% of the same series).[66, 69] Periodic upper gastrointestinal endoscopy with removal of gastric and duodenal polyps has been recommended as a means of early detection or prevention of gastric, duodenal, and periampullary cancers in these patients. This seems to be a reasonable approach, because the prognosis for these tumors is poor after symptoms develop.[69] However, there are few data to support the efficacy of surveillance in reducing the mortality from upper gastrointestinal malignancies in patients with familial adenomatous polyposis.

Gastric Polyps. Gastric mucosal polyps are uncommon and usually asymptomatic.[6, 8] They are most often discovered as incidental findings during radiographic or endoscopic evaluation of some other condition, but larger polyps may cause obstruction or bleeding. Approximately 25% of gastric polyps are adenomatous, and the remainder are hyperplastic.[70, 71] Adenomatous polyps are neoplastic and carry a recognized risk of malignancy related to size. Hyperplastic polyps are regenerative and have only a 0% to 2% potential for malignant change.[72, 73] Hyperplastic polyps have been associated with carcinomas elsewhere in the stomach in 4% to 28% of patients.[70, 71] The significance of this association is uncertain, because the figures come from retrospective analysis of surgical specimens and autopsy material in which the hyperplastic polyps were often incidental to the gastric cancer that led to the procedure. Whether hyperplastic polyps can predict which patients are at risk for later development of gastric cancer is unclear from these studies.

The ASGE panel recommends biopsy of all gastric polyps, with removal of pedunculated polyps and those causing obstruction or bleeding.[8] If biopsy shows a sessile polyp to be hyperplastic, excision and surveillance are not recommended. Polypectomy and surveillance are recommended for adenomatous polyps. This approach may require partial gastrectomy if the polyps are multiple, sessile, and larger than 2 cm. We agree with these guidelines and recommend yearly endoscopic surveillance after excision of adenomatous polyps, at least until no additional polyps are found by consecutive yearly examinations.

Gastric Resection. Gastric carcinoma has been reported in 2% to 8.7% of patients who have undergone gastric resection for benign ulcer disease after an average interval of 15 to 28 years.[6, 8, 74–79] This represents an increase over the expected lifetime risk for spontaneous gastric cancer in the United States of 1% to 1.7%.[6, 78] Gastric carcinoma has developed after both Billroth I and Billroth II reconstructions, although the incidence is probably higher after gastrojejunostomy.[77–80] Most postgastrectomy tumors are adenocarcinomas, but squamous cell cancer has also been observed.[81] Although carcinoma of the gastric remnant usually carries a poor prognosis, a high percentage of early treatable cancers has been reported by physicians employing regular endoscopic surveillance with multiple biopsies (Fig. 7–2).[82]

The ASGE panel does not recommend endoscopic surveillance for postgastrectomy patients, citing evidence from a large population-based study that showed no greater risk of gastric cancer death after gastrectomy for peptic ulcer disease than in the general population.[8] Because the general population in this study was from Scotland, where the death rate from gastric cancer is three times that in the United States, the study may confirm that postgastrectomy patients are at increased risk of developing gastric cancer.[83] By averaging risk over time, this study and a similar one from Minnesota may allow an early reduction in risk to mask a later increase.[84] When relative risk for gastric cancer is determined by five yearly intervals after gastrectomy, an initial reduction in risk is replaced by an increase after 15 to 25 years.[79, 85] We think that gastroscopy with random biopsies should be performed in asymptomatic patients beginning 15 years after gastrectomy, especially if gastrojejunostomy was performed. If dysplasia is identified on biopsy, yearly surveillance should be employed. If no dysplasia is encountered, yearly surveillance is probably not warranted.

Conditions of the Small Intestine

The small intestine is the least common site for gastrointestinal malignancies, accounting for only 3400 new cases and 950 deaths each year.[1] This low incidence and the relative inaccessibility of the jejunum and ileum to intubation have limited the role of endoscopy in evaluating tumors of the small bowel.

Newer techniques, such as push jejunoscopy, may succeed in forcing the endoscope up to 50 cm beyond the ligament of Treitz.[86] Regular intubation of the entire jejunum and ileum require longer endoscopes equipped with sheaths to prevent coiling within the stomach. One such instrument was reported to have reached a point 150 cm beyond the ligament of Treitz, but documentation was by x-ray measurement alone.[87] Even if equipment allowed easy endoscopic evaluation of the entire length of small intestine, there would be few conditions that would warrant such an examination for tumor surveillance. Other than familial polyposes, the only identified high-risk groups for malignant tumors of the small bowel are patients with the inherited autosomal dominant conditions of neurofibromatosis or Peutz-Jeghers syndrome.

Neurofibromatosis occurs in 1 of every 3000 live births, but only 11% of patients with this disease have gastrointestinal involvement, most commonly in the jejunum.[88] Most of these gastrointestinal tumors are benign neurofibromas, but as many as 15% can be malignant.[89] Because these lesions develop on the serosal surface of

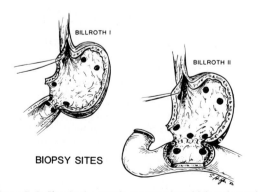

Figure 7–2. Sites in the gastric remnant for which endoscopic biopsy is recommended to identify early cancer.

the bowel and the mucosa is involved only as the enlarging mass pushes into it, endoscopic evaluation cannot detect early tumors in this disease.[90]

Peutz-Jeghers syndrome is a disease manifested by mucocutaneous pigmentation and gastrointestinal polyposis. Early in the course of the disease, complications arise from intussusception, bleeding, or obstruction from one or more of the large number of gastrointestinal hamartomas. After the age of 30, these hamartomas may undergo malignant degeneration. In one series of 72 patients, the chance of dying of cancer by the age of 57 was 48%.[91] Some physicians recommend removing as many polyps as possible by intraoperative enteroscopy when a patient with Peutz-Jeghers syndrome is explored for a complication of the disease.[92] Therapy can conceivably be carried out nonoperatively after endoscopes of sufficient length and maneuverability are available for total enteroscopy.

LOWER GASTROINTESTINAL TRACT

Risk and Detection of Malignancies

Cancers of the lower gastrointestinal tract are more suitable for screening than those of the upper gastrointestinal tract because they are more common and because they arise in preexisting lesions that can be removed before malignant transformation occurs. The relatively slower growth rate of these tumors permits longer intervals between examinations with less risk of interval tumor appearance or progression.

There were approximately 152,000 new cases of colorectal cancer in the United States in 1993, making this the third most common malignancy, after lung cancer and prostate cancer, in men and the second most common, after breast cancer, in women.[1, 93, 94] The overall survival from this disease is low, in large part because of the advanced stage at presentation.[94–96] More than 50% of patients have lymph node involvement or distant metastases, with 5-year survival rates of 46% and 5.4%, respectively, if symptoms develop before diagnosis.[97–99] If the tumor is confined to the bowel wall, as may be the case in as many as 90% of cancers detected by screening, the survival rates exceed 80% at 5 years.[99–101] Screening has the potential to improve survival by detecting tumors at an earlier, more treatable stage. Screening may also reduce

the incidence of cancer by allowing precancerous polyps to be removed before malignant transformation occurs. This has been suggested by studies of large numbers of patients for whom the incidence of invasive cancer has been lower than expected in the years after endoscopic removal of polyps.[102, 103]

Because most people screened never develop colorectal cancer, the tests employed should be simple, acceptable to patient and physician, safe, and reasonably accurate in predicting malignancy.[100, 101, 104] The group examined must also have a sufficiently high risk of disease that the small proportion of false-positive results inherent in most screening tests does not result in large numbers of additional examinations in normal people.[104–106] The risk for colorectal cancer is related to personal history, family history, and age, with the risk rising most sharply at age 50 (Table 7–2).[3, 93–95, 100, 105, 106] People younger than 50 years of age and lacking a family or personal history of cancer are considered to be at low risk of developing cancer. There is agreement that people in this risk category do not require screening. There is also agreement that people with personal risk factors, such as inflammatory bowel disease or familial conditions, such as familial polyposis, deserve some degree of endoscopic surveillance. Controversy exists about the appropriateness of screening people at average risk, those who are older than 50 years of age but asymptomatic and lacking a personal or family history associated with colorectal cancer.

In considering recommendations for early detection in people at average risk, some investi-

Table 7–2. RISK STATUS FOR COLORECTAL CANCER

Risk Status	Characteristics
Low risk	Age <50 years and no family history of early onset colorectal cancer or personal history of disease listed for high risk
Average risk	Age >50 years and asymptomatic
High risk	Personal history of adenoma or cancer in large bowel, inflammatory bowel disease, breast, ovarian, or endometrial cancer, radiation therapy
	Family history of sporadic colorectal cancer or adenoma, familial adenomatous polyposis, hereditary nonpolyposis, colorectal cancer syndromes, Gardner's, Turcot's, and Oldfield's syndromes

(From Young GP, Demediuk BH. The genetics, epidemiology, and early detection of gastrointestinal cancers. Curr Opin Oncol 4:728–735, 1992.)

gators differentiate between the clinical settings of screening and case finding.[100, 105, 106] Evidence of efficacy should be stronger before recommending a test for use in the general population (*i.e.*, screening) than is needed to recommend the same test for a patient seeking comprehensive medical evaluation from a physician (*i.e.*, case finding). The physician is better able to evaluate other evidence about the patient's health in the context of a complete examination, and the two-tier standard avoids the ethical issue of convincing large numbers of people who are otherwise well to undergo potentially harmful testing with little chance of benefit.

Mass Screening of Average-Risk Patients

The current recommendations of the American Cancer Society are for men and women older than 40 years of age to receive yearly digital rectal examinations and for people older than 50 years of age to undergo yearly fecal occult blood testing (FOBT) and a sigmoidoscopy every 3 to 5 years.[107] Only FOBT has been proven efficacious by a controlled clinical trial.[100] The other recommended screening techniques are unproven and may be based on theories of the distribution of colorectal cancer that are now considered out of date.

Fifty years ago, 50% of all colorectal cancers were within reach of the examining finger, and 67% were within the range of the rigid sigmoidoscope.[101, 108] Since that time, the distribution of colorectal cancers and polyps has shifted to the right side.[101, 109–111] The reasons for this are not clear but may reflect an aging population, because right-sided lesions appear later, or a greater diagnostic acumen in the detection of right-sided tumors. Whatever the reason, even flexible sigmoidoscopy to 60 cm can now detect only 55% of tumors.[6, 100, 101, 109–114]

Digital rectal examination, which has the advantages of simplicity, safety, and relative acceptability, is unlikely to detect more than 10% of all colorectal cancers.[100, 112] Rigid sigmoidoscopy can detect only 20% to 30% of tumors.[100, 101] Similarly, stool guaiac testing may fail to react in 35% to 50% of patients with colorectal cancers detected by other means.[99, 100, 112, 114, 115] By following the ACS recommendations, as many as 35% of patients with colorectal cancer may have their tumors missed, with most of the undetected tumors beyond the range of the sigmoidoscope. However, as a starting point, simple screening tests that detect as many as 65% of colorectal cancers early may be sufficient

to reduce the current death rate from this disease.

To determine if screening tests result in survival differences between patients randomly assigned to undergo screening or observation alone, prospective clinical trials are needed. There are five such trials underway, with more than 300,000 people enrolled, to examine the effectiveness of FOBT as a screening test for colorectal cancer in asymptomatic, average-risk men and women.[95, 100, 106, 116–122] The rate of positive test results has ranged from 1% to 2.4% in these studies, with adenomas or carcinomas detected in 24% to 58% of positive patients by means of further evaluation by colonoscopy or barium enema.[95, 100, 106] The carcinomas detected in this manner have been of an earlier stage than those that were eventually found in the control population. Dukes' stage A tumors accounted for 34% to 65% of cancers in the study population but for only 8% to 24% in the control group. The earlier stage of tumors detected by screening should result in a better outcome for the study population, but a survival advantage has so far been reported only for the smallest of the trials. In this study, a 43% reduction in mortality has been observed for the screened population after 10 years of follow-up.[100, 121] Another of the trials has shown a trend toward improved survival, which has yet to become statistically significant.[121] If this survival advantage is maintained and confirmed by the remaining three trials, the efficacy of FOBT screening as a means of reducing the mortality from colorectal cancer will be established. Until then, it can be argued that screening selectively detects the slowly growing tumors and that aggressive cancers appear in the intervals between screening sessions. Under such circumstances, early detection would not necessarily lead to improved survival (*i.e.*, length time bias). Earlier detection could also produce apparent improvements in survival by moving forward the date of diagnosis rather than altering the date of death (*i.e.*, lead time bias), although this would be unlikely in the case of colorectal cancer, for which the association of stage at diagnosis with prognosis is well established.[114]

Other studies of FOBT as a screening test have been largely descriptive in nature, showing an improvement in stage at diagnosis as evidence for the effectiveness of the test.[114, 123–126] The same flaws of length time and lead time bias affect the interpretation of these studies, but no concurrent control group is available to demonstrate an eventual survival advantage for the patients screened. Useful information can still be derived from these descriptive studies, such as the likely yield of polyps and cancers in a given population.[123–126] Gilbertson was able to use a descriptive study to demonstrate that the incidence of lower bowel cancer could be reduced to 15% of its predicted value in a study population after identification and removal of asymptomatic adenomatous polyps.[102, 103] In this case, a separate control group was not needed because the age-related incidence of colorectal cancer had already been established.

Trials of endoscopic screening have been less common and have usually involved relatively few patients.[127–131] This may reflect the difficulty in getting patients and physicians to invest the effort required for this type of screening when symptoms are lacking. Only one prospective clinical trial using the rigid sigmoidoscope to examine 20 cm of the colon and rectum has been reported. This study, which involved more than 10,000 persons, reported a twofold survival advantage for the screened population (2.3 vs. 5.2 deaths per 1000).[128] This advantage may have been due more to the counseling received by the study group than to the examination itself. The study design did not randomize patients to undergo sigmoidoscopic examination but rather to receive strong advice to do so. Patients were free to request this examination, even if they were in the control group. As a result, almost equal numbers of the study and control patients underwent sigmoidoscopy (30% and 25%, respectively), and most tumors in the two groups were discovered only after symptoms developed.[129] It is possible that the improved survival reflected a better understanding of the significance of symptoms by the study population after the counseling received.

Without data from clinical trials, case-control studies may offer an alternative method of documenting the effectiveness of endoscopic screening. In this type of study, previous exposure to the screening test is compared between patients who died of the cancer and the general population. A lower frequency of screening in the patients with fatal tumors provides evidence that the screening test has a protective effect against the disease. This effect was confirmed in a study of 261 patients from the Kaiser Permanente Medical Care Program who died of cancer of the distal colon and rectum between 1971 and 1988.[132] All had tumors that were within range of the rigid sigmoidoscope, but only 8.8% had undergone screening sigmoidoscopy. This contrasts with the 24% of 868 controls who were matched for age and sex, yielding an odds ratio of 0.30 for cases compared with controls. The protective effect was just as strong among patients whose last sigmoidoscopy was 9 to 10 years earlier. The results suggest that screening sigmoidoscopy can reduce the number of deaths due to cancers of the distal colon and rectum. They also suggest that examinations as infrequent as once in 10 years may be adequate.

The same study from Kaiser Permanente looked at patients dying of colon cancers above the level that could be reached by the rigid sigmoidoscope. For tumors at this level, there was no evidence that screening sigmoidoscopy offered any protection. This illustrates the concern that limiting endoscopic screening to the distal 20 cm of the gastrointestinal tract may not detect most colon cancers. The availability of 35- and 60-cm flexible sigmoidoscopes has extended the range of surveillance and improved the diagnostic yield of lesions 2.1- to 10-fold, with only minor increases in examination times and cost and no increase in morbidity or patient discomfort.[101, 133–135] Most of the additional lesions discovered are 21 to 35 cm above the level of the anus.[101, 106, 130] This means that the 35-cm scope may be the ideal instrument for screening. It has the advantage of being more acceptable to physicians and patients because it is easier to use and more comfortable than the rigid or the 60-cm flexible sigmoidoscope.[136, 137]

There has been little enthusiasm for using longer instruments for mass screening, because of the cost and physician time required.[6] Nevertheless, some physicians feel that the risk of right-sided lesions, especially after the age of 60, does justify routine colonoscopy for screening.[3, 138] Although colonoscopy can detect 94% to 97% of these neoplasms, barium enema may miss as many as one third.[2, 139–141] Conventional sonography is even less sensitive than contrast radiography, but hydrocolonic sonography, a technique that employs intraluminal water as a transmission medium to outline mucosal lesions, approaches the accuracy of colonoscopy in detecting colon cancers and polyps.[142] In a series of 300 symptomatic patients, ultrasonic examination that was carried out after relaxation of the colon with scopolamine-N-butylbromide and instillation of up to 1500 mL of water was able to identify 28 (97%) of the 29 cancers and 38 (91%) of the 41 polyps that were 7 mm or larger in diameter. Patient tolerance of the procedure, which took 15 minutes to complete, was good enough to consider this technique as a possible alternative to colonoscopy in asymptomatic patients. Lesions identified by hydrocolonic sonography still require endoscopic evaluation for removal and histologic characterization.

Because of the variety of screening tests available, the assessment of which combination and frequency of tests should have the greatest impact on survival at the least cost becomes a monumental task that is not suited to evaluation through prospective, randomized clinical trials. This has led to interest in mathematical models to identify the most favorable screening strategy. Modeling demonstrated that average-risk patients receive the greatest benefit at the least cost with annual FOBT and flexible sigmoidoscopy every 3 to 5 years.[112, 113, 143] Beginning this program at 50 years of age instead of 40 reduces costs by half with negligible effects on outcome. For patients with higher risks because of histories of colorectal cancer in first-degree relatives, complete colon evaluation with air-contrast barium enema every 3 to 5 years should be considered in place of sigmoidoscopy. Retaining flexible sigmoidoscopy in this schedule of evaluation improves effectiveness by another 11% to 13%. Colonoscopy can be substituted for the barium enema if cost is not a concern, eliminating the need for sigmoidoscopy to evaluate the lower colon and rectum.

If thorough colonic evaluation fails to reveal a source for the positive FOBT, it is probably unnecessary to examine the upper gastrointestinal tract unless there are symptoms. Gastric cancer developed in only 1 of 269 asymtomatic people who were followed for 2 to 8 years (median, 5 years) after an examination of the colon failed to identify a source for the occult fecal blood.[144] The patient who developed gastric cancer was not actually asymptomatic but had persistent dyspepsia 15 years after gastric resection for peptic ulcer disease. This patient had indications for gastroscopy quite independent of the FOBT results.

In our view, the data in favor of FOBT and flexible sigmoidoscopic screening for patients older than 50 years of age who are at average risk for colorectal cancer are strong enough to recommend that this be offered to all patients who come in for regular evaluation (i.e., case finding basis). The 35-cm flexible sigmoidoscope is probably adequate as a screening tool, but physicians skilled with the 60-cm instrument may identify enough additional pathologic tissue to justify the minor increments in time and discomfort associated with its use. Screening colonoscopy is not justified for the average-risk patient at this time. Whether these tests should be employed in a nationwide screening effort depends on the sources of funding available. Funding will undoubtedly be easier to justify if the survival data from the completed trials continue to support the efficacy of screening.

For first-degree relatives of patients with colorectal cancer, several studies indicate a risk of developing carcinoma of the colon or rectum as much as threefold higher than the incidence in the general population.[145] Similarly, patients with breast cancer may have a 1.2- to 1.6-fold increase in the expected risk of developing colorectal cancer.[146] Although these groups may be at high risk relative to the general population, the degree of increase does not justify major additions to the screening strategy already outlined. Nevertheless, substitution of colonoscopy or air-contrast barium enema every 3 to 5 years in place of flexible sigmoidoscopy seems warranted based on the predictions of mathematical modeling. This approach is especially recommended for first-degree relatives of patients with colorectal cancer because of the reported tendency of neoplastic polyps and cancers to develop beyond the 55-cm reach of the flexible sigmoidoscope.[145, 147–149]

Surveillance of High-Risk Groups
Index Malignancies

Index Carcinomas. The incidence of synchronous carcinomas of the colorectum is in the range of 2% to 10%.[110, 111, 150–161] Between 25% and 40% of patients with colorectal cancer have synchronous adenomas.[111, 150–156] After a cancer is discovered, the entire mucosal surface of the large bowel should be evaluated by colonoscopy.

Colonoscopy should probably be carried out before resection, unless obstruction by tumor limits intubation. Preoperative endoscopy provides the surgeon with an opportunity to alter the extent of surgical resection at the original procedure to include additional tumors not readily apparent on intraoperative palpation.[111, 154–156] This approach can reduce the likelihood that the patient will have an early recurrence because of missed lesions or require additional abdominal procedures. Some physicians have contended that preoperative endoscopy may spread cancer to more proximal sites, promoting local implantation or early distant spread.[152] Follow-up of patients evaluated by colonoscopy before resection has shown no evidence for increased rates of local or distant recurrence to substantiate such fears.[159]

If preoperative colonoscopy is not possible, the remaining colon should be evaluated by endoscopic means within 6 months of the operative procedure. Barium studies may miss as many as one third of synchronous cancers and two thirds of synchronous polyps.[110, 111, 159] Even if these lesions are identified by contrast studies, endoscopy may be necessary to provide histologic diagnosis of cancers or snare removal of polyps.

After all neoplastic lesions have been removed from the colon, patients need continued surveillance for metachronous lesions and anastomotic recurrences. Metachronous cancers develop in 0.8% to 4.6% of patients, and metachronous polyps occur in 21% to 54%, for a combined annual yield of 3 to 5 lesions per 100 patients.[160–166] Yearly endoscopic surveillance offers an ideal method of identifying and removing these lesions while they are early stage and curable, although biennial examination may be as effective. Most of these lesions occur during the first 4 to 5 years after resection of the original tumor.[166, 167] After that period, asymptomatic patients can probably be returned to yearly FOBT and endoscopic surveillance every 3 to 5 years, as recommended for patients at average risk. Periodic carcinoembryonic antigen (CEA) determination has been recommended as an additional method to identify patients in need of more intensive surveillance, but one analysis found the effect of CEA monitoring on survival to be negligible.[168–173]

Anastomotic recurrence may develop in 10% to 15% of patients after resection of a colorectal cancer, usually during the first 30 months postoperatively.[170–172, 174] When detected early by surveillance, recurrences can be resected for potential cure in 50% of patients, with 45% long-term disease-free survival.[174–176] When symptoms of pain, bleeding, or obstruction call attention to the recurrence, the chance of resection for cure is low.[166]

The portion of the lower gastrointestinal tract that is often overlooked in planning postoperative surveillance is the segment distal to a colostomy. Even when the original treatment plan calls for eventual closure of the stoma, years may pass with little further attention to the diverted segment as long as the patient is satisfied with the quality of life. Polyps and cancers may develop in the retained defunctionalized bowel, especially in patients whose original bowel resection was carried out to treat colorectal cancer.[177, 178] Inflammatory changes, probably caused by a nutritional deficiency, can occur, frequently without producing symptoms. Because these complications are amenable to treatment if detected in a timely manner, periodic surveillance of regions of colon or rectum that are not in continuity with the gastrointestinal tract for longer than 12 months is advisable. Experience with short-chain fatty acid irrigation suggests that the inflammatory changes can be reversed by supplying missing nutrients.[179]

Index Adenomas. Most carcinomas of the colon and rectum arise within preexisting adenomas.[180–184] Because the progression from adenoma to carcinoma can be interrupted by removing the neoplastic polyps before cells capable of invading the muscularis mucosae develop, endoscopic polypectomy holds promise as a measure that can reduce the incidence of colorectal cancer.[185] This potential has been demonstrated in at least one study in which removal of polyps lowered the incidence of subsequent carcinoma to 15% of the rate expected on the basis of historic controls.[102, 103]

Although the evidence that carcinomas arise in adenomas is strong, the evidence that polyps invariably progress to carcinoma is lacking. The fact that polyps are much more common than the incidence of carcinoma over a wide range of ages suggests that most polyps remain harmless over the life span of the affected persons.[186–188] Autopsy studies of asymptomatic patients show a prevalence of adenomas between 30% and 34% in 50- to 60-year-old patients, rising to 40% to 60% for those older than 70.[186, 189–192] The prevalence of cancer for these same age groups is 1.6% and 3%, respectively.[190, 192, 193] Even for polyps larger than 1 cm in diameter, in which high-grade dysplastic changes are most likely to occur, the cumulative risk of cancer developing at 5, 10, and 20 years is 2.5%, 8%, and 24%, respectively.[182, 194] At this rate of progression, a 75-year-old patient may not have a high enough prospect of benefit from the removal of smaller polyps to justify the risk, cost, and discomfort of endoscopic screening.

If a patient has one adenoma, there is a 2% to 4% chance that a synchronous cancer exists.[195–197] This prevalence is enough to justify total colonoscopy at the time the adenoma is discovered. Additional adenomas, which may be found in 60% of the patients, should be removed simultaneously.[195–199] After the colon has been cleared of lesions, a decision must be made whether follow-up evaluation is needed. The risk of additional adenomas and eventual carcinoma rises progressively to 60% and 7%, respectively, in patients with index adenomas after 15 years of follow-up, but not all types of polyps carry the same risk of later lesions.[200] To be most effective, colonoscopic surveillance must be tailored to suit the expected likelihood that a given patient will have recurrence. Objective data to help in formulating recommendations should become available after a multicenter, prospective trial of surveillance strategies after polypectomy, the National Polyp Study, is complete.[194, 197]

The main risk factor for subsequent adenomas after removal of neoplastic polyps is the multiplicity of lesions.[180, 196, 201–204] For patients with only one initial polyp, the risk of recurrence in

5 years is 28%. For those with more than four, the risk is 59%.[201] The risk of recurrence appears to be higher for men.[200, 205] High-grade dysplasia and associated carcinoma in a given polyp is related to the size of the polyp and to the degree of villous changes (Table 7–3).[194] Whether these changes also predict the likelihood that metachronous lesions will develop remains to be seen. Polyps that become large enough that they call attention to their presence tend to be of a higher grade and larger size than those discovered at autopsy.[194, 199] They also have a distribution that favors the left colon and rectum, with two thirds located beyond the splenic flexure. After the colon is cleared of neoplastic lesions, subsequent recurrences tend to mimic the histologic appearance and uniform geographic distribution typical of lesions observed as incidental autopsy findings.[185, 199, 207] After this status is achieved, an argument for returning to the level of surveillance recommended for patients at average risk for colon cancer can be made.

It seems reasonable to recommend that any patient with neoplastic polypoid lesions have them removed entirely at the time of first diagnosis. Early reevaluation, within 3 to 6 months, should be considered for any patient whose colon could still contain adenomas because of piecemeal removal or inadequate examination.[185, 198, 202, 206] After the colon is free of adenomas, patients with single, low-grade lesions can probably be adequately followed with yearly FOBT and flexible sigmoidoscopy every 3 years, as is recommended for average-risk patients. Consideration for colonoscopy in place of sigmoidoscopy to follow patients with dysplastic or large lesions of the colon proximal to the splenic flexure may appear reasonable, but there is no data to support this approach.[198, 202, 206, 208] Patients with multiple polyps found during the

initial assessment should be followed with yearly colonoscopy until only random tubular adenomas are encountered or until the patient is old enough (e.g., 75 to 80 years) that the likelihood of progression during the remaining life span of the patient is too small to justify the risk and expense of further endoscopic intervention.[186]

Hyperplastic polyps represent a regenerative rather than a neoplastic process. They do not have any malignant associations or potential.[199, 209] The suggestion that hyperplastic polyps in the rectosigmoid may serve as a marker for proximal adenomas has not been confirmed by studies using control patients without rectosigmoid abnormalities.[209–212] When patients with rectosigmoid hyperplastic polyps are compared with those with rectosigmoid adenomas and those without abnormalities, there is no difference in the prevalence of proximal adenomas between the patients with hyperplastic polyps and those with normal mucosa. In contrast, patients with distal adenomas were three times as likely to have proximal polyps as the control population. Surveillance of patients with hyperplastic polyps is inappropriate, and total colonoscopy on the basis of incidental hyperplastic polyps of the distal colon or rectum may be unwarranted.

Inflammatory Bowel Disease

Patients with long-standing ulcerative colitis have a well-recognized increase in the risk of developing colon cancer.[6, 95, 213–219] This risk varies according to the degree of colon involvement and the duration of illness. Only patients with symptoms of colitis for more than 8 years and whose disease extends proximal to the sigmoid colon, as determined by barium enema and endoscopy, are likely to develop cancer (Fig. 7–3).[6, 214–217, 220] The best estimate for this risk of developing colon cancer is 0.5% to 1.0% per year beginning 8 years after the onset of colitis, for a cummulative risk of 8% at 25 years.[215–217, 221] Patients with colitis limited to the left colon are only one fourth to one third as likely to develop cancer as those having pancolitis, primarily as a result of a prolongation of the cancer-free interval from 8 to 10 up to 15 to 20 years after the onset of symptoms.[215]

Cancers developing in the setting of long-standing colitis may be multiple or arise in areas of mucosa that lack polypoid changes to draw the attention of the examining physician. Endoscopic surveillance requires random histologic sampling of the entire length of affected colon. Typically, three to four biopsies are obtained for each 10 cm of colon.[223] The procedure is tedious and expensive, with no assurance that

Table 7–3. NATIONAL POLYP STUDY: ODDS RATIO FOR HIGH-GRADE DYSPLASIA IN ADENOMAS FOR COMBINED EFFECTS OF SIZE AND HISTOLOGY FROM THE LOGISTIC MODEL

Histology	Small (<0.5 cm)	Medium (0.6–1.0 cm)	Large (>1.0 cm)
Tubular	1.0	3.3	7.7
Villous A	2.7	9.0	21.0
Villous B	3.4	11.3	26.1
Villous C and D	8.1	27.1	62.7

(From O'Brien MJ, Winawer SJ, Zauber AG, et al. The National Polyp Study: patient and polyp characteristics associated with high-grade dysplasia in colorectal adenomas. Gastroenterology 98:371–379, 1990.)

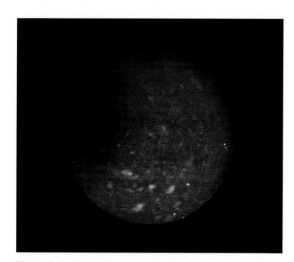

Figure 7–3. Sigmoidoscopic appearance of active ulcerative colitis, showing granular appearance with surface exudate.

an area of malignant change will not be missed. Pathologists frequently disagree in their assessments of dysplasia.[224] These drawbacks have encouraged some surgeons to propose prophylactic colectomy for all patients whose disease began before the age of 40, reserving endoscopic surveillance for those whose disease began between the ages 40 and 60.[214, 220, 221] The fact that surgical options have expanded to include the ileoanal J-pouch as an alternative to permanent ileostomy after total proctocolectomy makes this approach more palatable. Other studies, however, have demonstrated a low rate of conversion to dysplastic mucosa among most patients with ulcerative colitis who showed no dysplasia on initial endoscopic biopsy.[222, 225] If relatively low-risk persons can be identified and followed in a reliable fashion by endoscopic means, and if they prefer the periodic discomfort of endoscopy to that of prophylactic colectomy, endoscopic surveillance is the reasonable approach. Whether newer immunohistochemical markers can separate low-risk and high-risk patients remains to be seen.[226] The recommended interval between examinations is 2 years for patients with no sign of dysplasia on two consecutive annual examinations. This interval should be shortened to 6 to 12 months at the first sign of dysplasia, and colectomy is recommended after definite dysplasia is documented.

Patients who develop ulcerative colitis after the age of 60 do not require colectomy or surveillance. The risk of developing cancer for this group of patients is not greater than that of similarly aged patients without colitis. Patients with Crohn's disease of the large or small intestine have an increased risk of intestinal cancer

that is approximately one fourth that of patients with ulcerative colitis.[227] Cancer may develop in the small intestine and in the unaffected portions of the colon of these patients, making surveillance difficult. Although endoscopic surveillance is probably not indicated for them, prompt evaluation of new symptoms that could indicate malignancy is warranted.

Familial Cancer Syndromes

Between 10% and 20% of colorectal cancers occur in family settings.[228] Most of these involve clusters of two or more first-degree relatives without a clear pattern of inheritance, but 4% to 6% involve dominently inherited nonpolyposis or polyposis syndromes. The nonpolyposis variants (*i.e.,* hereditary nonpolyposis colorectal cancer [HNPCC] or Lynch syndromes I and II) are four to five times more frequent than the adenomatous polyposis variants (*i.e.,* familial polyposis, Gardner's syndrome, Turcot's syndrome).[229–231] Although people whose first-degree relatives have colorectal cancer have a 2- to 3-fold risk of developing cancer themselves, this risk does not justify more extensive screening than usually recommended, except the substitution of barium enema or colonoscopy for flexible sigmoidoscopy. People with hereditary cancer syndromes are at high risk and need aggressive screening beginning at an early age.

The key to identifying persons at high risk is a careful family history. Patients may be unaware of the extent of family involvement until their own symptoms stimulate the physician to inquire. Young patients with large numbers of polyps or multiple family members with colon cancer at an early age should alert the physician to include the family in the evaluation. If possible, a pedigree should be established to identify family members at highest risk.[232, 233] Genetic markers may help in this endeavor.[234, 235] It may be important to identify those at average risk to be able to limit screening to the people most likely to benefit.

In families with polyposis syndromes, screening should begin before the age of 20 (some recommend as early as age 10) and continue on a yearly basis until the age of 35.[236] Flexible sigmoidoscopy should provide sufficient information to identify those with the polyposis trait. Because most polyps are manifested by the age of 30, screening after age 35 can be reduced in frequency to that for average-risk patients (*i.e.,* yearly FOBT and flexible sigmoidoscopy every 3 years). If genetic markers are negative, sigmoidoscopy every 3 years until age 35 is more appropriate.

After the polyposis phenotype is discovered, prophylactic colectomy should be performed. This approach should probably entail a total protocolectomy with ileoanal anastomosis, because as many as 55% of patients develop polyps in the rectum, some with associated cancers, if this structure is not removed. Some success has been reported in causing polyps to regress with sulindac, a long-acting analog of indometha-cin.[237, 238] If this drug proves effective in clinical trials, periodic colonoscopic surveillance will undoubtedly play a larger role in the follow-up care of these patients.

Patients in families with HNPCC have a 50% risk of developing colorectal cancer at an age 15 to 20 years earlier than the general population. Screening should include full colonoscopy because of an excess of proximal tumors in HNPCC and should begin at the age of 25 or 5 years earlier than the earliest age at which cancer has been reported in the family group (whichever is earlier). An interval of 2 to 3 years between examinations has been recommended as long as the colon remains free of pathology. More frequent examination is warranted if adenomas are encountered. Subtotal colectomy is recommended as the management of carcinoma in these patients because of the high incidence of metachronous lesions. Some families with HNPCC have an increased risk of extracolonic cancers (*i.e.,* Lynch syndrome II), particularly carcinomas of the endometrium. Gynecologic screening tests should be included in the evaluation of these families but are not necessary for site-specific HNPCC (*i.e.,* Lynch syndrome I).

References

1. Boring CC, Squires TS, Tong T. Cancer statistics, 1993. CA Cancer J Clin 43:7–26, 1993.
2. Aldridge MC, Sim AJW. Colonoscopy findings in symptomatic patients without x-ray evidence of colonic neoplasms. Lancet 2:833–834, 1986.
3. Rex DK, Lehman GA, Hawes RH, et al. Screening colonoscopy in asymptomatic average-risk persons with negative fecal occult blood tests. Gastroenterology 100:64–67, 1991.
4. Habr-Gama A, Waye JD. Complications and hazards of gastrointestinal endoscopy. World J Surg 13:193–201, 1989.
5. Jarvinen HJ. Premalignant conditions of the gastrointestinal tract: a basis for selective screening programs. Ann Med 21:285–286, 1989.
6. Dent TL, Kukora JS, Buinewicz BR. Endoscopic screening and surveillance for gastrointestinal malignancy. Surg Clin North Am 69:1205–1225, 1989.
7. Nabeya K, Hanaoka T, Onozawa K, et al. Early diagnosis of esophageal cancer. Hepatogastroenterology 37:368–370, 1990.
8. American Society for Gastrointestinal Endoscopy. The role of endoscopy in the surveillance of premalignant conditions of the upper gastrointestinal tract. Gastrointest Endosc 34(Suppl):18S–20S, 1988.
9. Lightdale CJ, Winawer SJ. Screening diagnosis and staging of esophageal cancer. Semin Oncol 11:101–112, 1984.
10. Wychulis AR, Woolam GL, Andersen HA, et al. Achalasia and carcinoma of the esophagus. JAMA 215:1638–1641, 1971.
11. Feczko PJ, Ma CK, Halpert RD, et al. Barrett's metaplasia and dysplasia in postmyotomy achalasia patients. Am J Gastroenterol 78:265–268, 1983.
12. Agha FP, Keren DF. Barrett's esophagus complicating achalasia after esophagomyotomy: a clinical, radiologic, and pathologic study of 70 patients with achalasia and related motor disorders. J Clin Gastroenterol 9:232–237, 1987.
13. Goodman P, Scott LD, Verani RR, et al. Esophageal adenocarcinoma in a patient with surgically treated achalasia. Dig Dis Sci 35:1549–1552, 1990.
14. Bozymski EM, Herlihy KJ, Orlando RC. Barrett's esophagus. Ann Intern Med 97:103–107, 1982.
15. Stein HJ, Barlow AP, DeMeester TR, et al. Complications of gastroesophageal reflux disease: role of the lower esophageal sphincter, esophageal acid and acid/alkaline exposure, and duodenogastric reflux. Ann Surg 216:35–43, 1992.
16. Waring JP, Legrand J, Chinichian A, et al. Duodenogastric reflux in patients with Barrett's esophagus. Dig Dis Sci 35:759–762, 1990.
17. Haggitt RC. Adenocarcinoma in Barrett's esophagus: a new epidemic? Hum Pathol 23:475–476, 1992.
18. Collins BJ, Abbott M, Thomas RJS, et al. Clinical profile in Barrett's esophagus: who should be screened for cancer? Hepatogastroenterology 38:341–344, 1991.
19. Williamson WA, Ellis FH, Gibb SP, et al. Effect of antireflux operation on Barrett's mucosa. Ann Thorac Surg 49:537–542, 1990.
20. Oka M, Attwood SE, Kaul B, et al. Immunosuppression in patients with Barrett's esophagus. Surgery 112:11–17, 1992.
21. Soltero E, Cruz NI, Nazario CM, et al. Cholecystectomy and right colon cancer in Puerto Rico. Cancer 66:2249–2252, 1990.
22. Paraf F, Flejou JF, Potet F, et al. Esophageal squamous carcinoma in five patients with Barrett's esophagus. Am J Gastroenterol 87:746–750, 1992.
23. McArdle JE, Lewin KJ, Randall G, et al. Distribution of dysplasias and early invasive carcinoma in Barrett's esophagus. Hum Pathol 23:479–482, 1992.
24. Ovaska J, Miettinen M, Kivilaakso E. Adenocarcinoma arising in Barrett's esophagus. Dig Dis Sci 34:1336–1339, 1989.
25. Robertson CS, Mayberry JF, Nicholson DA, et al. Value of endoscopic surveillance in the detection of neoplastic change in Barrett's oesophagus. Br J Surg 75:760–763, 1988.
26. Hameeteman W, Tytgat GNJ, Houthoff HJ, et al. Barrett's esophagus: development of dysplasia and adenocarcinoma. Gastroenterology 96:1249–1256, 1989.
27. Duhaylongsod FG, Wolfe WG. Barrett's esophagus and adenocarcinoma of the esophagus and gastroesophageal junction. J Thorac Cardiovasc Surg 102:36–42, 1991.
28. Williamson WA, Ellis FH, Gibb SP, et al. Barrett's ulcer: a surgical disease? J Thorac Cardiovasc Surg 103:2–7, 1992.
29. Reid BJ, Weinstein WM, Lewin KJ, et al. Endoscopic biopsy can detect high-grade dysplasia or early ade-

nocarcinoma in Barrett's esophagus without grossly recognizable neoplastic lesions. Gastroenterology 94:81–90, 1988.

30. Li H, Walsh TN, Hennessy TPJ. Carcinoma arising in Barrett's esophagus. Surg Gynecol Obstet 175:167–172, 1992.

31. Riddell RH. Screening strategies in gastrointestinal cancer. Scand J Gastroenterol 25(Suppl 175):177–184, 1990.

32. Geisinger KR, Teot LA, Richter JE: A comparative cytopathologic and histologic study of atypia, dysplasia and adenocarcinoma in Barrett's esophagus. Cancer 69:8–16, 1992.

33. Shiozaki H, Tahara H, Kobayashi K, et al. Endoscopic screening of early esophageal cancer with the Lugol dye method in patients with head and neck cancers. Cancer 66:2068–2071, 1990.

34. Garewal HS, Sampliner RE, Fennerty MB. Flow cytometry in Barrett's esophagus: what have we learned so far? Dig Dis Sci 36:548–551, 1991.

35. Achkar E, Carey W. The cost of surveillance for adenocarcinoma complicating Barrett's esophagus. Am J Gastroenterol 83:291–294, 1988.

36. Blot WJ, Devesa SS, Kneller RW, et al. Rising incidence of adenocarcinoma of the esophagus and gastric cardia. JAMA 265:1287–1289, 1991.

37. Harris OD, Cooke WT, Thompson H, et al. Malignancy in adult coeliac disease and idiopathic steatorrhoea. Am J Med 42:899–912, 1967.

38. Swinson CM, Slavin G, Coles EC, et al. Coeliac disease and malignancy. Lancet 1:111–115, 1983.

39. Shaha A, Hoover E, Marti J, et al. Is routine triple endoscopy cost-effective in head and neck cancer? Am J Surg 155:750–753, 1988.

40. Atkinson D, Fleming S, Weaver A. Triple endoscopy: a valuable procedure in head and neck surgery. Am J Surg 144:416–419, 1982.

41. Atkins JP, Keane WM, Young KA, et al. Value of panendoscopy in determination of second primary cancer: a study of 451 cases of head and neck cancer. Arch Otolaryngol 110:533–534, 1984.

42. Atabek U, Mohit-Tabatabai MA, Rush BF, et al. Impact of esophageal screening in patients with head and neck cancer. Am Surg 56:289–292, 1990.

43. Nino-Murcia M, Vincent ME, Vaughan C, et al. Esophagography and esophagoscopy: comparison in the examination of patients with head and neck carcinoma. Arch Otolaryngol Head Neck Surg 116:917–919, 1990.

44. Neel HB. Routine panendoscopy—is it necessary every time? Arch Otolaryngol 110:531–532, 1984.

45. Appelqvist P, Salmo M. Lye corrosion carcinoma of the esophagus: a review of 63 cases. Cancer 45:2655–2658, 1980.

46. Isolauri J, Markkula H. Lye ingestion and carcinoma of the esophagus. Acta Chir Scand 155:269–271, 1989.

47. Goldman LP, Weigert JM. Corrosive substance ingestion: a review. Am J Gastroenterol 79:85–90, 1984.

48. Segel MC, Campbell WL, Medsger TA, et al. Systemic sclerosis (scleroderma) and esophageal adenocarcinoma: is increased patient screening necessary? Gastroenterology 89:485–488, 1985.

49. Sprung DJ, Gibb SP. Dysplastic Barrett's esophagus in scleroderma. Am J Gastroenterol 80:518–522, 1985.

50. Katzka DA, Reynolds JC, Saul SH, et al. Barrett's metaplasia and adenocarcinoma of the esophagus in scleroderma. Am J Med 82:46–52, 1987.

51. Li FP. Family cancer syndromes and clusters. Curr Probl Cancer 14:75–113, 1990.

52. Sons HU. Etiologic and epidemiologic factors of carcinoma of the esophagus. Surg Gynecol Obstet 165:183–190, 1987.

53. Wynder EL, Hultberg S, Jacobsson F, et al. Environmental factors in cancer of the upper alimentary tract: a Swedish study with special reference to Plummer-Vinson (Patterson-Kelly) syndrome. Cancer 10:470–487, 1957.

54. Strickland RG, Mackay IR. A reappraisal of the nature and significance of chronic atrophic gastritis. Am J Dig Dis 18:426–440, 1973.

55. Kurtz RC, Sherlock P. Carcinoma of the stomach. In: Berk JE, ed. Bockus' Gastroenterology. Philadelphia: WB Saunders, 1985:1278–1304.

56. Walker IR, Strickland RG, Ungar B, et al. Simple atrophic gastritis and gastric carcinoma. Gut 12:906–911, 1971.

57. Testoni PA, Masci E, Marchi R, et al. Gastric cancer in chronic atrophic gastritis: associated gastric ulcer adds no further risk. J Clin Gastroenterol 9:298–302, 1987.

58. Sipponen P, Kekki M, Siurala M. Atrophic chronic gastritis and intestinal metaplasia in gastric carcinoma. Cancer 52:1062–1068, 1983.

59. Asaka M, Kimura T, Kudo M, et al. Relationship of Helicobacter pylori to serum pepsinogens in an asymptomatic Japanese population. Gastroenterology 102:760–766, 1992.

60. Forman D, Newell DG, Fullerton F, et al. Association between infection with Helicobacter pylori and risk of gastric cancer: evidence from a prospective investigation. Br Med J 302:1302–1305, 1991.

61. Parsonnet J, Friedman GD, Vandersteen DP, et al. Helicobacter pylori infection and the risk of gastric carcinoma. N Engl J Med 325:1127–1131, 1991.

62. Nomura A, Stemmermann GN, Chyou PH, et al. Helicobacter pylori infection and gastric carcinoma among Japanese Americans in Hawaii. N Engl J Med 325:1132–1136, 1991.

63. Correa P. Is gastric carcinoma an infectious disease? N Engl J Med 325:1170–1171, 1991.

64. Laxen F. Gastric carcinoma and pernicious anaemia in long-term endoscopic follow-up of subjects with gastric polyps. Scand J Gastroenterol 19:535–540, 1984.

65. van Stolk R, Sivak MV, Petrini JL, et al. Endoscopic management of upper gastrointestinal polyps and periampullary lesions in familial adenomatous polyposis and Gardner's syndrome. Endoscopy 19:19–22, 1987.

66. Kurtz RC, Sternberg SS, Miller HH, et al. Upper gastrointestinal neoplasia in familial polyposis. Dig Dis Sci 32:459–465, 1987.

67. Iida M, Yao T, Itoh H, et al. Natural history of gastric adenomas in patients with familial adenomatosis coli/Gardner's syndrome. Cancer 61:605–611, 1988.

68. Jagelman DG, DeCosse JJ, Bussey HJR, et al. Upper gastrointestinal cancer in familial adenomatous polyposis. Lancet 1:1149–1151, 1988.

69. Beckwith PS, van Heerden JA, Dozois RR. Prognosis of symptomatic duodenal adenomas in familial adenomatous polyposis. Arch Surg 126:825–828, 1991.

70. Ming SC, Goldman H. Gastric polyps: a histogenic classification and its relation to carcinoma. Cancer 18:721–726, 1965.

71. Tomasulo J. Gastric polyps: histologic types and their relationship to gastric carcinoma. Cancer 27:1346–1355, 1971.

72. Adam YG, Efron G. Trends and controversies in the management of carcinoma of the stomach. Surg Gynecol Obstet 169:371–385, 1989.

73. Daibo M, Itabashi M, Hirota T. Malignant transfor-

mation of gastric hyperplastic polyps. Am J Gastro-enterol 82:1016–1025, 1987.

74. Orlando R, Welch JP. Carcinoma of the stomach after gastric operation. Am J Surg 141:487–490, 1981.

75. Perez D, Narayanan C, Russell JC, et al. Gastric carcinoma after peptic ulcer surgery. Am Surg 50:538–540, 1984.

76. Offerhaus GJA, vd Stadt J, Huibregtse K, et al. Endoscopic screening for malignancy in the gastric remnant: the clinical significance of dysplasia in gastric mucosa. J Clin Pathol 37:748–754, 1984.

77. Greene FL. Neoplastic changes in the stomach after gastrectomy. Surg Gynecol Obstet 171:477–480, 1990.

78. Eberlein TJ, Lorenzo FV, Webster MW. Gastric carcinoma following operation for peptic ulcer disease. Ann Surg 187:251–256, 1978.

79. Toftgaard C. Gastric cancer after peptic ulcer surgery: a historic prospective cohort investigation. Ann Surg 210:159–164, 1989.

80. Lundegardh G, Adami HO, Helmick C, et al. Stomach cancer after partial gastrectomy for benign ulcer disease. N Engl J Med 319:195–200, 1988.

81. Piper MH, Ross JM, Bever FN, et al. Primary squamous cell carcinoma of a gastric remnant. Am J Gastroenterol 86:1080–1082, 1991.

82. Sasako M, Maruyama K, Kinoshita T, et al. Surgical treatment of carcinoma of the gastric stump. Br J Surg 78:822–824, 1991.

83. Ross AHM, Smith MA, Anderson JR, et al. Late mortality after surgery for peptic ulcer. N Engl J Med 307:519–522, 1982.

84. Schafer LW, Larson DE, Melton LJ, et al. The risk of gastric carcinoma after surgical treatment for benign ulcer disease. N Engl J Med 309:1210–1213, 1983.

85. Offerhaus GJA, Tersmette AC, Giardiello FM, et al. Evaluation of endoscopy for early detection of gastric-stump cancer. Lancet 340:33–35, 1992.

86. Iida M, Matsui T, Itoh H, et al. The value of push-type jejunal endoscopy in familial adenomatosis coli/Gardner's syndrome. Am J Gastroenterology 85:1346–1348, 1990.

87. Barkin JS, Lewis BS, Reiner DK, et al. Diagnostic and therapeutic jejunoscopy with a new, longer enteroscope. Gastrointest Endosc 38:55–58, 1992.

88. Hochberg FH, Dasilva AB, Galdabini J, et al. Gastrointestinal involvement in von Recklinghausen's neurofibromatosis. Neurology 24:1144–1151, 1974.

89. Wander JV, Das Gupta TK. Neurofibromatosis. Curr Probl Surg 14:2–81, 1977.

90. Ishizaki Y, Tada Y, Ishida T, et al. Leiomyosarcoma of the small intestine associated with von Recklinghausen's disease: report of a case. Surgery 111:706–710, 1992.

91. Spigelman AD, Murday V, Phillips RKS. Cancer and the Peutz-Jeghers syndrome. Gut 30:1588–1590, 1989.

92. Panos RG, Opelka FG, Nogueras JJ. Peutz-Jeghers syndrome: a call for intraoperative enteroscopy. Am Surg 56:331–333, 1990.

93. Berg RL. Cancer prevention and screening in light of health promotion and prevention of disability for the second 50 years: a report from the Institute of Medicine of the National Academy of Science. Cancer 68:2511–2513, 1991.

94. Ransohoff DF, Lang CA. Screening for colorectal cancer. N Engl J Med 325:37–41, 1991.

95. Winawer SJ, Zauber AG, Stewart E, et al. The natural history of colorectal cancer: opportunities for intervention. Cancer 67:1143–1149, 1991.

96. Fleischer DE, Goldberg SB, Browning TH, et al. Detection and surveillance of colorectal cancer. JAMA 261:580–585, 1989.

97. Wood CB, Gillis CR, Hole D, et al. Local tumour invasion as a prognostic factor in colorectal cancer. Br J Surg 68:326–328, 1981.

98. Cappell MS, Goldberg ES. The relationship between the clinical presentation and spread of colon cancer in 315 consecutive patients: a significant trend of earlier cancer detection from 1982 through 1988 at a university hospital. J Clin Gastroenterol 14:227–235, 1992.

99. Knight KK, Fielding JE, Battista RN. Occult blood screening for colorectal cancer. JAMA 261:586–593, 1989.

100. Winawer SJ, Schottenfeld D, Flehinger BJ. Colorectal cancer screening. J Natl Cancer Inst 83:243–253, 1991.

101. Selby JV, Friedman GD. Sigmoidoscopy in the periodic health examination of asymptomatic adults. JAMA 261:594–601, 1989.

102. Gilbertsen VA. Proctosigmoidoscopy and polypectomy in reducing the incidence of rectal cancer. Cancer 34:936–939, 1974.

103. Gilbertsen VA, Nelms JM. The prevention of invasive cancer of the rectum. Cancer 41:1137–1139, 1978.

104. Weil J, Langman MJS. Screening for gastrointestinal cancer: an epidemiological review. Gut 32:220–224, 1991.

105. Young GP, Demediuk BH. The genetics, epidemiology, and early detection of gastrointestinal cancers. Curr Opin Oncol 4:728–735, 1992.

106. Winawer SJ, St John J, Bond J, et al. Screening of average-risk individuals for colorectal cancer. Bull WHO 68:505–513, 1990.

107. American Cancer Society. Update January 1992: the American Cancer Society guidelines for the cancer-related checkup. CA Cancer J Clin 42:44–45, 1992.

108. Hertz REL, Deddish MR, Day E. Value of periodic examinations in detecting cancer of the rectum and colon. Postgrad Med 27:290–294, 1960.

109. Greene FL. Distribution of colorectal neoplasms: a left to right shift of polyps and cancer. Am Surg 49:62–65, 1983.

110. Thorson AG, Christensen MA, Davis SJ. The role of colonoscopy in the assessment of patients with colorectal cancer. Dis Colon Rectum 29:306–311, 1986.

111. Isler JT, Brown PC, Lewis FG, et al. The role of preoperative colonoscopy in colorectal cancer. Dis Colon Rectum 30:435–439, 1987.

112. Eddy DM, Nugent FW, Eddy JF, et al. Screening for colorectal cancer in a high-risk population: results of a mathematical model. Gastroenterology 92:682–692, 1987.

113. Eddy DM. Screening for colorectal cancer. Ann Intern Med 113:373–384, 1990.

114. Simon JB. Occult blood screening for colorectal carcinoma: a critical review. Gastroenterology 88:820–837, 1985.

115. Letsou G, Ballantyne GH, Zdon MJ, et al. Screening for colorectal neoplasms: a comparison of the fecal occult blood test and endoscopic examination. Dis Colon Rectum 30:839–843, 1987.

116. Gilbertsen VA, McHugh R, Schuman L, et al. The early detection of colorectal cancers: a preliminary report of the results of the occult blood study. Cancer 45:2899–2901, 1980.

117. Winawer SJ, Andrews M, Flehinger B, et al. Progress report on controlled trial of fecal occult blood testing for the detection of colorectal neoplasia. Cancer 45:2959–2964, 1980.

118. Kronborg O, Fenger C, Sondergaard O, et al. Initial mass screening for colorectal cancer with fecal occult blood test: a prospective randomized study at Funen in Denmark. Scand J Gastroenterol 22:677–686, 1987.

119. Kewenter J, Bjork S, Haglind E, et al. Screening and

rescreening for colorectal cancer: a controlled trial of fecal occult blood testing in 27,700 subjects. Cancer 62:645–651, 1988.

120. Hardcastle JD, Thomas WM, Chamberlain J, et al. Randomized, controlled trial of faecal occult blood screening for colorectal cancer: results for first 107 349 subjects. Lancet 1:1160–1164, 1989.

121. Flehinger BJ, Herbert E, Winawer SJ, et al. Screening for colorectal cancer with fecal occult blood test and sigmoidoscopy: preliminary report of the colon project of Memorial Sloan-Kettering Cancer Center and PMI-Strong Clinic. In: Chamberlain J, Miller AB, eds. Screening for gastrointestinal cancer. Kirkland, WA: Hogrefe and Huber, 1988:9–16.

122. Kronborg O, Fenger C, Olsen J, et al. Repeated screening and rescreening for colorectal cancer with fecal occult blood test: a prospective randomized study at Funen, Denmark. Scand J Gastroenterol 24:599–606, 1989.

123. Morris JB, Stellato TA, Guy BB, et al. A critical analysis of the largest reported mass fecal occult blood screening program in the United States. Am J Surg 161:101–106, 1991.

124. Miller MP, Stanley TV. Results of a mass screening program for colorectal cancer. Arch Surg 123:63–65, 1988.

125. Khubchandani IT, Karamchandani MC, Kleckner FS, et al. Mass screening for colorectal cancer. Dis Colon Rectum 32:754–758, 1989.

126. Petrelli NJ, Palmer M, Michalek A, et al. Massive screening for colorectal cancer: a single institution's public commitment. Arch Surg 125:1049–1051, 1990.

127. Crespi M, Weissman GS, Gilbertsen VA, et al. The role of proctosigmoidoscopy in screening for colorectal neoplasia. CA Cancer J Clin 34:158–176, 1984.

128. Friedman GD, Collen MF, Fireman BH. Multiphasic health checkup evaluation: a 16-year follow-up. J Chronic Dis 39:453–463, 1986.

129. Selby JV, Friedman GD, Collen MF. Sigmoidoscopy and mortality from colorectal cancer: the Kaiser Permanente multiphasic evaluation study. J Clin Epidemiol 41:427–434, 1988.

130. Shida H, Yamamoto T. Fiberoptic sigmoidoscopy as the first screening procedure for colorectal neoplasms in an asymptomatic population. Dis Colon Rectum 32:404–408, 1989.

131. Luchtefeld MA, Syverson D, Solfelt M, et al. Is colonoscopic screening appropriate in asymptomatic patients with family history of colon cancer? Dis Colon Rectum 34:763–768, 1991.

132. Selby JV, Friedman GD, Quesenberry CP, et al. A case-control study of screening sigmoidoscopy and mortality from colorectal cancer. N Engl J Med 326:653–657, 1992.

133. Bohlman TW, Katon RM, Lipshutz GR, et al. Fiberoptic pansigmoidoscopy: an evaluation and comparison with rigid sigmoidoscopy. Gastroenterology 72:644–649, 1977.

134. Sarles HE, Sanowski RA, Haynes WC, et al. The long and short of flexible sigmoidoscopy: does it matter? Am J Gastroenterol 81:369–371, 1986.

135. Winawer SJ, Miller C, Lightdale C, et al. Patient response to sigmoidoscopy: a randomized, controlled trial of rigid and flexible sigmoidoscopy. Cancer 60:1905–1907, 1987.

136. Groveman HD, Sanowski RA, Klauber MR. Training primary care physicians in flexible sigmoidoscopy—performance evaluation of 17,167 procedures. West J Med 148:221–224, 1988.

137. Rodney WM. Flexible sigmoidoscopy and the despe-

138. Neugut AI, Forde KA. Screening colonoscopy: has the time come? Am J Gastroenterol 83:295–297, 1988.

139. Byrd RL, Boggs HW, Slagle GW, et al. Reliability of colonoscopy. Dis Colon Rectum 32:1023–1025, 1989.

140. Guillem JG, Forde KA, Treat MR, et al. The impact of colonoscopy on the early detection of colonic neoplasms in patients with rectal bleeding. Ann Surg 206:606–611, 1987.

141. Dodd GD. Imaging techniques in the diagnosis of carcinoma of the colon Cancer 67(Suppl):1150–1154, 1991.

142. Limberg B. Diagnosis and staging of colonic tumors by conventional abdominal sonography as compared with hydrocolonic sonography. N Engl J Med 327:65–69, 1992.

143. Byers T, Gorsky R. Estimates of costs and effects of screening for colorectal cancer in the United States. Cancer 70:1288–1295, 1992.

144. Thomas WM, Hardcastle JD. Role of upper gastrointestinal investigations in a screening study for colorectal neoplasia. Gut 31:1294–1297, 1990.

145. Meagher AP, Stuart M. Colonoscopy in patients with a family history of colorectal cancer. Dis Colon Rectum 35:315–321, 1992.

146. Harvey EB, Brinton LA. Second cancers following cancer of the breast in Connecticut 1935–82. Natl Cancer Inst Monogr 68:99–112, 1985.

147. Baker JW, Gathright JB, Timmcke AE, et al. Colonoscopic screening of asymptomatic patients with a family history of colon cancer. Dis Colon Rectum 33:926–930, 1990.

148. McConnell JC, Nizin JS, Slade MS. Colonoscopy in patients with a primary family history of colon cancer. Dis Colon Rectum 33:105–107, 1990.

149. Guillem JG, Forde KA, Treat MR, et al. Colonoscopic screening for neoplasms in asymptomatic first-degree relatives of colon cancer patients: a controlled, prospective study. Dis Colon Rectum 35:523–529, 1992.

150. Slater G, Aufses AH, Szporn A. Synchronous carcinoma of the colon and rectum. Surg Gynecol Obstet 171:283–287, 1990.

151. Dasmahapatra KS, Lopyan K. Rationale for aggressive colonoscopy in patients with colorectal neoplasia. Arch Surg 124:63–66, 1989.

152. Sollenberger LI, Eisenstat TE, Rubin RJ, et al. Is preoperative colonoscopy necessary in carcinoma of the colon and rectum? Am Surg 54:113–115, 1988.

153. Askew A, Ward M, Cowen A. The influence of colonoscopy on the operative management of colorectal cancer. Med J Aust 145:254–255, 1986.

154. Weber CA, Deveney KE, Pellegrini CA, et al. Routine colonoscopy in the management of colorectal carcinoma. Am J Surg 152:87–92, 1986.

155. Maxfield RG. Colonoscopy as a routine preoperative procedure for carcinoma of the colon. Am J Surg 147:477–480, 1984.

156. Pagana TJ, Ledesma EJ, Mittelman A, et al. The use of colonoscopy in the study of synchronous colorectal neoplasms. Cancer 53:356–359, 1984.

157. Finan PJ, Ritchie JK, Hawley PR. Synchronous and "early" metachronous carcinomas of the colon and rectum. Br J Surg 74:945–947, 1987.

158. Greenstein AJ, Heimann TM, Sachar DB, et al. A comparison of multiple synchronous colorectal cancer in ulcerative colitis, familial polyposis coli, and de novo cancer. Ann Surg 203:123–128, 1986.

159. Howard ML, Greene FL. The effect of preoperative endoscopy on recurrence and survival following sur-

gery for colorectal carcinoma. Am Surg 56:124–127, 1990.

160. Evers BM, Mullins RJ, Mathews TH, et al. Multiple adenocarcinomas of the colon and rectum: an analysis of incidences and current trends. Dis Colon Rectum 31:518–522, 1988.

161. Luchtefeld MA, Ross DS, Zander JD, et al. Late development of metachronous colorectal cancer. Dis Colon Rectum 30:180–184, 1987.

162. Carlsson G, Petrelli NJ, Nava H, et al. The value of colonoscopic surveillance after curative resection for colorectal cancer or synchronous adenomatous polyps. Arch Surg 122:1261–1263, 1987.

163. Nava HR, Pagana TJ. Postoperative surveillance of colorectal carcinoma. Cancer 49:1043–1047, 1982.

164. Kiefer PJ, Thorson AG, Christensen MA. Metachronous colorectal cancer: time interval to presentation of a metachronous cancer. Dis Colon Rectum 29:378–382, 1986.

165. Granqvist S, Karlsson T. Postoperative follow-up of patients with colorectal carcinoma by colonoscopy. Eur J Surg 158:307–312, 1992.

166. Juhl G, Larson GM, Mullins R, et al. Six-year results of annual colonoscopy after resection of colorectal cancer. World J Surg 14:255–261, 1990.

167. Brady PG, Straker RJ, Goldschmid S. Surveillance colonoscopy after resection for colon carcinoma. South Med J 83:765–768, 1990.

168. Sugarbaker PH, Gianola FJ, Dwyer A, et al. A simplified plan for follow-up of patients with colon and rectal cancer supported by prospective studies of laboratory and radiologic test results. Surgery 102:79–87, 1987.

169. Fantini GA, DeCosse JJ. Surveillance strategies after resection of carcinoma of the colon and rectum. Surg Gynecol Obstet 171:267–273, 1990.

170. Kelly CJ, Daly JM. Colorectal cancer: principles of postoperative follow-up. Cancer 70:1397–1408, 1992.

171. Rocklin MS, Slomski CA, Watne AL. Postoperative surveillance of patients with carcinoma of the colon and rectum. Am Surg 56:22–27, 1990.

172. Himal HS. Anastomotic recurrence of carcinoma of the colon and rectum: the value of endoscopy and serum CEA levels. Am Surg 57:334–337, 1991.

173. Kievit J, van de Velde CJH. Utility and cost of carcinoembryonic antigen monitoring in colon cancer follow-up evaluation: a Markov analysis. Cancer 65:2580–2587, 1990.

174. Buhler H, Seefeld U, Deyhle P, et al. Endoscopic follow-up after colorectal cancer surgery: early detection of local recurrence? Cancer 54:791–793, 1984.

175. Stulc JP, Petrelli NJ, Herrera L, et al. Anastomotic recurrence of adenocarcinoma of the colon. Arch Surg 121:1077–1080, 1986.

176. Ovaska J, Jarvinen H, Kujari H, et al. Follow-up of patients operated on for colorectal carcinoma. Am J Surg 159:593–596, 1990.

177. Haas PA, Fox TA. The fate of the forgotten rectal pouch after Hartmann's procedure without reconstruction. Am J Surg 159:106–111, 1990.

178. Haas PA, Fox TA, Szilagy EF. Endoscopic examination of the colon and rectum distal to a colostomy. Am J Gastroenterol 85:850–854, 1990.

179. Harig JM, Soergel KH, Komorowski RA, et al. Treatment of diversion colitis with short-chain-fatty acid irrigation. N Engl J Med 320:23–28, 1989.

180. Tierney RP, Ballantyne GH, Modlin IM. The adenoma to carcinoma sequence. Surg Gynecol Obstet 171:81–94, 1990.

181. Bedenne L, Faivre J, Boutron MC, et al. Adenoma-carcinoma sequence or "de novo" carcinogenesis? A study of adenomatous remnants in a population-based series of large bowel cancers. Cancer 69:883–888, 1992.

182. Stryker SJ, Wolff BG, Culp CE, et al. Natural history of untreated colonic polyps. Gastroenterology 93:1009–1013, 1987.

183. Olsen HW, Lawrence WA, Snook CW, et al. Risk factors and screening techniques in 500 patients with benign and malignant colon polyps: an urban community experience. Dis Colon Rectum 31:216–221, 1988.

184. Simons BD, Morrison AS, Lev R, et al. Relationship of polyps to cancer of the large intestine. J Natl Cancer Inst 84:962–966, 1992.

185. Atkin WS, Morson BC, Cuzick J. Long-term risk of colorectal cancer after excision of rectosigmoid adenomas. N Engl J Med 326:658–662, 1992.

186. Pollock AM, Quirke P. Adenoma screening and colorectal cancer: the need for screening and polypectomy is unproved. Br Med J 303:3–4, 1991.

187. Johnson DA, Gurney MS, Volpe RJ, et al. A prospective study of the prevalence of colonic neoplasms in asymptomatic patients with an age-related risk. Am J Gastroenterol 85:969–974, 1990.

188. Foutch PG, Mai H, Pardy K, et al. Flexible sigmoidoscopy may be ineffective for secondary prevention of colorectal cancer in asymptomatic, average-risk men. Dig Dis Sci 36:924–928, 1991.

189. Eide TJ, Stalsberg H. Polyps of the large intestine in northern Norway. Cancer 42:2839–2848, 1978.

190. Rickert RR, Auerbach O, Garfinkel L, et al. Adenomatous lesions of the large bowel: an autopsy survey. Cancer 43:1847–1857, 1979.

191. Vatn MH, Stalsberg H. The prevalence of polyps of the large intestine in Oslo: an autopsy study. Cancer 49:819–825, 1982.

192. Williams AR, Balasooriya BAW, Day DW. Polyps and cancer of the large bowel: a necropsy study in Liverpool. Gut 23:835–842, 1982.

193. Delendi M, Gardiman D, Riboli E, et al. Latent colorectal cancer found at necropsy. Lancet 1:1331–1332, 1989.

194. O'Brien MJ, Winawer SJ, Zauber AG, et al. The national polyp study: patient and polyp characteristics associated with high-grade dysplasia in colorectal adenomas. Gastroenterology 98:371–379, 1990.

195. Warden MJ, Petrelli NJ, Herrera L, et al. The role of colonoscopy and flexible sigmoidoscopy in screening for colorectal cancer. Dis Colon Rectum 30:52–54, 1986.

196. Wegener M, Borsch G, Schmidt G. Colorectal adenomas: distribution, incidence of malignant transformation, and rate of recurrence. Dis Colon Rectum 29:383–387, 1986.

197. Winawer SJ, Zauber AG, O'Brien MJ, et al. The national polyp study: design, methods, and characteristics of patients with newly diagnosed polyps. Cancer 70:1236–1245, 1992.

198. American Society for Gastrointestinal Endoscopy. The role of colonoscopy in the management of patients with colon polyps: guidelines for clinical application. Gastrointest Endosc 34(Suppl):6S–7S, 1988.

199. Church JM, Fazio VW, Jones IT. Small colorectal polyps: are they worth treating? Dis Colon Rectum 31:50–53, 1988.

200. Morson BC, Bussey HJR. Magnitude of risk for cancer in patients with colorectal adenomas. Br J Surg 72(Suppl):S23–S25, 1985.

201. Olsen HW, Lawrence WA, Snook CW, et al. Review of recurrent polyps and cancer in 500 patients with

initial colonoscopy for polyps. Dis Colon Rectum 31:222–227, 1988.

202. Holtzman R, Poulard JB, Bank S, et al. Repeat colonoscopy after endoscopic polypectomy. Dis Colon Rectum 30:185–188, 1987.

203. Nava H, Carlsson G, Petrelli NJ, et al. Follow-up colonoscopy in patients with colorectal adenomatous polyps. Dis Colon Rectum 30:465–468, 1987.

204. Woolfson IK, Eckholdt GJ, Wetzel R, et al. Usefulness of performing colonoscopy one year after endoscopic polypectomy. Dis Colon Rectum 33:389–393, 1990.

205. Kronborg O. Follow-up surveillance in patients with adenomas. J Gastroenterol Hepatol 6:552–553, 1991.

206. Kronborg O. Follow-up after removal of colorectal adenomas and radical surgery for colorectal carcinomas. Br J Surg 72(Suppl):S26–S28, 1985.

207. Ransohoff DF, Lang CA. Small adenomas detected during fecal occult blood test screening for colorectal cancer: the impact of serendipity. JAMA 264:76–78, 1990.

208. Williams CB. Polyp follow-up: how, who for and how often? Br J Surg 72(Suppl):S25–S26, 1985.

209. Provenzale D, Garrett JW, Condon SE, et al. Risk for colon adenomas in patients with rectosigmoid hyperplastic polyps. Ann Intern Med 113:760–763, 1990.

210. Provenzale D, Martin ZZ, Holland KL, et al. Colon adenomas in patients with hyperplastic polyps. J Clin Gastroenterol 10:46–49, 1988.

211. Blue MG, Sivak MV, Achkar E, et al. Hyperplastic polyps seen at sigmoidoscopy are markers for additional adenomas seen at colonoscopy. Gastroenterology 100:564–566, 1991.

212. Rex DK, Smith JJ, Ulbright TM, et al. Distal colonic hyperplastic polyps do not predict proximal adenomas in asymptomatic average-risk subjects. Gastroenterology 102:317–319, 1992.

213. Nugent FW, Haggitt RC, Gilpin PA. Cancer surveillance in ulcerative colitis. Gastroenterology 100:1241–1248, 1991.

214. Collins RH, Feldman M, Fordtran JS. Colon cancer, dysplasia, and surveillance in patients with ulcerative colitis. N Engl J Med 316:1654–1658, 1987.

215. Greenstein AJ, Sachar DB, Smith H, et al. Cancer in universal and left sided ulcerative colitis: factors determining risk. Gastroenterology 77:290–294, 1979.

216. Ekbom A, Helmick C, Zack M, et al. Ulcerative colitis and colorectal cancer: a population-based study. N Engl J Med 323:1228–1233, 1990.

217. Lashner BA, Silverstein MD, Hanauer SB. Hazard rates for dysplasia and cancer in ulcerative colitis: results from a surveillance program. Dig Dis Sci 34:1536–1541, 1989.

218. American Society for Gastrointestinal Endoscopy. The role of colonoscopy in the management of patients with inflammatory bowel disease: guidelines for clinical application. Gastrointest Endosc 34(Suppl):10S–11S, 1988.

219. Levin B. Inflammatory bowel disease and colon cancer. Cancer 70(Suppl):1313–1316, 1992.

220. Lennard-Jones JE. Compliance, cost, and common-sense limit cancer control in colitis. Gut 27:1403–1407, 1986.

221. Ransohoff DF. Colon cancer in ulcerative colitis. Gastroenterology 94:1089–1091, 1988.

222. Lashner BA. Recommendations for colorectal cancer screening in ulcerative colitis: a review of research from a single university-based surveillance program. Am J Gastroenterol 87:168–175, 1992.

223. Woolrich AJ, DaSilva MD, Korelitz BI. Surveillance in the routine management of ulcerative colitis: the predictive value of low-grade dysplasia. Gastroenterology 103:431–438, 1992.

224. Melville DM, Jass JR, Morson BC, et al. Observer study of the grading of dysplasia in ulcerative colitis: comparison with clinical outcome. Hum Pathol 20:1008–1014, 1989.

225. Brostrom O, Lofberg R, Ost A, et al. Cancer surveillance of patients with longstanding ulcerative colitis: a clinical, endoscopical, and histological study. Gut 27:1408–1413, 1986.

226. Saclarides TJ, Jakate SM, Coon JS, et al. Variable expression of p-glycoprotein in normal, inflamed, and dysplastic areas in ulcerative colitis. Dis Colon Rectum 35:747–752, 1992.

227. Greenstein AJ, Sachar DB, Smith H, et al. Patterns of neoplasia in Crohn's disease and ulcerative colitis. Cancer 46:403–407, 1980.

228. Stephenson BM, Finan PJ, Gascoyne J, et al. Frequency of familial colorectal cancer. Br J Surg 78:1162–1166, 1991.

229. Burt RW, Bishop DT, Cannon-Albright L, et al. Hereditary aspects of colorectal adenomas. Cancer 70(Suppl):1296–1299, 1992.

230. Lynch HT, Watson P, Smyrk TC, et al. Colon cancer genetics. Cancer 70(Suppl):1300–1312, 1992.

231. Lynch HT, Smyrk T, Watson P, et al. Hereditary colorectal cancer. Semin Oncol 18:337–366, 1991.

232. Cannon-Albright LA, Skolnick MH, Bishop DT, et al. Common inheritance of susceptibility to colonic adenomatous polyps and associated colorectal cancers. N Engl J Med 319:533–537, 1988.

233. Vasen HFA, Griffioen G, Offerhaus GJA, et al. The value of screening and central registration of families with familial adenomatous polyposis: a study of 82 families in the Netherlands. Dis Colon Rectum 33:227–230, 1990.

234. Leppert M, Burt R, Hughes JP, et al. Genetic analysis of an inherited predisposition to colon cancer in a family with a variable number of adenomatous polyps. N Engl J Med 322:904–908, 1990.

235. Paul P, Jagelman DG, Fazio VW, et al. Evaluation of polymorphic genetic markers for linkage to the familial adenomatous polyposis locus on chromosome 5. Dis Colon Rectum 33:740–744, 1990.

236. Burt RW. Familial screening. J Gastroenterol Hepatol 6:548–551, 1991.

237. Labayle D, Fischer D, Vielh P, et al. Sulindac causes regression of rectal polyps in familial adenomatous polyposis. Gastroenterology 101:635–639, 1991.

238. Waddell WR, Ganser GF, Cerise EJ, et al. Sulindac for polyposis of the colon. Am J Surg 157:175–179, 1989.

8

Endoscopic Management of Gastrointestinal Tract Foreign Bodies

Frederick L. Greene

Since the dawn of time, humankind has been intrigued by the variety of unusual substances and objects that could be ingested. Although aberrations of the psyche have led to most unusual ingestions (Fig. 8–1) and placement of objects through the rectal orifice, ancient physicians understood that therapeutic benefits could be produced by having patients ingest unusual foods and objects. In the time of Hippocrates, physicians encouraged their patients to drink heavy metal solutions, such as gold or calomel, to open obstructed areas of the gastrointestinal (GI) tract. Modern physicians continue to face patients who ingest unusual substances and objects, and surgeons are called on frequently to give opinions on management or to remove these objects by open or endoscopic means.

Management of foreign bodies of the upper GI tract has become easier for patients and physicians since the introduction of flexible endoscopy. During the 1980s, reports outlined the variety of techniques and accessory instruments developed for extraction.[1–3] Although rigid endoscopy was traditionally used for foreign body removal, the surgeon–endoscopist must continue to have experience in extraction through the rigid bronchoscope or esophagoscope.

Between 80% and 90% of inert objects, if small enough or blunt enough, can pass through the pylorus, the small bowel, the ileocecal valve, and into the rectum. Approximately 10% to 20% of these objects require endoscopic or open removal (Fig. 8–2). In considering the best approach for the removal or management of a

GI tract foreign body, the size, shape, and sharpness must be taken into account. Most objects are swallowed by children and pass through the GI tract unencumbered, creating distress only for the physicians and parents involved. Most of these objects are coins or portions of toys. Occasionally, patients ingest toxic materials, such as "button" or cylindric batteries or condoms filled with illicit drugs, such as cocaine.[4] The surgeon–endoscopist must become familiar with the radiographic appearance created by the objects, because the position and size on plain film may indicate the location of the foreign body. A coin lodged in the esophagus appears as a solid, opaque circle in an anteroposterior view (Fig. 8–3). A similar

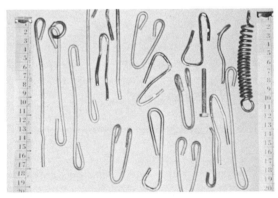

Figure 8–1. Multiple metallic fragments, consisting of springs, screws, and brackets, removed by an open surgical technique from the stomach of a patient in a psychiatric facility.

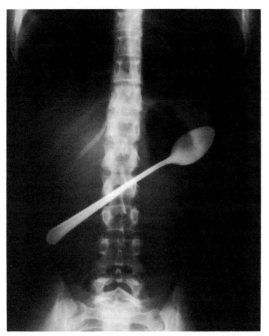

Figure 8–2. Impacted iced tea spoon in the stomach. Configuration of the spoon did not allow passage of a snare wire for extraction, and open surgical removal was needed.

view shows the edge of the coin when it is lodged in the larynx or trachea because of the configuration of the upper airway. This information enables the endoscopist to approach the proper orifice for safe extraction.

Foreign objects may become impacted because of a narrowing in the GI tract caused by benign or malignant disease. It is not unusual for bones, metal objects, and boluses of meat to become lodged in areas associated with stricture. The endoscopist must be skilled at identifying and removing the foreign material and must remember to biopsy or obtain brush cytologies from the area to avoid missing an important underlying process.

INDICATIONS FOR ENDOSCOPIC REMOVAL OF FOREIGN BODIES

After the diagnosis of a gastrointestinal tract foreign body is made and the location of the impaction or position of the object is confirmed, the physician must decide on the safest and most efficacious way to remove it. Endoscopic removal is indicated for any object located within the esophagus that creates obstruction with production of complete dysphagia and the possibility of aspiration. Foreign bodies identi-

fied in the esophagus should be removed to avoid complications such as aspiration and fistula formation. Gastric foreign bodies may allow a more elective approach, because these objects may pass through the pylorus and eventually traverse the entire gastrointestinal tract.

The nature of the foreign body is important in determining indications for endoscopic removal. Sharp or pointed objects should be removed as soon as possible, because the only other alternative may be to repair a perforation after the object disrupts the gastric wall. Some objects are followed radiographically for a long period and do not seem to move distally from the stomach into the small bowel. It is appropriate to approach these lesions endoscopically, because gastritis or ulceration may be caused by foreign body irritation, and healing can be realized only by removal of these objects. In patients with previous gastric resection and reconstruction, gastric bezoars can create problems. Most bezoars should be diagnosed and removed endoscopically.

If the foreign body has already traversed the pylorus and duodenum and has moved into the small bowel, it is prudent to continue a conservative approach with radiographic follow-up. Endoscopic removal may be possible if these objects do not continue to progress distally, but

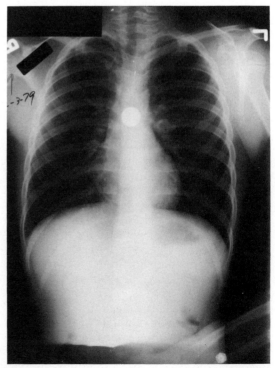

Figure 8–3. Posteroanterior chest x-ray film showing a classic picture of a coin in the esophagus of a child.

they usually require open celiotomy with simultaneous intraoperative peroral placement of a colonoscope for extraction. Some objects, especially pointed or unusually shaped objects, pass through the ileocecal valve and are retained in the wall of the colon. After a routine bowel preparation, colonoscopic identification and an attempt at removal is indicated. The bowel must be prepared for surgery and possible colotomy if endoscopic evaluation is undertaken. Impacted rectal foreign bodies may be amenable to endoscopic removal, but they usually have been resident for several days before the patient seeks medical care. Extraction through the rectum should be attempted under spinal or general anesthesia, and extraction often necessitates celiotomy and colotomy for complete removal.

FOREIGN BODIES IN THE STOMACH AND ESOPHAGUS

After the diagnosis of a foreign body in the esophagus or stomach is confirmed by radiographic or endoscopic means, an attempt to remove the offending object is reasonable if the endoscopist is skilled in the technique and if appropriate accessories are available for safe removal. The upper airway, including the larynx and pharynx, must be examined carefully, because additional objects or injury may be associated with esophageal or gastric foreign objects. To protect the upper airway, it may be appropriate to use a general anesthetic in the operating room. This approach allows conversion to open techniques if gastric or duodenal objects cannot be removed safely.

Depending on the foreign object, a variety of

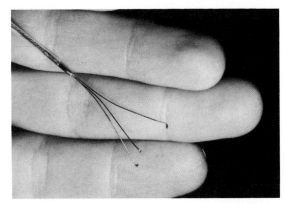

Figure 8–5. Grasping accessory, ideal for removal of meat or rounded metal objects from esophagus.

accessories to facilitate removal should be in the repertoire of the surgeon–endoscopist. If a circular coin is identified, a snare wire or grasper (Figs. 8–4 and 8–5) may be appropriate. These objects usually do not create a perforation, but the endoscopist must examine the mucosa carefully to ensure that an associated stricture or ulceration is not apparent. Patients often have fish or poultry bones impacted in the upper esophagus (Fig. 8–6). This is especially true in

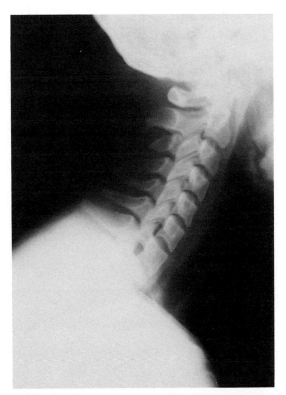

Figure 8–6. Chicken bone seen in the upper esophagus on a lateral x-ray film. There was no evidence of an air column outside the esophagus suggesting perforation.

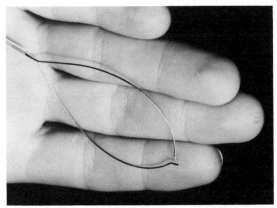

Figure 8–4. Snare wire used for extraction of coins or meat from esophagus.

Table 8–1. RADIOPACITY OF FISH BONES

Radiopaque	Faintly Radiopaque	Radiolucent
Bass	Salmon	Bluefish
Cod	Pike	Butterfish
Flounder		Mackerel
Fluke		Pompano
Gray sole		Trout
Haddock		
Halibut		
Porgy		
Red snapper		
Sea bass		
Striped bass		
Smelt		
White perch		

(Modified from Goldman JL. Fish bones in the esophagus. Ann Otol Rhinol Laryngol 60:957, 1951.)

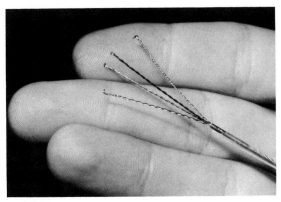

Figure 8–8. Serrated, heavy grasper used for removal of meat or a portion of bezoars from stomach.

patients who have dentures and who are unable to appreciate small bones during mastication. Most fish bones are radiopaque, but several varieties of fish have bones that are radiolucent (Table 8–1). The bone may penetrate the mucosa, and the endoscopist must search diligently for evidence of perforation. Preoperative antibiotics should be given at the time of removal of fish bones because of the high incidence of penetration.

Although most bony impactions occur at the level of the cricopharyngeus, bones may also become lodged in the middle and lower third of the esophagus. It is important to obtain radiographs of the upper neck and the chest to identify areas of abnormal fluid or air collections. Most of the bony objects are embedded in a way that allows easy extraction, because the sharp end of the bone usually trails when the proximal end of the bone is grasped with forceps and withdrawn through the esophagus. Alligator forceps (Fig. 8–7) or other forceps

with serrations can facilitate removal. After the bone is removed, the endoscopist must carefully inspect for mucosal disruption or associated stricture. Routine biopsy should be accomplished if there are unusual mucosal findings.

Impacted meat, the most frequent foreign body in adults, is a sign of the "steakhouse syndrome," which usually occurs in patients with associated stricture or narrowing of the middle or lower esophagus. Patients often have dribbling of saliva and substernal discomfort, which may mimic cardiac symptoms. This scenario should encourage early endoscopic evaluation, because dissolution with enzymatic agents or antispasmodics is generally unsuccessful and contraindicated.[5] The approach to boluses of meat is facilitated by using a therapeutic fiberoptic endoscope to allow appropriate suctioning and passage of accessories through the dual-lumen instrument. The meat impaction may be dislodged in a piece-meal approach using a serrated grasper or a polyp retriever (Fig. 8–8). Successful disimpaction necessitates multiple entries and withdrawals of the endoscope, and an overtube facilitates repeated passage of the endoscope (Fig. 8–9). Occasionally, the meat bolus is suctioned free of its impacted site in the esophagus using strong suction. Although some physicians have advocated sedation only, my

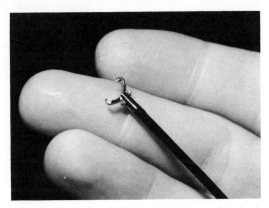

Figure 8–7. Grasping instrument, ideal for removal of coins or safety pins from esophagus or stomach.

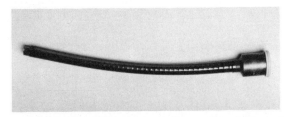

Figure 8–9. Overtube used to facilitate reintroduction of the endoscope or protection of esophageal mucosa when a pointed object is removed endoscopically.

colleagues and I have found that general anesthesia helps to reduce patient agitation and protects the airway.

A bolus of meat sometimes may be gently advanced through a narrow portion of the esophagus and positioned into the stomach for easy passage. This is usually a blind technique, and extreme caution should be used in trying to advance any impacted object in this area. Passage of a small flexible endoscope past the bolus of meat helps to assess the distal esophagus before gentle pushing into the stomach. After the meat is removed by a proximal withdrawal or distal push technique, the area of narrowing should be inspected carefully and biopsied to rule out malignancy. The physician commonly finds a peptic stricture, which can be dilated if edema and friability are not significant.

A variety of other objects may be found in the esophagus and stomach, and some can test the skill and ingenuity of the most experienced surgeon–endoscopist for safe removal.[6] Expertise with the rigid esophagoscope is still important, because the endoscope itself may provide a barrier in the removal of sharp or pointed objects without injury to the proximal esophagus during withdrawal. The use of modern fiberoptic endoscopic equipment, especially facilitated by video accessories, is suitable for removal of most foreign bodies in the esophagus and stomach. The endoscopist should make a "dry run" to practice grasping the type of object that will be found, using turning and sheathing maneuvers to protect the proximal GI tract during withdrawal (Fig. 8–10). This is especially true in the approach to open safety pins or other sharp objects. The advice given many years ago by Chevalier Jackson is still appropriate: "Advancing points puncture; trailing do not."[7]

Several forceps are appropriate for removing metallic objects of various shapes. Grasping forceps can secure the ring of an open safety pin. If the point of the safety pin is facing proximally in the esophagus, the pin can be reduced into the stomach and then turned to

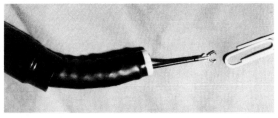

Figure 8–10. Close-up view of grasper, using a "dry-run" approach to remove a foreign body. Notice the overtube in a position that facilitates protection during withdrawal.

allow the open sharp point to be removed in a trailing fashion by the grasper. Another safe maneuver is to place a thin rubber hood over the end of the endoscope to cover sharp instruments such as razor blades and open safety pins during withdrawal. The important principle is to avoid removal of sharp objects endoscopically if the maneuver would encourage perforation. If the surgeon–endoscopist thinks that the risk of perforation is greater during removal of the object, open celiotomy should be performed.

Razor blades have been a favorite object for ingestion, especially in patients in psychiatric facilities and those incarcerated in penal institutions. The razor blade is usually a single-edge variety, because it can pass through the oropharynx without causing too much discomfort. The use of a piece of Latex as a protective hood on the end of the scope can protect the proximal esophagus during withdrawal of the razor blade. An alternative method is to place a balloon over the end of the fiberoptic instrument and to distend the esophagus by inflating the balloon, which protects the esophageal mucosa as the trailing razor blade is removed.

Endoscopists are gaining experience in removing the button batteries that are used in electronic equipment, watches, and hearing aids. These types of ingestions have occurred mostly in children, and characteristic radiographic findings are used to differentiate these foreign bodies from the usual ingested coin.[8, 9] Injury to the esophageal or gastric mucosa results from leaking of the strong alkaline material contained in the battery, which may create a fistula. Under general anesthesia, these objects can be removed using a through-the-scope balloon technique under direct vision. Retrieval with a basket or snare wire (Fig. 8–11) is appropriate for removal from the stomach. These small batteries usually pass benignly through the remainder of the GI tract if gastric removal is not possible.

After the removal of any foreign body from the esophagus, follow-up endoscopy or barium contrast studies should be obtained to rule out fistulization or perforation. Patients should be observed in the hospital for 24 to 48 hours to look for any signs of mediastinitis, suggested by crepitus in the neck, hoarseness, chest pain, or fever.

GASTRIC BEZOARS

The appearance of gastric bezoars is associated with previous partial gastric resection and reconstruction. Bezoar material has traditionally

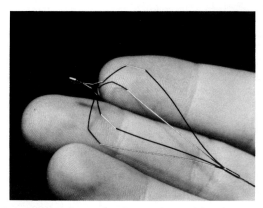

Figure 8–11. Wire basket that can be used for removal of round objects or button batteries.

been limited to vegetable matter, hair, or other ingested materials. The radiographic appearance of a bezoar is characteristic, but the definitive diagnosis is made endoscopically. The bezoar has the appearance of a large, irregular mass that includes amorphous material. The lesion may occupy the entire gastric remnant or may be movable within the remaining stomach. Trichobezoars or hair-filled concretions are quite firm and are not amenable to endoscopic disruption. Surgical resection through formal celiotomy is necessary for most trichobezoars.

Removal of bezoars containing vegetable material can be facilitated by instillation of enzymes that encourage dissolution of the phytobezoar. Dissolution can be facilitated using endoscopic graspers or polyp retrieval graspers, which hasten dissolution and eventual disruption of the bezoar. It is important to inspect the entire stomach or gastric remnant to identify areas of stricture, especially at the gastroenterostomy site.

FOREIGN BODIES IN THE SMALL INTESTINE

Because of the inability to easily pass small bowel endoscopes, foreign bodies that tend to lodge in the small bowel usually require removal by open celiotomy. Sharp objects should be removed before passage into the small bowel because of the higher rate of perforation after they reach the ileocecal valve. However, smooth foreign bodies can be "milked" into accessible areas of the colon or stomach for simultaneous endoscopic removal, avoiding enterotomy.[2] This should not be attempted with foreign bodies having sharp points or razor-like edges because of the possibility of further injury to the patient and operating surgeon. For foreign objects in

the proximal jejunum, a conventional colonoscope can be passed through the mouth and advanced well into the proximal or middle jejunum. This maneuver can remove the object without enterotomy and enables intraluminal detection of associated lesions such as strictures.

FOREIGN BODIES IN THE COLON

After a foreign object has reached the colon, it is likely that complete passage can be achieved through the rectum. Occasionally, especially in the case of sharply pointed objects, a foreign body becomes lodged in the colon and is removed only by surgical or endoscopic means. The splenic and sigmoid flexures are the usual areas where foreign bodies come to rest, but they can be reached easily with conventional endoscopic equipment. In approaching foreign bodies of the colon, complete bowel preparation should be accomplished, because celiotomy and colotomy may be the next step after unsuccessful endoscopic removal. The endoscopic removal itself may facilitate and hasten perforation, especially by sharp objects, and concomitant colotomy or colostomy depends on whether the colon is appropriately prepared. After condoms containing illicit drugs are identified in the colon, surgical removal should be undertaken, because the endoscopic removal may puncture the condom, causing rapid absorption of the drug.

Colonic foreign bodies can be removed using intravenous sedation alone in cooperative patients. Appropriate accessories must be available, including graspers, snare wires, and polyp retrievers.

FOREIGN BODIES IN THE RECTUM

The types of objects that find their way into the rectum of patients are legion and extraordinary.[10] Most of these objects are firmly impacted at the time of diagnosis and do not lend themselves to easy endoscopic extraction. The problem with impacted foreign objects results from pressure necrosis, which eventually leads to ulceration and perforation. Rigid proctoscopy is indicated if the object is above the examining finger. This study can determine whether surgical intervention or further endoscopic manipulation is indicated. The use of intravenous glucagon may facilitate extraction, but spinal anesthesia or general anesthetic techniques are usually needed to relax the anal sphincter. If

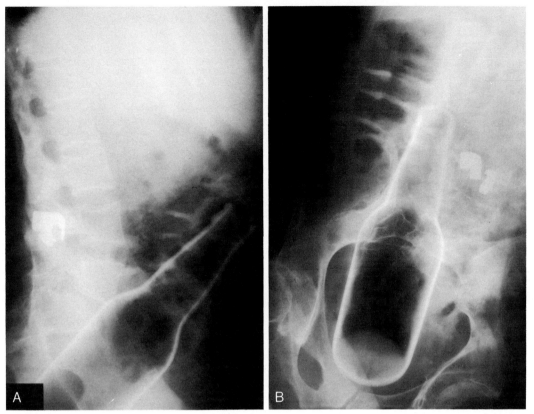

Figure 8–12. (A) Lateral and **(B)** anteroposterior view of impacted beer bottle in rectum and sigmoid colon. Endoscopic extraction was unsuccessful.

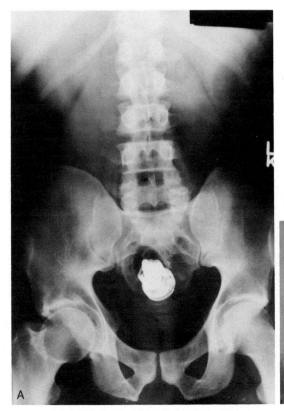

Figure 8–13. (A) Abdominal plain films show the metallic portion of a battery device associated with a plastic vibrator. **(B)** Plastic vibrator seen on the x-ray film in **A.** Removal of the vibrator was facilitated by manual palpation, followed by endoscopic and manual removal.

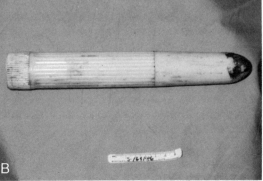

bottles and other cylindric devices are appropriately positioned, a snare wire may be the best fixation device to allow withdrawal. Most bottles are placed in the rectum with the narrow pointed end inserted first (Fig. 8–12). The large, flat bottom of a bottle or container may not allow placement of a snare wire or positioning of a grasper. Occasionally, manual palpation of the abdomen has been successful in advancing a smooth impacted foreign object toward the anus, enabling manual extraction (Fig. 8–13). The prudent surgical endoscopist should realize quickly whether endoscopic means will be successful for the removal of a rectal foreign body and, if not, should resort to traditional transabdominal approaches.

References

1. Webb W. Management of foreign bodies of the upper gastrointestinal tract. Gastroenterology 94:204–216, 1988.
2. Chung R. Removal of foreign bodies. In: Chung R, ed. Therapeutic endoscopy in gastrointestinal surgery. New York: Churchill-Livingstone, 1987:227–242.
3. Webb W. Endoscopic removal of foreign bodies of the esophagus and stomach. Probl Gen Surg 7:35–42, 1990.
4. Caruana DS, Weinbach B, Goerg D, et al. Cocaine packer ingestion. Ann Intern Med 100:73, 1984.
5. Cotton PB, Williams CB. Management of foreign bodies and polyps. In: Cotton PB, Williams CB, eds. Practical gastrointestinal endoscopy. Oxford: Blackwell Scientific, 1990:72–74.
6. Moussa SE, Tunuguntla K, Chan CH, et al. Endoscopic removal of an intact anti-reflux prosthesis 6 years after implantation. Gastrointest Endosc 36:525–527, 1990.
7. Jackson C, Jackson CL. Disease of the air and food passages of foreign body origin. Philadelphia: WB Saunders, 1937.
8. Votteler TP, Nash JC, Rudledge JC. The hazards of ingested alkaline disk batteries in children. JAMA 249:2504, 1983.
9. Maves MD, Lloyd TV, Carithers JS. Radiographic identification of ingested disc batteries. Pediatr Radiol 16:154, 1986.
10. Barone JE, Sohn N, Nealon TF. Perforations and foreign bodies of the rectum: report of 28 cases. Ann Surg 184:601, 1976.

9

Endoscopic Transintestinal Ultrasonography

Marc L. Eckhauser

Most gastrointestinal tumors have mucosal origins. Barium contrast studies and endoscopy have been the primary modalities employed for diagnosis, and transcutaneous ultrasound and computed tomography (CT) have been used for staging. Each of these modalities has its limitations. Endoscopic ultrasonography (EUS) is a marriage between two imaging modalities: fiberoptic endoscopy and real-time ultrasound. The introduction of high-frequency transducers into the intestinal lumen is a new approach for visualizing the intestinal wall architecture and the surrounding structures in extraordinarily fine detail. The most realistic applications for EUS appear to be in the staging of esophageal, gastric, and rectal malignancies. Information about transmural invasion, locoregional adenopathy, and distant metastases can be ascertained. The preservation of intact tissue planes around the tumor can aid in differentiating malignant from benign processes. The potential exists for detecting benign and malignant lesions in the biliary tract and pancreas, but additional clinical studies are required.

Indications for EUS are listed in Table 9–1. Although EUS is still in its infancy, it has proven capable of providing important information, particularly in the preoperative diagnosis and staging of malignant gastrointestinal tumors.

ULTRASOUND FUNDAMENTALS

As with any ultrasound technique, successful application and interpretation of EUS require an understanding of the principles involved in producing the image. Ultrasound refers to sound waves with frequencies greater than 20 thousand cycles per second (cps). Diagnostic ultrasound uses frequencies in the range of 1 to 20 million cps. Sound waves require a medium for transmission, and the physical properties of the medium, primarily compressibility and density, determine the velocity of the sound wave. Sound travels slowest in gases, at intermediate velocities in liquids and all body tissues except bone, and most rapidly in solids (Table 9–2). The velocity of a sound wave is inversely related to the compressibility of the conducting medium, which explains the poor penetration through gas. Density and compressibility are inversely proportional. An increase in density and a decrease in compressibility increase velocity. Acoustic impedance is a fundamental property

Table 9–1. INDICATIONS FOR ENDOSCOPIC ULTRASOUND

Staging of malignant tumors
  Esophagus
  Stomach
  Duodenum
  Pancreas
  Biliary tract
  Rectum
Differentiating benign from malignant submucosal lesions
  Esophagus
  Stomach
  Duodenum
  Rectum
Evaluation of enlarged gastric folds
Evaluation of extraluminal and anastomotic recurrences
  Esophagus
  Stomach
  Rectum

Table 9–2. VELOCITY OF SOUND IN
VARIOUS MEDIA

Medium	Velocity (m/sec)
Air	331
Water	1530
Fat	1450
Brain	1541
Liver	1549
Kidney	1561
Blood	1570
Muscle	1585
Bone	3050

of matter and is the product of the density and velocity of the sound wave in the medium. As the ultrasound wave passes from one tissue plane to another, the amount of reflection is determined by the impedance of the adjacent tissue. The greatest differences in impedance are seen when comparing air and soft tissue and comparing bone and soft tissue. Both interfaces reflect almost the entire ultrasound wave, allowing little or none of the wave to be transmitted.

Attenuation is the reduction in intensity as the sound wave propagates. Absorption, scattering, and reflection of the wave contribute to attenuation. The frequency of the sound wave is an important component that contributes to attenuation; the higher the frequency used, the greater is the amount of attenuation (Fig. 9–1). Ultimately, this translates into a reduction in the depth of tissue that can be imaged. The advantage of EUS over its transcutaneous equivalent resides in the use of high-frequency

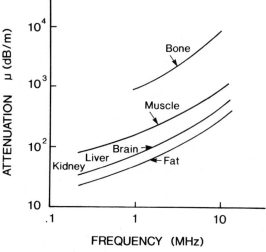

Figure 9–1. This graph depicts the relationship between frequency and attenuation. As the frequency (MHz) increases, so does attenuation (dB/m), and the end result is less penetration through tissue.

transducers, leading to exceptional resolution because the probe is directly adjacent to the tissue to be evaluated.

ENDOSCOPIC ULTRASOUND EQUIPMENT

GF-UM3 Ultrasound Gastrofiberscope

The Olympus GF-UM3 fiberscope and the endoscopic ultrasound system, the EU-M3, is the fourth generation of ultrasound endoscopes designed for transintestinal ultrasonography and the examination of structures adjacent to the esophagus, stomach, duodenum, and rectum. However, there is limited direct intraluminal visualization of the gastrointestinal tract, which necessitates a complete endoscopic examination before its application. The working length of the GF-UM3 is 1230 mm, and the distal tip housing the transducer is 13 mm in diameter (Fig. 9–2). The angle of view is 80°, with a forward-oblique viewing direction of 65°. Distal tip angulation is possible in the up or down position to 130° and to 90° in the left or right position. A 2-mm channel is available for biopsies.

The ultrasound system uses a piezoelectric transducer that rotates at 7.0 cps. The radial scanner is driven by a flexible shaft extending from a motor contained proximally in the endoscope. The radial scanner provides a 360° view and is at right angles to the shaft of the endoscope. The frequencies used are usually higher than those used for transcutaneous ultrasonography. Two frequencies are available, 7.5 MHz and 12 MHz, by flicking the frequency switch, and the focusing points are 30 mm and 25 mm, respectively. There are provisions for the attachment of a balloon at the distal tip to

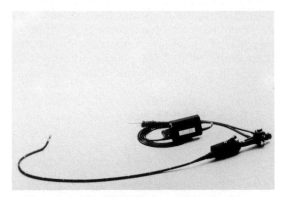

Figure 9–2. The GF-UM3 ultrasound endoscope.

cover the transducer so that de-aerated water can be used to maximize wave transmission and negate intestinal gas.

EU-M3 Endoscopic Ultrasound System

The EU-M3 endoscopic ultrasound system uses radial scanning with a rotating acoustical mirror and stationary transducer (Fig. 9–3). Radial scanning facilitates orientation within the body and provides a full 360° ultrasonic image. There is a choice between a 360° radial view and a 180° sectional view, forward and backward. The screen provides a bright, unflickering image and is graduated with a metric scale, simplifying the measurement of distances, area, and circumference. Data can be entered by the keyboard generator and displayed on the screen. The range of the monitored image can be adjusted from 6 to 18 cm. Gain and contrast knobs are located on the console for adjusting the intensity and contrast of the image. Partial modification of the echo volume is possible by using the sensitivity transducer control (STC) knob. If the sensitivity of the transducer is too high or

low, movement of the STC knob regulates the desired image strength. An image direction switch is used to reverse the right and left positions. The unit has freeze-frame capability, a special photographic monitor for polaroid film documentation, and capability for real-time documentation.

TECHNIQUE

The patient is prepared for endoscopy in the standard manner (see Chapter 4). A meticulous diagnostic endoscopic examination is performed first to delineate mucosal or intramural pathology, and biopsies and brushings are obtained at this time. After completing the diagnostic examination, the endoscope is withdrawn, and the GF-UM3 is inserted with digital guidance to assist passage of the rigid distal segment. The anticipated approach to existing pathology must be ascertained using the measurements on the working shaft of the instrument, because only a slide-by view is obtained with the forward-oblique viewing angle. The instrument is passed through the pylorus, using techniques similar to those employed during endoscopic retrograde cholangiopancreatography (ERCP). Seven standard viewing positions have been recommended for examination of the upper gastrointestinal tract: distal duodenum, duodenal papilla, duodenal bulb, gastric antrum, gastric corpus, gastric fundus, and distal esophagus (Fig. 9–4). Additional scanning positions may be necessary to define an area of specific interest.

The water-filled balloon method is used for studying the duodenum and esophagus, but direct apposition of the transducer in the esophagus is the optimal method for analysis in this area. The stomach is best studied by using the water immersion method, in which 300 to 500 mL of de-aerated water is placed in the lumen. When in position, the transducer is directed toward the target area, with an attempt to position the probe perpendicularly 3 cm from the area of interest. A multiecho pattern indicates an inadequate transducer–wall interface. The patient's position may be changed during the procedure to enhance transducer contact or to better image specific organs. Scan depths of 6, 9, 12, and 18 cm can be used. The 6-cm scan depth is best for esophageal, gastric, duodenal, and rectal wall imaging. The 9- and 12-cm ranges are best suited for visualizing retroperitoneal structures. A high-quality video recording of the real-time ultrasound examination is important, because it allows the examiner to document and

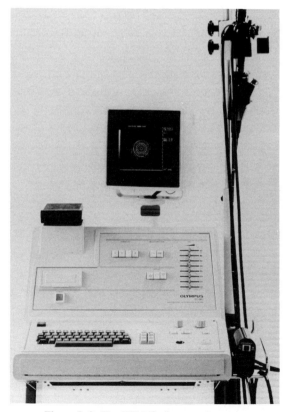

Figure 9–3. The EU-M3 ultrasound system.

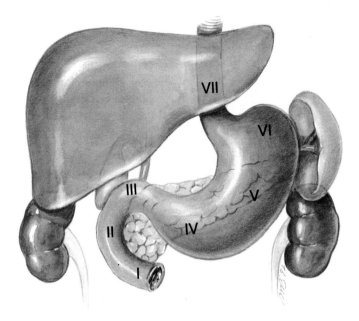

Figure 9–4. The seven standard positions necessary for a complete endoscopic ultrasound examination.

review findings, although polaroid documentation is also important for review purposes.

NORMAL GASTROINTESTINAL WALL MORPHOLOGY

High-frequency, high-resolution ultrasound produces precise images of the architecture of the gastrointestinal wall. Changes in wall thickness, obliteration of layers, and alterations in the characteristics of the tissue can be evaluated. EUS has repeatedly demonstrated a correlation between the imaged and the in vitro histologic five-layer structure of the gastrointestinal wall.[1-5] Figure 9–5 illustrates the wall morphology and corresponding ultrasound description. The first layer is echogenic and corresponds to the mucosa, and the second layer is hypoechoic and corresponds to the muscularis mucosae. A third echogenic layer is equivalent to the submucosa,

and the fourth hypoechoic stratum represents the muscularis propria. The fifth layer, which is hyperechoic, delineates the serosa (Fig. 9–6). Each histologic layer has been described as hyperechoic or hypoechoic, which is the ultrasound representation of interfaces between tissues of different densities.

Standard endoscopic evaluation of mucosal, submucosal, muscularis, and subserosal lesions is frequently not definitive. Biopsies are rarely diagnostic, particularly if the lesion is submucosal. Imaging modalities, including US, CT, plain films, and barium contrast studies, may

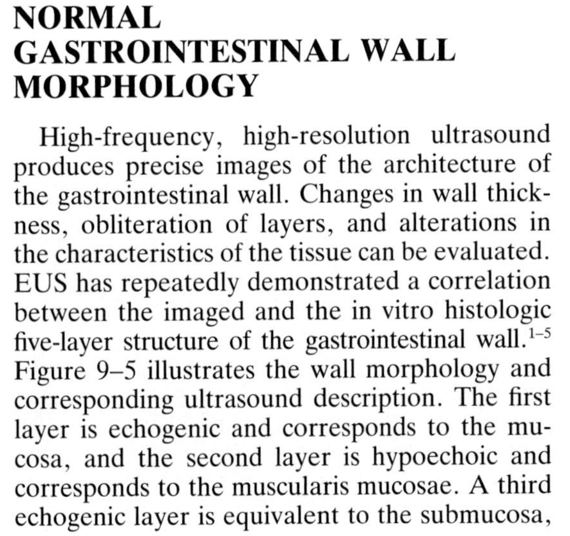

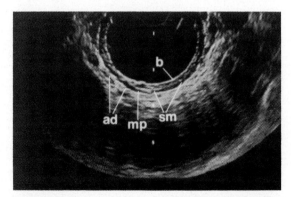

Figure 9–6. This endoscopic ultrasound examination illustrates the normal gastrointestinal wall architecture using the balloon method. The interface between the balloon (b) and mucosa is hyperechoic; the muscularis mucosa is hypoechoic; sm, submucosa (hyperechoic); mp, muscularis propria (hypoechoic); ad, serosa (hyperechoic). (From Tio T, Tytgat GNJ. Atlas of transintestinal ultrasonography. Aalsmeer, The Netherlands: Smith Kline and French, 1986.)

1st layer;
(border echo) } mucosa
2nd layer;
3rd layer; submucosa
4th layer; muscularis propria

5th layer; border echo + (serosa or adventitia)

Figure 9–5. Schematic illustration of the architecture of the gastrointestinal tract wall. The five layers are the morphologic equivalents to those seen by endoscopic ultrasound.

only suggest the presence of an intramural mass. EUS evaluation can, in a single examination, provide information not available from other imaging techniques. Although conventional imaging modalities may suggest intramural abnormalities if they are substantial in size, EUS can define the size, position, depth of wall penetration, and the margins of a lesion. The wall layer of origin may be delineated, suggesting a histologic diagnosis.

ENDOSCOPIC ULTRASONOGRAPHY OF THE UPPER GASTROINTESTINAL TRACT

Benign Lesions of the Esophagus and Stomach

Benign submucosal tumors are reasonably easy to recognize because of their well-defined margins, homogenicity, and absence of invasion into adjacent layers (Fig. 9–7). Yasuda and colleagues studied 83 patients with suspected intramural or extramural masses.[6] All submucosal tumors (50 patients) and extramural masses (33 patients) were diagnosed accurately. Through correlation with the examination of resected specimens, it was shown that EUS demonstrated the correct wall layer of origin in all cases. The researchers observed that differentiation between leiomyoma and leiomyosarcoma originating in the muscularis was difficult. EUS can also be used to delineate benign processes, such as polyps, varices, lipomas, aberrant pancreas, cysts, foveolar hyperplasia, and Menetrier's disease.[6–8] Before endoscopic resection of mucosal lesions, the vascularity and depth of invasion can be determined (Fig. 9–8). Tio and Tytgat[9] and Strohm and Classen[7] showed that the benignity of esophageal ulcers, Barrett's esophagus, and gastric ulcers could be determined by EUS (Fig. 9–9).

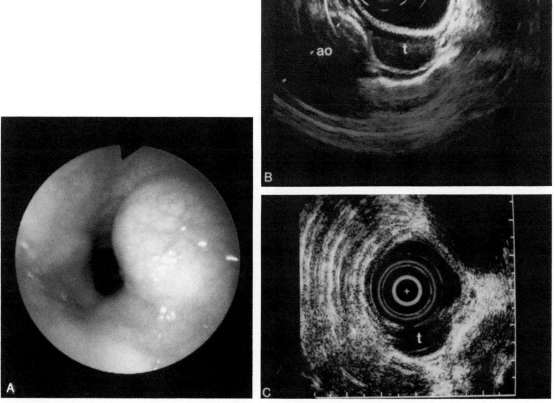

Figure 9–7. (A) An endoscopic view of a submucosal mass of the distal esophagus. **(B, C)** Endoscopic ultrasound demonstrates a homogeneous, well-demarcated mass in the esophageal wall. ao, aorta, t, tumor. (From Tio T, Tytgat GNJ. Atlas of transintestinal ultrasonography. Aalsmeer, The Netherlands: Smith, Kline and French, 1986.)

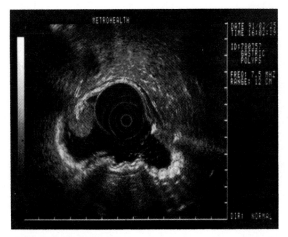

Figure 9–8. A large gastric polyp is shown by endoscopic ultrasound to be confined to mucosa and submucosa.

Figure 9–9. Endoscopic ultrasound demonstrates a small hypoechoic lesion in the mucosal and submucosal layers without penetration into the muscularis propria. u, ulcer; sm, submucosa; mp, muscularis propria. (From Tio T, Tytgat GNJ. Atlas of transintestinal ultrasonography. Aalsmeer, The Netherlands: Smith, Kline and French, 1986.)

Malignant Lesions of the Esophagus and Stomach

The extent of disease determines the likelihood of cure for patients with esophageal and gastric cancer. CT and transcutaneous ultrasonography have been used most frequently for preoperative staging. Many physicians display a nihilistic attitude about these malignancies. However, if a more aggressive approach consisting of surgery with or without preoperative chemotherapy or radiotherapy is to be adopted, more precise preoperative staging is mandatory. In most instances, the diagnosis of carcinoma is made by biopsy. In some cases, EUS may help

by demonstrating echogenic characteristics of malignancy.[9, 10] Inflammatory processes do not penetrate the muscularis propria, but malignancies commonly do. Benign and malignant lesions tend to be hypoechoic, but cancers are irregular, nodular, and invasive. The early cases of esophageal and gastric cancers are determined by their involvement of only the mucosa and submucosa (Fig. 9–10). Involvement of the muscularis propria indicates advanced disease as does the involvement of regional lymph nodes and adjacent structures (Fig. 9–11).

Spread to regional lymph nodes can be discerned by their hypoechoic pattern and sharp

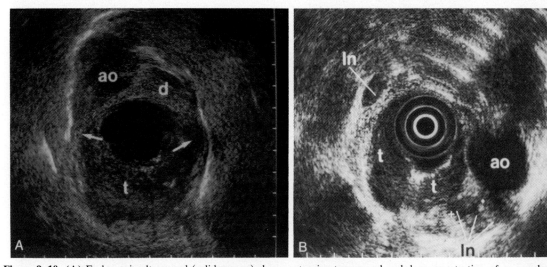

Figure 9–10. (A) Endoscopic ultrasound (solid arrows) shows extensive transmural and deep penetration of an esophageal tumor (t) into the adjacent diaphragm (d); ao, aorta. **(B)** Transmural invasion (t) with locoregional nodal metastases (ln) and apparent involvement of the aorta (ao) by an esophageal carcinoma. (From Tio T, Tytgat GNJ. Atlas of transintestinal ultrasonography. Aalsmeer, The Netherlands: Smith, Kline and French, 1986.)

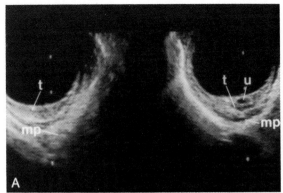 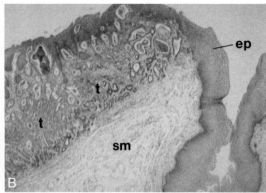

Figure 9–11. **(A)** On the left, endoscopic ultrasound demonstrates a superficial ulcerated (u) carcinoma of the esophagus (t) limited to the mucosa and submucosa. The muscularis propria (mp) is intact. **(B)** This figure depicts the histology from the resected specimen, showing extension into the submucosa (sm). t, tumor; ep, mucosa. (From Tio T, Tytgat GNJ. Atlas of transintestinal ultrasonography. Aalsmeer, The Netherlands: Smith, Kline and French, 1986.)

demarcation.[11, 12] Lymph nodes smaller than 5 mm in diameter may be imaged and are unlikely to be malignant.[11] Several series found that lymph nodes larger than 5 mm were positive for metastatic disease in 43% to 58% of patients.[11, 12] Ide[13] and Grimm[14] each identified mediastinal lymphadenopathy in 89% and 86% of patients, respectively. Lightdale demonstrated a concordance of 78% for EUS and 48% for dynamic CT when comparisons were made with surgical specimens.[15] A prospective study performed at the Memorial Sloan-Kettering Cancer Center compared preoperative staging of esophageal and gastric cancer using EUS, dynamic CT, and magnetic resonance imaging (MRI).[16] EUS was highly accurate in the assessment of depth of tumor invasion, with a sensitivity of 100%, compared with 80% for CT and 82% for MRI. EUS was slightly more sensitive (89%) in detecting lymph node metastases than CT (85%) or MRI (82%). A similar study performed by Tio and colleagues demonstrated the superiority of EUS over CT for the evaluation of depth of tumor invasion (89% vs. 59%) and assessment of regional lymph node metastases (80% vs. 51%) in patients with esophageal cancer.[17]

In a study by Lightdale, evaluation of the depth of tumor invasion in gastric cancers demonstrated a concordance with surgical pathology of 92% for EUS and 48% for CT.[18] In a prospective study, EUS was evaluated for use in diagnosing recurrences in the area of surgical anastomoses.[19] Twenty-one patients were studied with CT scans, which were considered to be negative. For the same patients, EUS had a sensitivity of 91% and specificity of 80% for diagnosing anastomotic recurrences.

Accurate staging of esophageal and gastric cancers by EUS may be thwarted by an existing stenosis, which prevents passage of the endoscope distal to the lesion. The ability to pass the endoscope beyond the lesion varies considerably (34–74%).[20, 21] Dilation of the stenotic area is possible but carries with it an increased risk of perforation.

EUS has been successful in demonstrating gastric wall abnormalities in patients with non-Hodgkin's lymphoma involving the stomach.[22] EUS was more accurate than endoscopy, barium meal, or CT in detecting and staging the tumors.[23] Nonresectability could reliably be determined before surgery based on detection of deep infiltration of the lesion into the surrounding structures. EUS was a sensitive modality for detection, staging, and follow-up after chemotherapy for non-Hodgkin's lymphoma (Fig. 9–12).

Endoscopic Ultrasound of the Pancreas and Biliary Tract

Pancreatic imaging, combining conventional ultrasonography, CT, pancreatography, and fine-needle aspiration is capable of delineating 90% to 95% of the abnormalities.[24] CT has been the best technique for defining the morphologic changes in severe pancreatitis but has an overall sensitivity of about 70% in chronic pancreatitis.[24] Although endoscopic retrograde pancreatography is the most specific method for diagnosing pancreatic ductal abnormalities, moderately severe parenchymal changes may exist with only minimal alterations in duct anatomy. EUS of the pancreas and biliary tract is difficult but potentially an extremely useful diagnostic modality because of its high-frequency

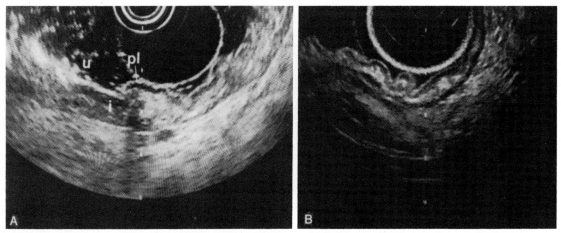

Figure 9–12. (A) Endoscopic ultrasound (EUS) may be useful for the staging of non-Hodgkin's lymphoma. This study demonstrates an ulcerative lesion (u), polypoid margins (pl), with transmural infiltration (i) and disruption of gastric wall architecture. **(B)** EUS may also be useful for follow-up after chemotherapy. This study shows the restoration of the normal gastric wall architecture after systemic chemotherapy. (From Tio T, Tytgat GNJ. Atlas of transintestinal ultrasonography. Aalsmeer, The Netherlands: Smith, Kline and French, 1986.)

resolution. The transduodenal and transgastric routes provide good access to the entire pancreas and biliary system.

Benign Lesions of the Pancreas

The endosonographic echo pattern of the normal pancreas is homogeneous and similar to that seen by conventional ultrasound. The pancreatic duct and side branches can also be visualized (Fig. 9–13). The best visualization of the pancreas is obtained from the duodenum, antrum, and body of the stomach. Lees applied EUS in 30 patients with suspected acute or chronic pancreatitis, and a definitive diagnosis was obtained for 23 patients.[24] For 7 patients, the study was a technical failure because it was impossible to advance the endoscope through the pylorus. Ten patients had a normal pancreatic tissue, evidenced by a smooth boundary, homogeneous texture, and normal ductal system. The ultrasound appearance of chronic pancreatitis was characterized by ductal changes that included increased caliber, irregularity of the lumen, visualization of ectatic side branches, increased echogenicity of the duct wall, increased thickness of duct wall echoes, intraluminal echoes, strictures, and pseudocyst for-

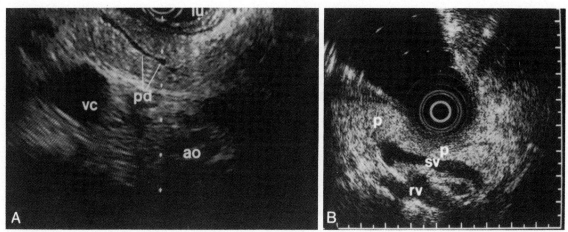

Figure 9–13. (A) A cross section through the stomach demonstrates a normal pancreas and pancreatic duct. Notice the homogeneous texture of the pancreas; vc, vena cava; pd, pancreatic duct; ao, aorta; lu = lumen. **(B)** The body and tail of the pancreas may be further visualized through the water-filled gastric corpus; p, pancreas; sv, splenic vein; rv, renal vien. (From Tio T, Tytgat GNJ. Atlas of transintestinal ultrasonography. Aalsmeer, The Netherlands: Smith, Kline and French, 1986.)

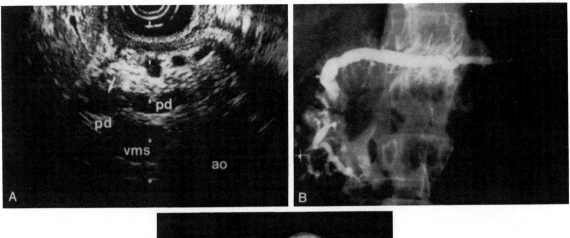

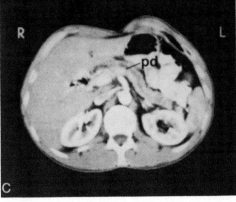

Figure 9–14. **(A)** Endoscopic ultrasound shows dilation of the pancreatic duct (pd), and the arrow points to an area of ductular narrowing. The ectatic side branches can be seen; ao, aorta; pd, pancreatic duct; vms, superior mesenteric vein. **(B)** The corresponding endoscopic retrograde cholangiopancreatogram demonstrates ductular narrowing in the pancreatic head with prestenotic dilatation. **(C)** The CT scan demonstrates ductular dilatation; pd, pancreatic duct. (From Tio T, Tytgat GNJ. Atlas of transintestinal ultrasonography. Aalsmeer, The Netherlands: Smith, Kline and French, 1986.)

mation (Fig. 9–14). In 6 patients, morphologic features such as periductal fibrosis, branch duct ectasia, and lobular inflammation were demonstrated by EUS and substantiated by operative specimens. Similar studies by Sivak[25] and Dancygier[26] have shown EUS to be a useful technique for visualizing benign morphologic changes of the pancreas. Dancygier also demonstrated the efficacy of EUS in diagnosing small benign tumors of the pancreas.[26]

Carcinoma of the Pancreas

There may be a role for EUS in the detection of pancreatic carcinomas while they are still small and resectable. Yasuda's study included 42 cases of pancreatic carcinoma with lesions as small as 2 cm identified.[27] Although thought to be as accurate as conventional ultrasound or CT for making the diagnosis of pancreatic cancer, these results have not been confirmed by prospective, randomized studies. In Sivak's series,

only 60% of pancreatic cancers were correctly diagnosed by EUS.[25] Technical problems accounted for the low diagnostic success rate. EUS may be more useful in accurately staging pancreatic carcinoma. Tio and Tytgat were able to determine the extent of disease and locoregional lymphadenopathy in 14 patients.[28] Carcinoma deeply infiltrating into surrounding structures and major blood vessels indicated nonresectability (Figs. 9–15 and 9–16). Clearly defined, well-circumscribed, hypoechoic tumors without distant lymphadenopathy indicated resectability (Fig. 9–17). Tio and colleagues staged 43 patients with a presumed diagnosis of pancreatic carcinoma after ERCP and EUS, with an overall accuracy for EUS of 92% when compared with the operative specimens.[29]

Lesions of the Biliary Tract

The optimal position for endosonography of the biliary tract is from the duodenum. Sonography of the papilla, gallbladder, and extrahe-

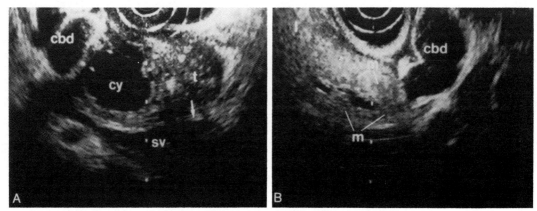

Figure 9–15. (A) Endoscopic ultrasound demonstrates an inhomogeneous tumor mass (t) with an anechoic cavity (cy) compressing the common bile duct (cbd). The tumor penetrates into the splenic vein (sv) *(arrow)*. **(B)** This figure illustrates a markedly dilated common bile duct (cbd) and probable liver metastases (m), which were subsequently found to be positive by aspiration cytology. (From Tio T, Tytgat GNJ. Atlas of transintestinal ultrasonography. Aalsmeer, The Netherlands: Smith, Kline and French, 1986.)

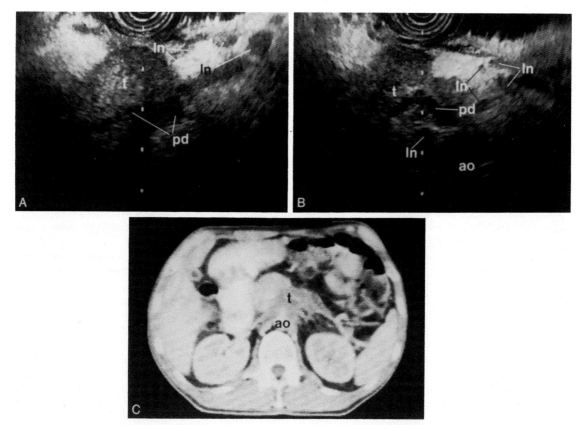

Figure 9–16. (A) Endoscopic ultrasound shows a round, hypoechoic mass (t) with compression of the pancreatic duct (pd); there are also enlarged lymph nodes (ln). **(B)** Another cross section demonstrates retroperitoneal spread adjacent to the aorta (ao), and positive lymph nodes (ln). **(C)** The corresponding CT scan shows a large pancreatic tumor (t) with involvement of the adjacent aorta (ao). (From Tio T, Tytgat GNJ. Atlas of transintestinal ultrasonography. Aalsmeer, The Netherlands: Smith, Kline and French, 1986.)

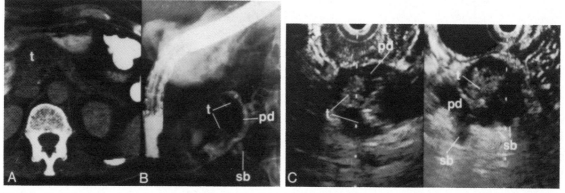

Figure 9–17. (A) CT scan showing enlargement of the pancreatic head suspicious for a malignancy (t). **(B)** An endoscopic retrograde cholangiopancreatogram demonstrating a dilated pancreatic duct (pd) with filling defects. **(C)** Endoscopic ultrasound scan showing an intraductular polypoid lesion (t) on a stalk originating from the wall of the pancreatic duct (pd); sb, side branches. (From Tio T, Tytgat GNJ. Atlas of transintestinal ultrasonography. Aalsmeer, The Netherlands: Smith, Kline and French, 1986.)

patic bile ducts is best performed using the balloon method. Yasuda reported 55 patients with disorders of the biliary tract and ampulla of Vater.[30] EUS was successful in visualizing the gallbladder (20 patients), extrahepatic bile ducts (23 patients), and papilla (12 patients). Seventeen tumors (i.e., 5 gallbladder, 5 common bile duct, 7 papilla) were correctly identified. Benign pathologic conditions (e.g., gallstones, cholesterolosis, polyps, papillitis) were also identified consistently. EUS was compared with conventional ultrasound, ERCP, CT, and angiography for the detection of tumors smaller than 30 mm in diameter. EUS interpretation was correct for 100% of patients, conventional ultrasound for

27%, ERCP for 100%, CT for 40%, and angiography for 36%.

EUS may also be useful in assessing the resectability of tumors of the bile duct and ampulla. Tio and Tytgat performed EUS in 20 patients with bile duct tumors (i.e., 12 proximal and 8 distal).[31] Endosonographic studies demonstrated intraductal masses, locoregional nodes, and infiltration of tumor into adjacent structures (Figs. 9–18 and 9–19). EUS accurately documented the extent of the tumor and the adjacent lymph node involvement as evidenced at the time of operation. EUS was complementary to ERCP and better than conventional ultrasound or CT for staging purposes.

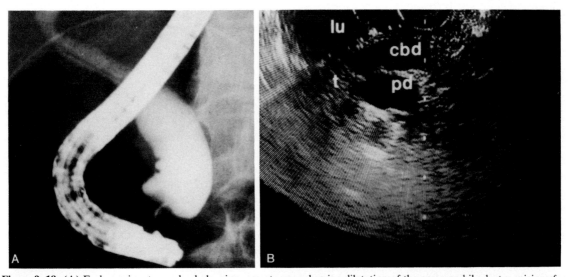

Figure 9–18. (A) Endoscopic retrograde cholangiopancreatogram showing dilatation of the common bile duct suspicious for a periampullary tumor. **(B)** Endoscopic ultrasound demonstrating dilatation of the common bile duct (cbd) and pancreatic duct (pd) due to a tumor mass (t) in the periampullary region; lu, lumen. (From Tio T, Tytgat GNJ. Atlas of transintestinal ultrasonography. Aalsmeer, The Netherlands: Smith, Kline and French, 1986.)

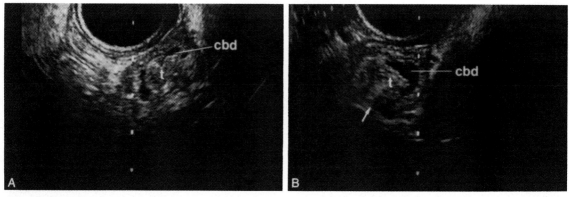

Figure 9–19. (A) A cross section through the distal common bile duct (cbd) showing an intraductular polypoid hypoechoic tumor (t), contrasting with the normal ductular wall on the contralateral side. **(B)** Another cross section demonstrates the tumor (t) originating from the common bile duct (cbd). (From Tio T, Tytgat GNJ. Atlas of transintestinal ultrasonography. Aalsmeer, The Netherlands: Smith, Kline and French, 1986.)

Tio and associates studied 33 patients preoperatively with EUS and correlated their results with the resected specimens according to the TNM (i.e., tumor, node, metastasis) classification.[32] The overall accuracy for common bile duct carcinoma and common hepatic duct carcinoma was 83% and 85%, respectively.

TRANSRECTAL ULTRASONOGRAPHY

The prognosis of rectal carcinoma has been correlated with the stage of the disease at the time of diagnosis. Preoperative staging traditionally relied on rectal examination, endoscopy, and CT. CT examination has various degrees of sensitivity in the staging of rectal cancer, ranging from 37% to 95%, and the accurate staging of the invasiveness of rectal carcinoma is less than optimal.[33–35] EUS initially was developed for the evaluation of prostatic and urinary tract malignancies.[36, 37] Transrectal ultrasonography was shown to be a more effective modality for the staging of rectal tumors, offering better information to determine the therapeutic approach (Fig. 9–20). A five-layer ultrasonographic pattern of the rectal wall has been documented experimentally and in vivo.[38] However, a limitation of transrectal ultrasonography is that 3- to 4-mm benign lymph nodes cannot be differentiated from pathologically involved nodes. Comparisons among blind transrectal ultrasound (BUS), ultrasound without

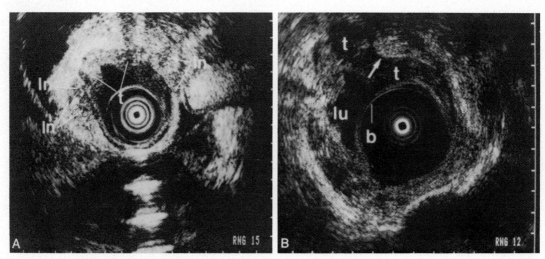

Figure 9–20. (A) This transrectal ultrasound scan demonstrates deep penetration of the tumor (t) into the perirectal fat. There are several enlarged lymph nodes (ln). **(B)** Transrectal ultrasound in this instance demonstrates a large mass (t) with penetration into the muscularis propria *(arrow)*. b, balloon; lu, lumen. (From Tio T, Tytgat GNJ. Atlas of transintestinal ultrasonography. Aalsmeer, The Netherlands: Smith, Kline and French, 1986.)

optics, and EUS have been performed. Each can provide clear visualization of the rectal wall and perirectal structures. Assessment of perirectal abnormalities may be superior using BUS because of the deeper penetration. The delineation of mucosal and submucosal lesions is diminished with BUS but is best seen with EUS because of the endoscopic guidance of the transducer. Adjacent lymph nodes appear to be better visualized by EUS.

Rifkin and colleagues compared endoscopic transrectal ultrasound with CT for the staging of invasive rectal cancer.[39] Fifty-one of 54 patients undergoing successful EUS also had CT scans. The rate of accurate demonstration of the tumor was 96% for EUS and 69% for CT. EUS also correctly identified perirectal fat invasion in 52 (96%) of 54 patients, but CT accurately delineated the pathology in only 55% of the patients. Lymph node status was accurately determined by EUS in 8 of 11 patients and by CT in 2 of 10 patients. Beynon and associates examined 100 patients with rectal adenocarcinoma preoperatively with EUS, and 50 patients also underwent CT examinations.[40] EUS was more accurate in detecting nodal involvement than CT (83% vs. 57%). The positive and negative predictive values for EUS were 78% and 89%, but for CT, they were 75% and 53%, respectively. Similar findings were confirmed by Tio and colleagues.[41]

THREE-DIMENSIONAL ENDOSCOPIC ULTRASOUND

Endoscopic ultrasound provides extraordinarily fine detail of gastrointestinal wall architecture and the association of adjacent structures to benign or malignant lesions. However, representation of ultrasound in real time or by still documentation is two dimensional. These two-dimensional images are abstract representations and may cause misinterpretation by the clinician. Three-dimensional (3D) imaging is relatively new and has been used in the planning of craniofacial surgery, neurosurgery, and orthopedic surgery.[42-44] Franceschi and coworkers applied 3D ultrasound in vascular surgery and demonstrated strong correlations with the pathologic specimens.[45] The same group applied 3D ultrasound to gastrointestinal neoplasms with remarkable results (Fig. 9–21).[46] There are several compelling aspects to this technique. After the image is created, the model may be cut and cross sections recreated in any plane, allowing for 3D visualization of invasion into adjacent structures (Fig. 9–22). Tumor volume in regional lymph nodes is thought to be a better predictor of long-term survival for patients with malignant melanoma.[47, 48] Tumor volume of gastrointestinal tumors can be determined preoperatively and provide additional or more accurate information relative to long-term survival than the currently employed parameters. Although work stations for 3D reconstruction of medical images has been costly, implementation of this system can now be done at a modest cost. Three-dimensional EUS of the gastrointestinal tract is experimental, but the potential for a more precise understanding of pathology exists.[45, 46]

CONCLUSION

EUS is a new technique that provides exceptional morphologic visualization of the gastrointestinal wall and adjacent structures. Imaging is performed from within the intestinal lumen,

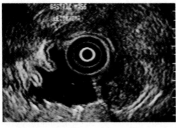 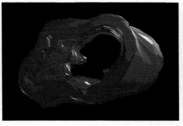 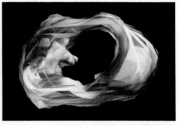

A   B   C

Figure 9–21. **(A)** Endoscopic ultrasound demonstrates a homogeneous and sharply demarcated submucosal mass in the stomach, typical for a leiomyoma. **(B)** This is an illustration of the three-dimensional reconstruction performed with computer enhancement. A suggestion of the lesion can be seen along the lesser curvature. **(C)** To better delineate the tumor, different shading techniques were used, and ultimately the stomach was rendered transparent and the tumor yellow. (From Franceschi D, Pritchard T, Eckhauser, M. Three dimensional reconstruction of gastrointestinal ultrasound. Surg Endosc, in press.)

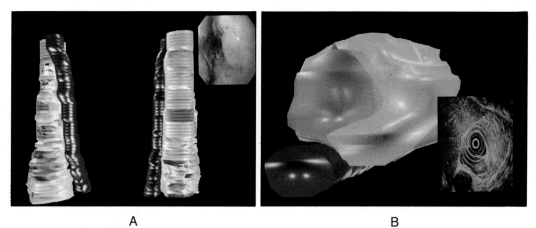

A   B

Figure 9–22. (A) This figure represents a reconstruction of an endoscopic ultrasound (EUS) scan performed to stage an esophageal carcinoma. An endoscopic view of the tumor can be seen in the inset. The reconstruction on the left is a view from the right side of the mediastinum. A view into the left mediastinum shows the large extent of tumor bulk (yellow) outside the esophagus. **(B)** Rotation of the reconstruction (rostral view) from the same patient. The inset represents a view of the EUS from which a part of the reconstruction was made. The tumor invades through the muscularis propria and abuts the aorta. The three-dimensional reconstruction demonstrates the extent of tumor outside the esophagus and its relationship to the aorta. (From Franceschi D, Pritchard T, Eckhauser, M. Three dimensional reconstruction of gastrointestinal ultrasound. Surg Endosc, in press.)

obviating some of the drawbacks encountered with its transcutaneous equivalent. EUS has demonstrated its efficacy over CT for the staging of gastrointestinal, biliary, and possibly pancreatic neoplasms. The anticipated refinement of the ultrasound probes and the computer-enhanced imaging will further increase our understanding of gastrointestinal disease processes.

References

1. Tio TL, Tytgat GNJ. Endoscopic ultrasonography of normal and pathologic upper gastrointestinal wall structure. Scand J Gastroenterol 21:27–33, 1986.
2. Silverstein F, Kimmey M, Martin R, Haggitt R, Mack L, Moss A, Franklin D. Ultrasound and the intestinal wall: experimental methods. Scand J Gastroenterol 21:34–40, 1986.
3. Aibe T, Fuji T, Okita K, Takemoto T. A fundamental study of normal layer structure of the gastrointestinal wall visualized by endoscopic ultrasonography. Scand J Gastroenterol 21:6–15, 1986.
4. Caletti GC, Bolondi L, Zani L, Labq G. Technique of endoscopic ultrasonography investigation: esophagus, stomach and duodenum. Scand J Gastroenterol 21:1–5, 1986.
5. Tanaka Y, Yasuda K, Aibe T, Fuji T, Kawai K. Anatomical and pathological aspects in ultrasonic endoscopy for GI tract. Scand J Gastroenterol 19:43–50, 1984.
6. Yasuda K, Nakajima M, Kawai K. Endoscopic ultrasonography in the diagnosis of submucosal tumor of the upper digestive tract. Scand J Gastroenterol 21:59–67, 1986.
7. Strohm WD, Classen M. Benign lesions of the upper GI tract by means of endoscopic ultrasonography. Scand J Gastrocnterol 21:41–46, 1986.
8. Gordon SJ, Rifkin MD, Goldberg BB. Endosonographic evaluation of mural abnormalities of the upper gastrointestinal tract. Gastrointest Endosc 32:193–198, 1986.
9. Tio TL, Tytgat GNJ. Endoscopic ultrasonography of normal and pathologic upper gastrointestinal wall structure. Comparison of studies in vivo and in vitro with histology. Scand J Gastroenterol 21:27–33, 1986.
10. Heyder N, Kaarmann H, Giedl J. Experimental investigations into the possibility of differentiating early from invasive carcinoma of the stomach by means of ultrasound. Endoscopy 19:228–232, 1987.
11. Tio TL, Tytgat GNJ. Endoscopic ultrasonography in analyzing periintestinal lymph node abnormality. Preliminary results of studies in vitro and in vivo. Scand J Gastroenterol 21:158–163, 1986.
12. Aibe T, Ito T, Yoshida T, et al. Endoscopic ultrasonography of lymph nodes surrounding the upper GI tract. Scand J Gastroenterol 21:164–169, 1966.
13. Ide H, Hanyu F, Murata Y, Fukui H, Ishii Y, Kaburagi Y, Yamada A. Multidisciplinary treatment of thoracic esophagus carcinoma based on preoperative staging. Gan To Kaguku Ryoho 15:589–596, 1988.
14. Grimm H, Sollano J, Hamper K, Noar M, Soehendra N. Endoscopic ultrasound (EUS) of esophago-gastric cancer: A new requirement for preoperative staging? Gastrointest Endosc 34:176–177, 1988.
15. Lightdale C, Botet J, Brennan M, et al. Endoscopic ultrasonography (EUS) compared to computerized tomography (CT) for pre-operative staging of gastric cancer. Gastrointest Endosc 35:154, 1989.
16. Botet JF, Lightdale CJ, Heelan RT, Brennan MF. Preoperative staging of esophageal cancer; comparison of endoscopic US and dynamic CT. Radiology 181:419–425, 1991.
17. Tio TL, Cohen PP, Coehne J, Udding FCA, Jager DH, Tytgat GNJ. Endosonography and computed tomography of esophageal carcinoma. Gastroenterol 96:1478–1486, 1989.
18. Lightdale CJ. Staging esophageal/gastric malignancy. Endoscopic ultrasonography update. New York: Olympus, 1988:58–61.

19. Lightdale CJ, Botet JF, Brennan MF, et al. Diagnosis of recurrent gastric cancer at the surgical anastomosis by endoscopic ultrasound. Gastrointest Endosc 34:179, 1988.

20. Dancygier H, Classen M. Endoscopic ultrasonography in esophageal diseases. Gastrointest Endosc 35:220–225, 1989.

21. Lightdale C, Botet J, Zauber A, Brennan M. Endoscopic ultrasonography compared to computed tomography for preoperative staging of esophageal cancer. Gastrointest Endosc 36:A191, 1990.

22. Tio TL, den Hartog Jager FC, Tytgat GNJ. Endoscopic ultrasonography of non-Hodgkin lymphoma of the stomach. Gastroenterology 91:401–409, 1986.

23. Tio TL, Jager DH, Tytgat GNJ. Endoscopic ultrasonography in detection and staging of gastric non-Hodgkin lymphoma. Scand J Gastroenterol 21:52–58, 1986.

24. Lees WR. Endoscopic ultrasonography of chronic pancreatitis and pancreatic pseudocysts. Scand J Gastroenterol 21:123–129, 1986.

25. Sivak MV, Kaufman A. Endoscopic ultrasonography of chronic pancreatitis in the differential diagnosis of pancreatic disease. Scand J Gastroenterol 21:130–134, 1986.

26. Dancygier H, Classen M. Endosonographic diagnosis of benign pancreatic and biliary lesions. Scand J Gastroenterol 21:119–122, 1986.

27. Yasuda K, Tanaka Y, Fujimoto S, et al. Use of endoscopic ultrasonography in small pancreatic cancer. Scand J Gastroenterol 21:143–150, 1986.

28. Tio TL, Tytgat GNJ. Endoscopic ultrasonography in staging local resectability of pancreatic and periampullary malignancy. Scand J Gastroenterol 21:135–142, 1986.

29. Tio TL, Tytgat GNJ, Cikot RJL, Houthoff HJ, Sars PRA. Ampullopancreatic carcinoma: preoperative TNM classification with endosonography. Radiology 175:455–461, 1990.

30. Yasuda K, Nakajima M, Kawai K. Technical aspects of endoscopic ultrasonography of the biliary system. Scand J Gastroenterol 21:143–150, 1986.

31. Tio TL, Tytgat GNJ. Endoscopic ultrasonography in staging local resectability of pancreatic and periampullary malignancy. Scand J Gastroenterol 21:135–142, 1986.

32. Tio TL, Cheng J, Wijers OB, Sars PRA, Tytgat GNJ. Endosonographic TNM staging of extrahepatic bile duct cancer: comparison with pathological staging. Gastroenterology 100:1351–1361, 1991.

33. Nicholls RJ, Mason AY, Morson BC, Dixon AK, Fry KI. The clinical staging of rectal cancer. Br J Surg 69:404–409, 1982.

34. Meyer JE, Dosoretz DE, Gunderson LL, Stark P, Kipans DB. CT evaluation of locally advanced carcinoma of the distal colon and rectum. J Comput Assist Tomogr 7:265–267, 1983.

35. Dixon AK, Fry KI, Morson BC, Nicholls RJ, Mason AY. Pre-operative computed tomography of carcinoma of the rectum. Br J Radiol 54:655–659, 1981.

36. Watanabe H, Mishina T, Ohe H. Staging of bladder tumors by transrectal ultrasonotomography and UI Octoson. Urol Radiol 5:11–16, 1983.

37. Rifkin MD, Kurtz AB, Choi HY, Goldberg BB. Endoscopic ultrasonic evaluation of the prostate using a transrectal probe: prospective evaluation and acoustic characterization. Radiology 149:265–271, 1983.

38. Boscaini M, Montori A. Transrectal ultrasonography: interpretation of normal intestinal wall structure for the preoperative staging of rectal cancer. Scand J Gastroenterol 1986;21:87–98.

39. Rifkin MD, McGlynn ET, Marks G. Endorectal sonographic prospective staging of rectal cancer. Scand J Gastroenterol 21:99–103, 1986.

40. Beynon J, McC Mortensen NJ, Foy DMA, Channer JL, Rigby H, Virjee J. Preoperative assessment of mesorectal lymph node involvement in rectal cancer. Br J Surg 76:276–279, 1989.

41. Tio TL, Coene PP, van Deiden OM, Tytgat GNJ. Coloretal carcinoma: preoperative TNM classification with endosonography. Radiology 4:165–170, 1991.

42. Koltai PJ, Wood GW. Three-dimensional CT reconstruction for the evaluation and surgical planning of facial fractures. Otolaryngol Head Neck Surg 95:10–15, 1986.

43. Virapongse C, Shapiro M, Gmitro A, Sarwar M. Three-dimensional computed tomographic reformation of the spine, skull, and brain from axial images. Neurosurgery 18:53–58, 1986.

44. Grasso G, Andreoni A, Romeo N, Cipriano R, Uzzielli G. Recent developments in imaging diagnosis in fractures of the acetabulum: the role of CAT and tridimensional reconstruction. Ital J Orthop Traumatol 16:79–91, 1990.

45. Franceschi D, Bondi JA, Rubin JR. A new approach for three-dimensional reconstruction of arterial ultrasonography. J Vasc Surg 15:800–804, 1992.

46. Franceschi D, Pritchard TJ, Eckhauser ML. Three dimensional reconstruction of gastrointestinal ultrasound. Surg Endosc (in press).

47. Cochran AJ, Wen D, Morton DL. Management of the regional lymph nodes in patients with cutaneous malignant melanoma. World J Surg 16:214–221, 1992.

48. Friedman RJ, Rigel DS, Kopf AW, et al. Volume of malignant melanoma is superior to thickness as a prognostic indicator. Preliminary observation. Dermatol Clin 9:643–648, 1991.

10

Endoscopic Management of Esophageal Varices

Greg V. Stiegmann

During the past decade, endoscopic therapy became the treatment of choice for bleeding esophageal varices in many medical centers. Surgical and radiologic treatments assumed secondary roles and were usually reserved only for patients who failed endoscopic treatment or for those who lived long distances from the treatment facility. Introduction of new endoscopic methods expanded the potential of endoscopic therapy. This chapter examines the endoscopic treatment techniques available in the United States for bleeding esophageal varices and compares results of such treatment with results of other therapy.

DEVELOPMENT OF ENDOSCOPIC THERAPY

Endoscopic treatment of esophageal varices was first performed in 1936 by Crafoord and Frenckner, who used quinine-uretan to inject and successfully treat the bleeding varices of a 19-year-old girl with portal vein thrombosis.[1] Clinical introduction of the portacaval shunt in the 1940s distracted interest from endoscopic treatment. Macbeth in Britain, Fearon and Sass-Kortsak in Canada, and Wodak in Austria continued to employ endoscopic sclerotherapy in the 1950s and 1960s.[2-4] Fearon and Sass-Kortsak demonstrated that sclerotherapy was useful for children with variceal hemorrhage, and Wodak introduced paravariceal injection techniques.[3, 4] Dissatisfaction with shunt and devascularization operations appeared in the 1970s. Interest in endoscopic sclerotherapy reemerged in 1973, when Johnston and Rodgers reported a 93%

success rate in controlling bleeding varices in 117 patients using sclerotherapy.[5] Wodak, Paquet, and Terblanche each presented convincing evidence that endoscopic sclerotherapy was a useful treatment for bleeding varices.[6-8]

Flexible endoscopes entered clinical use in the 1970s, and by the mid-1980s, flexible endoscopic sclerotherapy was widely employed for treatment of bleeding varices. Several controlled clinical trials compared sclerotherapy with medical or operative treatments.[9-20] Three new forms of endoscopic therapy were introduced during this decade. Endoscopic laser coagulation of varices was attempted and abandoned.[21] Endoscopic polymer injections were shown to be effective for control of active bleeding, although these methods have yet to be employed clinically in the United States.[22, 23] Mechanical endoscopic ligation of varices was introduced in 1986 in an attempt to provide a safer and more effective endoscopic treatment than injection sclerotherapy.[24]

ANATOMIC CONSIDERATIONS

Most variceal hemorrhage occurs in the distal esophagus, usually within 5 cm of the gastroesophageal junction. Bleeding from varices in the gastric fundus is the second most likely site and may occur in as many as 10% of patients.[25] Anatomic studies have shown that four layers of veins and a series of perforating veins constitute the venous drainage of the lower esophagus.[26-30] The deep and superficial submucosal channels normally travel through the submucosa of the stomach and esophagus beneath the muscularis mucosae. Just above the gastroesophageal junction, the veins of the submucosa traverse the muscularis mucosae and come to lay superficially covered only by the esophageal mucosal epithelium. This superficial location is maintained for a cephalad distance of 1 to 4 cm, at which point the vessels return to their normal location beneath the muscularis mucosae.

In portal hypertension, all of the venous channels in and around the distal esophagus are dilated. Kitano and colleagues showed that the deep submucosal veins enlarge to become giant varices.[27] Variceal bleeding is more common in the distal esophagus, because varices in this area are less protected than in other areas of the gastrointestinal tract. Major variceal hemorrhage may follow rupture of an enlarged deep submucosal channel (*i.e.,* varix). Lesser hemorrhage, which ceases spontaneously, may occur from the dilated intraepithelial or superficial submucosal veins.[27, 28] Perforating vessels that connect the paraesophageal veins with the intrinsic veins of the esophagus may contribute to massive hemorrhage and appear to play a role in the recurrence of varices in patients who have achieved initial eradication of varices by endoscopic methods.

ENDOSCOPIC SCLEROTHERAPY

Bleeding from esophageal varices may be controlled by injecting sclerosant directly into the venous channel (*i.e.,* intravariceal method), beside the channel (*i.e.,* paravariceal method), or a combination of both. Paravariceal sclerotherapy was described by Wodak and is employed by many European and Japanese endoscopists.[4, 6] Wodak thought esophagogastric varices helped decompress the portal venous system and that a protective fibrous cover could be induced by sclerotherapy to ensheath varices and prevent them from bleeding while permitting them to serve as collateral channels. Paravariceal injection is performed by injecting multiple aliquots (≤1 mL) of sclerosant on both sides of variceal channels in the distal 5 to 10 cm of the esophagus (Fig. 10–1). As many as 40 injections are made at 1-cm intervals from the gastroesophageal junction proximally.

Most North American endoscopists use direct intravariceal injections, performed by placing 1 to 5 mL of sclerosant into the lumen of the varix (Fig. 10–2). Injections are performed at or just above the gastroesophageal junction. Some endoscopists perform a second, more proximal

injection during the same treatment session. The goal of intravariceal sclerotherapy is thrombosis of the varix. Both paravariceal and intravariceal injection techniques are clinically effective, and only one study demonstrated superiority of one over the other.[31, 32] Sanowski and coworkers attempted intravariceal injections using sclerosant combined with radiopaque contrast agents followed by serial roentgenograms.[33] Forty-four percent of injections resulted in accumulation of contrast agent in the esophageal wall. Rose and colleagues reported similar findings with a greater propensity to use paravariceal injections if the injected varix was small.[34] The intravariceal injections demonstrated rapid passage of the contrast agent in a cephalad (42%) or caudad (14%) direction. These findings confirmed earlier work by Barsoum and indicate a potential cause of failure in the intravariceal technique in addition to the potential for complications resulting from systemic dissemination of sclerosant.[35]

Tetradecyl sodium (1–3% solution), sodium morrhuate (5% solution), and ethanolamine oleate (5% solution) are the most commonly employed sclerosing agents in the United States. Outside North America, ethanolamine oleate (5% solution) and polidocanol (1% solution) are used; polidocanol is usually employed for

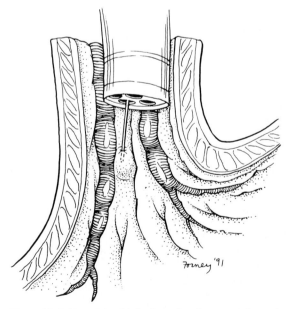

Figure 10–1. Paravariceal injection sclerotherapy performed with a flexible endoscope. The endoscopist injects small aliquots of sclerosant beside varices to induce a sheath of fibrous tissue around the veins to prevent bleeding. (From Stiegmann GV, Yamamoto M. Approaches to the endoscopic treatment of esophageal varices. World J Surg 16:1034–1041, 1992.)

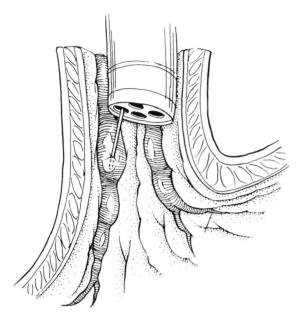

Figure 10–2. Intravariceal injection sclerotherapy performed with the flexible endoscope. The endoscopist injects up to 5 mL of sclerosant directly into the lumen of each esophageal varix. The goal of intravariceal therapy is thrombosis of the vein. (From Stiegmann GV, Yamamoto M. Approaches to the endoscopic treatment of esophageal varices. World J Surg 16:1034–1041, 1992.)

paravariceal injections. Tetradecyl sodium is a potent endothelial toxin that destroys the integrity of the endothelium and exposes highly thrombogenic subendothelial tissue.[36] Tetradecyl sodium in low concentrations may inactivate the physiologic anticoagulant protein C and cause platelet aggregation. Tetradecyl sodium was shown superior to sodium morrhuate and ethanolamine in two rodent studies.[37, 38] Jensen's group, in studies using dogs, found that ethanolamine, 95% ethanol, and 1.5% tetradecyl sodium were the most effective thrombogenic agents.[39–41] This group demonstrated ulcerations at the injection site in 90% of sites treated with 95% ethanol, 40% of sites treated with 1.5% tetradecyl sodium, 30% of sites treated with 5% sodium morrhuate, and at 10% of sites treated with a combination sclerosant consisting of 1% tetradecyl sodium, 32% ethanol, and saline. The most effective thrombogenic agents appear to result in the highest incidence of treatment site ulceration and have the greatest potential for producing complications, such as stricture and necrosis of the esophageal wall.

A trial by Kitano demonstrated the clinical superiority of ethanolamine oleate over polidocanol in reducing the incidence of rebleeding from sclerotherapy-induced ulcers and the number of treatment sessions required to eradicate varices.[42] Mortality rates between treatment groups did not differ. These researchers also compared ethanolamine with 2% tetradecyl sodium and found ethanolamine superior to the tetradecyl sodium solution but were unable to demonstrate a difference in mortality between the two treatment groups.[43] Sarin's group compared absolute ethanol with 50% ethanol and found that varices could be eradicated with fewer endoscopic sessions using absolute alcohol, but there was no significant difference in complications, rebleeding, or mortality rates between the two agents.[44] Lyons and colleagues found that patients treated with a combination sclerosant consisting of tetradecyl sodium, thrombin, and cefazolin fared better with regard to transfusion requirements and length of hospital stay than did those treated with 1% tetradecyl sodium.[45] None of these trials demonstrated a survival advantage for any sclerosant regimen. I recommend the endoscopist performing sclerotherapy select one of the available agents and become familiar with its characteristics and limitations. My colleagues and I currently employ 5% ethanolamine oleate.

Rigid endoscopic sclerotherapy is done with a large-caliber endoscope that has a longitudinal slot in the distal end to allow the varix to protrude into the lumen of the instrument. After injection, the endoscope is rotated to compress and tamponade the injected varix. The adjacent varix, which protrudes into the slot at the end of the instrument is then injected, and the process is repeated until all varices are treated. Bornman and associates showed there was no advantage to rigid endoscopic sclerotherapy compared with flexible endoscopic methods.[46] Increased risk of general anesthesia in the patient with compromised hepatic function and the greater chance for mechanical perforation with the rigid instrument offset any other benefits associated with the original technique of sclerotherapy. Rigid endoscopic sclerotherapy remains an effective method with which to treat infants and children in whom a general anesthetic is required regardless of the instrumentation employed.[47]

Flexible endoscopic sclerotherapy is performed in the awake, sedated patient. Those with active bleeding may benefit from use of an endoscopic overtube, which is preloaded over the endoscope before insertion of the endoscope into the esophagus. After visual confirmation that the endoscope is positioned in the patient's esophagus, the overtube is advanced into the esophagus using the endoscope as an obturator. The overtube allows multiple insertions and withdrawals of the endoscope, facilitates lavage of blood from the stomach and esophagus, and protects the patient's airway from tracheal aspiration.

Patients who are actively bleeding require precise delineation of the bleeding site. Examination of the esophagus, stomach, and duodenum is performed in all patients, with exception of those undergoing elective repeat treatment aimed at eradication of varices. Inspection of the body and fundus of the stomach should be performed at each elective endoscopic treatment session to detect development of gastric varices. Esophageal varices in a patient with upper gastrointestinal hemorrhage does not exclude other nonvariceal sources of bleeding, which must be carefully sought. In the patient with active or recent upper gastrointestinal bleeding, the detection of varices and identification of no other identifiable source of bleeding presumes a variceal source of hemorrhage.

Injection of varices in nonactively bleeding patients is begun near the gastroesophageal junction. In an actively bleeding patient with a discretely identified bleeding site, the actively bleeding varix, regardless of location, is treated first with insertion of the needle and injection of sclerosant below the site of bleeding if possible. The needle is inserted directly into the varix, and 1 to 5 mL of sclerosant are injected. Injections are continued at or near the gastroesophageal junction, beginning with the most gravity-dependent varix and proceeding in circumferential fashion to the least dependent. Three to five channels usually exist, and each should be treated with 1 to 5 mL of sclerosant. During a properly performed intravariceal injection, the varix should slowly balloon and blanch. Very rapid ballooning indicates that the sclerosant is being placed too superficially, between the epithelium and the variceal wall. Injections in this plane have the potential to result in ulceration over a nonthrombosed varix, which may result in delayed bleeding.

After completion of the injections at the gastroesophageal junction, the endoscope is retracted from 2 to 5 cm and the process repeated. Injections should not be done in the middle or proximal esophagus, because sclerosant may escape rapidly from a large varix into the azygos system and then into the pulmonary circulation.[48] Large volumes of sclerosant are usually required only at the first or second endoscopic treatment sessions. Progressively smaller volumes are needed as the varices diminish in size. The total sclerosant volume should seldom exceed 20 mL per treatment session or 5 mL per individual varix.

Elective endoscopic retreatment aimed at eradication of varices from the distal esophagus is often begun during the same hospitalization as for the acute bleed. Complete eradication of varices is desirable, but reduction of variceal channels to small venules is equally effective in preventing recurrent hemorrhage. Most investigators report an average of five to six endoscopic sessions are required to achieve eradication.[49] Most recurrent bleeds in sclerotherapy-treated patients occur before eradication of varices in the distal esophagus. Expeditious eradication of varices should result in a lower incidence of recurrent variceal hemorrhage. Two prospective trials compared 1-week intervals of repeat injections with 3-week intervals. Sarin and associates demonstrated a lower incidence of rebleeding and shorter time to initial variceal obliteration in patients treated at weekly intervals.[50] Westaby and colleagues were unable to demonstrate a significant difference in the incidence of recurrent hemorrhage and found that weekly treatments had to be postponed in 68% of patients during their study because of extensive mucosal ulceration.[51] High-risk (i.e., Child-Pugh C) patients were at greater risk for ulcer formation in this study, and our experience confirms a greater risk for deep mucosal ulceration and esophageal wall injury in these patients.[52] Flexibility in scheduling repeat endoscopic sclerotherapy is indicated. My colleagues and I frequently treat good-risk patients (i.e., Child-Pugh A and B) and those who appear less likely to adhere to a more protracted schedule of repeat injections on a 7- to 14-day cycle until varices are small or are completely eradicated.

Endoscopic sclerotherapy was compared with medical therapy in five prospective randomized trials that assessed control of acute bleeding and in eight that assessed long-term therapy and follow-up. Six trials compared operative treatment with sclerotherapy. Four of the five studies that compared sclerotherapy with medical management for the acute treatment of variceal bleeding demonstrated no advantage for sclerotherapy-treated patients in terms of prevention of early (i.e., within 40 days of index treatment) recurrent bleeding or improved survival.[9, 13, 14, 16, 53] Endoscopic sclerotherapy as employed in these trials does not appear to confer measurable advantage early in the course of variceal hemorrhage.[53]

Results of eight trials that compared serial endoscopic sclerotherapy with medical management for long-term treatment of variceal hemorrhage are summarized in Table 10–1. Survival in sclerotherapy-treated patients was significantly better than in medically treated patients in five trials, and the incidence of

Table 10–1. COMPARISON OF SERIAL SCLEROTHERAPY WITH MEDICAL THERAPY FOR LONG-TERM TREATMENT OF VARICEAL HEMORRHAGE

Investigation	Group	No. of Patients	No. Who Rebled	Rebleeding Episodes	Survival (%)
Barsoum[9]	ES	50	29*		70*
	C	50	13		48
Copenhagen[16]	ES	48	15	24*	68*
Early survivors	C	52	31	101	50
El-Zayadi[11]	ES	63	12*		85*
	C	55	18		71
Korula[12]	ES	63			50
	C	57			40
Paquet[13]	ES	21	4		67*
	C	22	7		33
Soderlund[14]	ES	57	32	50*	49
	C	50	33	99	34
Terblanche[17]	ES	37	14	43*	38
	C	38	20	73	37
Westaby[20]	ES	56	31	66*	68*
	C	60	49	125	47

Abbreviations: ES, endoscopic sclerotherapy; C, control.
*Significant differences between study cohorts.

recurrent bleeding was less in sclerotherapy-treated patients in four trials. The Cape Town study did not demonstrate improved survival, but patients in the control arm of that trial were treated with acute sclerotherapy to control active bleeding and then compared with the chronic sclerotherapy patients, who received acute therapy for active bleeding and chronic sclerotherapy to eradicate varices.[17] This trial suggested that results of "on demand" sclerotherapy treatment were similar to those of planned retreatment—an issue still not completely settled. Soderland and coworkers were unable to demonstrate a survival advantage in sclerotherapy-treated patients despite a significant reduction in the incidence of recurrent hemorrhage in that group, suggesting that death from hepatic failure or causes other than hemorrhage may play an important role in outcome.[14] Results from seven of the long-term studies cited have been assessed by meta-analysis.[54] Data from these trials indicated that endoscopic sclerotherapy, when compared with medical management, reduced the number of deaths by 15% to 25%.

Six prospective trials compared sclerotherapy with operative treatment.[10, 15, 18, 19, 55, 56] Cello's study was restricted to high-risk patients, and the surgical treatment consisted of portacaval shunt placement.[10] Planas' trial also employed central shunts but was not restricted to high-risk patients.[55] Cello's data initially suggested an economic advantage for sclerotherapy-treated patients, but this advantage diminished with time as many patients in the sclerotherapy arm rebled. Neither study showed one treatment superior to the other. The remaining trials compared patients initially treated by sclerotherapy with those initially treated with selective splenorenal shunt operations. Patients who failed sclerotherapy (definitions of failure varied) were submitted to salvage selective shunt operations. The incidence of salvage operations was higher in the Atlanta study than in the others.[19] The Atlanta data showed that survival and preservation of hepatic function were superior in patients initially treated with sclerotherapy, despite the fact that 31% eventually required a shunt operation. The Omaha and Barcelona groups did not demonstrate superiority of one technique over the other with regard to survival or preservation of hepatic function.[15, 18] Rikkers' group found costs between the two treatments to be similar and further emphasized the importance of proximity to treatment for patients undergoing sclerotherapy.[18] Several sclerotherapy patients who lived long distances from the treatment center experienced rebleeding and failed to make the trip in time for salvage therapy.

Endoscopic sclerotherapy is associated with a high incidence of minor complications (*i.e.*, those producing discomfort or symptoms but not requiring active treatment or prolonged hospitalization) and a significant incidence of major ones. Complications associated with sclerotherapy may occur as a result of the endoscopic procedure itself or of the injected sclerosant. Early local complications include mechanical perforation of the esophagus, which is seldom associated with injections performed using the flexible endoscope, but more often associated with the rigid endoscope.[15, 18] Aspiration pneumonia is more likely to occur in the setting of active variceal hemorrhage and may be prevented if endotracheal intubation or an endoscopic overtube is used. The overall incidence of pulmonary effects associated with sclerotherapy may reach 60% to 79%.[57] Most of the x-ray changes consisted of effusions, infiltrates, atelectasis, and mediastinal enlargement, which resolved without treatment. More serious pulmonary problems, including the adult respiratory distress syndrome, have been associated with sclerotherapy, but the incidence is low.[58] Temporary deterioration of pulmonary function after sclerotherapy using ethanolamine oleate was observed by Kitano and found to resolve within 7 days.[48] Other clinical investigations of pulmonary function in patients treated with tetradecyl sodium and sodium morrhuate failed to detect appreciable abnormalities.[59, 60]

Systemic effects of injected sclerosant include chest pain and fevers. Fever does not appear related to bacteremia, which occurs in 5% to 10% of patients.[61, 62] Sclerotherapy-associated bacteremia is not a significant hazard to most patients, but those who have prosthetic heart valves or other implanted devices (e.g., Denver shunt) should receive prophylactic antibiotic therapy. Some evidence points to a greater risk of bacterial peritonitis in patients with ascites treated with sclerotherapy, but these observations need confirmation.[63] Thrombotic complications, including paralysis resulting from thrombosis of the anterior spinal artery and portal and mesenteric venous thrombosis have been reported in a few cases.[64–66] Caletti and colleagues performed ultrasound examination of the portal venous system in 25 patients before initiation of sclerotherapy and after obliteration of their varices. They demonstrated no evidence of thrombosis or alteration in the caliber of the portal venous system.[67] In contrast, Hunter and coworkers observed portal vein thrombosis in 36% of a small series of patients who had undergone sclerotherapy and found histologic changes of intimal thickening of the portal vein in most of those in whom the portal vein remained patent. Controls had only a 10% incidence of these findings.[68] Studies by Jensen suggested a beneficial effect of sclerotherapy on portal hemodynamics, with sclerotherapy-treated portal hypertensive pigs demonstrating increased portal flow compared with control animals.[69] Korula and associates found portal pressure increased in response to eradication of varices in some patients but decreased in others, suggesting the effects of treatment may vary between patients.[70]

Ulceration at the site of injection occurs frequently and is more common in high-risk patients.[71] Shallow ulcers may signify an effective injection and are seen in as many as 94% of patients who have endoscopic reexamination of the esophagus within 24 hours and as many as 80% of those examined within 1 week after sclerotherapy.[50, 51, 72] Hemorrhage from sclerotherapy-induced ulcers or mucosal sloughing has been reported in 2% to 13% of patients.[73] Deep ulceration is associated with formation of esophageal strictures, a complication that occurs in 10% to 20% of patients undergoing serial sclerotherapy. Most sclerotherapy-induced strictures respond to bougienage. Deep ulcers often represent partial- or full-thickness esophageal wall necrosis, which may result in perforation. Esophageal necrosis and perforation occur in 1% to 6% of patients and should be suspected if persistent chest pain and pleural effusions develop after sclerotherapy. If suspected, water-soluble contrast studies should be done to determine if a leak exists. If contrast is visualized outside of the esophageal lumen and is contained in a cavity that drains freely back into the esophagus, conservative therapy with antibiotics, nasogastric drainage, and closed-tube thoracostomy is indicated and often successful. Free perforation is treated by thoracotomy and drainage, with or without esophagogastric exclusion.

The long-term sequelae of sclerotherapy include effects on esophageal motility and the potential for developing cancer. Abnormalities in esophageal motility and in lower esophageal sphincter pressures have been observed in some postsclerotherapy manometric studies.[74–76] Despite frequent esophageal strictures, sclerotherapy appears to result in little demonstrable long-lasting adverse effect on esophageal function. Six patients have developed carcinoma of the esophagus after serial sclerotherapy treatments.[77–79] Most had several other risk factors for developing this malignancy, and no conclusions regarding cause and effect can be drawn.

Prevention of the first variceal bleed is the goal of prophylactic sclerotherapy. Two thirds of patients with varices may never bleed, and preventive treatment of cirrhotics with varices who have never bled must be targeted at patients who are at high risk for bleeding.[80–82]

Three trials have shown a reduction in mortality in sclerotherapy-treated patients who had never bled compared with a medically treated cohort.[83–85] Two of the studies have been criticized because of a higher than expected incidence of hemorrhage in control patients and failure to employ the best available method of treatment in control patients who did bleed.[81] The third trial of Piai and colleagues consisted predominantly of patients with nonalcoholic cirrhosis and showed the benefit of prophylactic sclerotherapy only in high-risk (*i.e.,* Child B and C) patients.[84] Other trials and a meta-analysis demonstrated limited or no survival advantage for patients who had prophylactic treatment.[86–89] The Veterans Affairs Trial of prophylactic sclerotherapy compared with sham sclerotherapy was halted after interim analysis showed almost twice the mortality in patients who were treated with sclerotherapy.[87] Accurate identification of the patient who is at high risk for a first variceal bleed is not yet possible, and prophylactic sclerotherapy does not appear justified.

ENDOSCOPIC VARICEAL LIGATION

Endoscopic ligation of bleeding varices is performed using a device that is similar in concept to those employed for elastic band ligation of internal hemorrhoids. Endoscopic variceal ligation is done in a manner similar to sclerotherapy.[90] Survey esophagoscopy or esophagogastroduodenoscopy is done before attaching the device to the endoscope. An endoscopic overtube is inserted during the initial survey examination. After determining that varices are to be treated, the endoscope is removed and the ligating device attached. The first sites selected for ligation are the most distal. Subsequent ligations are done to adjacent varices at the same level or more proximally. The operator approaches the target varix under direct vision and positions the end of the ligating device in full 360° contact with the varix to be treated (Fig. 10–3). Endoscopic suction is activated, drawing the target tissue into the banding cylinder. When the banding cylinder is almost or completely filled, the operator pulls the trip wire, which is connected to the inner cylinder and runs through the endoscope working channel, moving the banding (inner) cylinder toward the endoscope and releasing the elastic "O" ring around the base of the target. After release of the endoscopic suction, the ligated varix is discharged from the banding cylinder. The endoscope is withdrawn, the spent inner cylinder removed and discarded, and a fresh inner cylinder loaded into the device. The endoscope is reinserted, and the process repeated until all variceal tissue in the distal 5 to 10 cm of the esophagus is treated. Five to eight individual ligations are done during the initial treatment in patients with large varices. Progressively fewer ligations are required during elective retreatments as the varices diminish in size and number. Actively bleeding varices are treated first if the site of bleeding can be defined. The endoscopist approaches the target and ligates the bleeding site, after which other channels are treated as previously described.

The effects of endoscopic variceal ligation on the esophagus and on varices were examined using the Jensen portal hypertensive canine model.[40, 91] Three to 7 days after ligation of varices, sloughing of the ligated tissue and shallow ulcers were observed at all treatment sites. Fourteen to 21 days after treatment, there were minimal residual varices and no evidence of full-thickness esophageal injury. Sites of previous shallow ulcers appeared healed, and microscopy showed full-thickness replacement of vascular structures in the submucosa with maturing scar tissue. An intense inflammatory response was observed, and reepithelialization of treated sites had occurred by 14 to 21 days. Between 50 and 60 days after ligation, the submucosa at treated sites was replaced by dense, mature scar tissue. The underlying muscular wall of the esophagus was consistently intact.

Endoscopic observations in the clinical setting paralleled those from the laboratory.[90] Soon after ligation, the ensnared tissue boluses filled much of the esophageal lumen and rapidly assumed a cyanotic hue. Examination 4 to 10 days after ligation showed tissue sloughing at treated sites, and the shallow ulcers were 10 to 12 mm in diameter and 1 to 2 mm deep. The ulcers appeared uniform and more superficial than many ulcers associated with endoscopic sclerotherapy. Between 14 and 21 days after ligation, treatment sites had healed. Shallow "divots" remained where variceal channels once were. The epithelium covering the divots appeared to be squamous on endoscopic observation, a finding confirmed by microscopic examination of autopsy specimens. Goff and associates compared patients who had undergone endoscopic ligation with those who had been treated by sclerotherapy and with untreated controls who had esophageal varices.[76] Patients treated with sclerotherapy had a greater incidence of stricture formation, but esophageal manometric studies did not show differences among the three groups.

Endoscopic ligation has been studied in one large, uncontrolled trial and is currently under evaluation in four multicenter prospective studies comparing ligation with sclerotherapy. An additional uncontrolled study of pediatric pa-

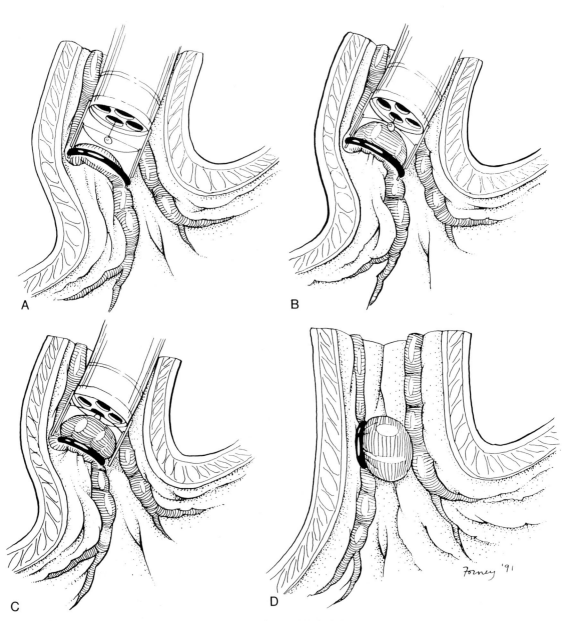

Figure 10–3. Endoscopic elastic band ligation of esophageal varices. **(A)** The endoscopist approaches the varix to be ligated and makes full contact with the end of the ligating device. **(B)** Endoscopic suction is activated, drawing the tissue to be ligated into the chamber. **(C)** After the chamber is filled (i.e., endoscopic "red-out"), the endoscopist pulls the trip wire, which moves the inner cylinder toward the endoscope and ejects the elastic O ring around the tissue bolus. **(D)** One varix has been ligated, and the endoscope has been removed for reloading and repeat ligation of the remaining varices. (From Stiegmann GV, Yamamoto M. Approaches to the endoscopic treatment of esophageal varices. World J Surg 16:1034–1041, 1992.)

tients is in progress. Our group studied 146 consecutive unselected patients with cirrhosis and variceal hemorrhage who were treated with endoscopic ligation for control of acute hemorrhage and had serial elective retreatments to eradicate varices.[92] Active variceal bleeding was controlled in 22 (96%) of 23 patients. Recurrent bleeding occurred in 47%. Eradication of varices was achieved in 79% of 125 patients who survived at least 30 days after entering the trial, with a mean of five endoscopic treatments. The overall survival rate was 74% at mean follow-up of 16 months. Only three treatment-related complications (i.e., two esophageal strictures and one meat impaction) were observed during this trial. Saeed and coworkers successfully treated a small group of patients who had recurrent bleeding after multiple sclerotherapy treatments, suggesting that the ligation technique may be useful in patients whose varices cannot be controlled by sclerotherapy.[93] Hall and associates reported successful control of bleeding in 16 infants and children treated with endoscopic ligation.[94]

Results from one completed multicenter trial and three ongoing prospective, randomized trials comparing endoscopic ligation with sclerotherapy are summarized in Table 10–2.[95-98] Three of the four trials showed ligation required significantly fewer treatments to eradicate varices than sclerotherapy. Complications were significantly diminished in ligation-treated patients in two of the three studies. The multicenter study found a significant survival advantage for ligation-treated patients, resulting primarily from a lower incidence of rebleeding and fewer deaths from complications.

Available data support several tentative conclusions about endoscopic ligation compared with sclerotherapy. Endoscopic ligation is at least as effective as conventional sclerotherapy

for control of active bleeding and prevention of rebleeding. All studies have shown that ligation requires fewer treatments to eradicate varices than sclerotherapy, and all have shown a lower incidence of recurrent bleeding for ligation. The significant survival advantage seen in the multicenter study resulted from a lower incidence of recurrent hemorrhage and fewer complication-related deaths. Endoscopic ligation appears to have a decided advantage over sclerotherapy with respect to the low incidence of treatment-related complications and fewer treatments needed to effect eradication of varices. These improvements may be associated with improved survival and a lower incidence of recurrent bleeding, but confirmation is necessary.

Recurrent hemorrhage in patients treated with sclerotherapy or ligation most often occurs before eradication of esophageal varices. Our group postulated that, by combining low-volume sclerotherapy with endoscopic ligation, eradication of varices could be accomplished rapidly while maintaining a low incidence of complications. Combination treatment is performed by ligating all variceal channels at the gastroesophageal junction and then performing intravariceal injections of 1 mL of sclerosant per varix 1 to 3 cm cephalad to the ligation sites (Fig. 10–4). Combination therapy should result in rapid eradication of varices because of the additive effects of mechanical stasis of ligation and intimal damage of sclerotherapy. Low volumes of sclerosant may result in fewer sclerosant-related local complications, and stasis in variceal channels may further inhibit widespread dissemination of sclerosant and minimize systemic sclerosant-related problems.

Two trials examined the combination of endoscopic ligation with low-volume sclerotherapy.[99, 100] Reveille and coworkers treated 46 unselected patients in a single-arm trial and

Table 10–2. COMPARISON OF ENDOSCOPIC LIGATION WITH ENDOSCOPIC SCLEROTHERAPY FOR THE TREATMENT OF ESOPHAGEAL VARICES

Investigation*	No. of Patients	Therapy	Patients Who Rebled (%)	Mean No. of Treatments to Eradicate Varices	Survival (%)	Complications† (%)
Multicenter[96]	65	ES	48	5	55*	20*
	64	EVL	36	4	72*	2*
El-Newihi[97]	19	ES	37	6*	95	68*
	20	EVL	25	4*	95	25*
Westaby[95]	40	ES	53	5*	NA	NA
	48	EVL	32	3*	NA	NA
Young[98]	13	ES	NA	6*	92	15
	10	EVL	NA	4*	90	0

Abbreviations: ES, endoscopic sclerotherapy; EVL, endoscopic variceal ligation; NA, not available.
*Results are from three ongoing trials and one concluded prospective, randomized trial; $p < 0.02$.
†Nonbleeding complications that required active treatment.

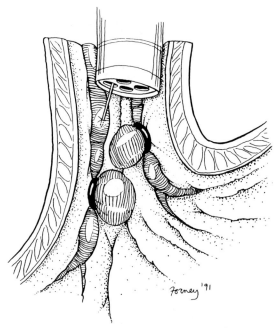

Figure 10–4. Combination ligation and low-volume sclerotherapy. The endoscopist ligates each varix at the gastroesophageal junction. The ligating device is then removed, and low volumes (e.g., 1 mL) of sclerosant are injected into each varix cephalad to the site of ligation. The combination of stasis and the low volume of chemical sclerosant appears to result in rapid eradication of varices while minimizing complications associated with conventional sclerotherapy, which uses larger volumes of sclerosant. (From Stiegmann GV, Yamamoto M. Approaches to the endoscopic treatment of esophageal varices. World J Surg 16:1034–1041, 1992.)

reported a mean of 2.1 endoscopic treatment sessions were needed to eradicate esophageal varices, compared with an average of four sessions for ligation alone and five to six for sclerotherapy alone. Survival and the incidence of recurrent bleeding and treatment-related complications compared favorably with those obtained using endoscopic ligation alone. Similar preliminary results have been reported from a prospective randomized trial in France that compared endoscopic sclerotherapy with combination ligation and low-volume sclerotherapy.[99]

CONCLUSION

Endoscopic treatment is accepted for initial and subsequent eradication of bleeding esophageal varices. Sclerotherapy, once performed with rigid endoscopes, is now done using flexible endoscopes in awake patients, often as an outpatient procedure. Endoscopic treatment does not confer a measurable survival advantage in the treatment of acute variceal hemorrhage, but serial treatment lowers the risk of recurrent hemorrhage and prolongs life. Primary treatment by endoscopic sclerotherapy appears to be equal or more effective than primary shunt therapy, even with a sclerotherapy failure rate of 10% to 30%. Despite these results, the incidence of rebleeding, treatment-related complications, and mortality in sclerotherapy-treated patients is high.

Endoscopic elastic band ligation eradicates varices more rapidly, causes fewer complications, and may be associated with better long-term survival than sclerotherapy. Additional trials are needed to confirm the efficacy of this new method and examine the role of endoscopic ligation in combination with low-volume sclerotherapy.

References

1. Crafoord C, Frenckner P. New surgical treatment of varicose veins of the esophagus. Acta Otolaryngol (Stockh) 27:422–429, 1939.
2. Macbeth R. Treatment of oesophageal varices in portal hypertension by means of sclerosing injections. Br Med J 2:877–880, 1955.
3. Fearon B, Sass-Kortsak A. The management of esophageal varices in children by injection of sclerosing agents. Ann Otol Rhinol Laryngol 68:906–909, 1959.
4. Wodak E. Osophagus varigen bei portaler hypertension: ihre therapie und prophylaxe. Wein Med Wochenschr 110:581–587, 1960.
5. Johnston GW, Rodgers HW. A review of 15 years' experience in the use of sclerotherapy in the control of acute hemorrhage from esophageal varices. Br J Surg 60:797–800, 1973.
6. Wodak E. Akute gastrointestinale blutung: resultate der endoskopischen sklerosierung von osophagusvarizen. Schweiz Med Wochenschr 109:591–596, 1979.
7. Paquet KJ, Oberhammer E. Sclerotherapy of bleeding oesophageal varices by means of endoscopy. Endoscopy 10:7–12, 1978.
8. Terblanche J, Northover JM, Bornman P, et al. A prospective evaluation of injection sclerotherapy in the treatment of acute bleeding from esophageal varices. Surgery 85:239–245, 1979.
9. Barsoum M, Bolous F, El-Rooby A, et al. Tamponade and injection sclerotherapy in the management of bleeding oesophageal varices. Br J Surg 69:76–78, 1982.
10. Cello J, Grendell J, Crass R, et al. Endoscopic sclerotherapy versus portacaval shunt in patients with severe cirrhosis and acute variceal hemorrhage: long-term follow-up. N Engl J Med 316:11–15, 1987.
11. El-Zayadi A, el-Din SS, Kabil SM. Endoscopic sclerotherapy versus medical treatment for bleeding esophageal varices in patients with schistosomal liver disease. Gastrointest Endosc 34:314–317, 1988.
12. Korula J, Balart L, Radvan G, et al. A prospective, randomized, controlled trial of chronic esophageal variceal sclerotherapy. Hepatology 5:584–589, 1985.
13. Paquet K-J, Feussner H. Endoscopic sclerosis and

esophageal balloon tamponade in acute hemorrhage from esophagogastric varices: a prospective controlled randomized trial. Hepatology 5:580–583, 1985.

14. Soderland C, Ihre T. Endoscopic sclerotherapy v. conservative management of bleeding oesophageal varices: a 5 year prospective controlled trial of emergency and long term treatment. Acta Chir Scand 151:449–456, 1985.

15. Teres J, Bordas JM, Bravo D, et al. Sclerotherapy vs. distal splenorenal shunt in the elective treatment of variceal hemorrhage: a randomized controlled trial. Hepatology 7:430–436, 1987.

16. The Copenhagen Esophageal Varices Project. Sclerotherapy after first variceal hemorrhage in cirrhosis: a randomized multicenter trial. N Engl J Med 311:1594–1600, 1984.

17. Terblanche J, Bornman P, Kahn D, et al. Failure of repeated injection sclerotherapy to improve long-term survival after oesophageal variceal bleeding: a five year prospective controlled clinical trial. Lancet 2:1328–1332, 1983.

18. Rikkers LF, Burnett DA, Volentine GD, et al. Shunt surgery versus endoscopic sclerotherapy for long-term treatment of variceal hemorrhage: early results of a randomized trial. Ann Surg 206:261–271, 1987.

19. Warren WD, Henderson JM, Millikan WJ, et al. Distal splenorenal shunt versus endoscopic sclerotherapy for long-term management of variceal bleeding: preliminary report of a prospective, randomized trial. Ann Surg 203:454–462, 1986.

20. Westaby D, Macdougall B, Williams R. Improved survival following injection sclerotherapy for esophageal varices: final analysis of a controlled trial. Hepatology 5:827–830, 1985.

21. Fleischer D. The Washington Symposium on Endoscopic Laser Therapy, April 18–19, 1985. Gastrointest Endosc 31:397–400, 1985.

22. Ramond MJ, Valla D, Gotlib JP, et al. Obturation endoscopique des varices oeso-gastriques par le Bucrylate. Gastroenterol Clin Biol 10:575–579, 1986.

23. Soehendra N, Nam VC, Grimm H, et al. Endoscopic obliteration of large esophagogastric varices with bucrylate. Endoscopy 18:25–26, 1986.

24. Stiegmann GV, Cambre T, Sun J. A new endoscopic elastic band ligating device. Gastrointest Endosc 32:230–233, 1986.

25. Trudeau W, Prindiville T. Endoscopic injection sclerosis in bleeding gastric varices. Gastrointest Endosc 32:264–268, 1986.

26. Butler H. The veins of the esophagus. Thorax 6:276–296, 1951.

27. Kitano S, Terblanche J, Kahn D, et al. Venous anatomy of the lower oesophagus in portal hypertension: practical implications. Br J Surg 73:525–531, 1986.

28. Hashizume M, Kitano S, Sugimachi K, et al. Three-dimensional view of the vascular structure of the lower esophagus in clinical portal hypertension. Hepatology 8:1482–1487, 1988.

29. Spence R. The venous anatomy of the lower esophagus in normal subjects and in patients with varices: an image analysis study. Br J Surg 71:739–744, 1984.

30. Vianna A, Hayes PC, Moscoso G, et al. Normal venous circulation of the gastroesophageal junction. Gastroenterology 93:876–889, 1987.

31. Kage M, Korula J, Harada A, et al. Effects of sodium tetradecyl sulfate endoscopic variceal sclerotherapy on the esophagus. A prospective clinical and histopathologic study. J Clin Gastroenterol 9:635–643, 1987.

32. Sarin S, Nanda R, Sachdev G, et al. Intravariceal versus paravariceal sclerotherapy: a prospective, controlled, randomized trial. Gut 28:657–662, 1987.

33. Sanowski RA. Venography during sclerotherapy. In: Sivak MV, ed. Endoscopic sclerotherapy of esophageal varices. New York: Praeger Special Studies, 1984:43–47.

34. Rose JDR, Crane MD, Smith PM. Factors affecting successful endoscopic sclerotherapy for esophageal varices. Gut 24:946–949, 1983.

35. Barsoum MS, Khattar NY, Risk-Allah MA. Technical aspects of injection sclerotherapy of acute oesophageal variceal hemorrhage as seen by radiography. Br J Surg 65:588–589, 1978.

36. Jacobson B, Franz R, Hurly E, et al. Mechanism of thrombosis caused by sclerotherapy of esophageal varices using sodium tetradecyl sulphate. Surg Endosc 6:4–9, 1992.

37. Blenkinsopp WK. Choice of sclerosant: an experimental study. Angiologica 7:182–186, 1970.

38. Reiner L. The activity of anionic surface active compounds in producing vascular obliteration. Proc Soc Exp Biol Med 62:49–54, 1946.

39. Jensen DM. Evaluation of sclerosing agents in animal models. Gastrointest Endosc 29:315–317, 1983.

40. Jensen DM, Machicado GA, Tapia JL. A reproducible canine model of esophageal varices. Gastroenterology 84:573–579, 1983.

41. Silpa JL, Jensen DM, Machicado GE. Efficacy and safety of agents for variceal sclerotherapy. Gastrointest Endosc 28:152–153, 1982.

42. Kitano S, Iso Y, Koyanagi N, et al. Ethanolamine oleate is superior to polidocanol (aethoxysklerol) for endoscopic injection sclerotherapy of esophageal varices: a prospective randomized trial. Hepatogastroenterology 34:19–23, 1987.

43. Kitano S, Iso Y, Yamaga H, et al. Trial of sclerosing agents in patients with oesophageal varices. Br J Surg 75:751–753, 1988.

44. Sarin SK, Nanda R, Sachdev G. Relative efficacy and safety of absolute alcohol as variceal sclerosants. Gastrointest Endosc 33:362–365, 1987.

45. Lyons SD, Sugawa C, Geller ER, et al. Comparison of 1% sodium tetradecyl sulfate to a thrombogenic sclerosant cocktail for endoscopic sclerotherapy. Am Surg 54:81–84, 1988.

46. Bornman P, Kahn D, Terblanche J, et al. Rigid versus fiberoptic endoscopic injection sclerotherapy: a prospective randomized controlled trial in patients with bleeding esophageal varices. Ann Surg 208:175–178, 1988.

47. Lilly JR. Endoscopic sclerosis of esophageal varices in children. Surg Gynecol Obstet 152:513–514, 1981.

48. Kitano S, Iso Y, Yamaga H, et al. Temporary deterioration of pulmonary functions after injection sclerotherapy for cirrhotic patients with esophageal varices. Eur Surg Res 20:298–303, 1988.

49. De Franchis R, Vitagliano P, Agape D, et al. Eradication of esophageal varices by endoscopic sclerotherapy: how much is enough? Gastrointest Endosc 34:395–399, 1988.

50. Sarin S, Sachdev G, Nanda R, et al. Comparison of two time schedules for endoscopic sclerotherapy: a prospective randomised controlled study. Gut 27:710–713, 1986.

51. Westaby D, Melia W, Macdougall B, et al. Injection sclerotherapy for oesophageal varices: a prospective randomised trial of different treatment schedules. Gut 25:129–132, 1984.

52. Perino L, Gholson C, Goff J. Esophageal perforation following fiberoptic variceal sclerotherapy. J Clin Gastrenterol 9:286–288, 1987.

53. Larson A, Cohen H, Zweiban B, et al. Acute esophageal variceal sclerotherapy: results of a prospective

randomized controlled trial. JAMA 255:497–500, 1986.

54. Infante-Rivard C, Esnaola S, Villeneuve JP. Role of endoscopic variceal sclerotherapy in the long-term management of variceal bleeding: A meta-analysis. Gastroenterology 96:1087–1092, 1989.

55. Planas R, Boix J, Broggi M, et al. Portacaval shunt versus endoscopic sclerotherapy in the elective treatment of variceal hemorrhage. Gastroenterology 100:1078–1086, 1991.

56. Spina GP, Santambrogio R, Opocher E. Distal splenorenal shunt versus endoscopic sclerotherapy in the prevention of variceal rebleeding. Ann Surg 211:454–462, 1990.

57. Saks BJ, Kilby AE, Dietrich PA, et al. Pleural and mediastinal changes following endoscopic injection sclerotherapy of esophageal varices. Radiology 149:639–642, 1983.

58. Monroe P, Morrow CF, Millen JE, et al. Acute respiratory failure after sodium morrhuate esophageal sclerotherapy. Gastroenterology 85:693–699, 1983.

59. Korula J, Baydur A, Sassoon C, et al. Effects of esophageal variceal sclerotherapy (EVS) on lung function. Arch Intern Med 146:1517–1520, 1986.

60. Bailey-Newton RS, Connors AF Jr, Bacon BR. Effect of esophageal variceal sclerotherapy (EVS) on gas exchange and hemodynamics in humans. Gastroenterology 89:368–373, 1985.

61. Brayko CM, Kozarek RA, Sanowski RA, et al. Bacteremia during esophageal variceal sclerotherapy: its cause and prevention. Gastrointest Endosc 31:10–12, 1985.

62. Camara DS, Gruber M, Barde CJ, et al. Transient bacteremia following endoscopic injection sclerotherapy of esophageal varices. Arch Intern Med 143:1350–1352, 1983.

63. Tank L, Estay R, Ovalle L, et al. Bacterial peritonitis and sclerotherapy for variceal hemorrhage. Gastrointest Endosc 38:200, 1992.

64. Ashida H, Kotoura Y, Nishioka A, et al. Portal and mesenteric venous thrombosis as a complication of endoscopic sclerotherapy. Am J Gastroenterol 84:306–310, 1989.

65. Seidman E, Weber AM, Morin CL, et al. Spinal cord paralysis following sclerotherapy for esophageal varices. Hepatology 4:950–954, 1984.

66. Thatcher BS, Sivak MV, Ferguson DR, et al. Mesenteric venous thrombosis as a possible complication of endoscopic sclerotherapy: A report of two cases. Am J Gastroenterol 81:126–129, 1986.

67. Caletti GC, Brocchi E, Zani L, et al. Sonographic evaluation of the portal venous system after elective endoscopic sclerotherapy of esophageal varices. Surg Endosc 1:165–167, 1987.

68. Hunter GC, Steinkirchner T, Burbige EJ, et al. Venous complications of sclerotherapy for esophageal varices. Am J Surg 156:497–501, 1988.

69. Jensen LS, Krarup N, Larsen JA, et al. Effect of endoscopic sclerotherapy of esophageal varices on liver blood flow and liver function. An experimental study. Scand J Gastroenterol 22:619–626, 1987.

70. Korula J, Ralls P. The effects of chronic endoscopic sclerotherapy on portal pressure in cirrhotics. Gastroenterology 101:800–805, 1991.

71. Choudhuri G, Agrawal BK, Tantry BV, et al. Post-sclerotherapy esophageal ulcers: a prospective analysis of their behavior. Indian J Gastroenterol 8:19–21, 1989.

72. Sarin SK, Nanda R, Vij JC, et al. Oesophageal ulceration after sclerotherapy—a complication or an accompaniment? Endoscopy 18:44–45, 1986.

73. Schuman BM, Beckman JW, Tedesco FJ, et al. Complications of endoscopic injection sclerotherapy: a review. Am J Gastroenterol 82:823–829, 1987.

74. Larson GM, Vandertoll DJ, Netscher DT, et al. Esophageal motility: effects of injection sclerotherapy. Surgery 96:703–709, 1984.

75. Snady H, Korsten MA. Esophageal acid clearance and motility after endoscopic sclerotherapy of esophageal varices. Am J Gastroenterol 81:419–422, 1986.

76. Goff JS, Reveille RM, Stiegmann GV. Endoscopic sclerotherapy versus endoscopic variceal ligation: esophageal symptoms, complications, and motility. Am J Gastroenterol 83:1240–1244, 1988.

77. Bochna GS, Harty RF, Harned RK, et al. Development of squamous cell carcinoma of the esophagus after endoscopic variceal sclerotherapy. Am J Gastroenterol 83:564–568, 1988.

78. Guillemot F, Bonniere P, Bretagne JF, et al. Esophageal cancer and endoscopic sclerosis of esophageal varices: a fortuitous association? Gastroenterol Clin Biol 12:858–861, 1988.

79. Nakamura R, Watanabe M, Sugimura Y, et al. Early esophageal cancer discovered 6 months after endoscopic injection sclerotherapy of esophageal varices. Gan No Rinsho 34:1190–1194, 1988.

80. Burroughs AK, D'Heygere F, McIntyre N. Pitfalls in studies of prophylactic therapy for variceal bleeding in cirrhotics. Hepatology 6:1407–1413, 1986.

81. Terblanche J. Sclerotherapy for prophylaxis of variceal bleeding. Lancet 1:961–963, 1986.

82. Terblanche J, Burroughs AK, Hobbs KEF. Controversies in the management of bleeding esophageal varices. N Engl J Med 320:1469–1475, 1989.

83. Paquet K-J. Prophylactic endoscopic sclerosing treatment of the esophageal wall in varices—a prospective controlled trial. Endoscopy 14:4–5, 1982.

84. Piai G, Cipolletta L, Claar M, et al. Prophylactic sclerotherapy of high risk esophageal varices: results of a multicentric prospective controlled trial. Hepatology 8:1495–500, 1988.

85. Witzel L, Wolbergs E, Merki H. Prophylactic endoscopic sclerotherapy of oesophageal varices: a prospective controlled study. Lancet 1:773–775, 1985.

86. Santangelo WC, Dueno MI, Estes BL, et al. Prophylactic sclerotherapy of large esophageal varices. N Engl J Med 318:814–818, 1988.

87. The Veterans Affairs Cooperative Variceal Sclerotherapy Study Group. Prophylactic sclerotherapy for esophageal varices in men with alcoholic liver disease: a randomized, single-blind, multicenter trial. N Engl J Med 324:1779–1784, 1991.

88. De Franchis R, Primignani M, Arcidiacono PG. Prophylactic sclerotherapy in high-risk cirrhotics selected by endoscopic criteria. Gastroenterology 101:1087–1093, 1991.

89. Ruiswyk JV, Byrd JC. Efficacy of prophylactic sclerotherapy for prevention of a first variceal bleed. Gastroenterology 102:587–597, 1992.

90. Stiegmann GV, Goff JS, Sun JH, et al. Technique and early clinical results of endoscopic variceal ligation (EVL). Surg Endosc 3:73–78, 1989.

91. Stiegmann GV, Sun JH, Hammond WS. Results of experimental endoscopic esophageal varix ligation. Am Surg 54:105–108, 1988.

92. Goff JS. Endoscopic variceal ligation. Can J Gastroenterol 4:639–642, 1990.

93. Saeed ZA, Michaletz PA, Winchester CB. Endoscopic ligation in patients who have failed sclerotherapy. Gastrointest Endosc 36:572–574, 1990.

94. Hall RJ, Lilly JR, Stiegmann GV. Endoscopic esoph-

ageal varix ligation: technique and preliminary results in children. J Pediatr Surg 23:1222–1223, 1988.

95. Westaby D. Prevention of recurrent variceal bleeding: endoscopic techniques. Gastrointest Endosc Clin North Am 2:121–136, 1992.

96. Stiegmann G, Goff J, Michaletz-Onody P, et al. Endoscopic sclerotherapy as compared with endoscopic ligation for bleeding esophageal varices. N Engl J Med 326:1527–1532, 1992.

97. El-Newihi H, Migicovsky B, Laine L. A prospective randomized comparison of sclerotherapy and ligation for the treatment of bleeding esophageal varices. [Abstract] Gastroenterology 100:A59, 1991.

98. Young M, Sanowski R, Raschke R. Comparison and characterization of ulcerations induced by endoscopic ligation of esophageal varices versus endoscopic sclerotherapy. [Abstract] Gastrointest Endosc 38:285, 1992.

99. Koutsomanis D. Endoscopic variceal ligation combined with low volume sclerotherapy: a controlled study. [Abstract] Gastroenterology 102:A835, 1992.

100. Reveille RM, Goff JS, Stiegmann GV, et al. Combination endoscopic variceal ligation (EVL) and low volume sclerotherapy (ES) for bleeding esophageal varices: a faster route to variceal eradication? [Abstract] Gastrointest Endosc 37:243, 1991.

11

Management of Nonvariceal Upper Gastrointestinal Bleeding

Choichi Sugawa and Anthony L. Joseph

Therapeutic endoscopy in selected patients identified during diagnostic examination has an important role in the treatment of patients with upper gastrointestinal hemorrhage.[1, 2]

Early endoscopy can accurately determine the precise cause of upper gastrointestinal hemorrhage and assess the risk of rebleeding and the need for surgical intervention.[3, 4] Accumulating evidence from Asia, Europe, and North America suggests that therapeutic endoscopy can significantly improve the clinical course of selected high-risk patients presenting with upper gastrointestinal hemorrhage.[5]

Endoscopic hemostasis is effective and relatively safe. It can be invaluable as definitive therapy for patients unwilling or unable to tolerate an operative procedure and for many patients in whom no previous history of ulcer disease exists. Endoscopic hemostasis can be used to control active bleeding so that a definitive operation may be performed electively, with lessened mortality and morbidity in patients with intractable ulcers and bleeding.[2] There are several effective endoscopic modalities for control of bleeding from nonvariceal upper gas-

trointestinal hemorrhage, including thermal contact, laser therapy, and injection therapy (Table 11–1).[1, 6–10] Other methods have been proposed, but they have not been widely accepted. This chapter reviews the current status of endoscopic therapy of nonvariceal upper gastrointestinal hemorrhage.

CAUSES OF UPPER GASTROINTESTINAL HEMORRHAGE

Upper endoscopy can give highly accurate and specific information about the source of bleeding. Most physicians report a diagnostic accuracy of 80% to 95%.[1, 11–13] Accuracy increases with the endoscopist's experience because persistent bleeding may obscure the site of hemorrhage and challenge the operator's technical ability.

The cause of upper gastrointestinal hemorrhage varies among series and depends on the nature of the admitting hospital, geographic area, and indigenous patient population. A sur-

Table 11–1. ENDOSCOPIC HEMOSTATIC METHODS

Proven Methods	Unproven Methods
Heater probe	Monopolar electrocoagulation
Bipolar (BICAP) or multipolar probe	Topical agents
Injection therapy	Ferromagnetic tamponade
Nd:YAG laser	Mechanical clips

Table 11–2. CAUSES OF UPPER GASTROINTESTINAL BLEEDING IN SELECTED SERIES

Series	No. of Patients	Esophageal Varices (%)	Mallory-Weiss Tear (%)	Peptic Ulcer (%)	Acute Gastric Mucosal Lesions (%)	Other (%)
Katz[14]	1429	16	3	25	44	12
Graham[15]	221	16	14	58	9	3
Himal[16]	334	6	1	62	18	13
Iglesias[17]	789	4	1	24	45	26
ASGE[18]	2097	15	8	45	30	21
Sugawa[1]	3549	13	10	32	33	12
Gostout[19]	342	10	6	44	12	28
Total	8761	13	7	36	33	11

vey of representative series is illustrated in Table 11–2.[1, 14–19]

Although individual series vary, peptic ulceration (with a slight preponderance of gastric over duodenal ulcers) generally is the most common cause, followed by acute gastric mucosal lesions (AGML), esophageal varices, and Mallory-Weiss tears. Other sources include esophagitis, tumors, vascular malformations, and gastric varices. Figure 11–1 depicts the distribution of causes of hemorrhage in the cumulative 8761 patients from the series in Table 11–2.

Acute Gastric Mucosal Lesions or Erosive Gastritis

In reported series, the incidence of AGML lesions ranges from 9% to 45%. An average of 33% was found in the series listed in Table 11–2. This condition is characterized by multiple superficial mucosal injuries. The lesions may penetrate deeper than the muscularis mucosae histologically and can be ulcers rather than erosions.

Absence of standardized nomenclature affects the comparative figures on the incidence of AGML or ulcer disease. Endoscopic changes in AGML include petechiae, red erosions, black erosions, red erosions with central blackening, and white-based erosions a few millimeters to 20 mm in diameter.[20] The mucosal lesions caused by "stress gastritis" secondary to trauma or sepsis usually occur in the proximal half of the stomach and spread to the distal stomach with increased severity.[21] Mucosal lesions associated with alcohol typically consist of red-based erosions that are usually located in the proximal half of the stomach.[20]

Gastric Ulcer

Peptic ulcers account for 24% to 62% of the causes of bleeding (see Table 11–2). We found

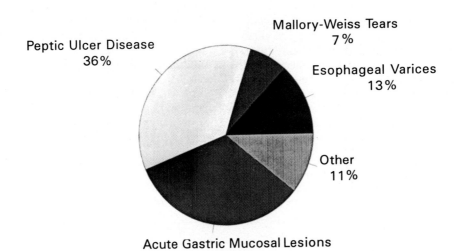

Figure 11–1. Causes of endoscopically diagnosed bleeding in 8761 patients.

that gastric ulcers were the cause of upper gastrointestinal bleeding in 19% of patients, compared with 14% of patients with bleeding secondary to duodenal ulcers in our inner city hospital setting.[2] An acute gastric ulcer is defined as a shallow crater with a sharp edge, no surrounding marginal swelling, and without fibrosis histologically. The chronic ulcer has a deep, often shaggy base with swelling of the ulcer edge and converging mucosal folds. It is important to examine the ulcer base to find an actively bleeding blood vessel and to record stigmata of recent bleeding (*e.g.*, adherent clot, protuberance or visible vessel) because these carry prognostic and therapeutic implications.

Duodenal Ulcer

In a review by Gostout, duodenal ulcer was the second most common cause of upper gastrointestinal bleeding (19.5%) after gastric ulcers (24%).[19] Duodenal ulcers may be difficult to visualize clearly because the duodenal bulb may be deformed and covered with blood. Careful local irrigation is essential to examine the ulcer and assess for stigmata of hemorrhage.

Varices

The incidence of bleeding esophageal varices ranges from 2% to more than 50%, depending on the geographic location. The higher rates come from China and Egypt and are attributable to endemic schistosomiasis. Care providers in an urban setting see more patients with AGML and esophageal varices.[2, 14] Early endoscopy is essential in determining that upper gastrointestinal bleeding is from esophageal varices. Complete examination of the esophagus, stomach, and duodenum must be performed to exclude another site of bleeding if the initial examination fails to reveal bleeding from varices. Large varices with red color signs are more prone to bleeding.[22, 23] Between 28% and 90% of patients with upper gastrointestinal bleeding who have esophageal varices actually bleed from them.[24–26] Of the 712 patients with varices in our series, 448 (63%) were bleeding from varices.[1]

Mallory-Weiss Syndrome

Mallory-Weiss tears accounted for bleeding in 1% to 14% of reported series (see Table 11–2). The Mallory-Weiss syndrome often is associated with alcohol abuse and is frequently preceded by nausea and vomiting. The offending laceration runs parallel to the long axis of the stomach and may extend proximally to the esophagogastric junction. The bleeding may be arterial or venous, and the manifestations may be trivial or catastrophic.[27]

Esophagitis

In our series, 184 of 3549 patients (5.2%) had severe esophagitis as the principal source of bleeding.[1] White plaques of various configurations, surrounded by an erythematous border with oozing blood, are the hallmarks of this entity.

Marginal Ulcer

Fifty-six of 3549 patients (1.6%) had bleeding marginal ulcers that were most often found on the jejunal side of the gastrojejunal anastomosis.[1] A few patients had deep ulcerations, but more often the lesions were shallow and contained clots. Thorough examination of the anastomosis is mandatory, because these ulcers are notoriously difficult to find.

Gastric Tumors

Fifty-five of a total of 3549 patients (1.5%) were bleeding from gastric tumors.[1] Bleeding in most of these patients was slow, resulting in melena and anemia.

Duodenitis

Duodenitis is diagnosed by scattered erosions and bleeding in association with a swollen erythematous mucosa. The distal duodenal bulb and proximal descending duodenum are typically involved. Duodenitis was responsible for 1.4% of the upper gastrointestinal bleeding in our series of 3549 patients.[1]

Angiodysplasia

Angiodysplasia (*i.e.*, vascular malformation) is identified infrequently in the upper gastrointestinal tract, but it is common in the large intestine. Patients with upper gastrointestinal bleeding caused by vascular malformations have an increased incidence of renal insufficiency.[28] Gastric antral vascular ectasia (*i.e.*, watermelon stomach) has been found predominantly in middle-aged women with iron-deficiency anemia. At endoscopy, broad, erythematous folds similar to the stripes of a watermelon are observed. Repeat treatments with laser and heater probe have been effective.[29]

Miscellaneous

A variety of other endoscopically diagnosed causes accounted for bleeding in 62 of 3549 patients (1.7%). These lesions included hematobilia, pancreatic pseudocysts, aortoduodenal fistulas following aneurysm surgery, duodenal diverticula, postoperative anastomotic bleeding, and duodenal varices.

PREDICTION OF FURTHER ULCER HEMORRHAGE

The strongest endoscopic predictor of persistent or recurrent bleeding is ongoing active bleeding (*e.g.,* arterial spurting, oozing) at the time of endoscopy (Table 11–3).[3, 4, 30–32] Eighty percent to 90% of the patients with active bleeding continue to bleed or rebleed. The presence of a discrete protuberance within the ulcer crater is important. This is referred to as a "visible vessel" or "sentinel clot." Some pigmented protuberances (*e.g.,* red, blue, purple) imply a high risk of rebleeding, even if they were not bleeding at the time of endoscopy.[31, 32] Pathologic studies indicate that such protuberances may represent a pseudoaneurysm of a penetrating artery or organized clot over a defect in an exposed artery. There is some disagreement about the prognostic significance of a white or a black protuberance. In a study employing endoscopic Doppler probes, a visible vessel or fresh clot with a positive Doppler signal rebled in 73% (8 of 11) of patients, but a Doppler-negative lesion rebled in only 13% (2 of 38) of patients.[33] A study using pulsed-wave Doppler confirmation of endoscopic stigmata found no bleeding in 28 Doppler-negative patients treated with H₂-antagonists alone. However, the natural history of endoscopically benign, Doppler-positive lesions is unclear.[34] It is generally agreed that a clean ulcer base or one that contains a flat, pigmented spot is associated with low frequency of rebleeding.

Multiple clinical risk factors can be used to predict the occurrence of continued or recurrent bleeding (see Table 11–3). Documented coagulopathy and the onset of bleeding in a patient already hospitalized for a related or concurrent

Table 11–3. CLINICAL AND ENDOSCOPIC FEATURES SIGNIFICANT FOR RISK OF REBLEEDING

Patient History
  Age >60 years
  Coexistent major organ system disease
  In-hospital onset
  Admission hemoglobin <8.0
Clinical Criteria
  Shock (systolic blood pressure <90)
  Transfusion requirements >5 U packed erythrocytes
  Coagulopathy
Endoscopic Findings
  Torrential hemorrhage
  Ulcer location in posterior bulb or high on lesser curvature
  Active spurting or oozing from base
  Pigmented protuberance (visible vessel)
  Adherent clot
  Doppler-positive lesion

medical condition are predictive of recurrent bleeding.[3, 4] In several studies, recurrent hemorrhage was significantly associated with age greater than 60 years, admission hemoglobin levels less than 8.0 g/dL, hematemesis on admission, and stigmata of recent hemorrhage seen on endoscopy.[3, 4, 35] Shock or hypotension on admission, combined with endoscopic findings of a visible vessel or stigmata of bleeding, significantly predicted rebleeding.[30, 36]

Bleeding is more likely to be massive and difficult to control and the incidence of rebleeding is greater if the ulcer is located on the inferior-posterior wall of the duodenal bulb (*i.e.,* near branches of the gastroduodenal artery) or high on the posterior wall of the lesser curvature (*i.e.,* near branches of the left gastric artery), but prepyloric ulcers have a much better prognosis.[37, 38]

INDICATIONS FOR ENDOSCOPIC INTERVENTION

Indications for endoscopic hemostasis include active bleeding from local lesions, such as peptic ulcers, AGML, esophagitis, Mallory-Weiss tears, and angiodysplasias (see Table 11–3).

Acute gastric and duodenal ulcer bleeding stop spontaneously in approximately 70% to 80% of patients without further intervention. It is therefore necessary to use endoscopic hemostatic therapy on selected patients who are most at risk of further hemorrhage. A National Institutes of Health (NIH) Consensus Conference held in 1989 was a forum for discussing such criteria.[3, 4] It was agreed that treatment should be directed at selected high-risk patients. Clinical factors that increase the risk of persistent or recurrent bleeding or death are rapid hemorrhage, manifested by shock, ongoing transfusion requirements, hematemesis or hematochezia; age older than 60 years; major associated diseases; in-hospital bleeding; and rebleeding episodes after admission (see Table 11–3).

Endoscopic findings of active arterial bleeding (e.g., spurting) or oozing from an ulcer are indications for treatment. Pigmented protuberances (e.g., visible vessels, sentinel clot) at the site of an ulcer are likewise an indication for treatment. Patients with ulcer craters that are clean or with flat pigmented spots do not require endoscopic hemostatic treatment. We attempt to treat all patients diagnosed with upper gastrointestinal bleeding who have clinical and endoscopic criteria placing them at high risk for rebleeding. Our objectives are to achieve permanent hemostasis, diminish the need for blood transfusion or operative intervention, and transform an emergent operation into an elective one.[2]

The Mallory-Weiss tear, which rarely bleeds persistently, is usually found at endoscopy to have arterial bleeding or a sentinel clot, which may require endoscopic hemostasis.

AGML and esophagitis usually cause minor hemorrhage. If major bleeding occurs in these lesions, there is a discrete ulcer with arterial bleeding or a sentinel clot in the lesion.

Many terms have been used to describe mucosal and submucosal vascular lesions: telangiectasia, arteriovenous malformation, and angiodysplasia. Endoscopic differentiation of these three lesions is seldom possible. Endoscopic treatment should aim at the submucosal level but avoid a full-thickness burn. A small lesion can be treated directly by endoscopic hemostasis. With a larger lesion, treatment proceeds from the periphery to the center of the lesion.

Treatment should be preceded by appropriate cardiovascular resuscitation and attempts to correct any coexisting coagulopathy. Removal of adherent clots (i.e., those resisting gentle washing) without evidence of active bleeding is not recommended unless surgical backup is available because of the risk of precipitating bleeding. Deep, bleeding ulcers on the posterior duodenal bulb or high lesser curvature are at high risk for major hemorrhage. Emergent surgical intervention may be necessary if endoscopic hemostasis is not possible, is unsuccessful, or precipitates uncontrollable bleeding. We are in agreement with the conclusions of an NIH Consensus Panel, which stated that a surgeon should be involved from the outset in the management team caring for the patient with upper gastrointestinal bleeding.[3, 4]

METHODS

Thermal Devices

Thermal devices are among the most commonly employed in endoscopic hemostasis. The localized heating causes tissue edema, shrinkage, protein denaturation, contraction of blood vessels, and tissue desiccation. A variety of endoscopic methods use the generation of heat to achieve hemostasis, including the monopolar probe, bipolar (BICAP) probe, the heater probe, and laser photocoagulation. Thermal energy is generated by conversion of electrical energy into optical frequencies (i.e., lasers), radio frequencies (i.e., electrocautery), or low frequencies (i.e., heater probe). BICAP and heater probes are contact thermal devices, and the endoscopist can attempt to compress a bleeding site (i.e., coaptation) before the application of thermal energy. This helps avoid the heat sink effect (i.e., loss of thermal energy to blood flowing away from the bleeding site), and effectively promotes protein bonding of the intimal surfaces.[39, 40]

Monopolar Electrocoagulation

One of the earliest techniques used in endoscopic hemostasis was the monopolar probe. The monopolar device employs a high-frequency current (1 MHz) that travels from the electrode through the patient's tissue toward a grounding plate attached to the patient. The current flow from the electrode to the tissue produces heat that coagulates protein, causing tissue contraction and vessel shrinkage. In typical usage, a Valley Laboratory electrosurgical unit is set on a coagulation dial setting of 5 to 7, or the Cameron-Miller coagulation unit set is on 5.[41, 42]

The monopolar probe is placed within 2 to 3 mm of the vessel in the ulcer base and activated for 2 to 3 seconds per application, as it is moved around the vessel in four to five applications. Most monopolar units are without liquid irrigation capabilities (i.e., dry). Simultaneous water irrigation capabilities (i.e., liquid electrocoagulation) can facilitate visibility and lessen adherence of the electrode to the treated site.

The success rate for control of upper gastrointestinal bleeding ranges from 80% to 96% in uncontrolled studies.[42] Controlled studies using liquid electrocoagulation demonstrated the effectiveness of monopolar coagulation in patients with peptic ulcer bleeding.[43, 44] Liabilities of monopolar electrocoagulation include the possibility of excessively deep tissue injury (*i.e.,* erosion), tissue adherence, and the need to periodically clean the tip of the probe as coagulum accumulates.[40, 41] A few perforations have been reported from Europe.[45] The unpredictability of the depth of injury produced by monopolar cautery precludes wide usage of this method. Monopolar electrocoagulation for endoscopic hemostasis has been virtually abandoned because it can produce deep tissue injury that risks perforation, and there are safer and more effective methods available.

Bipolar or Multipolar Electrocoagulation

The bipolar or multipolar probe (known commercially as BICAP) has three pairs of electrodes on its sides, and the tip forms a cylindric probe. If any pair of the electrodes is in contact with the tissue, electrocoagulation can be performed, allowing tangential application of the probe. A grounding plate is not necessary because the current flows between the two adjacent electrodes. Less deep tissue injury is incurred from the localized pathway, with a concomitant reduction in risk of perforation. The maximal depth of tissue coagulation is less than 3 mm. Irrigation of the target area is accomplished through a central opening in the probe. The maximal voltage from the BICAP power unit is limited to approximately 50 V. The maximal power output is 50 W, and the maximal tissue temperature attained is 100°C. As a result, deep tissue injury caused by arcing and erosion do not occur.

Large (3.2-mm) and small (2.4-mm) probes are available. Studies show that the 3.2-mm probe provides significantly better hemostasis than the 2.4-mm probe when the depth of tissue injury is equivalent.[46] Power source settings range from 1 to 10 for power and 1 second, 2 seconds, or continuous for timed delivery. The irrigation and coagulation modes are activated by means of a foot switch.

Placing the probe with firm pressure against the bleeding site or nonbleeding visible vessel helps obtain coaptive coagulation. Important factors in obtaining successful hemostasis include forceful application of the probe to the bleeding lesion and a prolonged period of coagulation.[47] Two techniques are employed to coagulate a vessel in an ulcer. One involves using a power setting of 7 on a 50-W generator, with several applications of 2-second bursts of energy. If bleeding continues or recurs, a second application of several bursts can be applied. The other technique uses a lower power setting (5 on a 50-W generator) with 5- to 10-second pulses, which allows slower, deeper heating before tissue desiccation occurs.[47] This technique produced better hemostasis in recent reports. The Gold probe (Microinvasive, Watertown, MA), a new multipolar electrocoagulation probe, has been shown to be comparable to the BICAP probe in recent studies.[48]

In controlled clinical trials, BICAP probes have shown promising, although sometimes conflicting, results. Two favorable studies evaluating the use of the BICAP in treatment of active upper gastrointestinal bleeding and in ulcers with nonbleeding visible vessels were reported by Laine.[49] The first study examined 44 patients with active bleeding at endoscopy, which is defined as persistent bleeding for more than 5 minutes of endoscopic observation. The second study included 75 patients with a nonbleeding visible vessel in a peptic ulcer.[50] These trials showed patients treated with BICAP to have significantly less need for emergency surgery, length of hospitalization, blood transfusion requirements, and hospital costs compared with controls. In both studies, a mean of more than 40 seconds of electrocoagulation (in 2-second pulses) per patient was given, with a setting of 5 on a 50-W BICAP power source. In the second trial, the BICAP precipitated bleeding in 7 of 38 patients treated. Continued BICAP coagulation controlled bleeding in 6 patients, but 7 patients required emergency surgery. No perforations occurred.

In four series reported from the United Kingdom, outcomes have not been as favorable as those reported by Laine.[51–54] Possible reasons for this discrepancy may be the inclusion of patients at low risk of further bleeding (*e.g.,* no stigmata) in the British studies, because the outcome in this group of patients is already quite good without intervention. Important differences in technique also exist between the British and Laine's studies. The British studies used much shorter periods of electrocoagulation, and three of four studies used the 2.3-mm probe. The optimal technique for bipolar electrocoagulation recommended by Laine[55] should include the use of the 3.2-mm probe, positioning of the tip of the endoscope en face as close as possible to the bleeding lesion, lower watt settings of 3 to 5 (*i.e.,* 15–25 W), and prolonged periods of coagulation.[55] Multiple 2-second pulses given in rapid succession appear to be as effective as a single, long pulse of identical duration. BICAP multipolar electrocoagulation has been used effectively to treat bleeding from angiomata and Mallory-Weiss tears.

Heater Probe

The heater probe is a thermal contact device that can be used to achieve hemostasis. The heater probe consists of an internal heating element covered by a teflon-coated aluminum cylinder, which can reach a maximal internal temperature of 250°C. Heat passes into the tissue by conduction, and no electrical current travels through the patient. A thermocoupling device maintains the tip at a constant temperature of 160°C until a preset amount of energy has been delivered. Three longitudinal channels near the tip allow irrigation of the target with a jet of water. Irrigation intensity and thermal energy delivered can be controlled by push buttons on the control box. The water also provides a liquid interface between the tissue and the probe to help avoid tissue adherence. The round tip of the heater probe is designed to allow the simultaneous application of heat and pressure (i.e., coaptive coagulation). Large (3.2-mm) and small (2.4-mm) probes are available.

Most physicians recommend initial tamponade at the visible vessel or site of bleeding, followed by coagulation with four or more 30-J pulses per station. Jensen and colleagues recommended techniques for heater probe hemostasis for different types of bleeding lesions.[56] They recommend fewer joules and total pulses for Dieulafoy's disease, Mallory-Weiss tears, and gastrointestinal angiomas (Table 11–4). It is important to maintain firm pressure on the bleeding site with the heater probe for sufficient periods, because each 30-J burst can take up to 8 seconds to deliver. After heater probe coag-

ulation, the protruding vessel appears flattened with a blanched area and cessation of hemorrhage. An alternative method of heater probe hemostasis is to coagulate in a circumferential manner, with eventual application of the heater probe to the visible vessel, avoiding instigation of further bleeding in treating larger lesions.

Johnston and associates reported encouraging results from a retrospective study using a heater probe in the treatment of major bleeding from peptic ulcer disease.[31] Seventy-four patients with bleeding ulcers were treated with the heater probe. Successful hemostasis was initially achieved in 97%, with an 18% rebleeding rate. Rebleeding was treated successfully in most patients, with a final success rate of 93%. There were no perforations attributed to heater probe treatment.

Fullarton and colleagues examined 630 patients presenting with upper gastrointestinal bleeding.[57] Of these, 166 (26%) had peptic ulcer disease. Of 43 patients, 20 were randomized to heater probe (18 with active bleeding, 2 with a visible vessel) and 23 patients to sham therapy (21 with active bleeding, 2 with a visible vessel). In actively bleeding ulcers, immediate hemostasis was achieved in 78% of patients treated with heater probe but in none of the patients receiving sham treatment. Significant rebleeding during hospitalization occurred in none of the 20 patients treated with the heater probe, and in 5 of the 23 in the control group. A single perforation occurred in the group treated with the heater probe. The researchers concluded that heater probe therapy could be effective in stopping acute bleeding and in the prevention of rebleeding. Lin and coworkers examined the efficacy of heater probe treatment versus medical therapy in 61 patients with nonbleeding visible vessels observed at the time of initial endoscopy for upper gastrointestinal bleeding.[58]

Table 11–4. RECOMMENDED HEATER PROBE TECHNIQUES

Lesion	Tamponade Pressure	Setting (Joules)	Pulses/ Tamponade Station	Site of Hemostasis
Chronic peptic ulcer	Very firm	30	4	Only on visible vessel
Acute ulcer or Dieulafoy's disease*	Firm	25	3	Only on bleeding point
Mallory-Weiss tear†	Moderate	20	2–3	Only on bleeding point
GI angiomas‡	Gentle	10	1–2	Entire angioma

*Treatment of visible vessel (actively bleeding or nonbleeding) only is recommended.
†Treatment of actively bleeding lesions only.
‡For treatment of all angiomas in the bowel segment causing GI bleeding.
Reprinted with permission from Jensen DM. Endoscopic coagulation therapy: heater probe. *In*: Sugawa C, Schuman BM, Lucas CE, eds. Gastrointestinal bleeding. New York: Igaku-Shoin, 1992: 298–313.

Patients were randomized to heater probe treatment (30) or medical management only (31). Patients treated by heater probe showed a statistically significant greater rate of ultimate hemostasis when specific subsets of patients with multiple clinical risk factors for rebleeding (*e.g.*, age >60 years, those presenting in shock, or those needing >500 mL of blood) were analyzed.

Laser Photocoagulation

Laser (*i.e., light amplification by stimulated emission of radiation*) energy differs from normal light sources in that the light is coherent, with all photons in phase at a given wavelength at which their energy is emitted. The intense monochrome light energy produced by a laser is directed through a flexible quartz silica fiber to photocoagulate the bleeding ulcers. Clinical studies have shown that Nd:YAG laser photocoagulation can effectively arrest bleeding secondary to peptic ulcer disease.

Endoscopic application of the laser depends on the ability of a flexible translucent conduit to transmit the light efficiently.[59] Fiber composition is usually crystalline quartz with an outer coating of silicon. The fiber is placed inside a teflon sheath that allows for a coaxial flow of CO_2 or H_2O to wash blood away from the lesion and protect the tip from overheating. These fibers are physically capable of transmitting light with a wavelength of approximately 250 to 2400 nm. This constraint limits which types of lasers can be adapted for endoscopic usage. The two lasers that fulfill this requirement and have had extensive clinical testing are the argon and neodymium:yttrium-aluminum-garnet crystal (Nd:YAG) lasers. The argon laser produces a bluish-green light with a wavelength of approximately 500 nm, which is strongly absorbed by red pigments, such as hemoglobin. The argon beam has little penetration power. It produces a shallow coagulative effect, with a depth of penetration of about 1 mm. The Nd:YAG laser, which emits light with a wavelength of 1060 nm in the near-infrared portion of the spectrum, produces a beam that is poorly absorbed by tissue chromophores and that can produce much greater depths of coagulation and injury. Because of its enhanced ability to coagulate tissue below the mucosal level, the Nd:YAG laser has largely supplanted the argon laser in the treatment of peptic ulcer disease, although the argon laser is preferred by some for treatment of vascular malformations, especially in the colon.

Generally recommended techniques involve a power setting on the laser of 50 to 100 W, with short bursts of 0.3 to 0.6 seconds. The endoscope is positioned approximately 0.5 to 1.5 cm from the lesion. The endoscopist typically initiates coagulation circumferentially around the vessel, observing for blanching of the tissue and trying to avoid vaporizing the tissue. After coagulation of the periphery, attention is directed to the bleeding focus. Bleeding can be iatrogenically induced, but this ceases with further endoscopic therapy in most cases. It behooves the operator to exercise caution with direct laser coagulation of bleeding ulcers located in the posterior duodenal bulb or high on the lesser curvature, because the procedure can elicit necrosis of the gastroduodenal or left gastric artery wall. These arteries are too large for effective endoscopic hemostasis and can bleed torrentially. Hemostasis is most effective when the ulcer can be approached en face with the laser, and this is more easily accomplished with gastric than with duodenal ulcers. Nd:YAG lasers have greater tissue penetration and more potential for perforation than other methods. Lasers are not easily transported, are expensive, and require a prolonged period of training for the endoscopist and technician–assistant.

Endoscopic laser hemostasis enjoyed significant popularity during the early and mid-1980s and numerous randomized, controlled studies were reported. Both Macleod and Rutgeerts and coworkers reported a decreased incidence of rebleeding and need for operation in patients treated with the Nd:YAG laser.[60, 61] Rohde and colleagues and Ihre and associates showed no benefit from laser treatment.[62, 63] Swain's group reported results in 1986 obtained from 138 bleeding peptic ulcer patients with stigmata of recent hemorrhage who were accessible to laser treatment.[64] Overall, 7 of 70 ulcer patients and 27 of 68 controls had further bleeding (p <0.001); 7 of 70 ulcer patients and 24 of 68 controls required surgery (p <0.001); and 1 of 70 ulcer patients and 8 of 68 controls died (p <0.05).

The outstanding results obtained in this study came from a group of superb gastroenterologists committed to and proficient in the use of the Nd:YAG laser. Even in expert hands, however, 19% of entrants into the study were unable to be treated by laser because of technical difficulties. A less sanguine assessment of endoscopic Nd:YAG treatment was published by Krejs and colleagues in 1987.[65] In a population of 174 patients (32 with active bleeding, 142 with stigmata of recent hemorrhage), no overall benefits over controls were observed in rebleeding, the need for operation or intensive care, and mean hospital stay. Proponents of Nd:YAG criticized the study for its low percentage of patients with active spurting hemorrhage (1%) and visible vessels (17%), because this might tend to dilute any real effect because most upper gastrointestinal bleeding stops spontaneously. Reports supporting Nd:YAG therapy have been published by Matthewson and colleagues in London and Eckhauser and Malangoni in Cleveland.[66, 67] The former group found a significant ($p < 0.05$) reduction in rebleeding and a numeric reduction (2% vs. 9%) in mortality in a controlled, randomized study. Although the Cleveland researchers were able to stop active bleeding in 35 (87.5%) of 40 patients, 4 patients rebled after laser therapy but responded to repeat endoscopic treatment. Hemostasis was not able to be achieved in 5 patients, and they required emergency surgery.

Although laser can provide effective hemostasis, its cost, lack of portability, and prolonged training time make it less attractive than some of the other modalities currently available. Increased portability, safety, miniaturization, and decreased cost of laser technology will be welcome, but these developments await advances in technical capabilities.

Injection Therapy

Injection sclerotherapy of esophageal varices (see Chapter 10) has been shown to be relatively safe and effective in the control of bleeding esophageal varices. This technique has been expanded to include nonvariceal bleeding lesions. Injection therapy is simple, inexpensive, and readily available, and it can be performed at the time of diagnostic endoscopy.[7, 9, 68–72]

Techniques

Table 11–5 lists several investigated injection methods. The technique and volume of injection therapy for bleeding lesions varies, depending on the type of sclerosing agents. All injections are made through a plastic or metal injector with a 23- to 25-gauge needle. The solution is injected at three or four sites about 1 to 3 mm from the vessel or lesion. The volume of injectate varies with the solution.

Sclerosing Agents

Epinephrine (1:10,000) Alone or Diluted with Normal Saline (1:10,000). This solution is made by mixing epinephrine (1:1000, 1 mL) with normal saline (0.9%, 9 mL). Between 1 and 3 mL of epinephrine (1:10,000) is injected into three or four sites around the blood vessel, with a total volume range from 6 to 12 mL. Hemostasis with epinephrine results from its vasoconstrictive properties on the submucosal or subserosal arteries, combined with a physical tamponade effect as it is injected with 3 to 4 mL of normal saline.[73] In a randomized, controlled study of epinephrine injection for actively bleeding ulcers, 68 patients with active bleeding from ulcers were divided into two groups of 34 patients.[74] The researchers concluded that endoscopic epinephrine injection was effective in stopping bleeding, and it significantly decreased transfusion requirements and the need for emergency surgery.

Hypertonic Saline-Epinephrine Solution. Three milliliters of a solution of 3.6% hypertonic saline plus 1:20,000 epinephrine is injected at three or four sites at the base of a bleeding vessel to a total dose of 9 to 12 mL. For bleeding lesions with extensive fibrosis, 1 mL of saline (7.2%) and epinephrine solution is similarly injected with a total dose of 3 to 4 mL. Repeat prophylactic injections are made at any visible vessel 24 or 48 hours after the initial hemostasis. Hypertonic saline prolongs the effects of epinephrine and adds tissue effects of hypertonic-

Table 11–5. INJECTED METHODS

Agent	No. of Sites	Total Dose (mL)
Epinephrine (1:10,000)[74]	2–4	6–12
Hypertonic saline (3.6%) + 1:20,000 epinephrine[75]	3–4	9–12
Absolute (98%) ethanol[69]	3–4	0.6–1.0
Epinephrine (1:10,000) + polidocanol (1%)[80]	3–4	5–12 5
Thrombin (100 IU) in 0.9% saline (3 mL)[81]	3–4	10–15
Sodium morrhuate (5%) + thrombin + dextrose (50%)[82]		3 2

ity, including tissue swelling, fibrinoid degeneration, and vessel wall thrombosis of the vessel lumen. Hirao and colleagues published results using hypertonic saline and epinephrine in 158 patients with peptic ulcer disease.[75] Permanent hemostasis was achieved in 93%. Only 1 of 128 patients who received prophylactic repeat injections required emergency surgery, and no complications were reported.

Absolute Ethanol. Dehydrated ethanol (98%) is injected, with a total dose of 0.6 to 1.0 mL, using a 1-mL disposable plastic tuberculin syringe.[69, 71] The ethanol is injected slowly in amounts of 0.1 to 0.2 mL per injection at three or four sites surrounding the bleeding vessel and 1 or 2 mm from the vessel. The mechanism of hemostasis is dehydration and fixation of the blood vessel and surrounding tissue. The resulting vascular wall degeneration, vasoconstriction, and endothelial cell destruction lead to local thrombosis.[76] Asaki and coworkers in Japan treated 332 patients, of whom 90% had peptic ulcer disease and 52% had exposed blood vessels.[68] Initial hemostasis was obtained in 330 patients (99%); rebleeding occurred in 20 (6%), and 3 (1%) developed perforations, which were not considered to be directly attributable to ethanol injection. In a review of our experience, we treated 75 patients with upper gastrointestinal hemorrhage, including 53 patients with peptic ulcer disease. Of 53 lesions actively bleeding at the time of endoscopic treatment, 52 were initially controlled. Rebleeding occurred in 3 of these patients. Definitive hemostasis was obtained in 50 (89%) of 56 actively bleeding lesions. Pascu and coworkers, in a randomized, controlled study, treated 145 patients with either active bleeding or stigmata of recent hemorrhage.[77] These patients were randomized to receive conventional medical therapy or to endoscopic hemostasis using absolute ethanol. Injection with absolute ethanol achieved hemostasis in 24 of 25 patients. Emergency surgery was not necessary in any of the patients in the injection group. The mortality rate was significantly lower in the injection group.

Epinephrine Followed by BICAP, Nd:YAG Laser, Heater Probe, Monopolar Electrocoagulation, or Polidocanol. Injection therapy has been combined with other hemostatic methods with good results. Epinephrine (1:10,000, 5–12 mL) is injected around the blood vessel to obtain initial hemostasis or decelerate bleeding by volume compression and vasoconstriction. Other hemostatic methods are applied to achieve definitive hemostasis by obliterating the vessel. Epinephrine injection has been combined with the Nd:YAG laser and BICAP. Rutgeerts and colleagues carried out a randomized trial comparing the efficacy of the Nd:YAG laser and BICAP in treating bleeding peptic ulcers.[78] All 50 bleeding lesions in each group were injected with 4 to 10 mL of epinephrine (1:10,000) before laser or BICAP application. After two sessions, the success rate was 88% in the laser group and 86% in the BICAP group. One perforation occurred in each group. Boix and coworkers combined injection of epinephrine with electrohydrocoagulation, followed by injection of polidocanol (1%).[79] They controlled 26 of 28 actively bleeding ulcers initially and 23 of 28 permanently in an uncontrolled study. No complications were reported. There are many reports on combined injection therapy using epinephrine (1:10,000) followed by polidocanol (1%) with good results.[80]

Thrombin in Normal Saline. Thrombin (100 IU) in normal saline (0.9%, 3 mL) is injected around the bleeding vessel until bleeding stops. This usually requires 10 to 15 mL of the solution. Fuchs and colleagues treated 47 patients with thrombin and normal saline.[81] Spurting bleeders were successfully treated in 7 of 10 patients. Ten (85%) of 13 patients with oozing lesions were permanently controlled. The rate of initial hemostasis was 96%. The injection method was ultimately successful in 75% of the cases, with no complications.

Other Sclerosing Agents. Adams used a mixture of sodium morrhuate (5%, 3 mL), thrombin (2 mL), and dextrose (50%) to sclerose and thrombose the bleeding vessel.[82] He reported successful hemostasis of bleeding peptic ulcers in 8 patients, with no complications.

Topical Agents

Four types of topical agents have been used to control bleeding: various clotting factors, cyanoacrylate tissue glues, microcrystalline collagen hemostat (MCH, Avitene), and metallic slurries as part of ferromagnetic tamponade. Because they cause minimal tissue damage, can reach diffuse lesions in the gastrointestinal tract, and require less precise localization of the bleeding site during administration, topical agents are theoretically attractive.[83] They would seem to have a place in the treatment of diffuse gastric mucosal lesions or as an addition to more well-established interventions, but definitive clinical studies have yet to be reported. Clinical series examining the use of topical agents have been poorly devised or have been too small to be of statistical significance. Their findings are frequently conflicting and inconsistent.

Mechanical Methods

Helicoidal metal "sutures" can be applied through the endoscope using a rotary motion.[84] Hemoclips (i.e., miniature metal clips 1.5 mm wide) can be applied to bleeding vessels through the biopsy channel of the endoscope by using a special flexible slip applicator. This technique becomes easier to perform with an improved clip and applicator. Although good results are reported from Japan, this method is seldom used in the United States. Use of the helicoidal suture, especially if it is absorbable, holds some promise, but it is untested.[84]

Taylor reported the use of a balloon for tamponade treatment of a bleeding duodenal ulcer.[85] A balloon is inserted over an endoscope and inflated to 2.5 cm in the duodenal bulb. The endoscope is then withdrawn, leaving the balloon impacted in the duodenal bulb. Three patients suffering from chronic duodenal ulcer bleeding were treated in this manner. Results were not impressive: 1 patient rebled, and 1 patient died. This treatment does not seem to be an effective means of controlling bleeding from vessels situated in the base of a deep ulcer.

COMPARATIVE STUDIES

Prospective randomized trials comparing methods of endoscopic hemostasis are listed in Table 11–6.

Laine published a randomized trial comparing BICAP with ethanol injection therapy in patients with actively bleeding ulcers and in those with a nonbleeding vessel.[86] BICAP and ethanol injection appeared equally effective and safe (Table 11–6) in 60 patients who had ulcers with active bleeding (26) or a nonbleeding vessel (34). He reported one delayed perforation 9 days after BICAP therapy.

In 1988, Woods and associates published results of a prospective trial comparing BICAP with injection therapy in 21 male patients.[87] They concluded that the heater probe and epinephrine injection are equally effective in controlling ulcer bleeding, and both are less successful in patients with large ulcers (>20 mm) or with significant orthostatic hypotension on admission.

Lin found the heater probe to be more effective than ethanol injection and more applicable in cases of spurting arteries and if tangential application was required.[88] He found that the ability to wash and compress the bleeding vessel simultaneously aided in identifying the vessel and in establishing hemostasis. A larger com-

Table 11–6. RANDOMIZED COMPARISONS OF ENDOSCOPIC HEMOSTATIC METHODS

Method 1/Method 2	No. of Patients	Initial Hemostasis (%)	Rebleeding (%)	Permanent Hemostasis (%)	Emergency Surgery (%)	Mortality (%)
BICAP/	14	100		94	6	3
ethanol inj[86]	12	83		90	7	3
BICAP/	11		28	72	0	9
ethanol inj[87]	10		20	80	10	10
Heat probe/	42	100	12	95	2	0
ethanol[88]	36	81*	22*	70	0	0
Heat probe/	45	98	18	91*	7	0
ethanol inj/	46	67*	7	67*	4	2
control[89]				52*	26*	15
Heat probe/	64	83	11		22	4
epineph[90]	68	96*	17		20	2
BICAP + epineph/	50	72	25	86	6	14
laser + epineph[78]	50	72	20	88	12	14
Hypert sal + epineph/	33	88	12	88	0	0
ethanol inj[91]	34	94	6	91	0	0
Nd:YAG/	44		20	80	20	2
heat probe/	57		28	72	22	10
control[66]	42		42	58	30	9
Heater probe/	32	93*	22*		3*	3
BICAP	30	90*	44		33	3
control[92]	32	20	72		41	9

*Significance by authors

Abbreviations: inj, injection; epineph, epinephrine; hypert sal, hypertonic saline.

Reprinted with permission from Steffes CP, Sugawa C. Endoscopic management of nonvariceal gastrointestinal bleeding. World J Surg 16:1025–1033, 1992.

parison with untreated controls confirmed the superiority of the heater probe to ethanol injection in terms of initial and permanent hemostasis, need for surgery, and mortality.[89]

Chung and colleagues found epinephrine injection to have a higher initial hemostasis rate than the heater probe, but the two methods were equivalent in terms of outcome.[90] However, they reported two perforations after two treatments with heater probes in two ulcer patients.

Rutgeerts and coworkers found that epinephrine injection followed by Nd:YAG laser or BICAP treatment achieved equivalent results.[78] He stressed the importance of multiple treatment sessions to obtain permanent hemostasis.

In 1986, Chen and associates compared the hemostatic effects of hypertonic saline-epinephrine solution and pure ethanol in 67 patients with nonvariceal gastrointestinal bleeding.[91] Thirty-three patients had saline-epinephrine and 34 patients had ethanol injections. There were no complications. The researchers suggested that the hemostatic effect was more effective with the ethanol injection in the group of patients with stigmata of recent hemorrhage, but the saline-epinephrine injection showed better results in patients with active bleeding.

The series by Matthewson and coworkers found that Nd:YAG treated patients had less rebleeding than those treated with a heater probe, but not significantly so.[66] Jensen and colleagues concluded that the heater probe was superior to BICAP in preventing rebleeding.[92]

COMPLICATIONS

Complications specific to endoscopic hemostasis are uncommon. Complications include induced acute hemorrhage, delayed hemorrhage, tissue necrosis, or perforation. The incidence of perforation has been low, with rates of 1% to 3% usually reported. Perforations have occurred with the use of monopolar electrocoagulation, laser, or heater probe; the injection of absolute ethanol or polidocanol; the use of epinephrine and laser and epinephrine and BICAP; or a combination of epinephrine, ethanol, and heater probe.[45, 57, 65, 68, 69, 78, 80, 89, 93] Extensive necrosis of the gastric mucosa and gastric necrosis have been reported after injections of epinephrine plus polidocanol and after ethanolamine oleate (12 mL), respectively.[94, 95] Pancreaticoduodenal necrosis has been reported after endoscopic injection of cyanoacrylate to treat bleeding ulcers in a very sick patient.[96] Induced bleeding is more common during ther-

mal therapy than with injection therapy. The rate of induced bleeding has been 5% to 30% in patients with visible vessels treated with thermal therapy. The incidence is slightly higher with lasers than with other contact devices.[78] Induced bleeding is also reported with injection therapy of epinephrine plus polidocanol.[97] Bleeding usually can be controlled with further endoscopic therapy. In the case of ulcers, hemostatic interventions occasionally induce bleeding from vessels damaged by injection or thermal therapy and by inadequate hemostasis of the original bleeding vessel.

The most common complications of endoscopic procedures are cardiopulmonary or are related to the sedation given.[98] Cardiopulmonary monitoring is important to avoid complications, especially in patients with severe gastrointestinal bleeding. We use blood pressure and continuous oxygen saturation monitoring by means of the pulse oximeter for all patients to avert these complications.[99]

RECOMMENDATIONS

There are an abundance of prospective, randomized trials showing comparable efficacy between thermal modalities and injection therapy for initial and permanent hemostasis, rate of rebleeding, transfusion requirements, need for emergency surgery, and mortality rates. Factors to be considered in comparing thermal and injection methods include efficacy, safety, cost, ease of use, and portability. A comparison of various endoscopic hemostatic modalities is shown in Table 11–7.

In 1989, a Consensus Conference held by the National Institutes of Health separated the various methods into three categories: most promising techniques, other techniques, and techniques not recommended. Multipolar electrocoagulation and heater probes were considered the most promising techniques. Nd:YAG laser and injection therapy were classified as other techniques. The drawbacks of Nd:YAG lasers are cost, lack of portability, and greater difficulty in learning the technique. The Conference considered that some agents used in injection therapy (e.g., sodium chloride plus epinephrine, ethanol) were promising for early control of bleeding, but that the current data were insufficient to warrant a specific recommendation. However, they thought that injection therapy warranted further study because of its technical ease of use, low cost, and promising results. The techniques not recommended included topical, argon laser, and monopolar coagulation.

Table 11–7. COMPARISON OF ENDOSCOPIC HEMOSTATIC MODALITIES

Parameter	Injection	Thermal Contact	Laser
Stop bleeding	Yes	Yes	Yes
Decrease in surgery	Yes	Yes	Yes
Reduce mortality	Yes	Yes	Yes
Cost	Least	Moderate	Expensive
Ease of use	Most	Intermediate	Least
Portability	Most	Intermediate	Least

Because of laboratory and clinical experience, we currently favor the combined use of epinephrine injection and heater probe.[2, 41, 70, 71, 73, 76, 100] Epinephrine injection is more effective for immediate hemostasis and preferable to ethanol injection because of greater overall effectiveness, lessened tissue damage and technical ease of use. The heater probe is preferred because of its low cost, portability, and effectiveness. We have also used BICAP electrocautery with success. Several hemostatic modalities should be available for use, depending on the anatomic location and type of bleeding ulcers. Our experience in upper gastrointestinal bleeding in an urban population has been that aggressive management, together with endoscopic hemostasis and surgery, based on clinical criteria and ulcer appearance results in a low overall mortality rate. In a series of over 500 admissions for upper gastrointestinal hemorrhage, we reported a surgical mortality rate of 3.7% for patients with bleeding peptic ulcers using this approach.[2]

CONCLUSION

Nonvariceal upper gastrointestinal bleeding continues to be a frequent and serious problem. Definition of the precise appearance and location of the source of bleeding by endoscopy gives important information about the cause and risk of rebleeding and the indications for surgery. It is difficult to champion a single method of endoscopic hemostatic therapy because of the contradictory outcome of studies, differences in population, patient exclusions, and differences in criteria for successful therapy. The nonerosive heater and BICAP probes are preferred. Injection therapy with epinephrine or sclerosing agents can be recommended as a safe, efficacious, and economical means of treatment and can be combined with a coaptive coagulation device. Several hemostatic modalities should be available for use, depending on the anatomic location and type of bleeding ulcers. The collaboration of skilled interventional endoscopists with their traditional surgical colleagues offers the patient with upper gastrointestinal bleeding the optimal probability of a successful outcome with minimal treatment-associated morbidity.

References

1. Sugawa C. Endoscopic diagnosis and treatment of upper gastrointestinal bleeding. Surg Clin North Am 69:1167–1183, 1989.
2. Sugawa C, Steffes CP, Nakamura R, et al. Upper GI bleeding in an urban hospital. Ann Surg 212:521–527, 1990.
3. NIH Consensus Conference. Therapeutic endoscopy and bleeding ulcers. JAMA 262:1369–1372, 1989.
4. NIH Consensus Statement. Therapeutic endoscopy and bleeding ulcers. Gastrointest Endosc 36:S62–S65, 1990.
5. Cook DJ, Guyatt GH, Salena BJ, et al. Endoscopic therapy for acute nonvariceal upper gastrointestinal hemorrhage: a meta-analysis. Gastroenterology 102:129–148, 1992.
6. Laurence BH, Cotton PB. Bleeding gastroduodenal ulcers: nonoperative treatment. World J Surg 11:295–303, 1987.
7. Sanowski RA. Endoscopic injection therapy for nonvariceal bleeding lesions of the upper gastrointestinal tract. [Editorial] J Clin Gastroenterol 11:247–252, 1989.
8. Steele RJC. Endoscopic haemostasis for non-variceal upper gastrointestinal haemorrhage. Br J Surg 76:219–225, 1989.
9. Sugawa C, Bradley SJ. Endoscopic sclerosis of non-variceal gastroduodenal hemorrhage. Probl Gen Surg 7:43–48, 1990.
10. Fleischer DE. Endoscopic control of upper gastrointestinal bleeding. J Clin Gastroenterol 12:S41–S47, 1990.
11. Dent TL. Diagnostic endoscopy. In Fidelian-Green RG, Turcotte JG, eds. Gastrointestinal hemorrhage. New York: Grune & Stratton, 1980:39–50.
12. Palmer ED. The vigorous diagnostic approach to upper gastrointestinal tract haemorrhage: a 23-year prospective study of 14,000 patients. JAMA 207:1477–1480, 1969.
13. Sugawa C, Werner MH, Hayes DF, et al. Early endoscopy: a guide to therapy for acute hemorrhage in the upper gastrointestinal tract. Arch Surg 107:133–137, 1973.
14. Katz D, Petchumoni CS, Thomas E, et al. The endoscopic diagnosis of upper gastrointestinal hemorrhage. Am J Dig Dis 21:182–189, 1976.
15. Graham DY, Davis RE. Acute upper gastrointestinal hemorrhage: new observations on an old problem. Am J Dig Dis 23:76, 1978.

16. Himal HS, Perrault C, Mzabi R. Upper gastrointestinal hemorrhage. Surgery 84:448–454, 1978.
17. Iglesias MC, Dourdourekas D, Adomavicious J, et al. Prompt endoscopic diagnosis of upper gastrointestinal hemorrhage: its value for specific diagnosis and management. Ann Surg 189:90–95, 1979.
18. Gilbert DA, Silverstein FE, Tedesco FJ, et al. The National ASGE Survey on upper gastrointestinal bleeding, III: endoscopy in upper gastrointestinal bleeding. Gastrointest Endosc 27:94–102, 1981.
19. Gostout CJ, Wang KK, Ahlquist DA, et al. Acute gastrointestinal bleeding. J Clin Gastroenterol 14:260–267, 1992.
20. Sugawa C, Lucas CE, Rosenberg BF, et al. Differential topography of acute erosive gastritis due to trauma or sepsis, ethanol and aspirin. Gastrointest Endosc 19:127–130, 1973.
21. Lucas CE, Sugawa C, Friend W, et al. Therapeutic implications of disturbed gastric physiology in patients with stress ulcerations. Am J Surg 123:25–34, 1972.
22. Lebrec D, DeFleury P, Rueff B, et al. Portal hypertension, size of esophageal varices, and risk of gastrointestinal bleeding in alcoholic cirrhosis. Gastroenterology 79:1139–1144, 1980.
23. Beppu K, Inokuchi K, Koyanagi N, et al. Prediction of variceal hemorrhage by esophageal endoscopy. Gastrointest Endosc 27:213–218, 1981.
24. DaGradi AE, Mehler R, Tan DTD, et al. Sources of upper gastrointestinal bleeding in patients with liver cirrhosis and large esophagogastric varices. Am J Gastroenterol 54:458–463, 1970.
25. McCray RS, Martin F, Amir-Ahmadi H, et al. Erroneous diagnosis of hemorrhage from esophageal varices. Am J Dig Dis 14:755–760, 1969.
26. Mitchell KJ, Macdougall BRD, Silk DBA, et al. A prospective reappraisal of emergency endoscopy in patients with portal hypertension. Scand J Gastroenterol 17:965–968, 1982.
27. Sugawa C, Benishek DJ, Walt AJ. Mallory-Weiss syndrome: a study of 224 patients. Am J Surg 145:30–33, 1983.
28. Clouse RE, Costigan DJ, Mills BA, et al. Angiodysplasia as a cause of upper gastrointestinal bleeding. Arch Intern Med 145:458–461, 1985.
29. Petrini JL Jr, Johnston JH. Heat probe treatment of antral vascular ectasia. Gastrointest Endosc 35:324–328, 1989.
30. Foster DN, Miloszewski KJA, Losowsky MS. Stigmata of recent hemorrhage in diagnosis and prognosis of upper gastrointestinal bleeding. Br Med J 1:1173–1177, 1978.
31. Johnston JH. Endoscopic thermal treatment of upper gastrointestinal bleeding: overview and guidelines. Endosc Rev 2:2–20, 1985.
32. Johnston JH. Endoscopic risk factors for bleeding peptic ulcer. Gastrointest Endosc 36:S16–S20, 1990.
33. Beckly DE. Prediction of rebleeding from peptic ulcer experience with an endoscopic Doppler device. Gut 27:96–99, 1986.
34. Kohler B, Riemann JF. The endoscopic Doppler: its value in evaluating gastroduodenal ulcers after hemorrhage and as an instrument of control of endoscopic injection therapy. Scand J Gastroenterol 26:471–476, 1991.
35. MacLeod IA, Mills PR. Factors identifying the probability of further haemorrhage after acute upper gastrointestinal haemorrhage. Br J Surg 69:256–258, 1982.
36. Bornman PC, Theodorou NA, Shuttleworth RD, et al. Importance of hypovolaemic shock and endoscopic signs in predicting recurrent haemorrhage from peptic ulceration: a prospective evaluation. Br Med J 291:245–247, 1985.
37. Hunt PS. Bleeding gastroduodenal ulcer: selection of patients for surgery. World J Surg 11:289–294, 1987.
38. Swain CP, Salmon PKR, Northfield TC. Does ulcer position influence presentation or prognosis of acute gastrointestinal bleeding? [Abstract] Gut 27:A632, 1986.
39. Jiranek GC, Silverstein FE. Introduction to endoscopic therapy for bleeding peptic ulcers. Gastrointest Endosc 36:S25–S29, 1990.
40. Johnston JH, Jensen DM, Auth D. Experimental comparison of endoscopic yttrium-aluminum-garnet laser, electrosurgery, and heater probe for canine gut arterial coagulation: importance of compression and avoidance of erosion. Gastroenterology 92:1101–1108, 1987.
41. Sugawa C, Shier M, Lucas CE, et al. Electrocoagulation of bleeding in the upper part of the gastrointestinal tract. A preliminary experimental clinical report. Arch Surg 110:975–979, 1975.
42. Papp JP. Monopolar and electrohydrothermal treatment of upper gastrointestinal bleeding. Gastrointest Endosc 36:S34–S37, 1990.
43. Freitas D, Donato A, Monteiro JG. Controlled trial of liquid monopolar electrocoagulation in bleeding peptic ulcers. Am J Gastroenterol 80:853–857, 1985.
44. Moreto M, Zaballa M, Ibanez S, et al. Efficacy of monopolar electrocoagulation in the treatment of bleeding gastric ulcer: a controlled trial. Endoscopy 19:54–56, 1987.
45. Koch H. Experimentelle untersuchungen und klinische erfahrungen sur electrokoagulation blutender lasionen im oberen gastrointestinaltrakt. Fortschr Endosk 4:69–71, 1973.
46. Morris DL, Brearley S, Thompson H, et al. A comparison of the efficacy and depth of gastric wall injury with 3.2- and 2.3-mm bipolar probes in canine arterial hemorrhage. Gastrointest Endosc 31:361–363, 1985.
47. Laine L. Bipolar/multipolar electrocoagulation. Gastrointest Endosc 36:S38–S41, 1990.
48. Laine L. Determination of the optimal technique for bipolar electrocoagulation treatment. An experimental evaluation of the BICAP and Gold probes. Gastroenterology 100:107–112, 1991.
49. Laine L. Multipolar electrocoagulation in the treatment of active upper gastrointestinal tract hemorrhage. A prospective controlled trial. N Engl J Med 316:1613–1617, 1987.
50. Laine L. Multipolar electrocoagulation in the treatment of peptic ulcers with nonbleeding visible vessels. A prospective, controlled trial. Ann Intern Med 110:510–514, 1989.
51. Brearley S, Hawker PC, Dykes PW, et al. Per-endoscopic bipolar diathermy coagulation of visible vessels using a 3.2 mm probe—a randomised clinical trial. Endoscopy 19:160–163, 1987.
52. Goudie BM, Mitchell KG, Birnie GG, et al. Controlled trial of endoscopic bipolar electrocoagulation in the treatment of bleeding peptic ulcers. [Abstract] Gut 25:A1185, 1984.
53. Kernohan RM, Anderson JR, McKelvey STD, et al. A controlled trial of bipolar electrocoagulation in patients with upper gastrointestinal bleeding. Br J Surg 71:889–891, 1984.
54. O'Brien JD, Day SJ, Burnham WR. Controlled trial of small bipolar probe in bleeding peptic ulcers. Lancet 1:464–467, 1986.
55. Laine LA. Bipolar multipolar electrocoagulation. In: Sugawa C, Schuman BM, Lucas CE, eds. Gastrointestinal bleeding. New York: Igaku-Shoin, 1992:314–323.

56. Jensen DM. Endoscopic coagulation therapy: heater probe. In: Sugawa C, Schuman BM, Lucas CE, eds. Gastrointestinal bleeding. New York: Igaku-Shoin, 1992:298–313.

57. Fullarton GM, Birnie GG, MacDonald A, et al. Controlled trial of heater probe treatment in bleeding peptic ulcers. Br J Surg 76:541–544, 1989.

58. Lin HJ, Lee FY, Kang WM, et al. A controlled study of therapeutic endoscopy for peptic ulcer with non-bleeding visible vessel. Gastrointest Endosc 36:241–246, 1990.

59. Hunter JG. Endoscopic laser applications in the gastrointestinal tract. Surg Clin North Am 69:1147–1166, 1989.

60. MacLeod IA, Mills PR, MacKenzie JF, et al. Neodymium yttrium aluminium garnet laser photocoagulation for major haemorrhage from peptic ulcers and single vessels: a single blind controlled study. Br Med J 286:345–348, 1983.

61. Rutgeerts P, Vantrappen G, Broeckaert L, et al. Controlled trial of YAG laser treatment of upper digestive hemorrhage. Gastroenterology 83:410–416, 1982.

62. Rohde H, Thon K, Fischer M, et al. Results of a defined therapeutic concept of endoscopic ND-YAG laser therapy in patients with upper gastrointestinal bleeding. Br J Surg 67:360, 1980.

63. Ihre T, Johansson C, Seligson U, et al. Endoscopic YAG-Laser treatment in massive upper gastrointestinal bleeding. Scand J Gastroenterol 16:633–640, 1981.

64. Swain CP, Kirkham JS, Salmon PR, et al. Controlled trial of Nd-YAG laser photocoagulation in bleeding peptic ulcers. Lancet 1:1113–1117, 1986.

65. Krejs GJ, Little KH, Westergaard H, et al. Laser photocoagulation for the treatment of acute peptic-ulcer bleeding. N Engl J Med 316:1618–1621, 1987.

66. Matthewson K, Swain CP, Bland M, et al. Randomized comparison of Nd YAG laser, heater probe, and no endoscopic therapy for bleeding peptic ulcers. Gastroenterology 98:1239–1244, 1990.

67. Eckhouser ML, Malangoni MA. Endoscopic intervention: a useful alternative to operation in the treatment of upper gastrointestinal hemorrhage. Am Surg 58:120–125, 1992.

68. Asaki S. Endoscopic hemostasis by local absolute ethanol injection for upper gastrointestinal tract bleeding—a multicenter study. In: Okabe H, Honda T, Ohshiba S, eds. Endoscopic surgery. New York: Elsevier, 1984:105–116.

69. Asaki S, Nishimura T, Satoh A, et al. Endoscopic hemostasis of gastrointestinal hemorrhage by local application of absolute ethanol: a clinical study. Tohoku J Exp Med 141:373–383, 1983.

70. Sugawa C, Fujita Y, Ikeda T, et al. Endoscopic hemostasis of bleeding of the upper gastrointestinal tract by local injection of ninety-eight percent dehydrated ethanol. Surg Gynecol Obstet 162:159–163, 1986.

71. Sugawa C. Injection therapy for the control of bleeding ulcers. Gastrointest Endosc 36:S50–S52, 1990.

72. Sugawa C, Schuman BM. Endoscopic injection therapy. In: Sugawa C, Schuman BM, Lucas CE, eds. Gastrointestinal bleeding. New York: Igaku-Shoin, 1992:347–357.

73. Whittle TJ, Sugawa C, Lucas CE, et al. Effect of hemostatic agents in canine gastric serosal blood vessels. Gastrointest Endosc 37:305–309, 1991.

74. Chung SCS, Leung JWC, Steele RJC, et al. Endoscopic injection of adrenaline for actively bleeding ulcers: a randomized trial. Br Med J 296:1631–1633, 1988.

75. Hirao M, Kobayashi T, Masuda K, et al. Endoscopic local injection of hypertonic saline-epinephrine solution to arrest hemorrhage from the upper gastrointestinal tract. Gastrointest Endosc 31:313–317, 1985.

76. Sugawa C, Fujita Y, Lucas CE, et al. Hemostatic effect of local intramural injection of dehydrated ethanol in the canine gastrointestinal tract. Gastrointest Endosc 35:28–32, 1989.

77. Pascu O, Draghici A, Acalovchi B. The effect of endoscopic hemostasis with alcohol on the mortality rate of nonvariceal upper gastrointestinal hemorrhage. A randomized prospective study. Endoscopy 21:53–55, 1989.

78. Rutgeerts P, Vantrappen G, Van Hootegem PV, et al. Neodymium-YAG laser photocoagulation versus multipolar electrocoagulation for the treatment of severely bleeding ulcers: a randomized comparison. Gastrointest Endosc 33:199–202, 1987.

79. Boix J, Planas R, Humbert P, et al. Endoscopic hemostasis by injection therapy and electrohydrocoagulation in high risk patients with active duodenal bleeding ulcer. Endoscopy 6:225–227, 1987.

80. Soehendra N, Grimm H, Stenzel M. Injection of nonvariceal bleeding lesions of the upper gastrointestinal tract. Endoscopy 17:120–132, 1985.

81. Fuchs KA, Wirtz HJ, Schaube H, et al. Initial experience with thrombin as injection agent for bleeding gastroduodenal lesions. Endoscopy 18:146–148, 1986.

82. Adams W. Endoscopic sclerosis of bleeding duodenal and antral ulcers. Gastrointest Endosc 30:A149, 1984.

83. Peura D. Topical therapy for the control of gastrointestinal bleeding. Gastrointest Endosc 36:S53–S55, 1990.

84. Escourrou J, Delvaux M, Buscail L, et al. First clinical evaluation and experimental study of a new mechanical suture device for endoscopic hemostasis. Gastrointest Endosc 36:494–497, 1990.

85. Taylor TV. Isolated duodenal tamponade for treatment of bleeding duodenal ulcer. Lancet 1:911–912, 1988.

86. Laine L. Multipolar electrocoagulation versus injection therapy in the treatment of bleeding peptic ulcers. A prospective, randomized trial. Gastroenterology 99:1303–1306, 1990.

87. Woods A, Sanowski RA, Waring JP, et al. Endoscopic therapy for gastric and duodenal ulcer bleeding: a comparison of BICAP coagulation versus ethanol sclerotherapy. Gastrointest Endosc 34:209, 1988.

88. Lin HJ, Tsai YT, Lee SD, et al. A prospectively randomized trial of heat probe thermocoagulation versus pure alcohol injection in nonvariceal peptic ulcer hemorrhage. Am J Gastroenterol 83:283–286, 1988.

89. Lin HJ, Lee FY, Kang WM, et al. Heater probe thermocoagulation and pure alcohol injection in massive peptic ulcer hemorrhage: a prospective randomized controlled trial. Gut 31:753–757, 1990.

90. Chung SCS, Leung JWC, Sung JY, et al. Injection or heat probe for bleeding ulcer. Gastroenterology 100:33–37, 1991.

91. Chen PC, Wu CS, Liaw YF. Hemostatic effect of endoscopic local injection with hypertonic saline–epinephrine solution and pure ethanol for digestive tract bleeding. Gastrointest Endosc 32:319–323, 1986.

92. Jensen DM, Machicado GA, Kovacs TOG, et al. Controlled, randomized study of heater probe and BICAP for hemostasis of severe ulcer bleeding. [Abstract] Gastroenterology 94:A208, 1988.

93. Bedford RA, van Stolk R, Sivak MV, et al. Gastric

perforation after endoscopic treatment of a Dieulafoy's lesion. Am J Gastroenterol 87:244–247, 1992.

94. Loperfido S, Patelli G, La Torre L. Extensive necrosis of gastric mucosa following injection therapy of bleeding peptic ulcer. Endoscopy 22:285–286, 1990.

95. Chester JF, Hurley PR. Gastric necrosis: a complication of endoscopic sclerosis for bleeding peptic ulcer. Endoscopy 22:287–288, 1990.

96. Vallieres E, Jamieson C, Haber GB, et al. Pancreatoduodenal necrosis after endoscopic injection of cyanoacrylate to treat a bleeding duodenal ulcer: a case report. Surgery 106:901–903, 1989.

97. Panes J, Forne M, Bagena F, et al. Endoscopic sclerosis in the treatment of bleeding peptic ulcers with a visible vessel. Am J Gastroenterol 85:252–254, 1990.

98. Hart R, Classen M. Complications of diagnostic gastrointestinal endoscopy. Endoscopy 22:229–233, 1990.

99. Steffes CP, Sugawa C, Wilson RF, et al. Oxygen saturation monitoring during endoscopy. Surg Endosc 4:174–178, 1990.

100. Sugawa C, Masuyama H. Comparison of endoscopic electrosurgical hemostasis in canine gastric serosal vessels. Gastrointest Endosc 31:169, 1985.

12

Endoscopic Evaluation of the Postoperative Stomach

Philip E. Donahue

If a patient has digestive problems after previous surgical interventions near the gastroesophageal junction, stomach, or juxtapyloric region, many factors may be relevant to the postoperative evaluation. A problem-oriented approach provides a framework for the evaluation of common complaints presented to the practitioner. I also consider postoperative complaints according to the type of surgical procedure employed. Both of these approaches have merit and often complement one another.

The goal is to develop a rationale for approaching any postoperative complaint in the context of all possible considerations. As physicians, we must be cautious in evaluating these patients, because there are problems that represent unique complications of previous surgical procedures or failure of the primary operation. There is always a possibility that the postoperative patient has developed an entirely new disease, presenting for the first time in the perioperative or postoperative period.

The information gained by means of the endoscope does not exist in a vacuum; the inside view is only part of a larger picture that includes all relevant diagnostic studies, a complete history and physical examination, and a master problem list synthesized and integrated by an experienced observer. This particular theme deserves frequent reiteration for any clinical setting in which postoperative patients are evaluated. Many of the patients' complaints can only be adequately evaluated by a surgeon, because the postoperative syndromes are sometimes recognizable only by someone who has had the opportunity to care for patients with similar presenting complaints.[1]

Because some problems are unique to a particular type of operation, part of this chapter focuses on the endoscopic findings after the common surgical procedures on the stomach. Each postoperative problem is mentioned in the context of the clinical diagnosis, anatomic location, specific radiologic findings, and endoscopic findings. In many cases, the examiner is able to predict the endoscopic finding, but surprises happen often enough to make the endoscopic examination mandatory.

PROBLEM-ORIENTED APPROACH

It is often relatively easy to formulate a list of possible explanations for postoperative dysphagia, if the physician has precise information about preceding operations. However, it is not unusual for patients to be confused about the details of previous operations.

Dysphagia

Dysphagia may be caused by mass lesions that interfere with aboral transit of liquids or solids. Commonly, these are neoplastic lesions near the cardia (Table 12–1). However, a variety of benign and malignant conditions may cause this symptom (see Table 12–1). The endoscopic findings depend on the pathology, and the practitioner, anticipating the types of problems that cause dysphagia, proceeds with a stepwise diagnostic approach that considers the interval between surgery and the patient's presenting

141

Table 12–1. DYSPHAGIA IN POSTOPERATIVE PATIENTS

Squamous cell cancer of esophagus
Adenocarcinoma of cardia
Bezoar
Paraesophageal (diaphragmatic) hernia
Acid or alkaline reflux (stricture?)
Anastomotic stricture
   Stenotic stapled anastomosis
   Recurrent cancer
   Recurrent ulceration
Mass lesions
   Mediastinal cyst
   Retroperitoneal cyst or mass
Diverticulum of esophagus or stomach
Motility disorder (*e.g.,* achalasia)

Table 12–2. CAUSES OF HEARTBURN TYPICAL OR ATYPICAL

Cardiac disease
Adenocarcinoma of cardia
Gastric atony
   Postvagotomy syndrome
   Diabetes mellitus
   Gastric ileus
Bezoar
Gastric outlet obstruction
   Recurrent ulcer
   Recurrent cancer
   Retroanastomotic hernia
   Gastrojejunal intussusception
Paraesophageal (diaphragmatic) hernia
Anastomotic stricture
   Stenotic stapled anastomosis
   Recurrent cancer
   Recurrent ulceration
Mass lesions
   Retroperitoneal cyst or mass
Pathologic gastroesophageal reflux

complaint. Depending on the urgency of the situation, it may be advisable to proceed with endoscopic examination directly. For example, if the patient presents with an acute illness, such as severe vomiting with electrolyte imbalance, it may be advisable to obtain an endoscopic examination before a barium meal. It is usually better to begin with a radiographic examination, because the postoperative stomach is especially challenging for endoscopic viewing. The problems are aggravated by distortion of the normal anatomy, difficulty in distending the stomach without a pyloric ring, or other abnormalities of the particular postoperative state. Each case requires an individual approach to the examination sequence.

In evaluating dysphagia, the physician should consider the aperture of the lesion that gives rise to the symptom. There is some discrepancy in the responses of patients to narrowing of the esophagus or esophagogastric junction. In some circumstances, especially in patients with benign strictures or narrowing of the esophagus, a lumen 15.9 mm in diameter (50 French) is required before all symptoms of dysphagia disappear. Patients with esophageal cancer may not have any symptoms until 90% of the esophageal lumen has been replaced by tumor. Persistent complaints of any degree of dysphagia should be considered as potentially serious.

Occasionally, there may be more than one explanation for a patient's dysphagia. For example, paraesophageal hernia, or diverticulum of the esophagus, may occur in a patient with achalasia of the esophagus. If one lesion is treated without knowledge of the other, the result will probably be a postoperative patient who still has serious complaints. Two problems facing the clinican are the subjective nature of the complaint and the absence of a definitive test for degree of dysphagia, factors that complicate many foregut problems.

Heartburn and Abdominal Pain

The most common cause of heartburn is uncomplicated gastroesophageal reflux, but the major concern for the practitioner is differentiating the possible causes listed in Tables 12–2 and 12–3. My colleagues and I always exclude cardiac causes, using at least an electrocardiographic examination. There is a place for the use of stress testing, up to and including stress and thallium examinations. The diagnostic considerations listed are not exotic diseases, but sometimes they are not obvious choices unless the possibility of a specific entity is entertained.

If postoperative reflux is a consideration, the

Table 12–3. CAUSES OF ABDOMINAL PAIN IN POSTOPERATIVE PATIENTS

Wound problems
   Hernia
   Suture material
   Neuroma (trigger points?)
Diseased hollow viscus
   Stomach or duodenum
   Biliary tract
   Colon
Pancreatic disorders
   Pancreatitis
   Pancreatic neoplasm
Functional disease
   Irritable colon
Degenerative disease (*e.g.,* arthritis)
Neoplastic lesion, primary or recurrent
Referred pain from extraabdominal site
   Cardiac disease
   Pulmonary disease
Dissecting aortic aneurysm

diagnostic approach is relatively simple. Documentation of an abnormal amount or duration of acid reflux can only be made with 24-hour pH testing. Because pH testing requires specific knowledge of the location of the lower esophageal sphincter (*i.e.,* the technician performing the test has to place the pH probe 5.0 cm above the sphincter), an esophageal motility test must be performed before the pH study.

The evaluation of a patient with heartburn often requires a barium meal and assessment of the stomach and duodenum, which can exclude gastric outlet obstruction, gastric stasis, or some unusual conditions that affect transit through the foregut. Other conditions identified by barium studies include intrinsic and extrinsic conditions that affect the potential for reflux, such as the physical relation of the gastric wall with the diaphragm. For example, a patient with paraesophageal hernia may have part or all of the stomach residing above the diaphragm, with various complaints including heartburn and dysphagia. The major concern for these patients, in whom reflux complaints may be quite mild,

is the recognition of the hernia, because the complications of a missed hernia are serious or lethal (Fig. 12–1).

An endoscopic examination often provides the only definitive way to observe, biopsy, and document problems such as dysplasia, infections or gastritis, phytobezoar or trichobezoar, recurrent cancer, and stomal ulcer. Some of the observations during endoscopy result in a diagnosis of exclusion, but there may not be a means of establishing the precise cause of symptoms. For example, the alkaline gastritis syndrome is notoriously difficult to document, and there is no certain means of establishing this diagnosis (Fig. 12–2). Monitoring of pH changes in the gastric corpus (*i.e.,* the frequency of acid to alkaline shifts at a point 5.0 cm below the gastroesophageal junction) can identify patients with excessive duodenogastric reflux as a primary or secondary problem.[2] The large number of patients with apparently unremarkable symptoms despite excessive amounts of reflux makes precise diagnosis difficult under the best of circumstances.

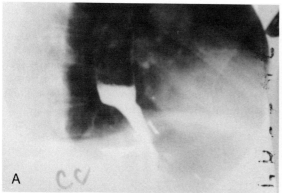

A

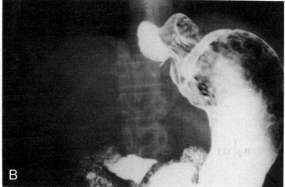

B

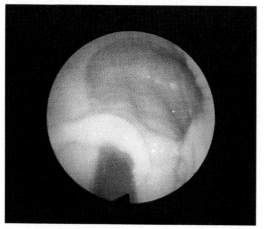

C

Figure 12–1. Paraesophageal hernia. **(A, B)** A barium meal shows the abnormal protrusion of the gastric fundus above the diaphragm. **(C)** The endoscopic view of a paraesophageal hernia reveals the gastroesophageal junction in the usual location and with a typical appearance.

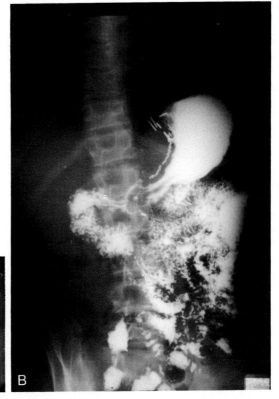

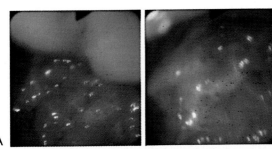

Figure 12–2. Alkaline gastritis syndrome. **(A)** An endoscopic view of the stomach shows diffuse erythematous gastritis in a patient with persistent bilious vomiting after vagotomy and antrectomy. **(B)** A barium meal shows a collection of barium, simulating an ulcer at the gastroduodenal anastomotic site.

Pain

Because pain is unusual after most surgical procedures, this unwelcome complaint requires particular attention (see Table 12–3). The systematic approach includes attention to the abdominal wall, local factors in and around the incision (*e.g.,* hernia, neuroma, painful suture material within the deep fascia), and intraabdominal abnormalities. Endoscopy is useful in patients suspected of duodenal ulcer and those with a history suggesting ulceration of the esophagus, stomach, or duodenum.

Because the differential diagnosis of postoperative pain includes many different organ systems, the examination must include a complete review of these systems. The patient often prefers to think that the symptoms are due to the surgical problem instead of a "new" disease. These patients require a systematic evaluation and a cautious interpretation of data from several sources. It is not possible to evaluate the gut as a single entity, ignoring other considerations, without increasing the chance for a missed diagnosis. Failure to approach patients in a systematic way can have serious consequences.

Experienced physicians and surgeons must provide these complex investigations within a cost-conscious framework, and they must properly inform patients about their conditions. In the United States, important diagnostic testing may not be performed because insurance companies will not pay for required testing. This especially affects the middle-class patients who may not otherwise be able to afford a series of diagnostic tests.

Bleeding

Bleeding is not uncommon in postoperative patients, although the real incidence of gastrointestinal bleeding in patients after surgery is unknown, because a thorough interpretation would include all degrees of bleeding after every operation performed (see Fig. 12–2; Fig. 12–3).[3] However, we focus on subsets of patients with previous operations, such as digestive tract surgery, operations on retroperitoneal solid organs, or vascular procedures that include the insertion of prosthetic materials (Tables 12–4 and 12–5). Another subset of patient with post-

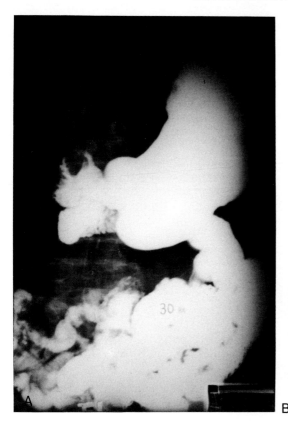

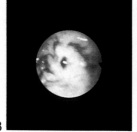

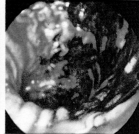

Figure 12–3. Recurrent ulcer after incomplete vagotomy by the Jaboulay procedure. **(A)** The radiograph shows an ulcer in the duodenum. **(B)** Endoscopic view shows a target lesion, which is at risk for recurrent bleeding. **(C)** The endoscopic Congo red test reveals that the anterior vagus nerve is intact, as shown by the rapid red-to-black color change on the anterior gastric wall.

operative bleeding is a product of the endoscopic era: patients with bleeding after one of the endoscopic operations to control bleeding or after polypectomy.

Postoperative bleeding after traditional operations is uncommon, as shown by the incidence of postoperative bleeding at the Cook County Hospital during the past 5 years. Of 15,600 operations on the General Surgery Service, 8 patients required reoperation for bleeding (0.05%). If only bleeding from suture lines, persistent ulcers, or from the gastric lumens are included, the number of reoperations falls to two (0.01%). These data do not include any of the patients operated on for nongastrointestinal disease.[3]

In reviewing a 20-year cohort of 40 patients who had recurrent bleeding as an indication for surgery, I included patients with traditional and endoscopic hemostasis or other endoscopic interventions (see Table 12–5). Endoscopic treatments are analogous to surgical procedures whose complications are considered similarly.

Endoscopic interventions for gastrointestinal bleeding have become the standard of practice in the United States during the past 10 years.[4–10] During the same time, urgent surgical interventions for bleeding have almost disappeared be-

cause of the availability and experience of well-trained physicians and surgeon–endoscopists.[11] Rebleeding after endoscopic treatment is more common than after surgical treatment. After surgical treatments, a rebleeding rate within 7 days or more than 1% to 2% may be excessive, but the rate of rebleeding after endoscopic treatment varies between 5% and 30%. Considering the average 10% operative mortality rate for emergency operations for gastrointestinal bleeding, these rates are quite acceptable.

Multiple lesions, which can account for the bleeding, are a common problem in many institutions. During a 1-year period at the Cook County Hospital, more than 20% of 600 patients examined initially for acute bleeding had more than one lesion documented as a possible source of bleeding. When one of multiple bleeding sites cannot be seen, subsequent decision making is compromised, and the potential for late postoperative bleeding rises (see Fig. 12–3).

If two potential sites of massive bleeding are identified at the original examination, extreme care must be used to determine which of the lesions may be more likely to contribute to the risk of morbidity, rebleeding, or death. Both of the potential sites are managed as separate and potentially lethal problems, until one or the

Table 12–4. GASTROINTESTINAL BLEEDING IN POSTOPERATIVE PATIENTS

Site of Bleeding	Specific Lesions	Endoscopic Treatment
Mouth	Arteriovenous malformations	+
	Telangiectasia	+
	Traumatic tears or lacerations	−
Oropharynx	Telangiectasia	+
Nose	Hypertension	−
	Telangiectasia	+
	Trauma	−
Nasopharynx	Trauma	
Esophagus	Esophagitis	+
	Esophageal varices	+
	Peptic ulceration	+
	Neoplasm	+
	Mallory-Weiss tear	+
Stomach	Acute gastric mucosal lesions	+
	Gastric ulcer	+
	Neoplasm	+
	Heterotopic tissue (*e.g.*, pancreas)	+
	Gastric varices	+
	Dieulafoy lesions	+
	Arteriovenous malformations	+
	Thrombocytopenia (any cause)	±
	Rupture of retrogastric aneurysm	
	Hereditary hemorrhagic telangiectasia	+
	Anastomotic bleeding	+
	Visible vessels ≤1.5 mm diameter	+
	Visible vessels >1.5 mm diameter	±
	Nasogastric tube-induced lesions	+
Duodenum or jejunem	Duodenal ulcer	+
	Duodenitis	+
	Neoplasm (*e.g.*, adenoma, carcinoma)	+
	Duodenal varices	+
	Aortoenteric fistula (atherosclerotic or graft-related)	
	Hemosuccus pancreaticus	
	Hemobilia	
	Telangiectasias	+
	Arteriovenous malformations	+
	Ulcerated diverticulum	
	Irritable bowel disease (*e.g.*, Crohn's disease)	
	Visible vessels ≤1.5 mm diameter	+
	Visible vessels >1.5 mm diameter	±

Table 12–5. DIFFERENTIAL DIAGNOSIS OF POSTOPERATIVE BLEEDING BY TIME AND SITE

A. Postoperative time bleeding is detected
  Suture line
    Handsewn (1–72 h; 7–12 d)
    Stapled (immediately; 7–12 d)
  Missed lesion (hours, days, or months later)
  Inappropriate operation (hours, days, or months)
  Wrong operation (hours to days)
  Persistence or recurrence of primary problem
    Technical failure of operation
    Progression of disease despite appropriate
      treatment
  Nonspecific response to stress
    Acute gastric mucosal lesion(s)
    Acute duodenal ulcer or perforative intestinal
      lesion
B. Bleeding sites that may be difficult to find or
    control
  Esophagus
    Atypical ulcers, diverticula, fistulas
    Rebleeding varices
    Coagulopathic diffuse bleeding
  Stomach
    Persistent arterial bleeding site
    High gastric ulcers
    Gastric varices with gastritis
    Coagulopathic diffuse bleeding
  Duodenum
    Persistent artery in ulcer base
    Bleeding from ampulla or Vater
    Aortoenteric fistula
    Atypical ulcer
    Advanced cancer of pancreas or duodenum
  Jejunem or ileum
    Arteriovenous anomalies or malformations
    Diverticula
    Diffuse infectious ulcers (*e.g.,* viral syndromes)
  Colon
    Arteriovenous malformations
    Diverticula
    Neoplastic lesions

C. Source of rebleeding in 40 patients (personal series)*
  Suture line (7)
    Handsewn (1)
    EEA anastomoses (gastrojejunostomy,
      jejunojejunostomy) (2)
    Gastrojejunostomy (2 sewn),† gastroduodenostomy
      (1 sewn), jejunojejunostomy (1 stapled)
  Ulcer site (3)
    Aortoesophageal fistula—monilia (1)
    Penetrating duodenal ulcer (progressive ulcer after
      vagotomy (gastric pH always > 5.0) (1)
    Multiple superficial ulcers (CMV?) through jejunem
      and ileum (1)
  Pseudoaneurysm or peripancreatic necrosis (3)
    Gastroduodenal artery (1)
    Left gastric artery (1)
    Splenic artery, after splenectomy (1)
  Unrecognized site (4)
    Anterovenous malformation of jejunem (1)
    Posterior pharynx or nasopharynx (*e.g.,* facial
      trauma) (1)
    Esophageal ulcer after sclerotherapy (1)
    Jejunal ulcer (1)
  Acute gastric mucosal lesions (3)
  Failure of endoscopic injection or thermal treatment (14)
    Gastritis (5)
    Duodenal ulcer (5)
    Duodenal ulcer (2)
    Mallory-Weiss tear (2)
  Bleeding from granulation tissue or small vessels (3)
  Duodenal ulcer (*e.g.,* reoperation, antrectomy) (1)
  Primary gastric resection for gastric ulcer (1)
  Left colon resection (*e.g.,* splenic flexure) (1)

*A personal series of patients treated over a 20-year period.
†Required endoscopic treatment.

other is shown to be the more dangerous and significant. Other sources of difficulty during endoscopic investigation are specific anatomic deformities, some of which may be the result of previous operations.

Stenosis of any luminal surface may be due to a variety of causes, but postoperative stricture is often caused by recurrent ulcer or tumor. Stenosis may occur as a result of fibrosis, neoplasia, or postoperative changes.

The experienced endoscopist can recognize when an examination is unsuccessful because of some of these factors and employ alternative means of diagnosis, such as side-viewing endoscopes to visualize the abnormality directly. It may be impossible to view the problem directly, and the clinician must consider other diagnostic means, including arteriography. The most important factor in the approach to the patient is the commitment to a global evaluation and the availability of a mature and experienced group of clinicians.[12–14]

Vomiting

The patient with vomiting must be evaluated for several primary possibilities in a systematic way (Table 12–6). This discussion focuses on the patients who had surgical procedures and does not address many of the more common conditions, including electrolyte imbalance, toxic effects of medications, and cholelithiasis and cholecystitis, except to stress that previous

surgical procedures such as truncal vagotomy do cause subsequent difficulties with gallbladder emptying and cannot be ignored in the evaluation of these patients. Similarly, patients with short bowel syndrome may have cholelithiasis caused or aggravated by a diminished enterohepatic circulation of bile. Vomiting in postoperative patients usually is related to some of the more common mechanical conditions and deserves cautious evaluation to discover these.

Patients who have had previous operations near the gastric cardia can have vomiting for several reasons. One of the preventable causes is postoperative diaphragmatic hernia, in which the esophageal hiatus is not closed at the primary operation. Because the negative intrathoracic pressure is a constant feature of the postoperative period, the gradual development or enlargement of a paraesophageal hernia is not surprising (see Fig. 12–1). The clinical symptoms associated with this condition range from none to severe dysphagia, pain, and vomiting

Table 12–6. CAUSES OF GASTRIC OUTLET OBSTRUCTION IN POSTOPERATIVE PATIENTS

Adenocarcinoma of cardia
Gastric atony
   Postvagotomy syndrome
   Motility disorder
   Diabetes mellitus
   Gastric ileus
Bezoar
Pyloric stenosis or channel ulcer
Duodenal stenosis, ulcer, or marginal ulcer
Recurrent cancer
Retroanastomotic hernia
Gastrojejunal intussusception
Pancreatic pathology
   Pancreatitis or abscess
   Pseudocyst
   Annular pancreas/duodenal stenosis
Duodenal tumor
Anastomotic stricture
Stenotic stapled anastomosis
Mass lesions
Retroperitoneal cyst or mass
Paraduodenal hernia

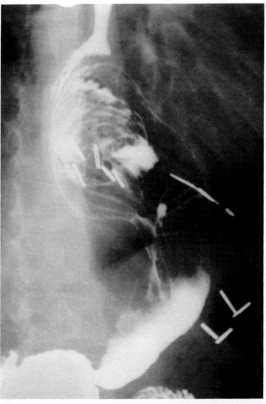

Figure 12–4. Slipped Nissen fundoplication. The barium study shows that the stomach has migrated into the thorax through the esophageal hiatus. This patient has a small ulcer at the point where the diaphragm traps the gastric wall. The patient also had intermittent gastric pain with bleeding. This problem is common if the esophageal hiatus is not closed securely after surgery in or near the gastroesophageal junction.

due to the incarcerated stomach syndrome. The patient may complain of dysphagia or symptoms consistent with gastroesophageal reflux.

If the patient is examined by an inexperienced endoscopist or if the condition is still somewhat early in its evolution, a small hernia may be difficult to detect, but a radiographic examination with barium can delineate this problem, demonstrating the utility of a comprehensive examination sequence (see Fig. 12–1). The pain and discomfort in this type of patient may be caused by several factors, including gaseous distention or peptic ulcers near the diaphragm (Figs. 12–4 and 12–5). If the underlying problem is not identified, the patient is subjected to symptomatic treatments that are doomed to failure. Mechanical causes (see Table 12–2 and Fig. 12–4) and nonmechanical causes must be considered in the differential diagnosis. For example, gastric atony due to vagus nerve injury may result in symptoms that are almost indistinguishable from those described earlier (see Table 12–6). The failure to recognize the root issue, whether it is gastric outlet obstruction, retroanastomotic hernia, marginal ulcer, or bezoar, may lead to infections and the possibility of a more serious complication (Figs. 12–6 through 12–12).

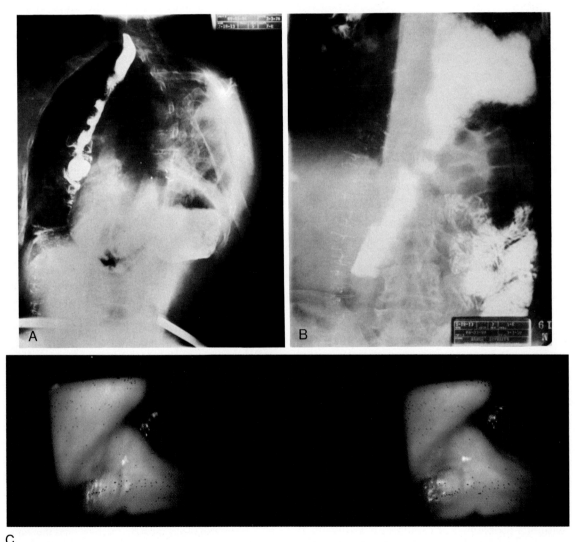

Figure 12–5. Gastric ulcer after colon interposition. Recurrent massive bleeding after colon interposition was caused by a large ulcer of the stomach, occurring where the stomach was narrowed by the diaphragm. **(A, B)** The radiographs did not reveal the bleeding site, but they did show the normal transit of barium. **(C)** The endoscopic views of the stomach revealed a deep ulcer that had caused pain in the ipsilateral acromioclavicular joint area (Kehr's sign) owing to diaphragmatic irritation.

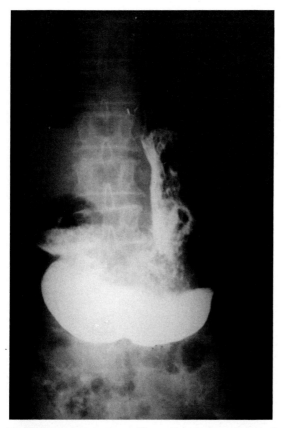

Figure 12–6. Gastric atony. The patient had symptoms of fullness 2 months after vagotomy was performed. The x-ray study shows barium, which remains in the stomach for prolonged periods without emptying.

Another group of problems must be considered when the primary operation was for a gastric cancer. In addition to the question of postvagotomy syndrome, these patients must be evaluated for residual or recurrent cancer.

Other problems interpreted as vomiting, such as frequent regurgitation after operations that destroy the lower esophageal and gastric components of the antireflux barrier, may be completely corrected by the construction of an effective antireflux mechanism. Table 12–6 indicates several problems that deserve careful consideration. Several of these conditions cannot be evaluated completely without endoscopic views, but most require the systematic evaluation described for other postoperative problems. Knowledge of any operation performed previously may provide immediate insight into the patient's problem. For example, if a Billroth II gastrectomy has been performed, retroanastomotic hernia (see Fig. 12–7), chronic afferent loop syndrome, gastrojejunal intussusception, and marginal ulcer are considerations. The ex-

perienced surgeon will be able to consider these situations and provide a systematic evaluation.

Knowledge of the indications for previous operations often provides insight into the cause of a later condition. For example, efferent loop syndrome in a patient with previous gastric cancer is usually due to carcinomatosis. A surgical procedure or laparoscopic evaluation is usually required to establish the diagnosis.

Weight Loss

Weight loss can be caused by countless medical problems if the frame of reference is the population at large. For an individual patient, weight loss usually has a specific cause, and the cause can usually be determined with confidence (Table 12–7).

Dumping

Gastric evacuation is hurried after any procedure that diminishes gastric volume, affects gastric adaptive responses to volume or increased intraluminal pressure, or interferes with the regulated gastric emptying controlled by the pyloric sphincter, osmoreceptors, and mechanical factors at the gastric outlet. It is difficult to quantitate the degree of dumping because of the subjective nature of the complaint, but it is relatively easy to identify the patient who is affected by severe dumping by his or her requirement for supine rest after meals and by the severity of the physiologic response to jejunal hyperosmolarity. Occasionally, the investigation may identify a correctible lesion (*e.g.*, the gastroileostomy shown in Fig. 12–13) in the course of evaluating a patient with this problem. For most patients with this problem, dietary measures and avoidance of liquids with meals generate symptomatic improvement, which further improves with time.

Table 12–7. CAUSES OF WEIGHT LOSS IN POSTOPERATIVE PATIENTS

Gastric remnant adenocarcinoma
Gastric stasis
Malabsorption syndrome
   Postvagotomy syndrome
   Motility disorder
   Diabetes mellitus
   Gastric ileus
Bezoar
Recurrent cancer

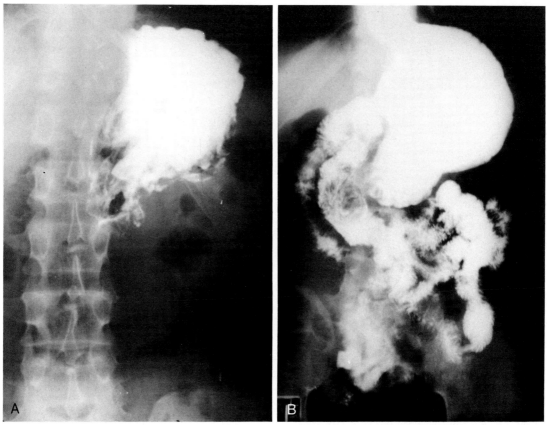

Figure 12–7. Retroanastomotic hernia. Barium meals on different days led to different conclusions. **(A)** The stomach does not empty, suggesting a mass lesion. **(B)** There is prompt emptying of the stomach. Endoscopic views were normal on two occasions. Because of persistent vomiting, the patient was explored and found to have a retroanastomotic hernia.

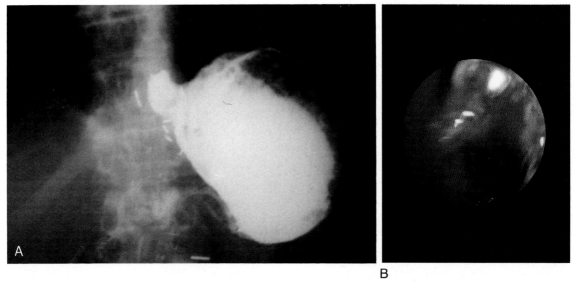

Figure 12–8. Gastric bezoar. **(A)** The radiograph suggests nonemptying of the stomach, with some evidence of filling defects in the stomach. **(B)** An endoscopic examination reveals phytobezoar material in the gastric lumen.

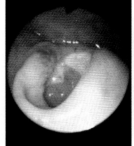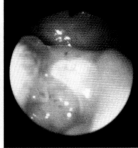

Figure 12–10. Endoscopic view of a gastroenterostomy. There are several circumferential ulcers, which bled and required endoscopic therapy.

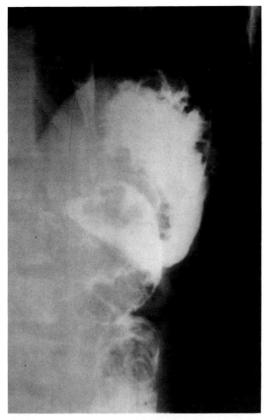

Figure 12–9. Jejunogastric intussusception. The barium meal shows an intraluminal filling defect after a previous gastroenterostomy. The endoscopic views showed edematous small bowel mucosa at the gastric outlet.

pregnancy, with or without aggravation by hyperemesis gravidarum, is a risk for mother and infant, and these patients require special consideration.

PROCEDURE-RELATED COMPLICATIONS

Many complaints can be ascribed to specific abnormalities in the postoperative period. One of the typical locations for this type of problem is the gastric cardia, especially after operations near the gastroesophageal junction. All the structures in the area should be systematically evaluated in developing a list of diagnostic considerations.

Chronic Cholelithiasis

It is not unusual for a patient with cholelithiasis to have marked vomiting and anorexia, with resulting weight loss. A similar problem in

Gastroesophageal Junction

Postoperative complaints involving the gastroesophageal junction are listed in Table 12–8.

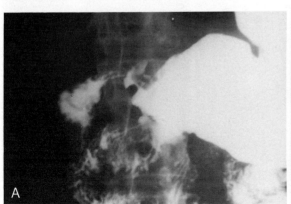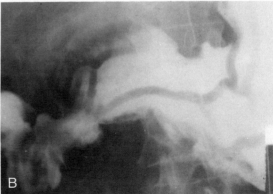

Figure 12–11. Marginal ulcers. **(A, B)** The radiographs of the distal stomach after gastroenterostomy show a deep ulcer on the afferent limb of the jejunem. This ulcer could not be seen with the panendoscope, but it was seen with the side-viewing endoscope.

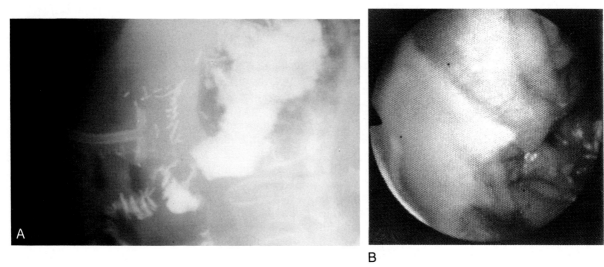

Figure 12–12. Marginal ulcers. **(A)** After pancreaticoduodenectomy, the radiographic view suggests edema on the seventh postoperative day. **(B)** Endoscopic examination shows a large ulcer at the gastric outlet, which eventually required surgical revision, probably due to ischemia of the gastric wall at the anastomotic site.

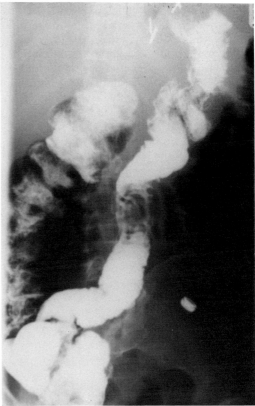

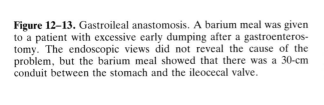

Figure 12–13. Gastroileal anastomosis. A barium meal was given to a patient with excessive early dumping after a gastroenterostomy. The endoscopic views did not reveal the cause of the problem, but the barium meal showed that there was a 30-cm conduit between the stomach and the ileocecal valve.

Table 12–8. POSTOPERATIVE COMPLAINTS INVOLVING THE GASTROESOPHAGEAL JUNCTION

Pleura
Diaphragm (hernia?)
Mediastinal lesion
Stricture or ulceration
Gastric pathology
Extrinsic pressure
   Surgical procedure
   Surgical prosthesis
Gastric atony

Operations for Control of Reflux

The operations that are performed commonly for reflux control include the Nissen fundoplication, the Belsey Mark IV procedure, the Hill gastropexy procedure, and others such as the Dor and Toupet operations. This discussion is limited to the first three, but the endoscopist should also be familiar with the Angelchik procedure and the endoscopic techniques used for the control of reflux disease.

Radiographic studies are especially important because several problems are unique to this group of patients, including strictured anastomosis, migration of the structures into the thorax caused by negative intrathoracic pressure, and partial unwrapping of antireflux procedures. The endoscopic view may not be specific, but in conjunction with information obtained from the radiographs, the endoscopic appearance is often much easier to interpret correctly (Figs. 12–14 and 12–15).[14, 15]

Operations for Cancer of the Esophagus or Stomach

Procedures for cancer usually include resection of the gastroesophageal junction, displacement or destruction of phrenoesophageal ligament, and construction of a sewn or stapled anastomosis between the stomach and esophagus. Alternatively, the stomach may be displaced into the thorax or the neck in the posterior mediastinum or the retrosternal position. The colon or jejunum may be interposed between the pharynx and proximal esophagus and the stomach. It is not unusual for patients to have several complaints, especially dysphagia and early satiety. These are expected and usual. If the patient complains of severe back pain or has hematemesis, a prompt endoscopic examination is mandatory. The fact that the patient has had a serious operation must be kept in mind, because recurrent cancer may be the source of the symptoms. When the endoscope is inserted into the stomach, it may be difficult to distend the stomach or interpret the examination because of retained food. The presence of a deep ulcer (2–4 cm) often indicates recurrent cancer, and the clinician should attempt to obtain tissue. The side-viewing endoscope can be extremely useful in assessing a patient who may have a small gastric remnant and absent pyloric ring.

Operations for Morbid Obesity

The commonly employed operations for morbid obesity are the vertical banded gastroplasty

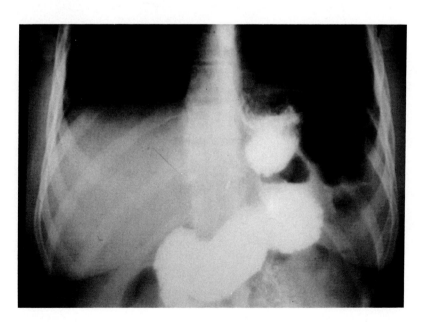

Figure 12–14. Slipped Nissen fundoplication (bucket-handle type). The patient had persistent discomfort after a Nissen fundoplication because the wrap had slipped, resulting in stomach plicated on stomach, an ineffective antireflux procedure. The radiographs show the waist-like constriction of the midcorpus of the stomach.

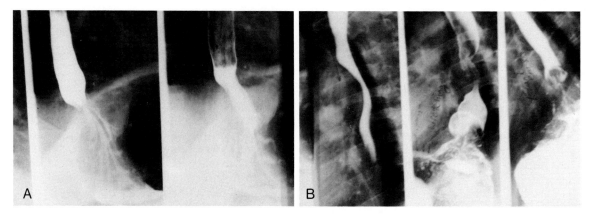

Figure 12–15. Telescoping of Nissen fundoplication. The endoscopic examination was normal, but the patient is disabled with severe postprandial vomiting. **(A)** The initial x-ray film shows a normal postoperative appearance of the cardia. **(B)** Ten seconds later, the patient retched in the radiographic suite, and the film shows unfolding of the wrap after incomplete fixation of the plicated fundus.

and the gastric bypass. These patients may have vomiting, bleeding, or pain, and they must be evaluated for the presence of ulcers, alkaline reflux syndromes, or strictured anastomoses. The endoscopist must be prepared to treat certain problems encountered endoscopically, such as anastomotic stricture after gastroplasty, which is easily treated by endoscopic dilation (Fig. 12–16).[12]

Operations for Chronic Pancreatitis

If the pancreatic duct is anastomosed directly to the stomach, as in patients with a modified Puestow procedure or cancer of the pancreas, the observer may see a reddened spot in the midcorpus of the stomach. Alternatively, one of the permanent suture materials may be found

in the corpus at the site of the suture between the capsule of the pancreas and stomach. This is similar to the finding that may be seen after cyst gastrostomy: after the cyst collapses, the sutures around the edge, which ensured hemostasis in the perioperative period, appear as a single line of sutures, many of which extend into the lumen of the stomach.

Gastric Corpus and Antrum

The most common cause for gastric resection is ulcer disease, although the popularity of nonresectional approaches for ulcer has resulted in fewer gastric resections being performed. In the West, ulcers are on the wane, with the widespread availability of effective antiulcer regi-

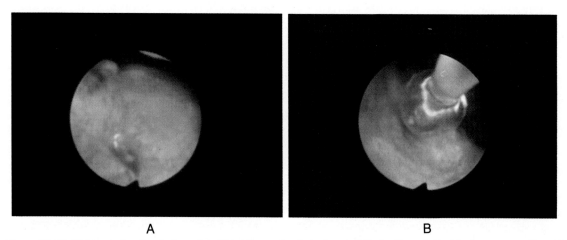

Figure 12–16. Stricture of gastroplasty outlet. **(A)** After gastroplasty for morbid obesity, a patient had severe vomiting. A suggestion of an outlet was seen where the gastric folds converged. **(B)** After passage of an endoscopic balloon dilation catheter, the outlet was successfully dilated to 15 mm in diameter, resulting in marked clinical improvement.

mens, and few gastric resections are performed for ulcers compared with 20 years ago.

Most ulcers of the stomach and duodenum require endoscopic evaluation at some point, whether medical or surgical treatments are being employed.[15] The goals of endoscopic examinations are to establish precise diagnosis, evaluate the risk of complications, and perform specialized diagnostic studies. The early diagnosis of gastric cancer, lymphoma, or premalignant lesions must be emphasized in the examination of high-risk patients. Screening is justified for any patient older than 15 years of age after gastric resection, for those from high-risk subgroups, or those with biopsy-proven atypia. Multiple blind biopsies of any area of abnormality and multiple, random, mucosal biopsies provide the only way to make a correct diagnosis. Cancers arise de novo, not as a complication of ulcer, but chronic ulcer scars should be biopsied to exclude cancer.[16, 17]

Any ulcer that is discovered must be evaluated in the context of the patient's history and ethnicity, previous operations, and other foregut pathology. Solitary ulcers that pose a risk of bleeding are recognized by stigmata such as a visible vessel or adherent platelet debris.

Postoperative Stomach

The postoperative stomach poses unique problems for the endoscopist. If pyloroplasty, distal resection, or gastroenteric anastomosis has been performed, the stomach is impossible to distend. The endoscopist quickly learns to follow the folds of the stomach toward the duodenal or jejunal mucosa, but it is sometimes hard to visualize the gastric wall. A small lesion hidden in the depth of a fold that cannot be flattened by gaseous distention may be missed.

Some postoperative changes are subtle and not obvious to the examiner. Adhesions in the right upper quadrant after cholecystectomy may "tent" the distal stomach into an unnatural position and contour, making entry into the duodenal bulb more difficult. This is usually not a problem for the seasoned endoscopist, but there is a remedy with the use of the side-viewing endoscope, which is ordinarily used only for retrograde studies of the pancreas and biliary tree.

With a side-viewing endoscope in place in the stomach, the gastric corpus can be stretched and distended by the physical contour of the endoscope. Because the side-viewing endoscopes are in their natural viewing position during this maneuver, the interior of the stomach is apparent. For bypassing the narrowing of a duodenal

ulcer or stenosis, the side-viewing scope can be insinuated blindly or with fluoroscopic assistance.

Follow-Up After Gastric Resection

For patients with gastric resections performed more than 10 years previously, the overall incidence of gastric cancer is increased, and the examiner should be aware of the utility of biopsy material in showing atypia or frank cancer. Because a stomach that is visually normal may harbor cancer, a liberal policy for biopsy should be encouraged. Although the incidence of cancer is low in gastric ulcer patients, there are "red flags" seen on biopsy that can predict the eventual appearance of gastric cancer, especially gastric epithelial dysplasia.[16, 17]

Gastroduodenostomy

The number of reconstructive gastroduodenostomies is large, but most retain common features that are of use to the endoscopic examiner. Among these is the lack of distensibility and suppleness of the original stomach. A double lumen at the gastric outlet is typical of the Jaboulay gastroduodenostomy reconstruction.

The examiner must be fully aware of the usual anatomic appearance and be prepared to exclude the other diagnostic considerations. Does this represent a double pylorus? Is there evidence of an ulcer that has affected the adjacent duodenum? Has an ulcer eroded into the common duct? Is there a chance that the second lumen is a result of tumor necrosis or another problem in a patient with a limited life expectancy? This latter problem is common in patients with far-advanced esophageal cancer, which continues to be a major problem in most urban centers in the United States and other countries. If an additional opening is seen in the proximal stomach, the diagnostic considerations include proximal gastric diverticula (i.e., true diverticula), outmoded reconstructions such as the Heyrovsky Grondahl esophagogastric anastomosis, and duplication cysts.

Incomplete Vagotomy

If the patient has a recurrent ulcer after any vagotomy, the question of incomplete vagotomy of the parietal cell mass must be considered. The endoscopic Congo red test (ECRT) for completeness of the vagotomy, which was developed and tested at the University of Illinois, Chicago, is still useful in locating missed or intact vagus nerve trunks.[18, 19] The ECRT consists of applying a solution of the indicator dye, Congo red, to the stomach and observing the gastric mucosa for a color change from red to black. Congo red is red at a pH greater than 3.0 and black at a pH less than 3.0. After gastric lavage with a dilute bicarbonate solution, the mucosa throughout the stomach is coated with a thin layer of the mixture. As acid is secreted in portions of the stomach, the Congo red undergoes a red-to-black color change; the antrum remains red, and the corpus and fundus appear entirely black. The period required for the color change is proportional to the rate of acid secretion, and the rate of secretion is faster if the vagus nerves are intact. The terminal branches of the vagus nerve are distributed to discrete regions of the stomach, and it is possible to differentiate between innervated and denervated portions of the stomach if there is a differential rate of secretion in these respective areas.

The requirements for a successful test include an endoscope, a solution of Congo red (0.5%) and bicarbonate (0.5–5.0%), a gastric mucosa that is actively secreting acid, and an experienced endoscopist. The test can be performed in outpatients without sedation or intraoperatively. When intraoperative tests are performed, subcutaneous pentagastrin (6 μg/kg) must be used as a secretagogue to overcome the acid-secretory depressant effects of general anesthetics. All histamine receptor antagonists are discontinued 12 hours before the test. We mix 2.5 g of Congo red dye with 500 mL of 0.5% $NaHCO_3$ (i.e., intraoperative, patient asleep) or 5.0% $NaHCO_3$ (i.e., outpatient, patient awake). The mixture eliminates technical difficulties in applying bicarbonate and Congo red separately and allows speedier performance of the test.

In unoperated patients, the red-to-black color change occurs almost immediately. After vagotomy of the parietal cell mass (i.e., truncal, selective, or highly selective), about 10 minutes elapse before the color change is seen. Patients with incomplete vagotomy have some areas of the stomach that turn black immediately (i.e., intact nerves) and others with the delayed or absent color change (i.e., postvagotomy). Further operative dissection is aimed at those areas of the stomach with the rapid acid secretion if the test is being performed intraoperatively.

After further operative dissection designed to complete the vagotomy, the test can be performed a second time (or more) as needed; each test requires 2 to 5 minutes for completion. If the ECRT is being performed in the outpatient clinic as part of the evaluation of a patient with recurrent duodenal ulcer, information can be gained about the intact vagus nerve branches in the stomach and their probable location (see Fig. 12–3).

The test is easy to perform, but endoscopic procedures performed perioperatively have special requirements, and physicians must be trained and gain experience before the test can be used with maximal efficiency. Compared with the other tests for completeness of vagotomy, it has the appeal of convenience, accuracy, and cost.

The ECRT has been useful when performing surgical vagotomy in patients with primary or recurrent duodenal ulcer.[20] When performing truncal vagotomy, we found many additional nerve fibers that would have remained undetected without the test.

In the evolution of highly selective vagotomy as an operative technique, findings at ECRT were the initial stimulus for a series of investigations that led to modifications of operative technique, resulting in our current technique of "extended highly selective vagotomy." The low recurrence rate (<2%) during an average 5-year follow-up achieved by this operation adds support for intraoperative testing for completeness of vagotomy.[21] This is especially true in training centers or for surgeons just beginning the practice of highly selective vagotomy. If we are to have excellent results with vagotomy performed laparoscopically, we should employ intraoperative testing to confirm its results. However, the use of a laparoscopic approach should make some of the sites of incomplete vagotomy accessible without a second laparotomy.

Division of Hepatic Vagus Nerves During Truncal Vagotomy

If the patient had a previous gastric resection accompanied by truncal vagotomy, biliary dyskinesia may have resulted. This is the inevitable result of sectioning the nerves that give coordinated contractile ability to the gallbladder; the usual result is a distended gallbladder with an enlarged volume. The inability of the gallbladder to empty normally can be identified with a cholecystokin infusion (Kinevac), which quantitates the ejection fraction of the gallbladder. Without this type of testing, the patient and the surgeon can expect a 50% chance for satisfaction after the operation.

CONCLUSION

The goals of endoscopic examinations in postoperative patients are similar to those in patients without previous operations: to establish a precise diagnosis, evaluate the risk of complications, and perform specialized diagnostic studies. Symptoms must be evaluated in the context of a patient's history and ethnicity, previous operations, and other foregut pathology. Endoscopic findings must be interpreted in light of additional information obtained from radiographs and specialized diagnostic studies.

The postoperative patients with digestive symptoms provide a challenge for the surgeon and a unique chance to exhibit diagnostic acumen in the interpretation of a problem. As with so many situations in medicine, a diagnosis will not be made unless it is first considered, and it will not be considered unless it is truly understood.

References

1. Donahue PE, Sugitani A. Gastrointestinal endoscopy and general surgical practice: surgical endoscopy versus surgeon endoscopists. Am Surg 57:330–333, 1991.
2. Stein HJ, Smyrk TC, Demeester TR, Rouse J, Hinder RA. Clinical value of endoscopy and histology in the diagnosis of duodenogastric reflux disease. Surgery 112:796–803, 1992.
3. Donahue PE. Approach to postoperative bleeding (rebleeding) after surgery for gastrointestinal bleeding or general abdominal procedures. In: Sugawa C, Schuman BM, Lucas CE, eds. Gastrointestinal bleeding. New York: Igaku-Shoin, 1992:419–430.
4. Donahue PE, Mobarhan S, Layden TJ, Nyhus LM. Control of upper gastrointestinal bleeding with a bipolar coagulation device. Surg Gynecol Obstet 159:113–118, 1984.
5. Chung SCS, Leung JWC, Sung JY, Lo KK, Li AKC. Injection or heat probe for bleeding ulcer. Gastroenterology 100:33–37, 1991.
6. Laine L. Determination of the optimal technique for bipolar electrocoagulation treatment. Gastroenterology 100:107–112, 1991.
7. Waring JP, Sanowski RA, Sawyer RL, Woods CA, Foutch PG. A randomized comparison of multipolar electrocoagulation and injection sclerosis for the treatment of bleeding peptic ulcer. Gastrointest Endosc 37:295–298, 1991.
8. Sugawa C, Steffes CP, Nakamura R, Sferra JJ, Sferra CS, Sugimura Y, Fromm D. Upper GI bleeding in an urban hospital. Etiology, recurrence, and prognosis. Ann Surg 212:521–526, 1990.
9. Hui WM, Ng MMT, Lok ASF, Lai CL, Lau YN, Lam SK. A randomized comparative study of laser photocoagulation, heater probe, and bipolar electrocoagulation in the treatment of actively bleeding ulcers. Gastrointest Endosc 137:299–304, 1991.
10. Lin HJ, Tsai YT, Lee SD, et al. A prospectively randomized trial of heat probe thermocoagulation versus pure alcohol injection in nonvariceal peptic ulcer hemorrhage. Gut 31:753–757, 1990.
11. Donahue PE. Gastroduodenal and non-variceal esophageal bleeding. In: Madden RL, ed. Problems in general surgery, vol 4. Philadelphia: JB Lippincott, 1987:332–346.
12. Strodel W, Knol J, Eckhauser F. Endoscopy of the partitioned stomach. Ann Surg 200:582–585, 1984.
13. Strodel W. Endoscopic examination in the evaluation of the postoperative stomach and duodenum. In: Donahue PE, ed. Problems in gastrointestinal endoscopy. Philadelphia: JB Lippincott, 1990:141–146.
14. Bowden TJ Jr, Hooks V, Mansberger A. The stomach after surgery: an endoscopic perspective. Ann Surg 197:637–640, 1983.
15. Donahue PE. Acute and chronic duodenal ulcers. In: Dent TL, Kukora JS, McCombs PR, Leibrandt TJ, eds. Surgical tips. Philadelphia: McGraw-Hill, 1988:381–398.
16. Lee S, Iida M, Yao T, Shindo S, Okabe H, Fujishima M. Long-term follow-up of 2529 patients reveals gastric ulcers rarely become malignant. Dig Dis Sci 35:763–768, 1990.
17. Lansdown M, Quirke P, Dixon MF, Axon AT, Johnston D. High grade dysplasia of the gastric mucosa: a marker for gastric carcinoma. Gut 31:977–983, 1990.
18. Kusakari K, Nyhus LM, Gillison EW, Bombeck CT. An endoscopic test for completeness of vagotomy. Arch Surg 105:386–391, 1972.
19. Donahue PE, Bombeck CT, Yoshida J, et al. The endoscopic Congo red test. Am J Surg 153:249–255, 1987.
20. Nyhus LM, Donahue PE, Krystosek RJ, Pearl RK, Bombeck CT. Complete vagotomy. Arch Surg 115:264–268, 1980.
21. Donahue PE, Richter HM, Liu KJM, Anan K, Nyhus LM. Experimental basis and clinical application of extended highly selective vagotomy for duodenal ulcer. Surg Gynecol Obstet 176:39–48, 1993.

13

Endoscopic Placement of Enteral Feeding Tubes

Bruce V. MacFadyen, Jr.

The use of intensive nutritional support to meet the metabolic nutrient requirements of critically ill patients has become standard medical treatment. Although intravenous hyperalimentation was the first successful nutritional method used to promote positive nitrogen balance and weight gain in critically ill patients unable to eat normally, intragastric and jejunal feedings have become the preferred technique for early and long-term nutritional support.[1, 2] The first surgical gastrostomy was proposed in 1837 by Egeberg and successfully performed in 1876 by Verneuil.[3] Although gastric decompression was the primary indication in these patients, intragastric feedings with blenderized diets were later infused for nutritional support. Some patients were unable to tolerate gastric feedings because of gastric outlet obstruction or gastroesophageal reflux and pulmonary aspiration.

Surgical jejunostomy was first used in 1878 in a patient with inoperable gastric malignancy, and indications expanded greatly over the next 50 to 60 years.[4, 5] Delaney and colleagues modified the surgical technique using a very small jejunostomy feeding catheter placed at laparotomy.[6] By using an elemental diet, positive nitrogen balance and weight gain were achieved. This technique was modified by others, with good nutritional results.[7, 8] Although there were few procedure-related complications in their series, operative mortality rates of 22% to 47% have been reported. The success of the procedure depends on the patients' ages, preoperative level of consciousness, type of anesthesia, and surgical method of jejunostomy.[9]

Diagnostic and therapeutic flexible endoscopy developed during the 1960s and 1970s and has been associated with a low incidence of complications. The application of this modality to gastric feedings was first described in 1980 by Gauderer and coworkers, who reported percutaneous endoscopic gastrostomy (PEG).[10] Several criteria have been used for PEG placement in patients who had intact gastrointestinal tracts and were unable to ingest sufficient nutrients orally to meet their metabolic requirements. These indications included neurologic diseases, head and neck cancers, advanced malignant diseases, impairment in deglutition, trauma, and severe cardiac or respiratory failure (Table 13–1). Parenteral nutrition has been preferred when complete bowel rest has been required or for nutritional supplementation of oral feedings. However, gastrointestinal feedings are advantageous because they maintain gastrointestinal mucosal integrity that protects against bacterial translocation in sepsis and in shock, and they decrease stress ulceration in the stomach.[11–14]

Because electrical bowel activity and peristalsis continue even after an abdominal operation, there are few reasons not to provide sufficient

Table 13–1. INDICATIONS FOR PERCUTANEOUS ENDOSCOPIC GASTROSTOMY

Neurologic impairment or decreased level of consciousness
Advanced malignant disease
Increased risk of gastric reflux and pulmonary aspiration
Gastroparesis
Gastric outlet obstruction
Anorexia and cachexia
Swallowing dysfunction
Gastric decompression and the need for concomitant enteral feedings

enteral nutrients through an intact gastrointestinal tract.[15] The indications for a percutaneous endoscopic jejunostomy (PEJ) tube are similar to those for PEG placement, and it is particularly useful in patients who are at risk for gastrointestinal reflux and pulmonary aspiration. Although parenteral nutrition effectively provides the caloric and protein needs of the patient, its cost, increased incidence of central venous catheter-related infections, metabolic complications, and development of gut atrophy secondary to bowel rest have led many physicians to prefer enteral nutrition, if the gastrointestinal tract is intact and functional. Although some of these complications have been observed with enteral feedings, they occur less frequently and are less severe than with parenteral nutrition.[7, 16] Enteral nutrients can be given through a nasogastric tube, gastrostomy, or a jejunal feeding tube instead of a central venous catheter. Which enteral feeding method is used depends on the patient's disease and the medical facilities that are available.

There are primarily five methods to insert a jejunal feeding tube (Table 13–2). The first type is the endoscopic placement of a duodenal or jejunal guidewire, followed by the advancement of a No. 8 to 12 French (2.6–4-mm) nasojejunal feeding tube over the guidewire under fluoroscopic control. The second method involves the placement of a No. 20 French (6.6-mm) silicone PEG tube through which a No. 8 French (2.6-mm) jejunal feeding tube is inserted and grasped by an endoscope and pushed or pulled into the duodenum. The third technique is the direct insertion of a PEJ tube into the jejunum using a No. 20 French PEG tube placement technique. The fourth method is the laparoscopic placement of a No. 8 to 12 French jejunal feeding tube, and the fifth type is direct surgical insertion of a feeding tube or small catheter by laparotomy distal to the ligament of Treitz into the jejunum.

The contraindications for PEJ tube placement are similar to those for a PEG (Table 13–3) and

Table 13–2. METHODS OF PERCUTANEOUS ENDOSCOPIC JEJUNOSTOMY TUBE PLACEMENT

Nasoenteral endoscopic placement of a jejunal feeding tube passed over a wire or under direct vision
A PEJ tube passed through a PEG tube and pushed or pulled into the duodenum
Direct endoscopic placement of a percutaneous endoscopic jejunostomy
Laparoscopic placement of a jejunal feeding tube or catheter
Jejunal feeding tube placement by means of a laparotomy

Table 13–3. CONTRAINDICATIONS FOR PERCUTANEOUS ENDOSCOPIC JEJUNOSTOMY PLACEMENT

Severe gastric and duodenal ulceration
Complete gastric outlet obstruction
Infected abdominal wall
Previous upper abdominal surgery
Ascites
Morbid obesity
Failure to transilluminate the endoscopic light in the anterior abdominal wall
Infection or neoplastic lesions of the stomach and jejunum
Massive hepatomegaly
Large gastric tumor
Proximal small bowel fistula

include gastric, duodenal, or jejunal ulceration and gastric outlet obstruction. Although pyloric dilation may be performed to allow passage of the endoscope and feeding tube, restenosis may occur, and an easier tube placement method may be the laparoscopic approach. An infected abdominal wall, previous upper abdominal surgery, ascites, and failure to transilluminate the endoscope light on the anterior abdominal wall may also contraindicate this technique, but nasojejunal tubes may be effective in these conditions. Infectious and neoplastic lesions of the stomach and proximal small bowel fistulas may contraindicate the use of PEG or PEJ and necessitate the use of intravenous hyperalimentation. If nutrition is required, successful PEG-PEJ placement can be accomplished in 95% of the patients.[17, 18]

ENDOSCOPIC PLACEMENT OF JEJUNAL FEEDING TUBES

Several techniques have been described for PEJ placement, but they have been difficult to perform. In 1984, Ponsky and Aszodi were the first to describe a PEG-PEJ method by which a standard No. 20 French latex PEG tube and a No. 8 French feeding tube were placed.[19] The endoscope was advanced into the stomach, and the endoscope light transilluminated on the anterior abdominal wall in the left upper quadrant of the abdomen. A needle and nylon suture were inserted through the abdominal and gastric walls and the nylon suture grasped by a snare placed through the accessory channel of the endoscope. The endoscope, snare, and nylon suture were then pulled out of the mouth. A 50-cm-long No. 8 French silicone feeding tube was used with a 2- to 3-cm 2-0 silk suture tied to the end of its 5-cm weighted mercury tip. The proximal end of the PEJ was inserted through the No. 20 French PEG tube crossbar and placed parallel to the PEG tube shaft, reinserted into the proximal PEG tube, and secured. The proximal end of the PEG tube was then tied to the nylon suture that had been brought out the mouth, and the PEG-PEJ tubes were pulled through the esophagus, stomach, and anterior abdominal wall and secured in place.

The endoscope was reinserted into the stomach, and rubber shod biopsy forceps were advanced through the accessory channel of the endoscope and used to grasp the silk suture on the mercury end of the PEJ tube. The biopsy forceps, PEJ, and endoscope were advanced to the pylorus, and the PEJ was pushed into the duodenal bulb. The PEG and PEJ tubes were separated externally. The PEG tube was used for gastric decompression, and the PEJ tube was used for feeding. In their original series of 10 patients, there was no morbidity or mortality, and gastroesophageal reflux was not observed.[19]

Strodel and colleagues reported a similar technique in which a No. 24 French (8-mm) 3-way Foley catheter was used to replace an established PEG tube.[17] A 50-cm-long No. 8 French silicone feeding tube with a weighted tip was advanced through the gastrostomy tube, and the weighted tip and endoscope were pushed through the pylorus into the duodenum under direct vision, with a biopsy forceps placed through the endoscope accessory channel. The advantages in this technique were the larger-diameter PEG tube, possibly less leakage around the PEG exit site on the abdominal wall, and PEJ placement in the duodenum under direct vision. One disadvantage with this technique has been retrograde PEJ tube withdrawal into the stomach as the endoscope was withdrawn through the pylorus. Intestinal peristalsis does not consistently advance the enteral feeding tube into the jejunum, and the so-called PEJ tube is more often a percutaneous endoscopic duodenostomy (PED) tube, which has been associated with a 30% to 40% incidence of gastroesophageal reflux and pulmonary aspiration.[20–22]

Because blind advancement of the nasoduodenal tube into the duodenum is often unsuccessful, a nasojejunal endoscopic placement technique was developed to minimize this problem and to avoid PEG placement and its potential complications. It was considered important to advance the PEJ tube consistently beyond the ligament of Treitz. In one technique, the endoscope was inserted into the duodenum and a 0.89-mm (0.035-in) wire was advanced into the duodenum or jejunum. The gastroscope was then removed and the wire brought out the mouth. A No. 12 to 14 French silicone, polyethylene, or polyurethane feeding tube was advanced over the wire and into the duodenum or jejunum. The wire was withdrawn and the tube transferred to the nose, and enteral feedings were usually started within 4 hours of the placement of the tube. Because the guidewire often produced a large loop in the stomach, this technique required fluoroscopy for tube placement, and consistent advancement into the jejunum was often difficult and time consuming. The No. 18 French (6-mm) polyethylene Kim tube (Kim Med Tech, Inc., Hughesville, PA) is the largest nasoenteral feeding tube used today, and it is passed over a 1.1-mm (0.045-in) guidewire that is endoscopically placed into the jejunum.[23] Although the wire can be placed accurately, tube positioning over the wire can be difficult and requires fluoroscopy for accurate placement. The wire looping problem in the stomach limits the use of nasoenteral feeding tubes to hospital units that have fluoroscopy.[24] Spontaneous tube passage into the duodenum is undependable.

The tube size is especially important in nasojejunal feeding tubes because of the greater irritation of the nasopharyngeal mucosa by the tube diameter and its material. In general, nasojejunal feeding tubes are used in patients who require enteral feedings for only 2 to 4 weeks, because ulceration of the nasopharyngeal mucosa often develops, especially with polyethylene tubes.

Two new techniques have been devised for the successful placement of PEG and PEJ tubes. In the first technique, a standard No. 20 French Ponsky-Gauderer silicone PEG tube was placed with the aid of a gastroscope with a 3.7-mm accessory channel.[25] After the PEG tube was inserted, a standard endoscopic biopsy forceps was advanced through the PEG tube into the gastric lumen and endoscopically grasped with an oval polypectomy snare passed through the endoscope accessory channel (Fig. 13–1). The endoscope and snare with the attached biopsy forceps were withdrawn extraorally, and the endoscope was reinserted into the fourth portion of the duodenum or proximal jejunum (Fig. 13–2). The jejunal feeding tube was fashioned from a 450-cm-long No. 8 French polyethylene nasobiliary tube (NBT) whose tip was cut in a half circle (Fig. 13–3), and additional holes were cut in the tube for feeding purposes. This tube was advanced through the accessory channel of the endoscope over an 0.89-mm guidewire and into the duodenum and advanced under direct vision into the jejunum (Fig. 13–4). As the endoscope

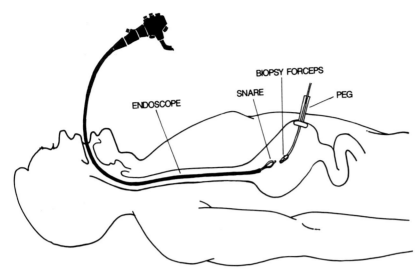

Figure 13–1. The endoscope with a polypectomy snare grasping the biopsy forceps is inserted through the percutaneous endoscopic gastrostomy (PEG) tube. (From MacFadyen BV Jr. Percutaneous endoscopic gastrostomy with jejunal extension. A new technique. Am J Gastroenterol 87:725–728, 1992.)

Figure 13–2. The biopsy forceps are positioned extraorally, and the endoscope is advanced into the fourth position of the duodenum or first part of the jejunum. (From MacFadyen BV Jr. Percutaneous endoscopic gastrostomy with jejunal extension. A new technique. Am J Gastroenterol 87:725–728, 1992.)

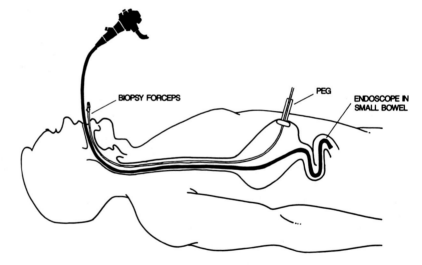

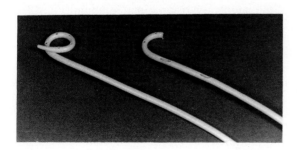

Figure 13–3. The tip of the nasobiliary tube has been cut into a half circle, and additional holes are added to allow easier flow of the enteral feeding. (From MacFadyen BV Jr. Concomitant placement of percutaneous endoscopic gastrostomy and jejunostomy. Surg Endosc 6:289–293, 1992.)

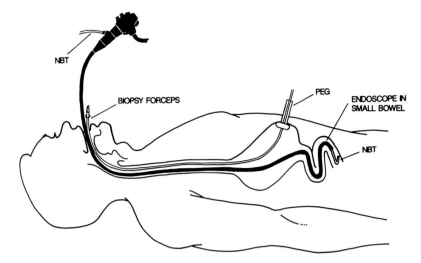

Figure 13–4. The endoscope is reinserted into the fourth part of the duodenum, and the nasobiliary tube (NBT) is advanced distally under direct vision. (From MacFadyen BV Jr. Percutaneous endoscopic gastrostomy with jejunal extension. A new technique. Am J Gastroenterol 87:725–728, 1992.)

was withdrawn, the NBT was pushed out into the jejunum through the endoscope channel and brought out of the mouth. The proximal end of the nasobiliary tube and the head of the biopsy forceps were joined end to end and secured with 2-0 silk suture (Fig. 13–5). The biopsy forceps was then pulled back through the gastrostomy tube (Fig. 13–6) with the PEJ tube and secured outside of the patient (Fig. 13–7). A small loop of NBT was left in the stomach, and a postoperative abdominal x-ray film confirmed the jejunal tube position distal to the ligament of Treitz (Fig. 13–8). Jejunal feedings were begun 6 to 12 hours after placement of the tube. Fluoroscopy was not necessary for accurate PEJ placement.

In this series of 12 patients, the average time for insertion of the PEG and PEJ was 26.2 minutes, and in 11 of the 12 patients, the jejunal tube remained functional for the first 8 weeks of placement.[25] In 2 patients (17%), the NBT clogged at 56 and 60 days, but both tubes were easily cleared of debris by inserting a 0.9-mm guidewire through the jejunal tube at the bedside. Gastroesophageal reflux and pulmonary aspiration did not occur in any of the patients, and they all received sufficient fluid and caloric nutrients without intravenous supplementation. There was no procedure-related mortality, but 1 patient died because of progressive malignant disease 4 weeks into the study.

In this series, the tip of the jejunal feeding tube was placed under direct vision by the endoscopist at least 40 to 50 cm beyond the pylorus without fluoroscopy. The primary reason for advancing the feeding tube into the jejunum was to prevent gastroesophageal reflux. As demonstrated by abdominal surgeons for many years, a 40- to 60-cm isoperistaltic Roux-en-Y loop of jejunum used after partial or total gastrectomy can prevent alkaline gastritis.[26] The application of this principle to the PEJ necessitated PEJ tube placement 40 to 50 cm beyond the pylorus. Because the duodenum is 20 to 25 cm long, the PEJ had to be placed an additional 20 to 30 cm beyond the ligament of Treitz into the jejunum. Although some surgeons have reported no reduction in gastroesophageal reflux and pulmonary aspiration after placement of other jejunal feeding tubes, jejunal tubes often

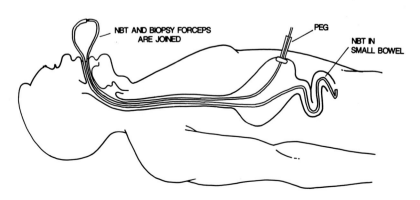

Figure 13–5. The nasobiliary tube (NBT) and biopsy forceps are joined extraorally with 2-0 silk suture. (From MacFadyen BV Jr. Percutaneous endoscopic gastrostomy with jejunal extension. A new technique. Am J Gastroenterol 87:725–728, 1992.)

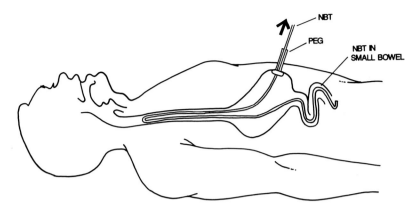

Figure 13–6. The biopsy forceps and nasobiliary tube (NBT) are pulled through the esophagus, stomach, and percutaneous endoscopic gastrostomy (PEG) tube. (From MacFadyen BV Jr. Percutaneous endoscopic gastrostomy with jejunal extension. A new technique. Am J Gastroenterol 87:725–728, 1992.)

Figure 13–7. The percutaneous endoscopic gastrostomy (PEG) and jejunostomy tubes are secured extraorally using a universal adaptor. The PEG tube can be attached to suction. (From MacFadyen BV Jr. Percutaneous endoscopic gastrostomy with jejunal extension. A new technique. Am J Gastroenterol 87:725–728, 1992.)

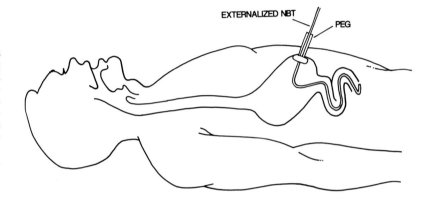

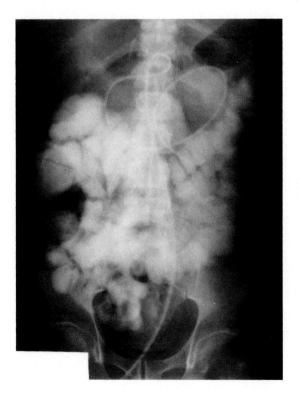

Figure 13–8. After the procedure, an abdominal x-ray film confirms that the nasobiliary tube is in the proximal jejunum 40 to 50 cm from the pylorus.

were not located in the jejunum initially, but rather in the duodenum.[20, 27, 28] Retrograde tube migration did not occur using the MacFadyen technique, although Wolfsen and coworkers observed an incidence of 15% in their patients.[25, 28] It appears that the feeding tube tip position distal to the ligament of Treitz may minimize retrograde tube migration and gastroesophageal reflux.

A modification of this PEJ placement used a No. 20 French silicone PEG tube and a No. 8 French silicone NBT as the PEJ tube.[29] The PEJ tube was initially placed through the 3.7-mm accessory channel of an upper endoscope and advanced into the jejunum 40 to 50 cm beyond the pylorus. The endoscope was withdrawn as the PEJ tube was advanced into the jejunum, and both were brought out of the mouth. The gastroscope was reinserted into the stomach, and a needle and nylon suture were then advanced through the abdominal and gastric walls and grasped with an endoscopic snare. The endoscope, snare, and nylon suture were withdrawn through the mouth, and the nylon suture was attached to a No. 20 French Ponsky–Gauderer PEG tube (Bard Interventional Products, Tewksbury, MA). The proximal end of the No. 8 French PEJ tube was inserted through the dome of the PEG tube, placed parallel to

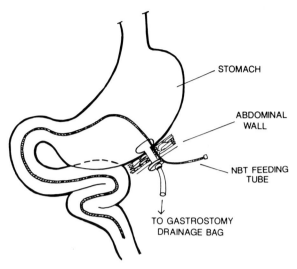

Figure 13–10. The percutaneous endoscopic gastrostomy tube is attached to suction, and the percutaneous endoscopic jejunostomy tube is used for enteral feeding. (From MacFadyen BV Jr. Concomitant placement of percutaneous endoscopic gastrostomy and jejunostomy. Surg Endosc 6:289–293, 1992.)

the PEG tube shaft, and reinserted close to the distal end of the PEG tube (Fig. 13–9). The tubes were sutured together with 2-0 silk suture and were then pulled through the esophagus, stomach, and anterior abdominal wall and secured in place (Fig. 13–10). In a series of 20 patients, the procedure required 59.3 minutes to be completed, and there was only one episode of pulmonary aspiration, which occurred in a patient in whom the PEJ tube had been accidentally pulled back into the duodenum. No fluoroscopy was used during PEG and PEJ placement, but the PEJ tip position was assured by a postoperative abdominal x-ray film. The major advantage of this method was simultaneous gastric decompression of the stomach and jejunal feedings.

Gustke and colleagues demonstrated that, when fluid was infused into the duodenum, there was significant reflux of feedings into the stomach.[30] However, this reflux greatly decreased when the fluid was infused 10 to 12 cm beyond the ligament of Treitz into the jejunum with a final tube tip position 30 to 40 cm beyond the pylorus. Bolus gastrointestinal feedings had a low incidence of reflux compared with continuous feedings. The data supported the fact that the placement of the PEJ tube 40 cm beyond the pylorus was extremely important to minimize gastroesophageal reflux and pulmonary aspiration.

A No. 8 French silicone or polyurethane PEJ tube is the standard feeding tube used with a

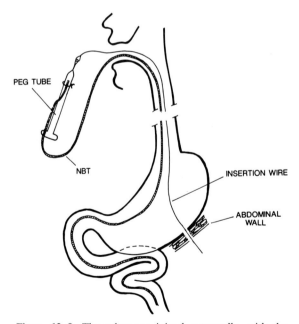

Figure 13–9. The tubes are joined extraorally, with the percutaneous endoscopic jejunostomy tube inserted through the dome of the percutaneous endoscopic gastrostomy (PEG) tube, placed parallel to the PEG tube shaft, reinserted, and secured. (From MacFadyen BV Jr. Concomitant placement of percutaneous endoscopic gastrostomy and jejunostomy. Surg Endosc 6:289–293, 1992.)

PEG. However, some investigators have expressed concern that the PEJ tube will clog after long-term use and have recommended larger tube diameters, ranging in size from 12 to 18 French in diameter. Although the large tubes may remain patent longer, there is greater difficulty in initial placement, and the larger tube is more likely to cause erosion of the gastrointestinal mucosa. In the more recent techniques of PEG and PEJ placement, the jejunal feeding tube was a modified nasobiliary polyethylene No. 8 French tube, although a technique is being developed for rapid insertion of a No. 12 French silicone PEJ tube.[25, 29]

Because most PEJ tubes are used in conjunction with a PEG tube, there is often a limitation of PEJ tube size, because the standard PEG tube is only 20 French in diameter and the internal diameter can accept only No. 8 to 10 French feeding tubes.

Most PEG tubes are made of silicone or polyurethane with a dome or crossbar that prevents the tube from being pulled out of the stomach. Other types of PEG tubes include a balloon catheter similar to the Foley catheter as has been advocated by Russell and colleagues and a silicone button tube (Bard Inc., Billerica, MA) that lies flush with the skin.[31] A No. 28 French silicone PEG tube (Sandoz Nutrition Biosystem, Minneapolis, MN) provides greater decompression of the stomach and allows placement through it of a larger-diameter jejunal feeding tube. This larger PEJ size should improve long-term patency rates and eliminate gastroesophageal reflux and pulmonary aspiration.

A PEJ tube has been directly inserted into the jejunum.[32] In this technique, the endoscope was advanced into the small bowel and its light visualized on the anterior abdominal wall. Direct insertion of a needle and wire into the jejunum was performed. The tube placement through the abdominal wall and jejunum was similar to a standard PEG technique. This technique may have some application after a gastric resection and Billroth II anastomosis, but there may be difficulty in passing a long endoscope consistently into the jejunum, having adequate light visualization on the anterior abdominal wall, and avoiding other intraabdominal organs. Although placement is technically feasible, consistent safety may be an issue.

The anesthetic requirements for most PEG and PEJ placements usually involve conscious sedation, and local anesthesia is used on the posterior pharynx and anterior abdominal wall. A combination of meperidine or alfentanil and diazepam, midazolam, or propofol is used.

These medications can be given safely, but patient monitoring of blood pressure, pulse, respiratory rate, and blood oxygen saturation are important. General anesthesia may be necessary in uncooperative patients, but it is not used frequently. With conscious sedation and local anesthesia, the PEG and PEJ procedure can be performed in any monitored inpatient or outpatient hospital unit.

With PEG, there was a 3% incidence of major complications, which included major wound infections, gastrocolic fistula, intraperitoneal leak of gastric contents, and peristomal enlargement.[33] Minor complications occurred in 13% of the patients in one series and included tube extrusion and minor wound infections. Gottfried and coworkers reported a 38% incidence of pneumoperitoneum after PEG placement.[34] Although those patients were asymptomatic, antibiotics or PEG revision may be necessary if abdominal symptoms develop.

Mortality rates associated with PEG and PEJ placement may be as high as 15% to 20%.[18, 29] In general, these are high-risk patients, and the cause of death is usually related to the underlying disease process and not to the procedure itself. The causes of death have included multiple organ failure, cardiopulmonary failure, disseminated carcinomatosis, aspiration pneumonia, and gastric perforation.[18, 29]

Problems with the feeding tube include tube complications such as clogging, retrograde tube migration, tube kinking, fracture of the mercury tip of the tube, and tube fracture. The overall incidence of complications was 53% to 84%.[18, 27, 28, 35] Tube occlusion was often related to the infusion of high-density feedings and crushed medication without appropriate irrigation after the infusions. Tube fracture was related to the weakness of the tube material, because it is in constant contact with gastric, pancreatic, biliary, and intestinal secretions (Table 13–4). Some of these complications may be decreased by using a No. 12 French or larger-diameter jejunal

Table 13–4. COMPLICATIONS OF PERCUTANEOUS ENDOSCOPIC GASTROSTOMY AND JEJUNOSTOMY

Pulmonary aspiration
Retrograde migration of the PEJ tube
Stomal leakage
Peristomal cellulitis
Gastroduodenal ulceration
Clogging of the PEJ tube
Gastrointestinal bleeding
Failure of nutritional support
Death

Table 13–5. PERCUTANEOUS ENDOSCOPIC JEJUNOSTOMY TUBE MANAGEMENT PLAN

Feeding Tube
  Use a 12- to 14-F diameter silicone or polyurethane tube.
  Place the PEJ tube 40 to 50 cm beyond the pylorus.
  Use a weighted or balloon tube tip.
  Change tube if it clogs or every 3 to 6 months.
Feedings
  Do not infuse crushed medications.
  Use a low-viscosity, high-flow tube feeding; an elemental diet is probably the best.
  Use frequent, small bolus infusions to help minimize reflux.
  Place the jejunal feeding tube 40 to 50 cm beyond the pylorus.
  Flush the feeding tube with water after each bolus feeding.

Table 13–7. CAUSES OF GASTROESOPHAGEAL REFLUX

An incompetent gastroesophageal sphincter
Gastric dilation
Inability to handle oropharyngeal secretions
Decreased pulmonary protective reflexes
Decreased gastrointestinal motility and ileus
Continuous feedings
Neurologic injury causing decreased swallowing, esophageal motility, and decreased gastric emptying
Continued pulmonary aspiration if there is a history of preoperative gastroesophageal reflux and pulmonary aspiration

feeding tube and by replacing the jejunal tube every 3 to 6 months. A PEJ tube management plan is outlined in Tables 13–5 and 13–6.

Although PEG is an easier and simpler procedure to perform, gastroesophageal reflux is more likely to develop, and pulmonary aspiration may occur in 50% to 70% of patients who have decreased levels of consciousness.[36] Various causes of gastroesophageal reflux and pulmonary aspiration are listed in Table 13–7. Cole and colleagues documented that the PEG lowers the gastroesophageal sphincter pressure and retards gastric emptying, and they have advocated advancing the feeding tube into the small bowel.[37] PEJ placement may minimize this problem, especially if it is placed through a PEG, and the PEG is used for gastric decompression. The PEJ feeding tube concept is based on the observation that reflux in a 40- to 50-cm Roux-en-Y segment of jejunum is minimal, and this has been corroborated in surgical jejunostomies in which gastroesophageal reflux and pulmonary aspiration were not observed.[6, 7, 26] However, Adams and associates reported gastroesophageal reflux after surgical jejunostomies.[38] In patients who had PEG and PEJ placement, Kadakia and colleagues found in a series of 79 patients that those who had preoperative pulmonary aspiration continued to have pulmonary aspiration even after PEG and PEJ tube place-

Table 13–6. MANAGEMENT OF AN OBSTRUCTED ENTERAL FEEDING TUBE

Advance a 0.9-mm (0.035-in) guidewire through the tube.
Flush the tube with cranberry juice, meat tenderizer, cola, or urokinase or streptokinase.
Brush out the tube.
Exchange the feeding tube.

ment, and their overall incidence of pulmonary aspiration was 11.9%.[18] The exact location of the tip of the PEJ tube was not stated, and it may have been that the intestinal feeding tube was in the duodenum, increasing the likelihood of gastroesophageal reflux.[20, 21] Oropharyngeal incompetence was not evaluated and may have been a cause of pulmonary aspiration.[39] DiSario and coworkers observed a 70% incidence of PEJ-related complications, of which 67% were due to pulmonary aspiration, and in this series, the feeding tube placement was more often in the duodenum than in the jejunum.[20, 27] Wolfsen and associates reported a 5% incidence of aspiration with PEG tubes and 17% incidence with PEJ tubes, but two series found a 38% incidence of aspiration if the PEJ tube was in the stomach or duodenum.[21, 22, 28] Patterson and Kozarek observed no aspiration with PEJ tubes in the jejunum, but 11.1% of patients with PEG tubes alone had aspiration.[40] These data emphasize that accurate tube placement 40 to 50 cm beyond the pylorus is important in decreasing gastroesophageal reflux.

Another contributing cause for gastroesophageal reflux and pulmonary aspiration is retrograde migration of the jejunal feeding tube, which has been observed to occur in 15% of patients.[28] The cause of retrograde migration may be initial placement in the duodenum and lack of distal tube progression because of paralytic ileus. A second cause may be related to inadvertent tube withdrawal by the patient while turning in bed. Third, a high-pressure continuous enteral infusion may increase the pressure at the tip of the feeding tube and cause it to curl and propagate in a retrograde manner. Because gastroesophageal reflux is potentially the most serious complication of the PEG-PEJ technique, various factors should be considered to prevent it from occurring: a functional gastrointestinal tract; absence of pylorospasm or gastric outlet obstruction; coordinated oropharyngoesophageal motility; placement of the feeding tube 40 to 50 cm beyond the pylorus; use of bolus feedings; a weighted or balloon tip of the tube to prevent retrograde migration; change of the tube every 3 to 6 months; and evaluation of the cause of pulmonary aspiration before PEG and PEJ placement. If these factors are incorporated in the enteral tube management of these patients, the incidence of gastroesophageal reflux and pulmonary aspiration can be greatly decreased.

LAPAROSCOPIC PLACEMENT OF GASTRIC AND JEJUNAL FEEDING TUBES

Although percutaneous endoscopic methods for PEG and PEJ placement suffice in most patients, a transabdominal approach may be required if there is pharyngeal, esophageal, or gastric outlet obstruction. In the past, obstruction would have required a laparotomy, but these tubes can be placed laparoscopically.[6–8]

Laparoscopic gastrostomy has been described by Edelman and colleagues, who used a percutaneous technique similar to the endoscopic method reported by Russell and coworkers.[31, 41] In the series of six laparoscopic gastrostomies by Edelman's group using CO_2 or nitrous oxide insufflation of the abdomen under local anesthesia and sedation, an 18-gauge needle and guidewire were inserted into the stomach, the tract dilated to a No. 16 French diameter, and a No. 14 French Silastic feeding tube with a 10 mL balloon at its tip introduced into the stomach.[41] The balloon was inflated with 5 to 10 mL of saline and pulled up against the anterior abdominal wall. No morbidity or mortality occurred with this technique.

This technique was modified by Murphy and colleagues, who used insufflation of the abdomen and placed trocars.[42] The stomach was distended with air through a nasogastric tube and grasped through a 5-mm right upper quadrant port and brought up to the left upper quadrant abdominal wall. Through a 10-mm left upper quadrant trocar, the stomach was regrasped, and two sutures were inserted transabdominally into the stomach around the left upper quadrant trocar and tied externally. The cutting stylet of the 10-mm trocar was reintroduced and used to puncture the stomach and then removed. Through this gastrotomy, a No. 28 French Malecot tube (C.R. Bard, Inc., Billerica, MA) was advanced through the trocar into the stomach, and the tube was pulled up

against the anterior abdominal wall. Although the results of this technique have not been reported, it appears that its advantage is that a large gastrostomy tube is used for gastric decompression or passage of a large-diameter jejunal feeding tube. This laparoscopic technique may have limited usefulness, because a No. 28 French PEG tube can be endoscopically inserted more quickly and at less cost.

Gastric outlet obstruction and a history of pulmonary aspiration often necessitate the laparoscopic insertion of a jejunal feeding tube. After CO_2 insufflation of the abdomen, a 10-mm trocar and laparoscopic camera are inserted, and 5-mm trocars are placed in the upper midline of the abdomen and in the left upper quadrant lateral to the rectus muscle.[43] The jejunum is grasped with a bowel clamp 20 to 30 cm distal to the ligament of Treitz and brought up to the anterior abdominal wall in the left upper quadrant. A 2-cm incision is made in the skin, muscle, and peritoneum in this region, and the bowel is regrasped through the incision and externalized. A 6- to 8-mm diameter pursestring suture is applied on the antimesenteric border of the jejunum, an 18-gauge needle and guidewire are introduced through the pursestring suture into the bowel, and the tract is dilated to a No. 16 French diameter. A No. 14 French Russell (Cook Critical Care, Bloomington, IN) gastrostomy feeding tube is advanced over the wire into the jejunum, and the balloon is inflated with 3 to 5 mL of sterile saline. The purse-string suture is tied around the feeding tube, and the tube is covered with intestinal wall for 2 cm in a Witzel technique. The bowel is sutured to the anterior abdominal wall, and muscle and skin are closed over the tube. Jejunal feedings are started within 12 to 24 hours after surgery. In a series of 20 patients, no gastroesophageal reflux, pulmonary aspiration, leakage around the tube, or deaths have occurred.[43] In a variation of this technique, the jejunum is brought up to the left upper quadrant abdominal wall, a needle inserted percutaneously, the tract dilated, and a jejunal tube placed directly.[43] Either technique is easy to perform and is associated with few complications.

In another laparoscopic method of providing jejunal feedings, a loop of jejunum distal to the ligament of Treitz is brought through a 2- to 3-cm incision in the left upper quadrant anterior abdominal wall.[43] The jejunum is divided externally, and a 40-cm Roux-en-Y limb of jejunum is created. The jejunostomy is sutured to the muscle fascia and skin in the left upper quadrant. Tube feedings can be started shortly after the procedure. Reflux of feedings on the anterior abdominal wall can occur, and this technique has limited applications because other methods are effective. However, it does minimize reflux into the stomach and eliminates the possibility of retrograde tube migration into the duodenum or stomach.

Enteral feedings offer significant advantages over parenteral nutrition. The PEG-PEJ technique is the simplest, most consistently effective, and least expensive method to provide gastric decompression, jejunal feeding, and reduction in gastroesophageal reflux and pulmonary aspiration. The tip of the PEJ tube must be placed in the jejunum 40 to 50 cm distal to the pylorus, and the tube position must be verified by abdominal x-ray films before starting tube feedings. If a PEG-PEJ procedure cannot be done, laparoscopic placement is a successful technique that is associated with low morbidity and mortality.

References

1. Dudrick SJ, Wilmore DW, Vars HM, et al. Long-term total parenteral nutrition with growth, development, and positive nitrogen balance. Surgery 64:134–142, 1968.
2. Dudrick SJ, Wilmore DW, Vars HM, et al. Can intravenous feeding as the sole means of nutrition support growth in the child and restore weight loss in an adult? An affirmative answer. Ann Surg 169:974–984, 1969.
3. Mamel JJ. Percutaneous endoscopic gastrostomy. Am J Gastroenterology 84:703–710, 1989.
4. Rosenak S, Hollander F. Surgical jejunostomy for alimentation. Clinics 3:638–662, 1944.
5. Wolfer JA. Jejunostomy with jejunal alimentation. Ann Surg 101:708–725, 1935.
6. Delany HM, Carnevale NJ, Garvey JW. Jejunostomy by a needle catheter technique. Surgery 73:786–790, 1973.
7. Page CP, Ryan JA, Haff RC. Continue catheter administration of an elemental diet. Surg Gynecol Obstet 142:184–188, 1976.
8. Feldtman R, Archie J Jr. Modification of the needle-catheter jejunostomy. Am J Surg 143:389–390, 1982.
9. Matino JJ. Feeding jejunostomy in patients with neurological disorders. Arch Surg 116:169–171, 1981.
10. Gauderer MWL, Ponsky JL, Izant RJ Jr. Gastrostomy without laparotomy: a percutaneous endoscopic technique. J Pediatr Surg 15:872–875, 1980.
11. Deitch EA, Berg R, Specian R. Endotoxin promotes the translocation of bacteria from the gut. Arch Surg 122:185–190, 1987.
12. Baker JW, Deitch EA, Ma L, et al. Hemorrhagic shock indices bacterial translocation from the gut. J Trauma 28:896–906, 1988.
13. Pingleton SK, Hadzima S. Enteral alimentation and gastrointestinal bleeding in mechanically ventilated patients. Crit Care Med 11:13–16, 1983.
14. Lally KP, Andrassy RJ, Foster JE, et al. Evaluation of various nutritional supplements in the prevention of stress-induced gastric ulcers in the rat. Surg Gynecol Obstet 158:124–128, 1984.
15. Carmichael MJ, Weisbrodt NW, Copeland EM. Effect of abdominal surgery on intestinal myoelectric activity in the dog. Am J Surg 133:34–38, 1977.
16. Hoover HC, Ryan JA, Anderson EJ, Fischer JE. Nutritional benefits of immediate postoperative jejunal feeding of an elemental diet. Am J Surg 139:153–159, 1980.
17. Strodel WE, Eckhauser FE, Dent TL, Lemmer JQ. Gastrostomy to jejunostomy conversion. Gastrointest Endosc 30:35–36, 1984.
18. Kadakia SC, Sullivan HO, Starnes E. Percutaneous endoscopic gastrostomy or jejunostomy and the incidence of aspiration in 79 patients. Am J Surg 164:114–118, 1992.
19. Ponsky JL, Aszodi A. Percutaneous endoscopic jejunostomy. Am J Gastroenterology 79:113–116, 1984.
20. Lewis BS. Perform PEJ, not PED. Gastrointest Endosc 36:311–312, 1990.
21. Miller KS, Tomlinson JR, Sahn SA. Pleuropulmonary complications of enteral tube feedings. Two reports, review of the literature and recommendations. Chest 88:230–233, 1985.
22. Winterbauer RH, Durning RB, Barran E, McFadden MC. Aspirated nasogastric feeding solution detected by glucose strips. Ann Intern Med 95:67–68, 1981.
23. Kim IG. Endoscopic guided intubation of long nasointestinal decompression tube. Surg Gynecol Obstet 161:282–284, 1985.
24. Alzate GD, Coons HG, Elliott J, Carey PH. Percutaneous gastrostomy for jejunal feeding: A new technique. AJR 147:822–825, 1986.
25. MacFadyen BV Jr, Catalano MF, Raijman I, Ghobrial R. Percutaneous endoscopic gastrostomy with jejunal extension: a new technique. Am J Gastroenterol 87:725–728, 1992.
26. Brintnall ES, Daum K, Womack NA. Maydl jejunostomy. Arch Surg 65:367–372, 1952.
27. DiSario JA, Foutch PG, Sanowski RA. Poor results with percutaneous endoscopic jejunostomy. Gastrointest Endosc 36:257–260, 1990.
28. Wolfsen HC, Kozarek RA, Ball TJ, et al. Tube dysfunction following percutaneous endoscopic gastrostomy and jejunostomy. Gastrointest Endosc 36:261–263, 1990.
29. MacFadyen BV Jr, Ghobrial R, Catalano M, Raijman I. Concomitant placement of percutaneous endoscopic gastrostomy and jejunostomy. Surg Endosc 16:289–293, 1992.
30. Gustke RF, Varms RR, Soergel KH. Gastric reflux during perfusion. Gastroenterology 59:890–895, 1970.
31. Russell TR, Brotman M, Norris F. Percutaneous gastrostomy: A new simplified and cost-effective technique. Am J Surg 184:132–137, 1984.
32. Shike M, Wallach C, Likier H. Direct percutaneous endoscopic jejunostomies. Gastrointest Endosc 37:62–65, 1991.
33. Larson DE, Burton DD, Schroeder KW, DiMagno EP. Percutaneous endoscopic gastrostomy. Gastroenterology 93:48–52, 1987.
34. Gottfried EB, Plumser AB, Clair MR. Pneumoperitoneum following percutaneous endoscopic gastrostomy. Gastrointest Endosc 32:397–399, 1986.
35. Kaplan DS, Murthy UK, Linscheer WG. Percutaneous endoscopic jejunostomy: long-term follow-up of 23 patients. Gastrointest Endosc 35:403–406, 1989.
36. Burtch GD, Shatney CH. Feeding jejunostomy (vs. gastrostomy) passes the test of time. Am J Surg 53:54–57, 1987.
37. Cole M, Smith J, Molnar C, et al. Aspiration after percutaneous gastrostomy. Assessment by TC-99m labelling of the enteral feed. J Clin Gastroenterol 9:90–95, 1987.

38. Adams MB, Seabrook GR, Quebbeman EA, et al. Jejunostomy: a rarely indicated procedure. Arch Surg 121:236–238, 1986.
39. Huxley EJ, Viroslav J, Gray WR, Pierce AK. Pharyngeal aspiration in normal adults and patients with depressed consciousness. Am J Med 64:564–568, 1978.
40. Patterson DJ, Kozarek RA. Comparison of percutaneous endoscopic gastrostomy alone versus PEG with jejunal feeding tube. Gastrointest Endosc 33:176, 1987.
41. Edelman DS, Unger SW. Laparoscopic gastrostomy. Surg Gynecol Obstet 173:401, 1991.
42. Murphy C, Rosemurgy AS, Albrink MH, Carey LC. A simple technique for laparoscopic gastrostomy. Surg Gynecol Obstet 174:424–425, 1992.
43. MacFadyen BV Jr, Wolfe BM, McKernan JB. Laparoscopic management of the acute abdomen, appendix, and small and large bowel. Surg Clin North Am 72:1169–1183, 1992.

14

Percutaneous Endoscopic Gastrostomy and Jejunostomy

Jeffrey L. Ponsky

PERCUTANEOUS ENDOSCOPIC GASTROSTOMY

Percutaneous endoscopic gastrostomy (PEG) was first described in 1980. It offered an endoscopic alternative to laparotomy for establishing long-term enteral access.[1] The technique is based on the principle of endoscopic guidance of gastrointestinal puncture and the subsequent fixation of the intestinal tract to the abdominal wall. In addition to permitting the establishment of a gastrostomy without the necessity for laparotomy, the procedure can be performed in an endoscopy unit, obviating the need for an operating room and general anesthesia. Since the early descriptions of the method, modifications in technique and technology have enhanced the options of the endoscopist and added to the ease and safety with which the procedure is performed.[2] Percutaneous endoscopic jejunostomy (PEJ) was developed as an extension of the gastrostomy technique.[3]

Indications and Contraindications

The predominant indication for PEG is the need for long-term enteral alimentation in a patient unable to swallow. This includes children and adults with permanent or progressive neurologic disorders, such as birth asphyxia, demyelinating disease, amyotrophic lateral sclerosis, and multiple sclerosis. It also includes patients with the inability to eat after cerebrovascular accidents. Another group of patients frequently benefitted by gastrostomy placement are those with malignancies of the upper aerodigestive tract. Additional indications for PEG placement have been the need for gastric decompression in cases of gastric atony or carcinomatosis, the necessity for replacement of bile or administration of unpalatable medications, as a route for alimentation after severe facial trauma, and for providing supplemental nighttime feedings in patients with inflammatory bowel disease. PEJ was originally thought to be useful for providing alimentation in patients with gastroesophageal reflux and aspiration, but evaluation of results reveal this to be a poor use of the method.[4] Patients with gastric atony often benefit from the concomitant gastric decompression and jejunal feeding provided by PEJ.

PEG and PEJ are contraindicated in patients with critical illness, ongoing infection, malnutrition, abdominal sepsis, and multiple organ system failure. It is in these patients that the worst results are to be expected. Patients with a short life expectancy or uncertain prognosis should be fed by nasoenteric tube until their condition improves and the long-term course becomes more apparent. Previous abdominal surgery, including partial gastrectomy, is not a contraindication, as long as the rules for safe placement of the tube are followed.[5] Patients requiring peritoneal dialysis are not good candidates for PEG. PEG can be safely performed in those with ventriculoperitoneal shunts, if the shunt tubing is avoided.

171

Technique

PEG requires three steps: endoscopic examination of the stomach with localization of the
correct puncture site; transabdominal gastric
puncture and passage of a suture or wire; and
gastrostomy tube positioning. Three approaches
incorporating these steps have become popular.
For each, the patient is prepared by fasting for
at least 8 hours before the procedure. The
abdomen is sterilely prepared and draped, and
a single preoperative dose of a parenteral antibiotic is administered. The patient is placed in
the supine position, and the mouth is cleansed
with an antiseptic solution.

In the pull technique, the gastroscope is introduced into the stomach and an examination
performed to ensure that concomitant problems,
such as gastric outlet obstruction or acute ulceration, are not present. The instrument is positioned in the body of the stomach, proximal to
the gastric angle, and the room lights are turned
down. A survey of the abdominal wall for the
site of best transillumination is performed. If
such a site cannot be easily detected, it may be
useful to apply pressure with a finger in the left
upper abdomen to see if the light becomes
visible. Transillumination of the abdominal wall
is one of the most crucial steps in the performance of PEG. It indicates that the stomach and
abdominal walls are opposed without any intervening tissue. After this point is selected, local

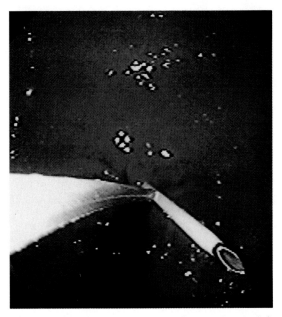

Figure 14–2. A polypectomy snare is tightened around the needle before its inner sheath is removed.

anesthesia is infiltrated in the skin, and an
incision about 1 cm long is made.

Finger pressure applied to the abdominal wall
by the assistant should result in a clear indentation within the stomach's lumen (Fig. 14–1).
The endoscopist uses a polypectomy snare to
surround the indentation, in preparation for
grasping the puncturing needle as it enters the
stomach. After the endoscopist and assistant
agree on the site and the snare is properly
positioned, the puncture is performed. The
sheathed needle is thrust across the opposed
gastric and abdominal walls into the gastric
lumen. The endoscopist tightens the snare
around the needle's shaft, and the needle is
removed from the sheath (Fig. 14–2). A long
suture or wire is then passed through the sheath
into the gastric lumen. The snare is loosened
and applied selectively to the suture (Fig. 14–
3). The endoscope and suture are pulled from
the patient's mouth. The suture or wire is affixed
to the tapered end of the gastrostomy tube, and
pulling commences at the abdominal end of the
suture. The tube is pulled down the esophagus
and into the stomach until the tapered end is
seen to emerge from the abdominal wall (Fig.
14–4). The gastroscope is reinserted and positioned above the mushroom head of the tube to
observe its progress as it is pulled into position.
Traction is ceased when the head of the catheter
just touches the gastric mucosa (Fig. 14–5). The
gastroscope is then removed. An outer crossbar
is applied to maintain position of the tube and

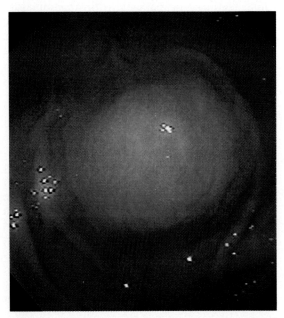

Figure 14–1. Finger pressure applied to the abdominal wall at the site of best transillumination should produce a clear indentation in the gastric lumen.

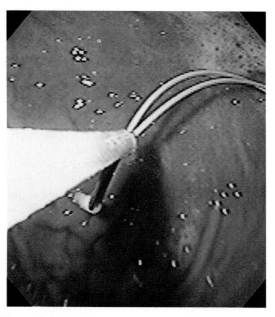

Figure 14–3. The snare is repositioned and selectively tightened around the suture.

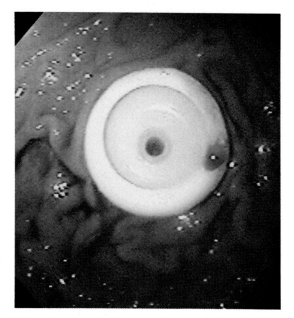

Figure 14–5. The head of the catheter is allowed to lightly contact the gastric mucosa.

prevent its distal migration where it might obstruct the pyloric channel. The crossbar need not be tight against the skin, and evidence suggests that only loose approximation of the gastric and abdominal walls is necessary (Fig. 14–6).[6] Excessive tension does not produce a better tract and may lead to tube migration through the abdominal wall and cause local ischemia with subsequent infection. Tube feedings are usually begun the day after the procedure.

A modification of the technique described by Saks and Vine involves the use of a guidewire rather than a suture.[7] The puncture site is selected as previously described, and a long guidewire is passed into the stomach and captured

with a snare. After it is out of the mouth, it is used as a trolley wire over which a gastrostomy catheter with a long, firm, tapered end is pushed (Fig. 14–7). The wire is held taut, and the tube is pushed over it until it emerges from the abdominal wall (Fig. 14–8). It is then pulled the rest of the way into the stomach, and its position is assessed with the gastroscope, as described with the pull method.

Russell and Brotman described a method for performing the PEG using the principles often associated with the placement of central venous lines.[8] The gastroscope is used to select the site for the gastrostomy as described with the other techniques. The stomach is punctured with a

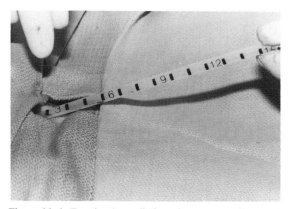

Figure 14–4. Traction is applied on the suture until several inches of the tube emerge from the abdominal wall.

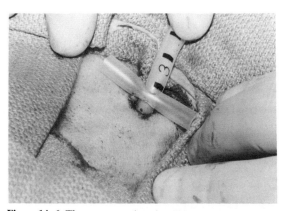

Figure 14–6. The outer crossbar should be positioned several millimeters from the skin to avoid tension, which may produce ischemia in the underlying tissue.

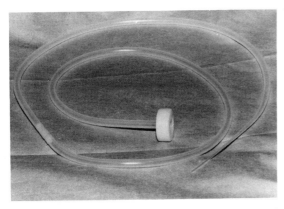

Figure 14–7. A gastrostomy tube with a long, firm, tapered end, which was designed for an "over the wire" technique.

short guidewire, and the gastroscope is used to observe this process. The needle is removed, and an introducer with overlying peel-away sheath is advanced over the wire into the stomach (Fig. 14–9). The introducer is removed, and a Foley balloon catheter is passed through the sheath and inflated (Fig. 14–10). The sheath is then removed (Fig. 14–11). Because a gastroscope remains in the stomach to observe the entire placement, a second passage is not required. Because the tube is not pulled down through the esophagus, there is less risk of seeding the abdominal wall with bacteria.

Results and Complications

With the maturation of the PEG procedure came numerous reports documenting the re-

sults. It became clear that the various method modifications were all acceptable. The pull and the push techniques are similar in their incidence and variety of associated complications.[9] The introducer technique is also effective and is associated with a lower rate of abdominal wall infection, but gastric wall separation and peritonitis are more frequent with this technique.[10]

The most frequent complication after PEG is infection of the abdominal wall. In most cases, this is caused by tracking oral bacteria into the abdominal wall. The administration of preoperative antibiotics for prophylaxis seems warranted to reduce the incidence of this problem.[11] After an abscess of the abdominal wall becomes apparent, rapid incision and drainage should be carried out to prevent necrotizing fasciitis. Although small infections can usually be managed without sacrificing the gastrostomy, more serious infections may require tube removal and site debridement. Abdominal wall infection is often the result of local tissue ischemia caused by excessive tension on the outer crossbar. Loose initial application of the crossbar limits the frequency of the problem.

Separation of the gastric and abdominal walls with resultant peritoneal soilage can occur early after PEG placement. This is almost always a result of excessive traction on the gastrostomy tube with tissue breakdown in the gastric wall. Peritonitis secondary to escape of the gastric contents may occur after this episode. Alternatively, the situation may be heralded by only an elevation of the leukocyte count and a temperature elevation. If separation is suspected, plain films of the abdomen should be obtained. Pneu-

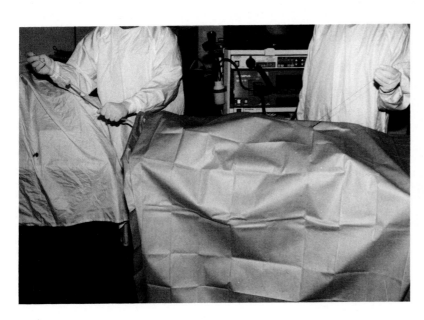

Figure 14–8. The wire is held taut at both ends as the tube is advanced over it.

moperitoneum may indicate a leaking site, but alone, it is not proof, because pneumoperitoneum is common after uncomplicated PEG procedures and may persist for weeks after the procedure.[12] Water-soluble contrast material should be introduced into the gastrostomy tube to ascertain whether there is a leak into the peritoneal cavity. If a leak is verified and signs of peritonitis exist, abdominal exploration and lavage are indicated. If clinical signs are minimal, a trial of nasogastric suction and intravenous antibiotics is usually reasonable. Separation can also occur if a physician or patient pulls the gastrostomy tube out of the stomach before a tract has completely formed. A trial of nasogastric suction and intravenous antibiotics is worthwhile. If clinical deterioration occurs, exploration, with repair and lavage, must be performed.

Gastrocolic fistula has occasionally occurred after PEG.[13] It is probably the result of transcolonic puncture at the time of the initial procedure or caused by pinching of the colonic wall between the stomach and abdominal wall with subsequent fistula formation. The condition often presents with voluminous diarrhea after feedings, and it may be noticed only if the tube becomes positioned in the colonic lumen after a tube change. Barium enema or instillation of contrast into the stomach through the gastrostomy tube can reveal the diagnosis. Fortunately, this complication is rarely serious and responds

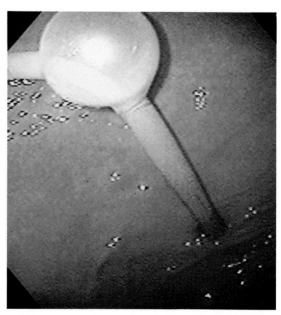

Figure 14–10. After the sheath is within the gastric lumen, the introducer is removed, and a balloon catheter is inserted.

rapidly with closure of the fistula after removal of the gastrostomy tube. Careful transillumination of the abdominal wall at the time of site selection for the PEG can help to prevent this occurrence.

Aspiration of gastric contents with resultant pneumonia can occur after PEG. Initial impressions that PEG might prevent gastroesophageal reflux have not been borne out. Feedings should be started in a progressive fashion after PEG, and residual gastric volumes should be checked to avoid gastric distention. Diarrhea after the procedure may indicate a need to dilute or change the feeding solution. Although the technical aspects of PEG are simple, the potential for serious complications exists, and careful

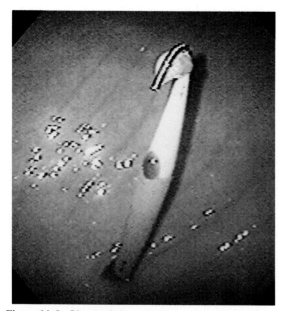

Figure 14–9. Observed through the gastroscope, the introducer and overlying sheath are advanced into the gastric lumen over a guidewire.

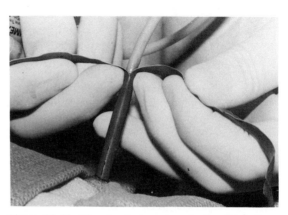

Figure 14–11. The sheath is removed after the balloon catheter is securely in place.

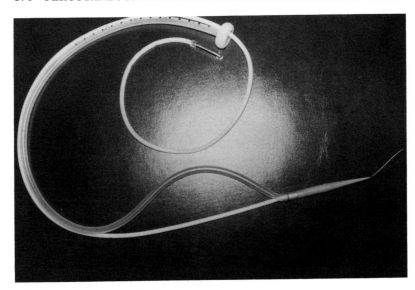

Figure 14–12. A modified tube with a gastrostomy port and a parallel jejunal lumen is designed for percutaneous endoscopic jejunostomy.

patient follow-up after the procedure is necessary for optimal results.

PERCUTANEOUS ENDOSCOPIC JEJUNOSTOMY

When it is desirable to feed the patient distal to the stomach, a PEJ may be established to provide gastric decompression and simultaneous delivery of nutrients to the small intestine. The procedure is performed just as PEG, but a two-lumen tube is used. A gastric lumen permits decompression of the stomach, and a smaller, longer tube is used for alimentation.

Initial descriptions of the technique involved the use of parallel tubes fixed together.[14] The gastrostomy portion is placed in a standard PEG fashion. The longer jejunal feeding tube is placed endoscopically into the duodenum and allowed to progress into the proximal jejunum (Fig. 14–12). This method does not prevent gastroesophageal reflux and aspiration of gastric contents, but it is effective in patients with gastric atony. The method suffers from the frequent plugging and the need for replacement of the jejunal feeding tube. Some endoscopists have developed modifications that attempt to use a larger-bore feeding tube. New tube designs offer improvements in results with this method.

Skin-Level Devices

Gauderer introduced the important concept of a skin-level gastrostomy device.[15] Some pa-

tients requiring PEG are functional but are limited in their activities by the social stigma of an indwelling abdominal tube. A skin-level device with an antireflux valve permits a cosmetic solution to gastrostomy feedings (Fig. 14–13). The device is also useful as a solution to the skin problems occurring around the gastrostomy tube. Stomal enlargement secondary to pivoting of the tube or leaking around the tube may be dealt with by removal of the original tube and insertion of a skin-level device.[16] Adaptations of this device permit placement at the time of the initial gastrostomy.

Ethical Considerations

Percutaneous endoscopic gastrostomy has provided a simple and effective means of providing nutrition in patients unable to swallow.

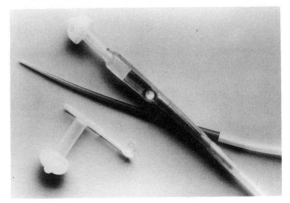

Figure 14–13. A skin-level device may be inserted through the gastrostomy site after the tract is mature or placed at the time of gastrostomy creation.

The procedure has become a frequent indication for the performance of endoscopy. Review of mortality figures after the procedure indicate that it is often performed in patients with short life expectancies or in those with critical illnesses.[17] A decision to perform PEG should be predicated on a reasonable expectation of continued survival. Patients with terminal conditions or multisystem organ failure are rarely benefited by PEG and are most likely to experience a poor outcome after the procedure. The performance of a feeding gastrostomy indicates a commitment to prolonged enteral nutritional support. Withdrawal of established nutritional support has significant ethical and legal implications.[18] Careful consideration of each case and critical patient selection can ensure the best outcome.

References

1. Gauderer MWL, Ponsky JL, Izant RJ Jr. Gastrostomy without laparotomy. A percutaneous endoscopic technique. J Pediatr Surg 15:872–875, 1980.
2. Ponsky JL, Gauderer MWL. Percutaneous endoscopic gastrostomy: a non-operative technique for feeding gastrostomy. Gastrointest Endosc 27:9–11, 1981.
3. Ponsky JL, Aszodi A. Percutaneous endoscopic jejunostomy. Am J Gastroenterol 79:113–116, 1984.
4. DiSario JA, Fiutch PG, Sanowski RA. Poor results with percutaneous endoscopic gastrostomy. Gastrointest Endosc 36:257–260, 1990.
5. Stellato TA, Gauderer MWL, Ponsky JL. Percutaneous endoscopic gastrostomy following previous abdominal surgery. Ann Surg 200:46–50, 1984.
6. Mellinger JD, Simon IB, Schlecter B, Lash RH, Ponsky JL. Tract formation following percutaneous endoscopic gastrostomy in an animal model. Surg Endosc 5:189–191, 1991.
7. Sacks BA, Vine HS, Palestrant AM, et al. A non-operative technique for establishment of a gastrostomy in the dog. Invest Radiol 18:485–487, 1983.
8. Russell TR, Brotman M, Forbes N. Percutaneous gastrostomy: a new simplified and cost-effective technique. Am J Surg 148:132–135, 1984.
9. Hogan RB, DeMarco DC, Hamilton JK, et al. Percutaneous endoscopic gastrostomy: to push or pull, a prospective randomized trial. Gastrointest Endosc 32:253–258, 1986.
10. Foutch GP. Complications of percutaneous endoscopic gastrostomy and jejunostomy, recognition, prevention, and treatment. Gastrointest Endosc Clin North Am 2:231–248, 1992.
11. Jonas SK, Neimark S, Panwalker AP. Effect of antibiotic prophylaxis in percutaneous endoscopic gastrostomy. Am J Gastroenterol 80:438–440, 1985.
12. Plumser AB, Gottfried EB, Clair MR. Pneumoperitoneum after percutaneous endoscopic gastrostomy. Am J Gastroenterol 79:440–441, 1984.
13. Strodel WE, Ponsky JL. Complications of percutaneous gastrostomy. In: Ponsky JL, eds. Techniques of percutaneous gastrostomy. New York: Igaku-Shoin, 1988.
14. Aszodi A, Ponsky JL. Percutaneous endoscopic jejunostomy. In: Ponsky JL, ed. Techniques of percutaneous gastrostomy. New York: Igaku-Shoin, 1988.
15. Gauderer MWL, Picha GJ, Izant RJ Jr. The gastrostomy "button"—a simple, skin-level nonrefluxing device for long-term enteral feedings. J Pediatr Surg 19:803–805, 1984.
16. Gauderer MWL, Olsen MM, Stellato TA, et al. Feeding gastrostomy button: experience and recommendations. J Pediatr Surg 23:24, 1988.
17. Wolfsen HC, Kozarek RA, Ball TJ, et al. Long-term survival in patients undergoing percutaneous endoscopic gastrostomy and jejunostomy. Am J Gastroenterol 85:1120–1122, 1990.
18. Wolfsen HC, Kozarek RA. Percutaneous endoscopic gastrostomy: ethical considerations. Gastrointest Endosc Clin North Am 2:259–269, 1992.

15

Endoscopic Retrograde Cholangiopancreatography

Jeffrey L. Ponsky

Maladies of the pancreas and biliary tree have traditionally been the domain of the general surgeon, yet precise means for evaluating these organs have been elusive. In the past, exploratory laparotomy frequently offered the only avenue for accurate assessment and treatment of pancreaticobiliary conditions. In 1968, McCune and associates reported the first endoscopic cannulation of the ampulla of Vater, with visualization of the pancreatic and biliary ductal systems.[1] Since the introduction of endoscopic retrograde cholangiopancreatography (ERCP), it has become an indispensable component of diagnosis of and therapy for the pancreaticobiliary system. The emergence of high-quality imaging techniques such as ultrasonography, computed tomography, and percutaneous transhepatic cholangiography has been revolutionary in assisting the surgeon in the approach to these organ systems, yet none has diminished the importance of ERCP.

INDICATIONS FOR ENDOSCOPIC RETROGRADE CHOLANGIO-PANCREATOGRAPHY

One of the earliest uses of ERCP was in evaluating the cause of jaundice and, in cases in which obstruction was present, defining the site and nature of the blockage. ERCP is useful in evaluating cases of suspected stones following cholecystectomy and potential cases of biliary tract or pancreatic malignancy.[2] Preoperative evaluation of the pancreatic ductal system prior to surgery for chronic pancreatitis or pseudocyst was an early indication for endoscopic pancreatography, and the method was also used to evaluate the pancreas after surgical decompression of the ductal system. With the development of a therapeutic capability, the use of ERCP in the total care of the patient with pancreatic or biliary disease has increased dramatically. The method has been effective in the management of common bile duct calculi, biliary strictures, bile leaks after surgery, and tumors of the bile duct.[3] It also allows careful inspection of the duodenum and assessment of irregularities of the ampulla of Vater. Therapeutic ERCP has also played an important role in the approach to pancreatic carcinoma, pseudocyst, acute and chronic pancreatitis, pancreatic duct calculi, and pancreas divisum.[4] Although some may argue the relative merits of ERCP versus computed tomography and ultrasonography, each method provides its own unique advantages and limitations and these modalities should be used in a complementary fashion. It is usually appropriate to obtain a noninvasive imaging study prior to the performance of ERCP. The latter will help to define the anticipated anatomy and may predict the need for therapeutic intervention.

Percutaneous transhepatic cholangiography is highly successful in revealing the anatomy of the biliary tree and may be extended to offer a therapeutic dimension. It is particularly useful when there is intrahepatic biliary dilation but is more difficult to perform in normal-sized ducts. The method may offer increased risk in the presence of coagulopathy or ascites and fails to offer visualization of the ampulla of Vater or the pancreatic duct. Once again, this technique may complement ERCP and may be particularly useful in demonstrating the intrahepatic ductal system when common duct obstruction is complete and an ERCP shows only the lower portion of the system. In a number of cases, the methods are complementary and may be used sequentially or in concert to supply information or perform a therapeutic maneuver.[5]

Contraindications to Endoscopic Retrograde Cholangiopancreatography

Although ERCP is extremely valuable and minimally invasive, it has the potential to cause complications and may be contraindicated in certain situations. Patients with hemodynamic instability are poor candidates for ERCP, as are those with florid sepsis. Such patients may quickly undergo decompensation during the procedure. It is preferable to stabilize the patient prior to the intervention. Severe acute pancreatitis may be exacerbated by the performance of ERCP, and the procedure is generally avoided in the initial phase of the disease, unless there is the suspicion that gallstones are the cause and the endoscopist is prepared to intervene therapeutically to alleviate the obstruction.[6] More recently, some authors have attempted pancreatic duct stenting for acute pancreatitis, but this procedure is not widely accepted or practiced at present.[7] Patients with coagulopathy or portal hypertension are poor candidates for endoscopic sphincterotomy, as massive hemorrhage may occur subsequent to division of vessels in the ampullary wall.

Previous gastric surgery may make the performance of ERCP difficult or impossible. In the presence of a Bilroth II reconstruction, it is necessary to approach the ampulla by way of the afferent loop. Although this is frequently accomplished, it renders the procedure more difficult, and therapeutic maneuvers are more complicated in this position. A Roux-en-Y gastrojejunostomy makes ERCP nearly impossible, as the Roux limb is generally too long to allow access to the papilla in a retrograde fashion.

Finally, ERCP should not be attempted by an endoscopist untrained in the technique. The examination is perhaps the most complex of all endoscopic procedures, and complications may result from unskilled manipulation around the papilla. Although the method is not as difficult to perform as was perceived in the initial years after its introduction, skill and success with the procedure are clearly related to practice and experience.[8]

PREPARATION OF THE PATIENT

As with all endoscopic procedures in the upper gastrointestinal tract, it is best that the patient fast for 6 to 8 hours prior to the procedure to ensure an empty stomach. Any hemodynamic instability, dehydration, or electrolyte abnormalities should be corrected prior to the procedure. When therapy is anticipated and any question of poor liver function or bleeding tendency is entertained, a coagulation profile should be obtained and abnormalities addressed prior to the procedure. When biliary obstruction is probable, as in the jaundiced patient or one with gallstone pancreatitis, preoperative parenteral antibiotics should be given.

ERCP is performed in a suite with fluoroscopic capability, most often in the radiology department. Therefore, it is imperative to ensure that all safety and monitoring equipment is present and functional prior to the procedure. Frequently, it is beneficial to place the patient's head at what is normally considered the foot of the fluoroscopy table to provide adequate room for the endoscopy instruments at the patient's head. In this situation, it is helpful if the equipment permits the fluoroscopic image to be reversed.

The procedure is commenced with the patient in the left lateral decubitus position, similar to that for upper gastrointestinal tract endoscopy. Some endoscopists prefer to begin with the patient's left arm behind them, as this facilitates turning the patient to the prone position after the duodenum is entered.

Posterior pharyngeal anesthesia is obtained with topical anesthetic spray, and intravenous sedation is administered. In addition, glucagon or atropine, or both, are commonly used to diminish duodenal peristalsis during attempts at cannulation of the ampulla of Vater.

TECHNIQUE OF ENDOSCOPIC RETROGRADE CHOLANGIO-PANCREATOGRAPHY

A side-viewing duodenoscope is used for the performance of ERCP (Fig. 15–1). This instrument is longer than a standard forward-viewing

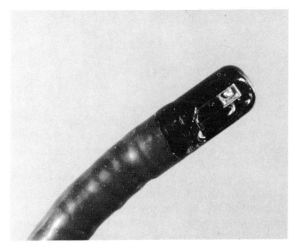

Figure 15–1. A side-viewing duodenoscope.

panendoscope, and its visual field is perpendicular to the long axis of the endoscope. The side-viewing design hinders introduction by direct vision and examination of the esophagus. The instrument is gently introduced first into the pharynx and then into the esophagus. It is advanced slowly into the gastric lumen. The esophagogastric junction can be easily recognized and its lumen followed into the stomach. Once in the stomach through further introduction of the instrument, there is a tendency to retroflex the scope and view the fundus (Fig. 15–2). This occurs as the angle of the stomach is reached. When this retroflexed view is noted, the scope should be pulled back a bit and its tip deflected downward to visualize and enter the gastric antrum. This will reveal the antrum and the pyloric orifice. With downward deflection of the tip maintained, the scope is advanced to the pylorus. When the pylorus is at hand, the tip of the instrument is slowly lifted, and gentle pressure is applied. This will align the tip with the pyloric channel and allow the scope to enter the duodenal bulb. The mucosa of the duodenal bulb can be noted to have a soft and slightly villous appearance. In order to advance the duodenoscope from the bulb into the descending duodenum, it is necessary to turn the instrument to the right and posteriorly. This is achieved with a right turn at the control head of the scope and rightward deflection of the control knob. The anatomy here may be slightly variable, and force should never be applied when advancing the scope in a blind fashion. When direct visualization of the lumen is possible, it provides the safest means for scope advancement.

Once the descending duodenum is entered, it is useful to roll the patient to the prone position so that the ampulla of Vater can be rotated into optimal position for cannulation. The major papilla is usually noted to be a vertical bulge breaking the line of the otherwise horizontal duodenal folds (Fig. 15–3). It often first presents in the 10 o'clock position. The minor papilla,

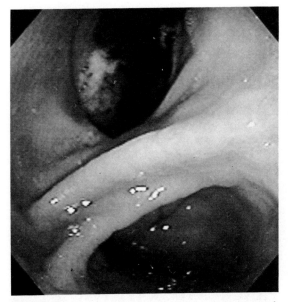

Figure 15–2. A view from the antrum of the stomach through the side-viewing scope permits the endoscopist to view the cardia and antrum simultaneously. Deflection of the tip downward will guide the instrument toward the pylorus.

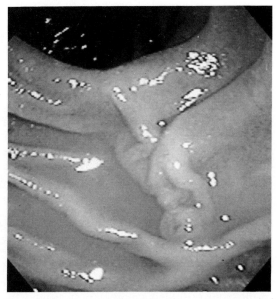

Figure 15–3. The ampulla of Vater appears as a vertical fold, crossing the horizontal semicircular folds of the duodenal mucosa. The orifice of the ampulla usually appears as a red, finely reticulated discoloration at the tip of the papilla.

when present, is typically noted to be slightly proximal to the major papilla in the 1 o'clock position. When the descending duodenum is first entered, the instrument typically follows a curve around the greater curvature of the stomach before entering the duodenum. This is the "long scope" position (Fig. 15–4). In most cases, this is not the most advantageous position for accurate cannulation, and it is usually best to deflect the tip of the instrument upward and pull gently backward on the instrument once the scope is at the papilla. This reduces the gastric loop and brings the shaft of the instrument along the lesser curvature of the stomach and the tip of the scope closer to the papilla. This "short scope" posture is generally most advantageous for accurate cannulation (Fig. 15–5). In some instances, however, one will find that attempts in the "short scope" position will fail and that the "long scope" position will provide success.

Once the papilla is identified and the scope shortened, small precise adjustments can be made to achieve an en face approach to the ampullary orifice. This orifice is usually recognized by a soft villous surface with a reticulated pattern. A variety of cannulas are available for penetration of the papilla. The standard cannula may have a straight tip or a slight taper. It is introduced gently into the ampullary orifice, and contrast medium is injected with fluoroscopic monitoring. When no ductal filling is noted, the cannula may be repositioned to enter the desired duct. Generally, the pancreatic duct orifice is at the 1 o'clock position within the papilla, whereas that of the bile duct is in the 11 o'clock position.

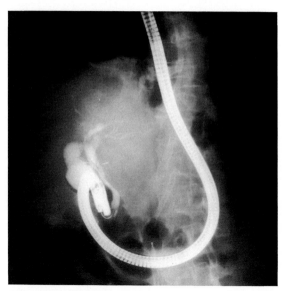

Figure 15–4. The scope is seen in the "long" position. This offers less control of the tip but may be advantageous for selective cannulation in certain cases.

There may be a thin septum between the openings, and elevation of the cannula as it is introduced into the ampulla will facilitate entering the upper opening, usually the bile duct. It should be kept in mind that the bile duct courses parallel to the duodenal wall and is best entered with an approach from below the papilla aiming upward, whereas the pancreatic duct courses perpendicular to the duodenal wall and may be best approached by a direct en face route. Although these approaches are generally correct, each case is unique, and the endoscopist

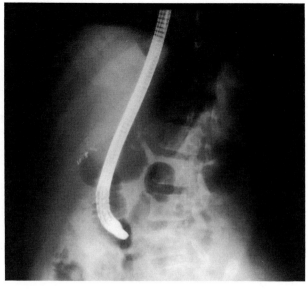

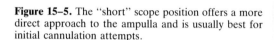

Figure 15–5. The "short" scope position offers a more direct approach to the ampulla and is usually best for initial cannulation attempts.

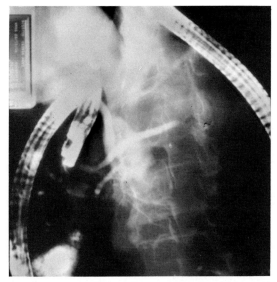

Figure 15–6. Overfilling of the ventral pancreatic duct with "acinarization" of the ventral pancreatic parenchyma is noted in this patient with a pancreas divisum. The dorsal duct was filled by a separate injection through the minor papilla.

must frequently try a number of approaches to obtain selective cannulation of each duct. When cannulation is achieved, the injection of contrast medium should be slow and measured, particularly in the pancreatic system. Excessive injection of the pancreatic duct, as evidenced by visualization of the glandular substance (acinarization) should be avoided, as it frequently produces pancreatitis (Fig. 15–6). When a need for therapy is anticipated, the procedure may begin with a double-channel papillotome. This will permit cannulation and injection through one channel, and subsequent division of the sphincter by means of the wire in the second channel, without the need for a catheter change. If a standard cannula is used and the need for therapy is encountered, a wire may be introduced through its lumen deep into the selected duct. The cannula is then removed, and a papillotome, or stent, is substituted.

DIAGNOSTIC ASPECTS OF ENDOSCOPIC RETROGRADE CHOLANGIO-PANCREATOGRAPHY

Although the technical aspects of ERCP are demanding and challenging, it is vital that the films obtained be subjected to careful scrutiny. It must be remembered that the goal of the

procedure is the correct assessment and treatment of the condition at hand, and *not* cannulation of the desired duct. The endoscopist must become skilled at interpreting variations in pancreatic and biliary anatomy and in recognizing subtle abnormalities. It is inappropriate that this function be relegated to the radiologist, although consultation with a radiologist is useful.

Bile duct anatomy is most familiar to the surgeon. Normal anatomy is not difficult to identify (Fig. 15–7). Stones are easily noted in the common duct but occasionally may be obscured in intrahepatic biliary radicals (Fig. 15–8). Subtle pruning of the intrahepatic biliary tree may indicate a parenchymal process such as cirrhosis or a tumor. Strictures can be isolated or multiple and signify benign or malignant conditions (Fig. 15–9). Congenital anomalies such as a choledochal cyst should be recognized. Consideration of future operative intervention may dictate that particular views be obtained or specific diagnostic or therapeutic maneuvers be carried out.

Pancreatic duct abnormalities may be less familiar to the surgeon. Tortuosity and dilation of the system is characteristic of chronic pancreatitis (Fig. 15–10). A small ductal system with ectatic clubbing of secondary side branches may also indicate chronic pancreatitis. Calculi are occasionally noted within the ductal system and on occasion may be approached endoscopically. Areas of ductal encasement or narrowing may signify the presence of a malignant process. Pseudocyst of the pancreas is not uncommon, and multiple pseudocysts may occur along the gland. Many pseudocysts fill with contrast medium as injection is performed. Infection of these cysts is a potential complication and must be kept in mind.

Pancreas divisum is an anatomic variant in which embryologic division of the pancreas persists, the head of the gland being drained

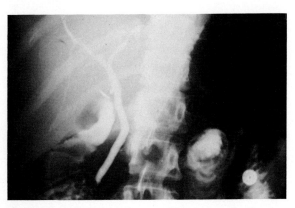

Figure 15–7. Normal biliary anatomy in a patient following cholecystectomy.

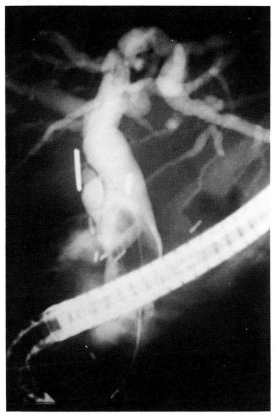

Figure 15–8. A large gallstone is noted in the common bile duct and is surrounded by a wire basket.

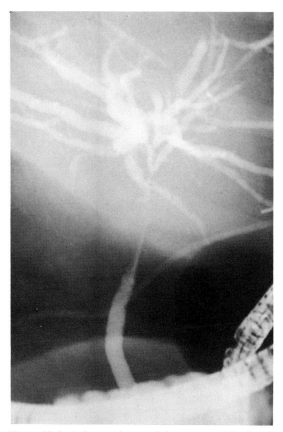

Figure 15–9. A long stricture of the common bile duct in its midportion, secondary to extrinsic compression by tumor.

through the major papilla and the body and tail through the persistent duct of Santorini at the more proximal minor papilla. Injection at the major papilla in the usual fashion will fill only the head of the gland. The condition can be recognized by the rapid arborization of the ductal system as it leaves the duodenum. If information regarding the body and tail of the gland is needed, it is necessary to attempt cannulation of the minor papilla, which is more challenging and requires the use of a tapered or needle-tip catheter. If obstruction is present at the minor papilla in such cases, pancreatic changes may be noted in the body and tail of the gland, whereas injection at the major papilla reveals a normal ductal system in the pancreatic head.

THERAPEUTIC ENDOSCOPIC RETROGRADE CHOLANGIO- PANCREATOGRAPHY

Prior to the introduction of endoscopic sphincterotomy, the use of ERCP was somewhat

limited in spite of its tremendous value as a diagnostic tool. This was because many of the potential findings at ERCP required prompt intervention. The inability to decompress an obstructed ductal system following the injection of contrast material may produce or exacerbate biliary sepsis. Since the description of endo-

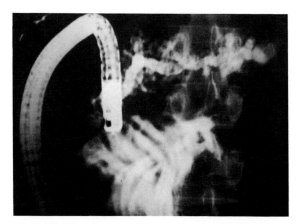

Figure 15–10. A pancreatogram demonstrating a dilated and tortuous pancreatic duct indicative of chronic pancreatitis.

scopic sphincterotomy, therapeutic dimensions to ERCP have developed rapidly and permit a great variety of interventions, including extraction of biliary and pancreatic duct calculi, dilation and stenting of biliary and pancreatic duct strictures, and drainage of pancreatic pseudocysts (see Chaps. 6, 16, and 17).

TRAINING IN ENDOSCOPIC RETROGRADE CHOLANGIO-PANCREATOGRAPHY

Instruction in ERCP should take place in the setting of a comprehensive endoscopic training program. Prior to performing ERCP, the trainee must be skilled in the performance of routine upper endoscopy and colonoscopy and should spend time practicing the manipulation of a side-viewing endoscope. Initial attempts at ERCP must be closely supervised and may begin with maneuvers necessary to advance the scope into the duodenum and position it en face with the ampulla of Vater. Once these manipulations are familiar, attempts at cannulation may begin. The novice must practice "selective" cannulation of each duct and learn to advance the catheter deeply into the ductal system in preparation for training in therapeutic interventions.

Diagnostic ERCP should be well in hand prior to commencement of attempts at therapeutic ERCP. The latter requires skill and confidence at selective ductal cannulation, a comprehensive knowledge of ductal anatomy, and an understanding of potential complications.

References

1. McCune WS, Shorb PE, Moscowitz H. Endoscopic cannulation of the ampulla of Vater: a preliminary report. Ann Surg 167:752, 1968.
2. Furguson RD, Sivak MV. Indications, contraindications, and complications of ERCP. In: Sivak MV, ed. Gastroenterologic Endoscopy. Philadelphia: WB Saunders, 1987:581–598.
3. Huibregtse K, Kimmey MB. Endoscopic retrograde cholangiopancreatography, endoscopic sphincterotomy and stone removal, endoscopic biliary and pancreatic drainage. In: Yamada T, ed. Textbook of Gastroenterology. Philadelphia: JB Lippincott, 1991:2266–2292.
4. Soehendra N, Grimm H, Schreiber H. Endoscopic transpapillary drainage of the pancreatic duct in chronic pancreatitis. Dtsch Med Wochenschr 111:727, 1986.
5. Robertson DAF, Hacking LN, Birch S, et al. Experience with a combined percutaneous and endoscopic approach to stent insertion in malignant obstructive jaundice. Lancet 2:1449, 1987.
6. Davidson BR, Neoptolemos JP, Carr-Locke DL. Endoscopic sphincterotomy for common bile duct calculi in patients with gallbladder in situ considered unfit for surgery. Gut 29:114, 1988.
7. Fuji T, Amano H, Harima K, et al. Pancreatic sphincterotomy and pancreatic endoprosthesis. Endoscopy 17:69, 1985.
8. Bilbao MK, Dotter CT, Lee TG, et al. Complications of endoscopic retrograde cholangiopancreatography (ERCP). A study of 10,000 cases. Gastroenterology 70:314, 1976.

16

Endoscopic Retrograde Cholangiopancreatography and the Management of Common Bile Duct Stones

Jeffrey L. Ponsky

Endoscopic cannulation of the ampulla of Vater was first suggested by McCune in 1968.[1] Subsequent advances in technology and technique made the procedure commonplace and indispensable in the diagnosis and therapy of biliary and pancreatic disease. Perhaps most dramatic has been the impact of endoscopic retrograde cholangiopancreatography (ERCP) on the approach to the management of choledocholithiasis. Two decades ago, the suspicion of biliary ductal stones was clearly an indication for operative intervention to prevent sepsis, cirrhosis, and pancreatitis. Although surgical clearance of the common duct remains a "gold standard," endoscopic evacuation of ductal stones is most often the preferred treatment.[2]

INDICATIONS

The primary indication for ERCP with sphincterotomy is retained or recurrent common bile duct stones after cholecystectomy. Although not all patients with this problem are suited for endoscopic therapy, most can be completely relieved of their stones and spared laparotomy.[3] Acute pancreatitis has often been cited as a contraindication to ERCP, but if the suspected cause is an impacted gallstone in the distal bile duct, endoscopic sphincterotomy and relief of obstruction may be effective therapy.[4,5] Cholangitis presenting with fever, chills, and jaundice can be rapidly assessed by ultrasound and ERCP. The source of sepsis, the obstructed bile duct, can be cleared with sphincterotomy and stone extraction.

ERCP has been used to evaluate patients in whom stones are suspected before laparoscopic cholecystectomy.[6] Findings suggesting ductal calculi include jaundice, elevated results of liver function tests, associated pancreatitis, and evidence of ductal dilation on ultrasound examination. The actual predictive value of these examinations is not high, and a significant number of the subsequent endoscopic cholangiograms obtained are negative. However, when stones are identified, they can usually be removed endoscopically, allowing the surgeon to perform laparoscopic cholecystectomy without the necessity of clearing the common duct.

Much discussion centers on the merits of treating stones identified by cholangiography at the time of laparoscopic cholecystectomy by postoperative endoscopic sphincterotomy.[7] Although the success rate of stone removal is high (>90%), the attendant complication rate (10%) cannot be ignored. Developments in laparoscopic management of common duct stones will considerably enhance the surgeon's ability to deal with unsuspected stones identified at the time of operation.[8]

185

PATIENT EVALUATION AND PREPARATION

If the diagnosis of choledocholithiasis is entertained, initial evaluation of the patient should include a thorough history and physical examination. Conditions producing similar manifestations, such as hepatitis, drug-induced jaundice, and toxin exposure, should be excluded. Laboratory examinations must include an assessment of liver function and basic hematologic parameters. If severe liver injury is suspected, clotting abnormalities should be sought.

Radiologic imaging studies are useful in evaluating the bile ducts before endoscopic intervention. Most useful is a sonogram of the liver, biliary tree, and pancreas. Ultrasound can provide information about the caliber of intrahepatic and extrahepatic bile ducts, cholecystolithiasis and cholecystitis, and pancreatic head pathology. This examination should precede endoscopic intervention. Radionuclide imaging of the biliary system can provide information about the patency of the cystic and common duct but offers little about bile duct anatomy. Computed tomography is less useful than ultrasound in assessing the anatomy of the common bile duct, but it may offer an advantage in examining the pancreas.

The patient should fast for 8 hours before ERCP. Intravenous access is mandatory for administration of medications and fluid, and antibiotics should be administered before the procedure in jaundiced patients or those with suspected ductal obstruction. A careful discussion of the potential risks and benefits of the intervention with the patient and family should be part of the preoperative routine. Intravenous sedation is administered, usually with topical anesthesia applied to the posterior pharynx. Additional medications include atropine and glucagon to inhibit motility and enhance relaxation of the ampullary sphincter.

TECHNIQUE

Every therapeutic ERCP should be immediately preceded by a careful diagnostic examination. A side-viewing duodenoscope is used for ERCP. After passing the instrument into the second portion of the duodenum, the endoscopist should shorten the loop of scope in the stomach so that the instrument comes to lie along the lesser gastric curvature and is en face with the ampulla of Vater (Fig. 16–1).[9] A standard ERCP cannula can be used to cannulate the ampulla and obtain the diagnostic confir-

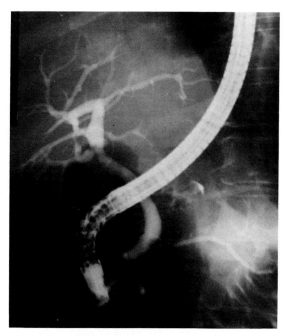

Figure 16–1. The duodenoscope should be withdrawn so that it comes to lie along the lesser curvature of the stomach. This "short-scope" position offers the most control for cannulation of the ampulla.

mation of choledocholithiasis (Fig. 16–2). The diagnostic cannula is then removed and replaced with a sphincterotome, a cannula with an electric wire for cutting (Fig. 16–3). If the diagnosis is likely, it is useful to use a cannula through which a guidewire may be passed after selective cannulation of the duct is achieved. This allows the endoscopist to maintain access to the duct while the diagnostic cannula is removed and replaced with a therapeutic one. A double-channel sphincterotome is required for the "over the wire" replacement (Fig. 16–4). Some endoscopists prefer to perform the initial ERCP with the double-channel sphincterotome. It allows fine tip maneuvers that can facilitate a difficult cannulation, and injection is easily carried out through the second channel. If stones are found, the sphincterotome is in a good position for therapy without the need for a catheter exchange.

After the endoscopic cholangiogram is obtained, a judgment must be made about whether endoscopic sphincterotomy and stone extraction provides the most appropriate therapy. Although most stones can be removed endoscopically, some ducts are best managed by surgical clearance and biliary-enteric drainage. If endoscopic therapy seems the best choice, the therapeutic dimension of the procedure is commenced.

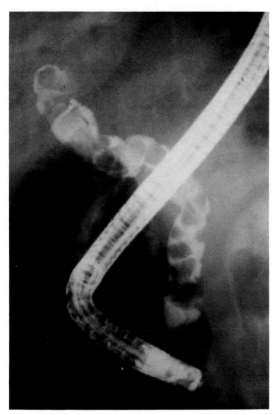

Figure 16–2. Diagnostic endoscopic retrograde cholangio-pancreatography confirms the diagnosis of choledocholithiasis.

The endoscopist must ascertain that the sphincterotome is correctly positioned within the common bile duct. If direct cannulation cannot be achieved, alternative methods of entry are available, such as precut papillotomy, in which the cutting wire is positioned where the ductal orifice is expected to be and attempts are made to cut into the lumen of the duct. This technique is associated with a greater risk of complications and should only be attempted by very experienced endoscopists and after all other methods are exhausted.[10]

In the usual case, after selective cannulation is achieved, blended cutting and coagulation current are applied in short bursts. The cutting wire is positioned in the duct only so far as the endoscopist is willing to cut. A white line of desiccation should be seen in the path of intended incision just before tissue separation. The incision is made at about the 12 o'clock position on the papilla. An incision farther to the right of this point increases the risks of perforation and pancreatitis. The incision should be made progressively, in short bursts, and carried no farther than the visible intramural

portion of the common bile duct. Division more cephalad risks hemorrhage and perforation. The eventual size of the sphincterotomy must be predicated on the dimensions of the stones to be removed and on the length of available intramural bile duct.

Many stones spontaneously pass after sphincteric division. In the past, it was the practice of some endoscopists to wait for several days after sphincterotomy and repeat the examination to see if the duct was clear. If stones remained, attempts were made to extract them. Most practitioners now prefer to attack stones immediately after the sphincterotomy. The sphincterotome is removed and replaced with a biliary basket or balloon catheter (Fig. 16–5). Small stones frequently pass with irrigation of the duct, and larger ones require capture in a basket or removal by traction behind a balloon. Multiple passes of these tools are occasionally required to clear the duct.

If stones are too large to be removed through the sphincterotomy incision, several techniques may be applied to extract them. Most useful is the mechanical lithotriptor (Fig. 16–6). If a stone is encircled with a basket but cannot be retrieved or crushed, it may be necessary to remove the handle from the basket wire and then the endoscope before beginning the lithotripsy process. A stout metal sheath is then passed over the basket and cranked tight under fluoroscopic guidance until the sheath comes in contact with the stone. Further tension is applied to the crank until the stone is crushed (or the basket breaks). If mechanical lithotripsy is required, a lithotriptor designed for passage through the endoscope channel can be employed. In such cases, the basket with overlying sheath is initially used to surround the stone.

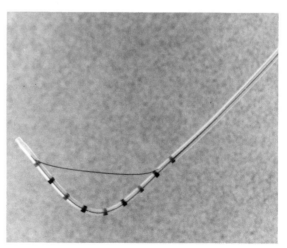

Figure 16–3. A single-channel sphincterotome with a cutting wire.

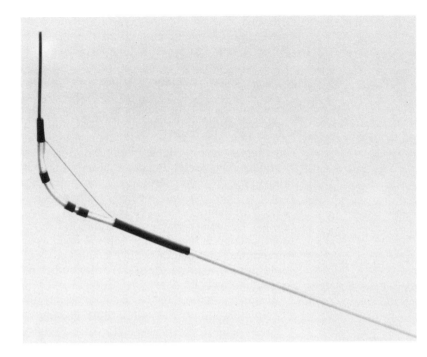

Figure 16–4. A double-channel sphincterotome allows "over-a-wire" placement and is useful in achieving difficult cannulations because its tip may be manipulated to seek an orifice and a wire can be passed through it.

Figure 16–5. A balloon catheter can be passed up the duct and inflated proximal to a stone. It is then pulled downward to deliver the stone through the sphincterotomy.

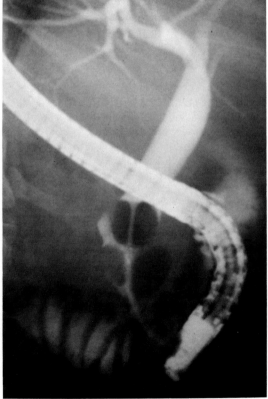

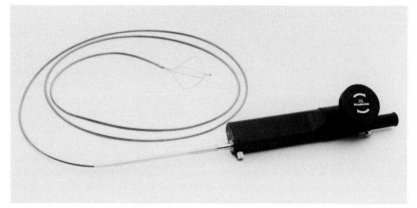

Figure 16-6. A mechanical lithotriptor can be used to surround large or difficult stones and crush them.

After the stone is captured under radiographic control, the crank is tightened, and the stone is crushed. Fragments may be removed with irrigation, basket, or balloon. Mechanical lithotripsy is safe and effective and has a relatively low cost. It can be used to remove most large stones. There are some stones that may be large or difficult to capture, and these may require more sophisticated and costly methods of extraction.

Smaller-caliber fiberscopes permit peroral cholangioscopy.[11] These instruments are delivered into the biliary tree by means of a mother–daughter scope combination (Fig. 16–7). The technique usually requires the performance of a generous sphincterotomy, although new, smaller instrumentation is being developed that may reduce the size of the required ampullary opening. After it is in the bile duct, the "baby" scope can be maneuvered proximally into the biliary tree. The right and left hepatic ducts and some of their branches are often accessible. Stones can be treated with pulse-dye laser lithotripsy or with electrohydraulic fragmentation. These modalities require direct visualization for best results, and the fibers that deliver the energy are delivered through the channel of the baby scope. This method is expensive and somewhat cumbersome.

Laser lithotripsy usually employs the pulse-dye laser with a wavelength of 504 nm. This energy form delivered directly to the stone surface has been effective in fragmenting stones.[12] Urologists use laser lithotripsy to fragment ureteral stones. Bile duct injury is minimal if aberrant direction of the laser light occurs. Another means of delivering the laser energy to the stone is through the use of special stone baskets that possess a central channel through which the laser fiber is passed after the stone is entrapped. Fluoroscopic observation guides the lithotripsy as it proceeds. These lasers are costly, and some lack portability, which limits their usefulness.

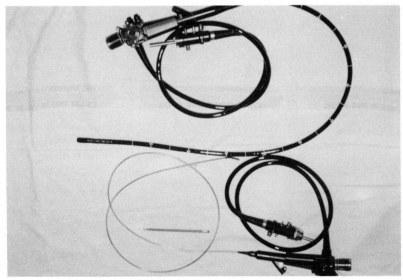

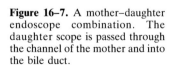

Figure 16-7. A mother–daughter endoscope combination. The daughter scope is passed through the channel of the mother and into the bile duct.

Their cost may be rationalized by sharing among specialties.

Electrohydraulic lithotriptors destroy stones by producing an electric spark in the liquid medium at the stone's surface. The fiber and the stone must be in direct contact for effective fragmentation to occur. The fiber can be brought into contact with the stone by means of a baby scope, or special baskets and balloons with central channels may be employed. This form of energy can produce serious harm to the bile duct wall if it is aberrantly directed. Perforation of the bile duct can occur. Newer generations of these instruments promise lower energy settings and greater safety.

MANAGEMENT OF REFRACTORY STONES

Most common bile duct stones can be removed without difficulty by ERCP with endoscopic sphincterotomy. A small percentage tax the endoscopist and resist extraction. The reasons for the resistance include difficult ampullary anatomy, as may occur if the ampulla resides within a duodenal diverticulum, or inability to successfully cannulate the bile duct. In such instances, consideration should be given to surgical exploration of the duct. At other times, the location of the stone (Fig. 16–8) or the ductal configuration itself may be troublesome (Fig. 16–9). Tortuous bile ducts may result from scarring after biliary surgery. There may be traction on the bile duct at the site of a former T-tube or drain insertion, resulting in sharp angulation of the duct. This may cause difficulty when attempts are made to extract stones in the proximal ducts. If no urgency exists, months may be allowed to elapse before further manipulation, and this may result in a straightening of the duct. An alternative approach for difficult ducts is a combined percutaneous transhepatic-endoscopic approach.

If attempts to access the duct endoscopically are frustrated by tortuosity of the duct or difficult anatomy, the radiologist can help by transhepatic puncture of the biliary tree. A long guidewire can be passed through the ductal system into the duodenum. The wire can be grasped with a snare through the endoscope, and a sphincterotome and extraction tools can be used over the wire until the duct is cleared.

Another frustrating problem is that of stones lying proximal to a ductal stricture. The stricture may be the result of surgical injury or sclerosing cholangitis. After sphincterotomy, balloon catheters can be used to dilate the stricture before attempts at stone extraction. For fragments too large for extraction after sphincterotomy, it is important to ensure ductal drainage until the biliary tree is totally cleared by inserting a stent or nasobiliary drain. Extracorporeal shock wave lithotripsy (ESWL) in selected cases can reduce the size of bile duct stones and allow the fragments to pass through a sphincterotomy.

In some elderly and extremely infirm patients, removal of multiple large stones may be difficult or otherwise require surgical intervention. In these cases, despite the endoscopist's inability to clear the duct of stones, a large stent can maintain patency of the biliary tree and prevent cholangitis. Although not solving the problem

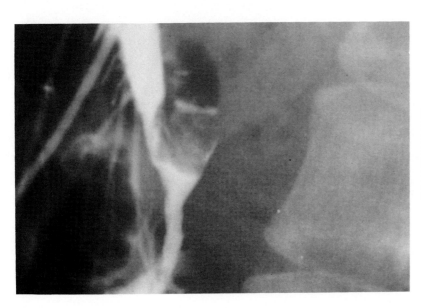

Figure 16–8. A large stone is impacted in a low-lying cystic duct junction, and it is difficult to extract. Extracorporeal shock wave lithotripsy, laser lithotripsy, or electrohydraulic lithotripsy may be useful in fragmenting these stones.

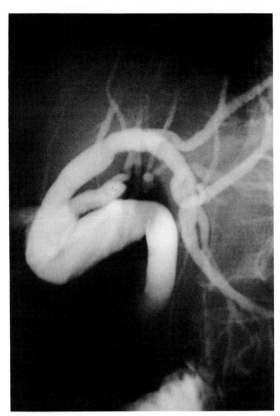

Figure 16–9. A tortuous common bile duct may be the result of postsurgical scarring, frequently after a T-tube has been in place. This may render stone extraction by endoscopic retrograde cholangiopancreatography difficult or impossible.

of biliary lithiasis, the stent can provide significant palliation of the cholangitis. Stent changes at intervals of 3 to 6 months are necessary to avert recurrent cholangitis secondary to stent occlusion.

CONCLUSION

Endoscopic therapy has become a sophisticated and reliable approach to the management of choledocholithiasis. Diagnostic ERCP can confirm the clinical suspicion of bile duct stones, and therapy can be immediately implemented by means of endoscopic sphincterotomy and stone extraction. An ever-increasing array of therapeutic tools have permitted the extraction of all but the most refractory stones. If the stones cannot be removed, biliary decompression can usually be accomplished. These methods do not supplant traditional approaches to biliary therapy, but they broaden the options of the hepatobiliary surgeon (see Chap. 17).

References

1. McCune WS, Shorb PE, Moscovitz H. Endoscopic cannulation of the ampulla of Vater: a preliminary report. Ann Surg 167:752, 1968.
2. Ponsky JL. Endoscopic sphincterotomy for recurrent or persistent biliary calculi. In: Fry DE, ed. Reoperative surgery of the abdomen. New York: Marcel Decker, 1986.
3. Venu RP, Geenen JE. Overview of endoscopic sphincterotomy for common bile duct stone. In: Kozarek RA, ed. Endoscopic approach to biliary stones. Gastointest Endosc Clin North Am, 1:1, 1991.
4. Shaffer RD. Indications and contraindications for the use of endoscopic retrograde cholangiopancreatography. In: Stewart ET, Vennes JA, Geenen JE, eds. Atlas of endoscopic retrograde cholangiopancreatography. St. Louis: CV Mosby, 1977.
5. Neoptolemos JP, London N, Slater ND, et al. A prospective study of ERCP and endoscopic sphincterotomy in the diagnosis and treatment of gallstone acute pancreatitis. A rational and safe approach to management. Arch Surg 121:6, 1986.
6. Phillips EH, Carroll BJ. New techniques for the treatment of common bile duct calculi encountered during laparoscopic cholecystectomy. In: Berci G, ed. Problems in general surgery. Laparosc Surg 8:3, 1991.
7. Reddick EJ, Olsen D, Alexander W, et al. Laparoscopic laser cholecystectomy and choledocholithiasis. Surg Endosc 4:3, 1990.
8. Petelin JB. Laparoscopic approach to common duct pathology. Surg Laparosc Endosc 1:1, 1991.
9. Ponsky JL. Endoscopic sphincterotomy. In: Atlas of surgical endoscopy. Chicago: Mosby Year Book, 1991.
10. Cotton PB. Precut papillotomy—a risky technique for experts only. [Editorial] Gastrointest Endosc 35:6, 1989.
11. Ponsky JL, Scheeres DE, Simon I. Endoscopic retrograde cholangioscopy: an adjunct to endoscopic exploration of the common bile duct. Am Surg 56:235–237, 1990.
12. Ponchon T, Gagnon P, Valette PJ, et al. Pulsed-dye laser lithotripsy of bile duct stones. Gastroenterology 100:6, 1991.

17

Endoscopic Techniques of Sphincterotomy

Ali Ghazi and Harry S. Himal

HISTORY

The first successful cannulation of the papilla of Vater through a flexible endoscope was reported in 1968 by McCune and associates.[1] They used an end-viewing endoscope and successfully visualized the pancreatic duct. This achievement led to the development of a side-viewing endoscope with the ability to cannulate selectively either the pancreatic duct or the common bile duct. In 1970, Oi[2] was the first to report the visualization of the common bile duct. Since then, many groups have reported on large series of patients undergoing endoscopic retrograde cholangiopancreatography (ERCP).[3, 4]

In 1974, endoscopic papillotomy for common bile duct stones was first reported by Classen and Demling in Germany[5] and by Kawai and associates in Japan.[6] The terms endoscopic papillotomy and endoscopic sphincterotomy have been used synonymously, but most authors today prefer the term endoscopic sphincterotomy, because it denotes the true nature of the procedure. ERCP and endoscopic sphincterotomy are routinely carried out for the diagnosis and treatment of pancreatic and biliary diseases in most major institutions today.

This chapter outlines the indications, technique, and necessary equipment for endoscopic sphincterotomy. Case histories are also presented to demonstrate the use of these techniques in the care and management of patients with biliary or pancreatic diseases.

INDICATIONS

The indications for endoscopic sphincterotomy can be divided into two main categories:

I. Endoscopic Sphincterotomy for Benign Diseases of the Biliary and Pancreatic Ducts
   A. Common bile duct stones
   B. Ascending cholangitis
   C. Sphincter of Oddi dysfunction
   D. Benign stricture of either the papilla of Vater or the distal common bile duct
   E. Benign stricture of the pancreatic duct
   F. Pancreatic duct stones
II. Endoscopic Sphincterotomy for Malignant Diseases of the Pancreas and Bile Ducts, With the Insertion of Large Endobiliary Stents
   A. Carcinoma of the pancreas, invading and obstructing the common bile duct
   B. Carcinoma of the common bile duct
   C. Carcinoma of the ampulla of Vater
   D. Klatskin tumor
   E. Carcinoma of the gallbladder, invading and obstructing the common bile duct
   F. Metastatic carcinoma at the junction of the hepatic ducts, causing obstructive jaundice

Some of these conditions will now be discussed.

Common Bile Duct Stones

The most common indication for endoscopic sphincterotomy is choledocholithiasis, especially in patients who have had previous cholecystectomy. The success rate for clearance of the common bile duct with endoscopic sphincterotomy and stone extraction exceeds 90%, and symptoms are improved in close to 95% of patients.

The procedure is more difficult to perform in patients with multiple large stones or large duodenal diverticula, or in those who had a Billroth II gastrectomy. The size and number of stones may create technical problems for the endoscopist. The average stone measures 10 to 12 mm in diameter and is usually removed by performing an adequate papillotomy and extracting the stone with the appropriate basket or balloon. However, multiple large stones require a longer papillotomy, which increases the risk of bleeding or perforation. In addition, large stones may require two or three endoscopic sessions to completely clear the common bile duct.

Stones greater than 20 mm are handled by mechanical lithotripsy, with removal of smaller fragments by balloon extraction followed by saline irrigation of the bile duct.

Recently, endoscopic sphincterotomy has been proposed for patients with common bile duct stones and cholelithiasis.[7-10] Most studies include older patients with significant cardiopulmonary disease. Follow-up studies in these patients show that they die of nonbiliary diseases. Younger patients would require cholecystectomy within a short time.[11]

Case History

A 73-year-old man was admitted to the hospital for chronic cholecystitis, cholelithiasis, and choledocholithiasis. Initially, he was admitted to another hospital with urinary retention and elevated levels of alkaline phosphatase. The patient underwent a workup consisting of a sonogram and computed tomography (CT) of the abdomen, which revealed common bile duct stones. On June 15, the patient underwent an ERCP, which demonstrated multiple common bile duct stones (Fig. 17–1). An endoscopic papillotomy was performed, and three stones were extracted. Another large stone remained in the common bile duct. A No. 10 French double-pigtail stent was inserted in the common bile duct to prevent common bile duct obstruction (Fig. 17–2). On June 24, a repeat ERCP revealed the persistent large common bile duct stone. This stone was grasped and fragmented using a basket and mechanical lithotripsy. The residual fragments were removed with an endoscopic balloon. The completion cholangiogram showed that the common bile duct was cleared of all stones (Fig. 17–3). The patient was discharged the following day and has remained asymptomatic.

After successful clearance of the common bile duct stones, the gallbladder can be handled by one of the following methods:

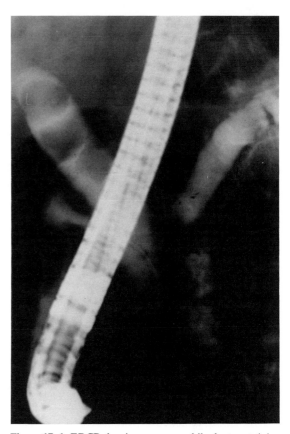

Figure 17–1. ERCP showing a common bile duct containing multiple large calculi.

1. The gallbladder could be removed by laparoscopy with the patient under general anesthesia.

2. In very elderly patients, no further therapy is necessary.[11]

3. If the gallbladder causes symptoms, and the patient cannot tolerate general anesthesia, cholecystostomy and stone extraction are possible under local anesthesia.

Sphincterotomy is not always necessary for stone extraction. Small stones can be removed with endobiliary techniques through an intact papilla either by balloon dilation[12] or through medication to relax the smooth muscle of the sphincter.[13]

Cholangitis

Acute cholangitis occurs in about 5% to 10% of patients with common bile duct stones and is associated with a mortality rate of greater than 10%.[14, 15] At present, there are three methods to treat acute cholangitis if the patient does not

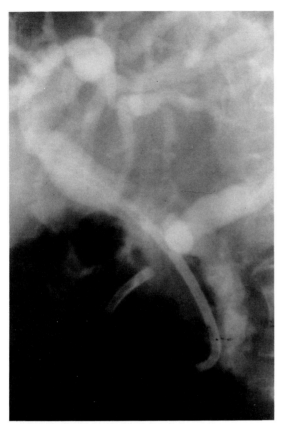

Figure 17–2. Same patient as in Figure 17–1 after removal of three smaller stones. A double-pigtail stent is inserted into the common bile duct to prevent obstruction by the remaining large calculus.

respond to conservative treatment: emergency surgery, percutaneous transhepatic drainage of the biliary tree, and endoscopic sphincterotomy.

For many years, emergency surgery was carried out in those patients who did not respond to conservative therapy. However, surgery is associated with a greater than 10% operative mortality rate.[14–16] Percutaneous transhepatic drainage of the biliary system is associated with significant morbidity and mortality.[17] Furthermore, a second procedure must be performed to remove the common bile duct stones and prevent recurrent cholangitis.

Endoscopic sphincterotomy has an important role in the treatment of acute cholangitis. Urgent endoscopic sphincterotomy and stone extraction will resolve the septic process and cure the problem.[16] Leese and colleagues[18] compared endoscopic sphincterotomy with surgery for acute cholangitis and concluded that endoscopic sphincterotomy is the procedure of choice. However, early surgery still has a role if there is no significant improvement.[19]

Sphincter of Oddi Dysfunction

Dysfunction of the sphincter of Oddi is a poorly understood condition in which there is abnormal anatomic and functional stenosis of the sphincter. Patients with this condition continue to have biliary-type pain even after cholecystectomy. The diagnosis rests on a combination of clinical symptoms, laboratory data, and special tests. The important features are:

- Biliary-type upper abdominal pain
- Elevated liver function tests, specifically alkaline phosphatase levels
- Dilation of the biliary tree seen either by sonography or ERCP
- Abnormal common bile duct emptying seen by ERCP or technetium-HIDA scanning
- Abnormal morphine-neostigmine provocation test
- Manometric pressure studies of the sphincter of Oddi that may demonstrate high phasic pressure waves with a mean amplitude of 130 mm Hg above baseline values

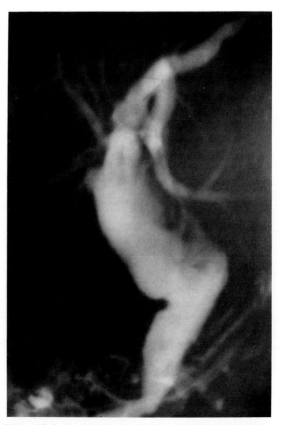

Figure 17–3. Same patient as in Figure 17–2 after lithotripsy of the large remaining stone. A dilated common bile duct without a filling defect is present.

Various groups have defined and treated patients with sphincter of Oddi dysfunction. Geenen[20] reported on a group of 10 patients with sphincter of Oddi dysfunction. Nine of the 10 patients had elevated baseline sphincter of Oddi pressure, and all underwent either endoscopic or surgical sphincterotomy. Follow-up studies demonstrated that all patients were relieved of their pain and had normal liver function studies. Farup and Tjora[21] reported on 5 patients with sphincter of Oddi dysfunction and demonstrated that all patients had satisfactory results after endoscopic sphincterotomy. However, one must exercise caution with this syndrome, and further detailed studies should be carried out before endoscopic sphincterotomy is recommended as the treatment of choice for patients suspected of having sphincter of Oddi dysfunction.

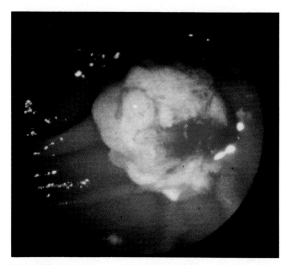

Figure 17–4. A 2.5-cm multinodular carcinoma of the papilla of Vater.

Tumors of the Ampulla of Vater

Benign and malignant tumors of the ampulla of Vater may cause distal common bile duct obstruction. In older patients and in those individuals not medically suitable for extensive surgery, endoscopic sphincterotomy may relieve the obstruction and could be considered an appropriate method of treatment.[22]

Case History

A 79-year-old woman was first seen for painless obstructive jaundice. She had no fever or chills. Her appetite was poor but she denied weight loss. Physical examination revealed mild jaundice and no other abnormal findings. Laboratory studies revealed the following values: white blood cell count, 12,000 mm³; hemoglobin, 12.1 g/dL; hematocrit, 33%; total bilirubin, 4 mg/dL; direct bilirubin, 1.9 mg/dL; alkaline phosphatase, 1300 IU/L; SMA-6 within normal limits. A CT scan of the abdomen showed markedly dilated intrahepatic and dilated common bile ducts, with a distended gallbladder, and a probable 2-cm mass present at the distal portion of the common bile duct. An ERCP was performed, revealing a 2 × 2.5 cm tumor of the papilla of Vater, with a normal pancreatic duct, and a very dilated common bile duct (Fig. 17–4). Biopsy of this tumor revealed a well-differentiated infiltrating adenocarcinoma (Fig. 17–5).

An endoscopic papillotomy was done and a No. 10 French biliary stent was placed (Fig. 17–6). The patient's jaundice resolved gradually,

and she suffered no complications from this procedure. She was discharged home 2 days later and has been followed on an ambulatory basis for more than 2 years. She has undergone two to three stent changes per year and is free of jaundice or any other symptoms.

Malignant Obstruction of the Common Bile Duct

The relief of jaundice should be one of the goals in patients with malignant obstruction of the common bile duct. Unresectable carcinoma of the pancreas, cholangiocarcinoma, or obstruction secondary to metastasis to the confluence of hepatic ducts can be managed by endoscopic sphincterotomy and placement of endobiliary stents.[23, 24] Larger stents (No. 10 French or larger) need less frequent replacement for obstruction but do require an endoscopic sphincterotomy.

Case History

A 72-year-old man was admitted to the hospital with a chief complaint of painless jaundice of 3 weeks' duration, with recent onset of mild epigastric discomfort. Physical examination revealed overt jaundice. He was afebrile with stable vital signs. Abdominal examination revealed no mass, no ascites, and normal bowel sounds. Laboratory studies revealed the following: leukocytosis (white blood cell count, 11,500 mm³); hyponatremia (129 mEq/L); alanine ami-

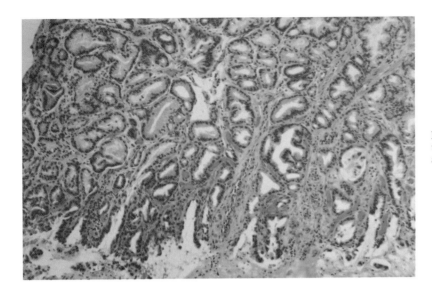

Figure 17–5. Biopsy of the mass of the papilla of Vater demonstrated a well-differentiated carcinoma.

notransferase levels, 314 IU/L; aspartate aminotransferase levels, 367 IU/L; alkaline phosphatase levels, 1085 IU/L; total bilirubin levels, 42.5 mg/dL; direct bilirubin levels, 29 mg/dL;

amylase levels, 103 IU/L. A sonogram and CT scan of the abdomen revealed a mass in the head of the pancreas. An ERCP was performed, revealing a stricture of the main pancreatic duct resulting from a neoplastic mass in the head of the pancreas, which invaded and obstructed the common bile duct (Fig. 17–7). An endoscopic papillotomy was done without complication and a No. 10 French, 8-cm straight biliary stent was inserted over a guidewire through the stricture in the common hepatic duct (Fig. 17–8). This established adequate bile drainage.

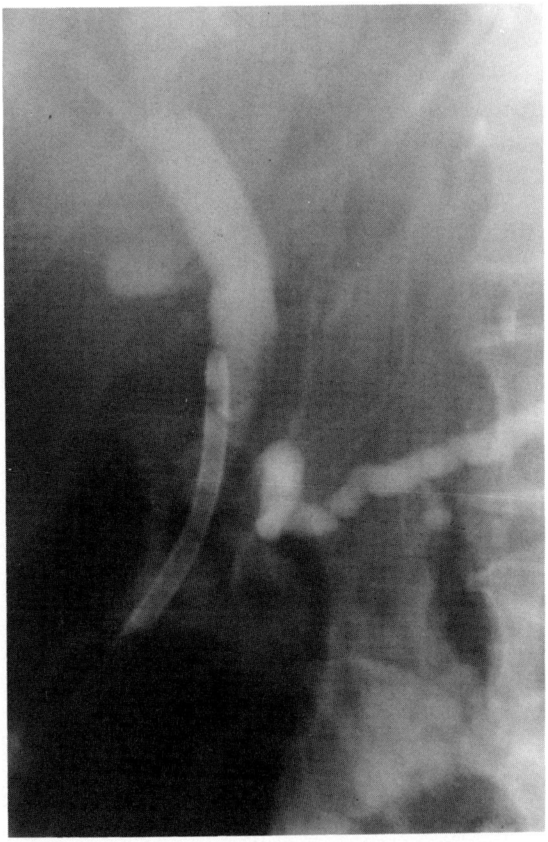

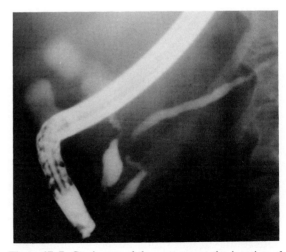

Figure 17–7. Carcinoma of the pancreas at the junction of the head and body of the pancreas invading and obstructing the common bile duct. Note the normal caliber of the common bile duct below the stricture in contrast to the dilation seen above the stricture.

Figure 17–6. After papillotomy, a straight No. 10 French biliary stent is inserted into the common bile duct.

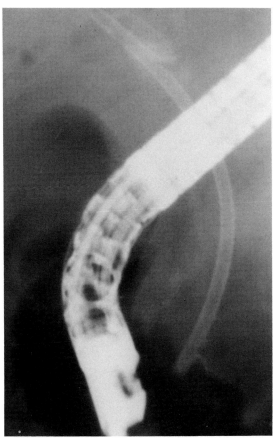

Figure 17–8. Same patient as in Figure 17–7 with a straight biliary stent in the common bile duct, bypassing the obstruction.

"Sump" Syndrome

Patients with choledochoenterostomy may harbor stones, sludge, or ingested debris, which occasionally accumulates in the common bile duct distal to the choledochoenterostomy. This can lead to cholangitis, pancreatitis, or malabsorption (Sump syndrome). Endoscopic sphincterotomy is curative in most cases.[25, 26] One should be very careful in making such a diagnosis because sometimes the presence of air can be misinterpreted as sludge or a stone. In addition, the presence of food debris may be a temporary phenomenon and may pass if the opening of the choledochoenterostomy is of adequate size.

Foreign Bodies

Foreign bodies in the common bile duct are rare. There are scattered reports of parasites in the bile duct. Endoscopic sphincterotomy and basket extraction have been successful in relieving the resulting cholangitis or pancreatitis.[27, 28]

CONTRAINDICATIONS

There are a few contraindications to endoscopic sphincterotomy, including abnormal clotting and bleeding tendencies that cannot be corrected. Recent myocardial infarction and severe chronic obstructive pulmonary disease are relative contraindications. Conversely, acute pancreatitis or cholangitis due to common bile duct stones may be an indication for endoscopic removal of the stone or insertion of a biliary stent if the patient is not improving with conservative management. Acute pancreatitis is also a relative contraindication unless it is due to common bile duct stones. It is usually better to wait and see if the pancreatitis resolves and the patient improves. However, without improvement, one may treat this situation through insertion of a biliary stent, or if the patient can tolerate a longer procedure, endoscopic sphincterotomy and extraction of the stone.

INSTRUMENTATION

Duodenoscopes

To perform ERCP and endoscopic sphincterotomy, a side-viewing duodenoscope is a necessity. Proper visualization of the papilla of Vater is not possible with a panendoscope. Most duodenoscopes can achieve the task of cannulation of the papilla, but to perform adequate instrumentation of the common bile duct for extraction of stones either with a balloon or basket, one may need instruments with a larger working (biopsy) channel—either a 3.8-mm channel or a 4.2-mm working channel. Most companies produce duodenoscopes with 2.8-mm and larger working channels. We highly recommend that every endoscopy suite own and maintain more than one working duodenoscope. If budget restraints do not allow the purchase of two or three duodenoscopes, we suggest the following duodenoscope, which is now available. This instrument has an 11.3-mm diameter distally and a large 3.8-mm channel, which allows insertion of a stent as large as a No. 10 French. The depth of view is from 5 to 100 mm. Tip deflection is 130° up and down with 120° right to left. Because of its narrow body and flexibility, this scope is tolerated more easily by the patient, and most problems can be handled with this duodenoscope. On the other hand, an en-

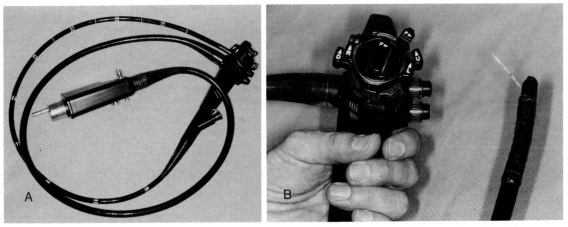

Figure 17–9. (A) A video duodenoscope. **(B)** Close-up view of the video duodenoscope. The control unit is similar to that in fiberoptic instruments.

doscopist who prefers larger diameter stents would prefer a scope with a 4.2-mm channel.

The video duodenoscope is an advance in technology and has good to excellent resolution. It is built with a high-resolution monochrome change-couple device with the traditional ability of the fiberoptic scopes, but it provides lifelike images (Fig. 17–9). In teaching institutions, it

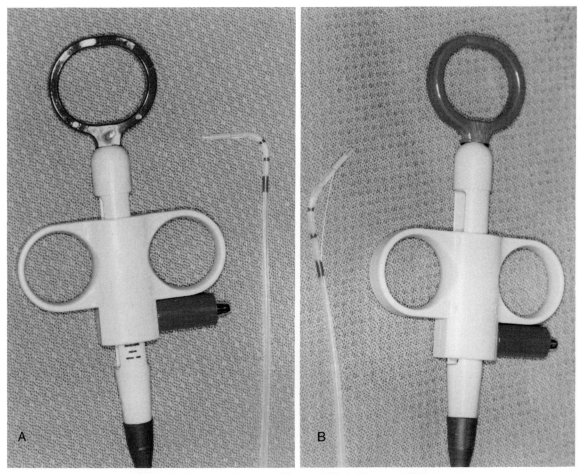

Figure 17–10. (A) A 20-mm papillotome. **(B)** A 30-mm papillotome.

provides a tool for education by allowing more than one viewer to observe the procedure. It also allows a nurse assistant and all other members of the team to view and actively participate in the instrumentation and progress of the procedure. These videoscopes also possess the ability to store information and photographs that may help the endoscopist to recall information on a given patient and compare the healing progress of any given lesion. There is still a need for better instruments, and there will be future duodenoscopes with additional qualities to make cannulation and instrumentation easier.

Sphincterotomes

There are numerous sphincterotomes available from different manufacturers. Most of the sphincterotomes are of the "pull-type," which was originally designed by Demling and Classen.[5] The main difference is in the length of exposed wire, which varies from 20 to 30 mm (Fig. 17–10). We use the shorter 20-mm sphincterotome when the common bile duct is 10 mm or narrower and a 30-mm sphincterotome when the duct is 15 mm or wider. Any measurement in between is based on the individual case.

A new sphincterotome, the cannulotome (Fig. 17–11), has several advantageous qualities that make sphincterotomy less complicated. The catheter size is only No. 6 French, the exposed wire is 25 mm and, most important, the contrast medium does not leak from the proximal point of the exposed wire. Therefore, this instrument could serve as a cannula for ERCP and endoscopic papillotomy. Some situations require special papillotomes. When cannulation is difficult and the catheter is finally in the common bile duct, it is easier to insert a long wire deep into the common bile duct prior to removing the cannula. An over-the-wire papillotome can then be inserted over this long wire, which makes access to the common bile duct easier. The long wire is then removed, and papillotomy is performed by bringing the handle of the papillotome to the cutting position. Another special papillotome is the Billroth II sphincterotome or sigmoid type of sphincterotome. Regular papillotomes are not appropriate for use in patients who have had a Billroth II gastrectomy. Since the instrument approaches the papilla from below, the usual papillotomes cannot and should not be used for sphincterotomy. Instead, one uses the sigmoid type of sphincterotome, which puts the incision into the papilla in a different plane than the usual 11 o'clock position (Fig. 17–12).

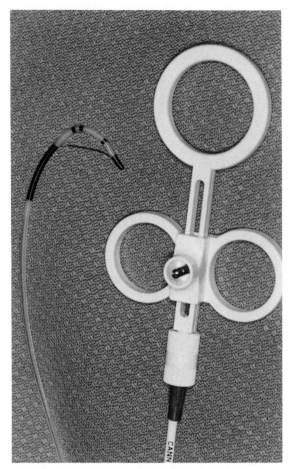

Figure 17–11. A cannulotome in cutting position.

The distal end of the papillotome, called the nose, requires some discussion. We believe the nose of the papillotome should not be very long, since the purpose of the tip of the papillotome is to prevent the exposed wire of the papillotome from touching the inside of the wall of the common bile duct while the sphincterotome is in the cutting position. If this end is too short, the wire may be in contact with the wall of the common bile duct and cause an accidental burn or perforation, or both. If the tip is too long, it will prevent it from bending, thus making a good contact impossible. We believe a 4 to 5-mm nose is adequate; longer tips may make the insertion of the papillotome into the duct much harder, whereas a short nose (less than 2 mm) may lead to perforation.

Finally, the electrosurgical unit should be one that transmits a high radiofrequency current. Most endoscopists prefer a blend mode (cutting with a mild coagulation effect). One must be familiar with the different settings and operation of the electrosurgical unit used. In our institu-

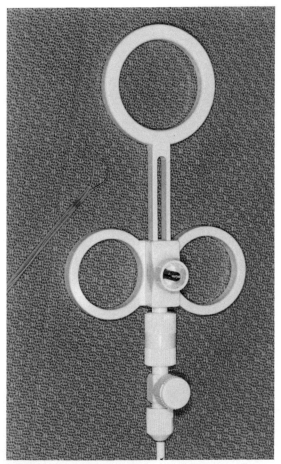

Figure 17–12. A sphincterotome for a patient who has had a Billroth II gastrectomy. Note the difference between this and a regular papillotome. This is also called a sigmoid papillotome and is used only for Billroth II gastrectomy patients.

tion, we use the same electrosurgical units (Valleylab SSE2L, Boulder, CO) for sphincterotomy that we use for polypectomy. For the latter procedure, we choose a coagulation current of 3 to 3.5, but for sphincterotomy we choose a cutting current of 4.5 to 5 in blend mode. Before the start of any planned endoscopic sphincterotomy, all necessary papillotomes and connections between electrosurgical units and papillotomes should be tested to make sure they are functioning properly and ready for use. Different manufacturers have different connecting wires from the electrosurgical units to the papillotome's handle. Both the endoscopist and the nurse assistant must be familiar with all of the equipment and accessories. There is no time to find a proper wire or connector when a papillotome is in place. Nothing could be more troublesome or embarrassing than an aborted procedure because of missing parts or a malfunction of the instrument. Therefore, both the nurse assistant and the operator must check not only for safety but also for proper functioning of all instruments, including the electrosurgical unit, papillotomes, and duodenoscopes. The radiology equipment should be of the highest quality. The fluoroscopic resolution should enable one to see even the smallest catheters or wires without any difficulty. Having radiology equipment in the endoscopy suite is much preferred to borrowing space in the radiology department. In addition, a radiograph developer is an integral part of the equipment. In our institution, two rooms are equipped with radiology equipment and a third room is equipped with C-arm fluoroscopy.

TECHNIQUES OF ENDOSCOPIC SPHINCTEROTOMY

Patient Preparation

In preparation for ERCP and papillotomy, the patient is asked to fast for a minimum of 8 hours prior to the procedure. An intravenous infusion is started for hydration, sedation, and administration of antibiotics, which are given if there is biliary obstruction or common bile duct stones. Antibiotics are given 2 hours prior to the procedure and continued for two doses 8 and 16 hours after the procedure.

The patient's pharynx is sprayed or the patient is asked to gargle with a topical anesthetic (lidocaine, 2% to 4%). The patient is then placed on a radiology table in the prone decubitus position with the right side up. Fluoroscopy is performed to ensure that no contrast medium remains in the gastrointestinal tract from prior radiologic examination. A mouthguard is placed between the teeth, not only to keep the mouth open but also to prevent biting of the duodenoscope. The patient is now sedated with diazepam, 5 to 10 mg, and nalbuphine hydrochloride (Nubain), 10 mg, both given intravenously. Additional medication can be given until the patient is asleep and adequately relaxed. The duodenoscope is introduced into the oropharynx. The patient is asked to swallow while gentle pressure is exerted as the duodenoscope is passed into the esophagus. The scope is passed through the stomach and pylorus into the first and second portions of the duodenum. Visualization of the papilla occurs when the duodenoscope is in a loop position (Fig. 17–13). Glucagon, 1 mg intravenously, is now given to decrease duodenal peristalsis and possibly relax the sphincter of Oddi.

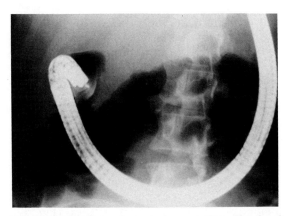

Figure 17–13. Duodenoscope in loop position. The tip of the instrument is in the duodenum and the loop is along the greater curvature of the stomach.

Cannulation in the loop position will allow visualization of one or the other duct. For selective cannulation, the scope should be brought into the straight position. This is done by turning the right-left knob forward and locking it, then torquing the scope clockwise with the right hand while the scope is pulled back. This should bring the scope into the straight position (Fig. 17–14). The papilla is now ready for cannulation, and the position is called the en face position.[10] This position makes selective cannulation easier and increases the chance of successfully cannulating either the common bile duct or the pancreatic duct in more than 90% of the cases. To cannulate the pancreatic duct, the endoscopist directs the catheter to the 1 o'clock position and approaches the papilla from a low position without significant elevation of the cannula elevator. To cannulate the common bile duct, the cannula should be directed to the 11 o'clock position, and while the cannula elevator is pushed upward, the orifice of the papilla is approached from the high position. Contrast medium should be injected only under fluoroscopic control, with gentle pressure. Three to 5 mL of diatrizoate meglumine and diatrizoate sodium (Hypaque) will fill the pancreatic duct, and up to 15 ml or more is needed to fill the common bile duct. The amount of contrast medium and the injection pressure must be kept low to decrease the incidence of pancreatitis and cholangitis, which can occur from ductal overdistention and excessive filling, especially in the presence of distal obstruction.

Endoscopy Team

The endoscopy team should consist of the endoscopist, an endoscopy nurse, and an en-

doscopist's assistant (who can be an endoscopy fellow, surgical resident, or a physician's assistant trained in endoscopic procedures). It cannot be adequately emphasized that the experience of the team has the greatest impact on the safe and successful outcome of this procedure. The presence of a radiologist is a valuable addition to the team; if this is not possible, a radiology technician is essential.

Technique of Endoscopic Papillotomy

After placing the patient in a semiprone position with the right side up and the left arm behind the patient, sedation is carried out with a combination of nalbuphine, diazepam, and midazolam HCl, as needed. The diathermy unit is checked and the proper setting is chosen. Our recommendation is that all diathermy units in any given hospital be the same, making recognition and operation easier and thus possibly preventing electrical accidents and injury to the patient. The current is in the blend mode and

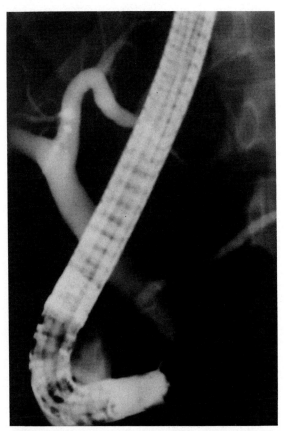

Figure 17–14. Duodenoscope in straight position. The papilla is cannulated in this position, and both the common bile duct and pancreatic duct are visualized.

is applied in short bursts. The papillotomy is done with the cutting current in the blend mode. The coagulation current may be used for hemostasis when minor bleeding is present.

In our practice, an end-viewing upper endoscope, preferably of pediatric size, is used to check the esophagus and stomach and to empty any remaining gastric contents or secretions. This should not take more than 1 or 2 minutes. At this point, the endoscopist chooses a therapeutic side-viewing scope with a 3.8- or 4.2-mm working channel if removal of a stone or insertion of a large biliary stent is planned. These scopes have larger diameters and make insertion more difficult, but the better resolution, size of the biopsy channel, and strength of the cannula elevator make the tradeoff worthwhile.

The introduction of the scope into the esophagus is somewhat blind, but it should be gentle and without any undue force. If there is any resistance to the insertion of the scope, it should be withdrawn and an upper endoscopy performed to rule out esophageal obstruction or the presence of a large Zenker's diverticulum. After all abnormalities are ruled out, the same (or smaller) diameter side-viewing scope is inserted and advanced into the stomach. Insertion through the pylorus is different from that using an end-viewing scope (see Chap 16). After reaching the second portion of the duodenum and straightening out the scope, the papilla is brought to an en face position.[10] Cannulation is performed with a regular cannula, documenting the presence of stones or any other pathologic condition of the common bile duct.

Once the ERCP is completed, the cannula is removed, and if there is a need for papillotomy, a proper papillotome is reintroduced through the biopsy channel and advanced into the common bile duct. Proper placement of the papillotome in the common bile duct should be permanently documented by fluoroscopy or, better, by a radiograph. The smaller bile duct requires a 20-mm papillotome; for the larger bile duct, a longer 30-mm papillotome would be more appropriate. If access to the common bile duct was difficult, the endoscopist should leave the cannula in place and insert a long wire through the cannula into the common bile duct and then remove the cannula. This will allow the use of the wire-guided papillotome and easier access for insertion of the papillotome into the common bile duct. Once the papillotome is in the common bile duct, the long wire is removed before the papillotomy is attempted. At this time, one must be absolutely certain that the patient is not in contact with any metal

and is properly grounded before application of cutting current is carried out.

To perform a sphincterotomy, one must withdraw the sphincterotome from the common bile duct until a small portion of the wire of the papillotome is visible in the duodenum. The gastrointestinal surgical assistant will pull the handle of the papillotome slowly to the cutting position. Care should be taken not to pull too much, causing acute angulation of the tip of the papillotome. Once the papillotome is in the cutting position, an incision is made in the papilla of Vater, starting from the center and continuing to the 11 o'clock position (Fig. 17–15). This is the safest position for papillotomy, but sometimes the papillotome cannot be brought into this exact position. Consequently, the cut may be positioned between the 11 and 12 o'clock positions, which is acceptable. The length of the cut should be between 10 and 15 mm. This incision should be made slowly and deliberately in stepwise fashion with small bursts of cutting current. The electrosurgical unit's pedal should be tapped repeatedly, with short contact. The pedal should not be held down for a long time, causing an uncontrolled and possibly misdirected incision. In other words, the endoscopist must control the length and direction of the incision. If the incision strays toward the 10 o'clock position or past the 12 o'clock position, the papillotome must be readjusted before proceeding with any further cutting. The cutting current always should be set on the blend mode, and the incision should *never* be directed beyond the 12 o'clock position. Extension of the incision toward the 1 o'clock position may cause either excessive bleeding or pancreatitis, which is most likely thermal in nature.

The length of the incision should be tailored to the size of the stone that is present in the common bile duct. If a stone has been present in the common bile duct for a long time, the intraduodenal portion of the duct bulges into the lumen of the duodenum. When this bulge is visible, especially if the distance between the orifice of the papilla and the transverse duodenal fold is long, the papillotomy is safe, and one may make a longer incision. In contrast, if the distal common bile duct is not dilated, and there is a large stone in the common bile duct, the endoscopist should be aware of the discrepancy between the size of the stone and the diameter of the duct. At times, a stone in the basket may become impacted in this narrow distal portion of the common bile duct. The majority of stones can be removed through a 10-mm incision, but stones greater than 15 mm require a longer

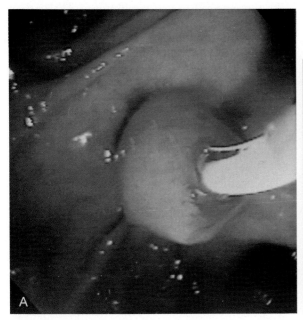
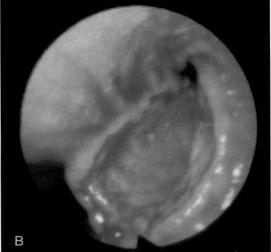

Figure 17–15. (A) A normal, but large, papilla with papillotome in place. **(B)** A 10-mm fresh papillotomy without bleeding or perforation.

incision. Extending the incision beyond the transverse duodenal fold will increase the chance of perforation. If the stone is too large, lithotripsy should be considered. If this is not possible, the endoscopist may place a biliary stent and reevaluate the patient for possible surgical removal of the stone. The key points for successful sphincterotomy are that (1) the endoscopist should not proceed if the direction of the incision is incorrect and (2) the papilla must always remain in view while an incision is being made. If conditions are not optimal (*i.e.*, too much peristalsis, poor visibility due to secretion or bleeding, patient's discomfort or lack of cooperation), the procedure should be stopped until all problems are corrected and optimal conditions are once again achieved. If this is not possible, it is better to stop the procedure and try the next day under more favorable conditions.

Once the papillotomy is completed, the endoscopist should evaluate the situation, and if no complications are present, proceed with the removal of the stone. To remove an average-sized stone, it is easier to use an extraction balloon (Fig. 17–16). This catheter is primed with contrast medium and the balloon is tested for air leakage. The extraction balloon catheter is inserted through the biopsy channel and, under fluoroscopic observation, is advanced past the stone in the proximal common bile duct. The balloon is inflated with care to prevent its

overdistention beyond the diameter of the duct. Overdistention not only causes pain for the patient but also makes removal of the balloon difficult. Once the balloon is inflated, the endoscopist slowly pulls it back toward the duodenum. If the size of the papillotomy is adequate, one may observe the delivery of the stone into the duodenum through the scope or the monitor. If this maneuver does not bring the stone through the papillotomy, one must consider the use of a basket. In this case, the size of the basket needs to be adjusted to the size of the stone. The basket should be primed with contrast material. After insertion of its tip above the stone, the basket is opened under fluoroscopic control. It is pulled back slowly until the stone is in the basket. At this time, the gastrointestinal surgical assistant closes the handle of the basket until the stone is trapped inside it (Fig. 17–17). Sometimes the basket may slip to the side of the stone without grabbing it. This maneuver may then have to be repeated several times until the stone is trapped in the basket. Care must be taken not to crush the stone by applying excessive force to the handle. Once the stone is caught, it is pulled back into the duodenum. It may be extracted by removing the duodenoscope containing the basket and stone. If there are several stones to be removed, the basket should be opened in the duodenum and the stone can be dropped, allowing it to pass by way of the gastrointestinal tract.

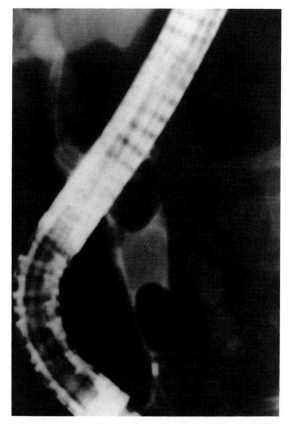

Figure 17–16. A dilated common bile duct with a large stone in the proximal duct. The filling defect in the distal common bile duct is a balloon catheter. This balloon now serves to block the distal duct to prevent the escape of contrast media into the duodenum. Once the stone's position is demonstrated, the balloon should be deflated. After pushing the balloon above the stone, the balloon is reinflated and used as an extraction balloon, pulling the stone in front of it and delivering it into the duodenum.

Any discrepancy between the size of the stone and the length of the incision should be corrected. In extending the papillotomy incision, it is important to remember the transverse duodenal fold, which should be the upper limit of the incision. Extension of the incision beyond this fold may increase the chances of perforation. At this time, a word of caution is in order. If there are too many stones, or the conditions are not favorable, one should insert a double-pigtail stent into the common bile duct and terminate the procedure for that day. The larger stones should be dealt with by more experienced endoscopists or, if necessary, surgical common bile duct exploration.

In 5% to 10% of cases, deep insertion of the papillotome into the common bile duct cannot be achieved; therefore, papillotomy cannot be done. The following techniques are available to remedy this situation: (1) over-the-wire papil-lotomy and (2) precut papillotomy. If bile duct visualization can be achieved only with impaction of the cannula, and the catheter cannot be advanced deeply enough into the common bile duct, one may try to insert a wire through the impacted cannula into the common bile duct. The insertion of the wire should be handled by a trained assistant familiar with fluoroscopy visualization and positioning of the wire. Once the wire is pushed up into the common bile duct, the cannula is removed. An over-the-wire papillotome is inserted into the common bile duct. The position of the papillotome is further documented by injecting contrast material into the common bile duct. If the papillotome is properly positioned in the duct, the handle is pulled back, and the papillotomy is completed.

The precut technique is needed in about 5% of cases. In these patients, one can visualize the pancreatic duct, but the common bile duct cannot be seen despite different maneuvers and trials with different catheters. In this situation, the endoscopist may resort to cutting the papilla of Vater from outside. This is done by using a straight papillotome or a needle knife papillotome (Fig. 17–18). This procedure is demand-

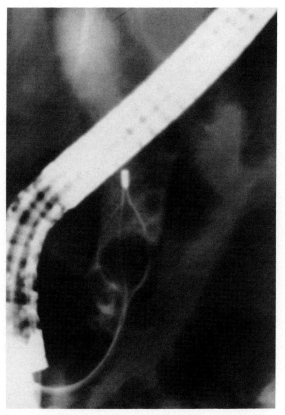

Figure 17–17. A large stone is grasped by a basket before it is pulled and delivered into the duodenum.

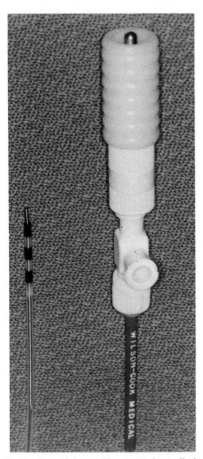

Figure 17–18. A straight papillotome, also called a needle knife. This is used for precut papillotomy.

ing, requiring a higher level of skill, and should be done only by endoscopists who have mastered endoscopic papillotomy. In performing precut papillotomy, the tip of the straight papillotome is inserted into the orifice of the papilla. An incision is started from the center toward the 11 o'clock position. The aim is to incise the anterior wall of the ampulla of Vater deeply enough to uncover the orifice of the common bile duct, but not so deeply as to go through the wall of the duodenum and cause perforation. The incision should be carried out slowly and should be between 5 and 8 mm in length. This is not a formal papillotomy but is used to find the orifice of the common bile duct for insertion of the papillotome. In our institution, the precut papillotomy is performed when the presence of the common bile duct stone is demonstrated by other means, such as sonography, and the insertion of a cannula or a papillotome into the common bile duct is not possible. The best approach is to perform the precut papillotomy and admit the patient for a 24 to 48-hour waiting period, which allows the edema to subside and the coagulated tissue to slough. This gives the endoscopist a clearer view of the papilla, making the cannulation of the common bile duct easier. Once the regular papillotome is inserted into the common bile duct, the papillotomy is carried out in routine fashion. The underlying theory behind carrying out a precut papillotomy is that the majority of patients have a common orifice for the common bile duct and the pancreatic duct, and the two ducts are separated by 1 to 2 mm. In a small number of patients, the two ducts are separated by a distance of 3 to 4 mm; in this situation, the common bile duct opens in the ampulla in a more cephalad position. Therefore, cannulation from a distally situated papilla becomes very difficult. Unroofing the ampulla by precutting techniques exposes the orifice of the common bile duct in the ampulla, making the papillotomy easier.

Transhepatic Assisted Endoscopic Sphincterotomy

In less than 2% to 3% of patients with known common bile duct stones, cannulation and sphincterotomy are unsuccessful, even in expert hands. One technique available in this instance is the percutaneous transhepatic insertion of a guidewire into the bile duct and through the papilla into the duodenum.[32] The wire is grasped by a snare or grasping forceps and is brought out through the mouth. The endoscope is reinserted over the wire, and after reaching the papilla in a straight position, an over-the-wire papillotome is inserted into the common bile duct. The wire is pulled back into the channel, and sphincterotomy is performed in the usual manner. This method of papillotomy carries the added risks and complications of percutaneous transhepatic insertion, including bile peritonitis and bleeding from the puncture site of the liver.

Endoscopic Sphincterotomy in Patients with Billroth II Gastrectomy

In patients who have undergone a Billroth II gastrectomy, the papilla of Vater is approached in a retrograde fashion through the afferent loop. Therefore, the longer the afferent loop, the less the chance of reaching the papilla. Today's surgeons should remember that the Billroth II gastrojejunostomy should be placed as close to the ligament of Treitz as possible.

ERCP in patients who have undergone Billroth II operations should first be tried with a side-viewing endoscope.[29-31] If this fails, the use of an end-viewing endoscope may allow the endoscopist to get through the afferent loop and reach the papilla. However, the lack of a cannula elevator and the usual loop position of the scope may make selective cannulation of the bile duct impossible. If the cannulation is successful and a papillotomy is indicated, a specially made Billroth II papillotome should be used. There is a greater risk of bleeding and perforation with endoscopic sphincterotomy in this situation, and this procedure should be performed only by an experienced endoscopist.

COMPLICATIONS OF ENDOSCOPIC SPHINCTEROTOMY

The major complications of endoscopic sphincterotomy are bleeding, perforation, pancreatitis, and cholangitis if the bile duct is not cleared of the stone.[4, 7, 9] Hemorrhage from the sphincterotomy site occurs in 2% of cases and in most cases stops with conservative therapy. In 1% of patients, bleeding is significant and may require transfusion and possible surgery to control the bleeding. Duodenal perforation is heralded by abdominal pain following the procedure, which may radiate to the back. It is associated with fever, leukocytosis, and intolerance to oral intake. Free air may not be present in the peritoneal cavity because most perforations are retroperitoneal, but the perforation is usually confirmed by contrast radiology. Most perforations respond to antibiotic therapy, intravenous fluid, and nasogastric suction. Some do require surgery, either for drainage of an abscess or closure of the perforation.[33]

Hyperamylesemia and pancreatitis are relatively common, occurring in about 7% of cases, but only 3% of these patients experience severe pancreatitis, requiring hospitalization. It usually develops after repeated injection of contrast material into the pancreatic duct but can occur after sphincterotomy without contrast injection into the pancreatic duct. Epigastric pain associated with nausea and vomiting shortly after the procedure points to the diagnosis, and a rise in serum amylase levels will confirm it. With conservative therapy, resolution occurs within 2 to 5 days. Acute pancreatitis develops rarely and results in prolonged hospitalization. Conservative therapy is always the treatment of choice. Surgical intervention is rarely, if ever, indicated.

Cholangitis usually develops because of stones remaining in the common bile duct. Endobiliary stent insertion into the common bile duct and antibiotic therapy may minimize the risk. However, recurrence of cholangitis will inevitably develop unless the stones are ultimately removed.[17, 19]

Stone and basket impaction is a rare occurrence that can be resolved either by mechanical lithotripsy or by extending the papillotomy incision. In doing so, one must cut the handle of the basket with a wire cutter and remove the endoscope. An assistant should hold the basket (which is still protruding through the mouth). Again the duodenoscope is inserted along the basket and advanced into the duodenum. The papilla is found and the papillotomy incision is enlarged using a new papillotome so that the stone may be removed with the impacted basket.[33] On rare occasions, the impacted basket may require surgical removal.

The mortality rate of endoscopic sphincterotomy is around 1% to 2%. It usually occurs in elderly patients following duodenal perforation, significant hemorrhage, severe pancreatitis, or cholangitis. Early recognition and administration of appropriate treatment minimizes mortality.

CONCLUSION

ERCP and endoscopic sphincterotomy have made the management of biliary and pancreatic diseases easier and treatment much simpler. In our lifetime, we have seen a revolution of a tremendous magnitude and a total change in the handling of retained, residual, or re-formed common bile duct stones. A secondary surgical exploration of the common bile duct for stones always carries a higher morbidity and mortality than primary common bile duct exploration. Today, with the advent of endoscopic sphincterotomy, the morbidity and mortality of stone extraction is possibly less than with surgical removal. The hospital stay is shorter, the recovery and return to work is much quicker and, most important, the patient suffers less pain. Because of the shorter hospital stay and faster recovery, cost savings are beyond question and may help to reduce overall health care costs.

In an environment of minimal-access surgery with laparoscopes, it is our recommendation that all general surgeons be involved in learning and performing endoscopic procedures, possibly adding endoscopic sphincterotomy to their armamentarium for managing pancreatic and biliary diseases.

References

1. McCune WS, Shorb PE, Moscovitz H. Endoscopic cannulation of the ampulla of Vater: a preliminary report. Ann Surg 167:752–754, 1968.
2. Oi I: Fiberduodenoscopy and endoscopic pancreatocholangiography. Gastrointest Endosc 17:59–62, 1970.
3. Gaisford WD. Endoscopic retrograde cholangiopancreatography in the diagnosis of jaundice. Am J Surg 132:699–704, 1976.
4. Bilballo MK, Dotter CT, Lee TG. Complications of endoscopic retrograde cholangiopancreatography (ERCP): a study of 10,000 cases. Gastroenterology 70:314–320, 1976.
5. Classen M, Demling L. Endoskopische sphincterotomie der papilla vateri und steinextraktion aus dem ductus choledochus. Dtsch Med Wochenschr 99:496–497, 1974.
6. Kawai K, Akasaka Y, Murakami K, et al. Endoscopic sphincterotomy of the ampulla of vater. Gastrointest Endosc 20:148–151, 1974.
7. Safrany L. Duodenoscopic sphincterotomy and gallstone removal. Gastroenterology 72:338–343, 1977.
8. Peiter JJ, Bayer HP, Mennicken C, Manegold BC. Results of endoscopic papillotomy: a collective experience from nine endoscopic centers in West Germany. World J Surg 2:505–511, 1978.
9. Selfert E. Long-term follow-up after endoscopic sphincterotomy. Endoscopy 20:232–235, 1988.
10. Ghazi A, Washington M. Endoscopic diagnosis and management of diseases of the pancreas and hepatobiliary tract. Probl Gen Surg 7:1610–1674, 1990.
11. Surick B, Ghazi A. Endoscopic papillotomy while the gallbladder is in situ. Am Surg 58:657–660, 1992.
12. Staritz M, Poralla T, Dormeyer HH, et al. Endoscopic removal of common bile duct stones through the intact papilla after medical sphincter dilatation. Gastroenterology 88:1807–1811, 1985.
13. Staritz M, Ewe K, Meyer Z, Buschenfelde KH. Endoscopic papillary dilatation (EPD) for the treatment of common bile duct stones and papillary stenosis. Endoscopy 15:197–198, 1983.
14. Boey JH, Way LH. Acute cholangitis. Ann Surg 191:264–270, 1980.
15. Andrew DJ, Johnson SE. Acute suppurative cholangitis, a medical and surgical emergency. Am J Gastroenterol 54:141–154, 1970.
16. Thompson JE, Tompkins RK, Longmire WP. Factors in management of acute cholangitis. Ann Surg 195:137–145, 1982.
17. Gogol HK, Runyon BA, Volpicelli R, Palmer RC. Acute suppurative obstructive cholangitis due to stones: treatment by urgent endoscopic sphincterotomy. Gastrointest Endosc 33:210–213, 1987.
18. Leese T, Neoptolemos JP, Baker AR, Locke-Carr DL. Management of acute cholangitis and the impact of endoscopic sphincterotomy. Br J Surg 73:988–992, 1988.
19. Himal HS, Lindsay T. Ascending cholangitis: surgery versus endoscopic or percutaneous drainage. Surgery 108:629–634, 1990.
20. Geenen JE. New diagnostic and treatment modalities involving endoscopic retrograde cholangiopancreatography and esophago-gastroduodenoscopy. Scand J Gastroenterol 77 (Suppl):93–106, 1982.
21. Farup PG, Tjora S. Sphincter of Oddi dysfunction. Scand J Gastroenterol 24:956–960, 1989.
22. Hulbregtse K, Tytgat GNJ. Carcinoma of the ampulla of Vater: the endoscopic approach. Endoscopy 20:223–226, 1988.
23. Siegel JH, Snady H. The significance of endoscopically placed prostheses in the management of biliary obstruction due to carcinoma of the pancreas: results of nonoperative decompression in 277 patients. Am J Gastroenterol 81:634–641, 1986.
24. Tytgat GN, Huibregste K. Intestinal endoprostheses. Dig Dis Sci 31(9)(Suppl):675–765, 1986.
25. Tanaka M, Ideda S, Yoshimoto H. Endoscopic sphincterotomy for the treatment of biliary sump syndrome. Surgery 93:264–267, 1982.
26. Marbet UA, Stalder GA, Faust H, et al. Endoscopic sphincterotomy and surgical approaches in the treatment of the "sump syndrome." Gut 28:142–145, 1987.
27. Mitchell R, Kerr R, Barton J, Schmidt A. Biliary obstruction secondary to shrapnel. Am J Gastroenterol 86:1531–1534, 1991.
28. Veerappan A, Siegal JH, Podany J, et al. Fasciola hepatica pancreatitis: endoscopic extraction of live parasites. Gastrointest Endosc 37:473–475, 1991.
29. Staritz M, Porolla T, Dormeyer HH, Bushchenfelde KHM. Endoscopic removal of common bile duct stones through the intract papilla after medical sphincter dilation. Gastroenterology 88:1807–1811, 1985.
30. Safrany L, Neuhaus B, Portocarrero G, Krause S. Endoscopic sphincterotomy in patients with Billroth II gastrectomy. Endoscopy 12:16–22, 1980.
31. Osnes M, Rosseland AR, Aabakken L. Endoscopic retrograde cholangiography and endoscopic papillotomy in patients with a previous Billroth II resection. Gut 27:1193–1198, 1986.
32. Shorvon PJ, Cotton PB, Mason RR, et al. Percutaneous transhepatic assistance for duodenoscopic sphincterotomy. Gut 26:1373–1376, 1985.
33. Mustard R Jr, MacKenzie R, Jamieson C, Haber GB. Surgical complications of endoscopic sphincterotomy. Can J Surg 27:215–217, 1984.
34. Wurbs D. Endoscopic papillotomy. Scand J Gastroenterol 77(Suppl):107–114, 1982.

18

Intraoperative Biliary Endoscopy

George Berci

OPEN CHOLECYSTECTOMY AND CHOLEDOCHOLITHOTOMY

In a few years, laparoscopic cholecystectomy and laparoscopic choledocholithotomy will largely replace open surgery of common bile duct (CBD) stones. The surgical community should become acquainted with this technique. Since the first choledochotomy by Courvoisier, surgeons have been frustrated by the inability to clear all bile ducts of calculi by instrumental manipulations.[1] This limitation is the result of the blind nature of the operative procedure. The true incidence of retained stones can be assessed only by a postoperative T-tube cholangiogram. The disappointingly high failure rate (5–10%) revealed by these examinations continues to hound biliary surgeons throughout the world, and the failure of surgeons to adopt this direct method for the diagnosis and retrieval of biliary calculi must be attributed to technologic inadequacies.

Instrumentation

A primitive instrument was described in 1922 by Bakes, who used a simple illuminated speculum without the optical or irrigating system and a mirror.[2] The instrument was introduced into the incised distal duct to observe the lumen. It did not gain wide acceptance. McIver designed a right-angle cystoscope in 1941, but the substandard visualization did not promote wider dissemination.[3] It remained for Wildegans to popularize biliary endoscopy in Europe with the introduction in 1953 of improved instrumentation. This scope still uses the standard lens system and the distal electric globe. The advantage was the 60° angled configuration of the shaft.[4]

With the advent of the Hopkins optical system, my colleagues and I developed a compact, right-angled, rigid choledochoscope in 1971. It was simple to use but still required some apprenticeship.[5] It took more than a decade until choledochoscopy was accepted. The flexible scope was later employed for the same purposes. It was easy to couple to a television camera and produce a large image that can be seen by both eyes from an optimal distance. Because four hands are required in using the video technique, the movements of the surgeon and assistants must be coordinated. The operator introduces the instrument, and the assistant advances the basket; both together pull out the entrapped stone through the incision.

Irrigation System

A Fenwal pressure irrigation system, commonly used for emergency transfusions, provides appropriate distention and clearing of the duct required for inspection. Commercially available plastic containers preloaded with sterile, normal saline are placed within this Fenwal pressure bag. A pressure of 150 to 200 mm Hg ensures adequate delivery of the perfusion fluid.

Accessories

Most important is the 1.3-mm (No. 4 French) Segura-type basket, which is advanced under visual control, if possible, beyond the stone, opened up, and pulled back. With some manipulation, the stone can be delivered into the incision. A 4-F vascular balloon catheter is important for advancing it through the sphincter into the duodenum and withdrawing it under visual control with some deflation to ensure that no stone is left in the sphincter area. A stone can be retrieved into the incision with a balloon if it is inflated beyond the stone. The recently developed pulse-dye lasers or electrohydrolic lithotriptors with a small probe can help in cases of impacted calculi.

INTRAOPERATIVE CHOLANGIOGRAPHY

Intraoperative cholangiography (IOC) should be performed routinely for several reasons. The anatomy of the cystic duct and its drainage (*i.e.,* 17% drains only from the lateral side into the common bile duct), the configuration and size of the stone, the size of the duct, the location of calculi, and sphincter function are important. We advocated fluorocholangiography for 14 years before it was accepted. If the appropriate equipment is being used, the injection can be completed in 3 minutes, and in another 5 minutes, the films can be shown. A completion cholangiogram after the removal of stones can confirm the success of the examination.

There is only one absolute indication of choledocholithotomy: stone palpation. Patients with abnormal preoperative liver function tests can have up to 50% negative cholangiograms because the stone passed in the interim period. Operative cholangiography can decrease significantly the unnecessary exploration of the CBD. Additional data is available in other publications.[6-8]

INTRAOPERATIVE BILIARY ENDOSCOPY DURING OPEN COMMON BILE DUCT SURGERY

After the cholangiogram is performed and the CBD is located, stay sutures are inserted into the anterior wall, and the CBD is opened between traction sutures. This facilitates a safe incision and avoids injury of the underlying structures (*e.g.,* portal vein). The sterile choledochoscope is prepared and connected to the irrigation and lighting systems. The attached television camera's white balance and focus are checked. For open choledocholithotomy and choledochoscopy, it is essential to mobilize (*i.e.,* Kocher maneuver) the duodenum, because in most cases, the distal CBD enters the duodenum in a slight curvature. During choledochoscopy, the operator working from the patient's left side keeps the duodenum mobilized with one hand. The distal CBD is placed on stretch, making it easier to examine the sphincter area. The choledochoscope is introduced into the proximal ductal system first, and each larger entry of the ducts in this area is observed. If no stones are discovered, the instrument is removed and reintroduced into the distal ductal system, but it is crucial that the distal duct, with the help of the mobilized duodenum, should be kept on stretch. Stay sutures can be crossed by the weight of attached mosquito forceps on each side and can help to close the incision around the scope to avoid leakage. If a stone is discovered, the basket is introduced, and the stone entrapped and removed.

In the case of multiple calculi, a smaller stone can be hidden in the cystic stump, escaping detection endoscopically or radiologically. It is advisable in cases with multiple calculi (*i.e.,* large number of small faceted stones), after the duct is cleared and no additional stones are endoscopically seen, to remove the ligature from the cystic stump and introduce a soft catheter into the CBD and rescope the patient. If stones were hidden in the stump, they are pushed into the CBD, seen through the choledochoscope, and removed.

The choledochotomy incision is closed by interrupted sutures around the inserted T-tube. We prefer tube drainage instead of primary closure. This provides an emergency exit in case of missed stones, which can be removed through the T-tube tract in 4 to 6 weeks. This is the safest method for removing retained calculi without splitting the sphincter, and it can be performed as an outpatient procedure. The incidence of retained stones after a properly performed intraoperative choledochoscopy can be decreased to 3% or less, which is acceptable. Ninety-five percent of this residual group can be removed through the T-tube tract as an outpatient procedure without mortality or significant morbidity.[9]

The technique of biliary endoscopy can be readily learned, and the important anatomic landmarks are easily identified. Unlike endoscopic examinations of other organs, there is no complex anatomy to master. The changes to be recognized are limited to calculi in most cases. The atraumatic nature of the choledochoscope is demonstrated by the absence of injury to the ducts and the low rates of cholangitis and pancreatitis after intraoperative biliary endoscopy.

There are two groups of patients: those with suspected stones and those with unsuspected stones.

Suspected Stones

Patients with suspected stones can present a history of recurrent colicky attacks. During an attack, the color of the urine may become dark, and liver function tests can be elevated. The ultrasound examination may display the CBD as normal or dilated.

Because of the history and the assumption that there is a stone, preoperative endoscopic retrograde cholangiography (ERC) can be attempted, and if the stone is confirmed, papillotomy can be performed, the stone evacuated, and the patient's gallbladder removed laparoscopically a few days later.

An alternative is to perform a laparoscopic cholecystectomy, confirm the stone with intraoperative cholangiography, and leave the stone behind. The stone is removed in the postoperative period by endoscopic papillotomy.

The third alternative is to refrain from performing preoperative ERC. The patient has an IOC during laparoscopic cholecystectomy, and the stone is removed laparoscopically.

Unsuspected Stone

Patients with unsuspected stones have no symptoms and no elevated liver function tests, but as many as 5% can harbor calculi in the CBD. There are alternatives for treating with this problem during laparoscopic cholecystectomy.

In one approach, the stone is left behind and is removed in a postoperative period with endoscopic sphincterotomy (ES). If the stone is very small, the operator can wait and observe the patient until symptoms develop.

ENDOSCOPIC RETROGRADE CHOLANGIOGRAPHY

ERC examination is extremely useful for selected patients. If an elderly, high-risk patient with cholangitis, jaundice, or septicemia is admitted with an established diagnosis of cholelithiasis, the CBD can be drained endoscopically or a papillotomy performed. If the patient's condition improves significantly in the next 24 to 48 hours, laparoscopic cholangiography can be performed. (See Chap. 17.)

ERC or ES is an important diagnostic tool in stone disease or other abnormalities of the extrahepatic biliary system. Not every patient's CBD can be cannulated. The successful cannulation rate is between 85% and 95%. It carries a morbidity rate of 8% to 10%. Perforation of the retroduodenal part of the CBD can occur, producing a severe arterial bleeder that requires immediate attention. There are difficulties in cannulation if there is a diverticulum of the duodenum adjacent to the ampulla. Some of these serious complications can be treated conservatively by transfusion or observation in the intensive care units. Approximately 25% of these patients need emergency surgery. The mortality rate of ES in the best hands is between 0.5% and 1%. Late strictures after sphincterotomy can occur in 2% to 5% of patients, with reforming of stones and partial stricturing in 6% to 10%. Despite the appealing advantages of ERC, the drawbacks of increased morbidity and mortality must be taken seriously.[10]

The aim of a CBD stone removal procedure should be to treat and cure the patient in one session, to reduce the risks of morbidity and mortality. If the surgeon is well trained and experienced in biliary surgery but not skilled in laparoscopic lithotomy, and it is a difficult case, there is nothing wrong in converting a laparoscopic procedure to an open choledocholithotomy, removing the stone, and leaving a T-tube in to solve the problem. We found that in 1200 cases of open cholecystectomy, 50% of the patients were younger than 60 years of age, with an 8% incidence of CBD stones.[11] There were no deaths in the group. The other half were older than 60 and included high-risk patients with an 18% incidence of CBD stones. Open choledocholithotomy was performed, and the overall mortality rate was 1.3%, with a 3% rate of retained stones. The retained stones were removed in the postoperative period through the T-tube tract.

Laparoscopic choledocholithotomy needs skills that can be obtained by surgeons who are already familiar with laparoscopic cholecystectomy. There are a few extra instruments required, such as dilating balloons, guidewires, a small choledochoscope or ureteroscope, a second TV camera, and stone retrieval baskets that can be advanced through the flexible scope. It is difficult to remove an impacted calculus with a basket or balloon. A pulsed-dye laser (from the department of urology) can be used, or a much less expensive electrohydraulic lithotriptor (also employed in urology) can be used to disintegrate the stone for endoscopic removal of the fragments.

CBD surgery requires modern fluorocholangiogram equipment, and the procedure should not be performed without having the necessary radiologic assistants available. The outdated mobile units are not suitable. They extend significantly the operating time, and the films obtained are substandard. Surgeons should use a mobile, digitized fluoroscope with permanent documentation facilities. The image is optimal. The injection of contrast material can be completed in 2 to 3 minutes. The anatomy, cystic duct configuration, location of the stone, size of the duct, drainage of the duct into the duodenum, and anomalies could be immediately discovered, and the technique of the operation could be tailored according to the findings. Important steps are recorded on a hard disk and printed in the form of films or hard copies after cholangiography is completed. These are presented to the operator for final analysis. Manipulations of the basket position in the CBD, if the endoscopic view is not satisfactory, can be completed using the fluoroscopic appearance.

A completion cholangiogram should be performed on the table to ensure that the ductal system is stone free and that no extravasation (*i.e.,* perforation of ductal system) has occurred.

REMOVAL OF A CBD STONE THROUGH THE CYSTIC DUCT DURING LAPAROSCOPIC CHOLECYSTECTOMY

A cystic duct cholangiogram is performed at the beginning of the procedure, after the duct is secured. The stone is localized. If the stone is small (2–3 mm) and the drainage of the duct is relatively straight into the duodenum without sharp angulations, several tests can be applied. The anesthesiologist administers 1 mg of glucagon intravenously. After 1 or 2 minutes of observation, warm saline is injected through the indwelling cholangiocatheter, and attempts are made to flush the little stone through the relaxed sphincter. This result can be obtained by exchanging the cholangiocatheter over the guidewire to a balloon catheter. Inflate the catheter, and pass it through the relaxed sphincter with the stone in front into the duodenum. A checkup cholangiogram can confirm the successful attempt.

If the stone is larger or if there are multiple stones, the cholangiocatheter is exchanged over a guidewire. The flexible scope attached to an irrigation system (*i.e.,* Fenwal pressure bag with prewarmed saline at a pressure of 150 mm Hg) is introduced over the guidewire through the cystic duct into the CBD.

If the cystic duct is too small, a dilating balloon is advanced over the guidewire. The balloon is 40 mm long and 5 mm in diameter. These balloons have radiomarkers on both ends, and the position of the balloon is easily seen fluoroscopically. One end is visible outside the cystic duct, and the other radiomarker is seen in the CBD area. The balloon is slightly inflated, observing the manufacturer's instructions, to the correct atmospheric pressure, kept there for a few minutes, and then released and withdrawn over the guidewire. The scope is advanced over the guidewire through the dilated cystic duct into the CBD, and the guidewire is removed. The irrigation system is opened, the duct is dilated, and the stone is brought into view.

There are electronic beam-splitting arrangements that allow the operator to see simultaneously the introduced choledochoscope through the laparoscope and the intraluminal appearance of the CBD on the other half of the screen. A small, Segura-type basket is advanced through the instrument channel, and through the coordinated movements of the operator and the assistant, the stone is entrapped and withdrawn through the cystic duct (Fig. 18–1), secured, and removed with a laparoscopic grasper through one of the operating ports. The assistant must be well trained, because choledocholithotomy is a team event.

After the stones are removed, the cholangiocatheter is reintroduced into the opening of the cystic duct. A cholangiogram is made, and if no stones are detected, the cystic duct is closed by hemoclip or endoloop. There are other alternatives for draining the CBD. The surgeon reintroduces the cholangiocatheter and secures it with an endoloop. This catheter is left in position and brought out in the flank. Another drainage catheter is placed in the subhepatic space. The cholangiocatheter remains open 24 hours for drainage.

Placing an indwelling, small catheter through the cystic duct has certain advantages. The CBD can be drained in the first 24 hours, and the intraluminal pressure, after manipulations, can be decreased. Spasms or edema can occur after repeated basket maneuvers. The catheter can be plugged before discharge, and the patient can be sent home with instructions and a small tube attached to the skin. On the eighth post-

VIA CYSTIC DUCT

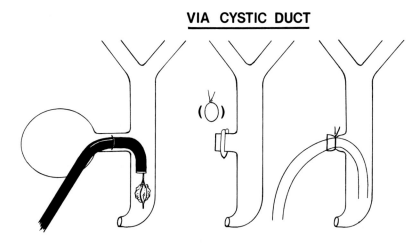

PROXIMAL DUCT VISUALIZATION ??

+ SEPARATE DRAINAGE ?

Figure 18–1. Schematic diagram of stone removal from the common bile duct through the cystic duct with a flexible scope. After the scope is removed, the cystic duct can be clipped or tied. The cystic duct can be also drained by leaving an indwelling catheter in the common bile duct for 24 hours. The patient is sent home with a plugged tube, and 8 days after surgery, a cholangiogram is performed. If the results are negative, the catheter can be pulled in a few days. If a missed stone is found, a guidewire can be advanced through the ampulla to help the endoscopist find the papilla and perform a sphincterotomy. Separate drainage is advised.

operative day, a tube cholangiogram can be made to ensure that the duct is stone free. In another week, the catheter can be pulled. If there is no distal obstruction, the stump is closed. If a missed stone is discovered, a guidewire can be introduced into the duodenum, and the papillotomy is facilitated by knowing the exact location of the papilla because of the exiting guidewire. If there are difficulties with the guidewire, methylene blue can be injected.

Most CBD stones are removed through the cystic duct, and the CBD is left with a closed cystic stump. Years of careful follow-up are required to obtain data about the incidence of retained stones. This technique is only a few years old, and more experience is required to see which of the alternatives should be selected. A disadvantage of the endoscopic examination of the CBD through the cystic duct is that the endoscope usually cannot be turned toward the common hepatic duct, and the proximal hepatic ductal system cannot be visualized, which means that 4% to 6% of these patients have stones that can escape endoscopic detection and be retained.

DIRECT COMMON BILE DUCT EXPLORATION WITH THE LAPAROSCOPE

The dilated CBD is incised after its location is verified by IOC and meticulous dissection. The choledochoscope is introduced through this incision into the CBD. In this case, the proximal and the distal duct can be visualized. The calculi

are removed, and a folded T-tube is inserted. The opening of the anterior CBD wall is closed with a few stitches around the T-tube and brought out in the flank (Fig. 18–2). A separate drain tube is inserted in the subhepatic space.

An alternative is to open the dilated duct, remove the stones with a scope, introduce a catheter through the cystic stump, and transfix it with an endoloop. The common bile duct is primarily closed (see Fig. 18–2).[12] A completion cholangiogram is obtained. Small catheters (*e.g.,* 4 or 5) are brought out in the flank, and

VIA CBD

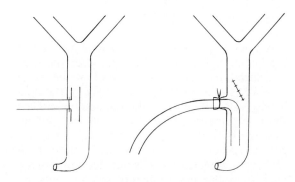

+ SEPARATE DRAINAGE

Figure 18–2. Schematic diagram of the direct laparoscopic approach of the common bile duct. In the left drawing, a T-tube is positioned after the duct is cleared of stones. In the right drawing, an incision is made in the common bile duct (CBD). The stones are cleared endoscopically, and the CBD is closed, but a tube is placed in the cystic duct, affixed, and brought out for drainage. A postoperative cholangiogram can be performed in this case.

the ductal system is drained for the first 24 hours. The patient is sent home with a plugged tube. If a missed stone is discovered, a T-tube or smaller indwelling tube can be left in position for 4 to 6 weeks until a tract is formed, and the missed stone can be removed through the dilated tract.

CONCLUSION

We do not yet know which method is better for removing CBD stones. The dissection or opening of the CBD is technically more difficult, but it is more precise because of the possibility of examining the proximal and distal ductal system and providing drainage. If the CBD is open, an additional subhepatic drain is advantageous. With these techniques, most CBD stones can be removed in one operative session without resorting to another postoperative procedure (*e.g.,* ERC and ES) and increasing the risk of complications.

The various laparoscopic choledocholithotomy techniques are only a few years old, and more time is required to evaluate the results. Each technique must be tailored to the particular anatomy of the patient, the available instrumentation, and the skills of the operator.

References

1. Courvoisier LG. Casuistische Beitrage zur Pathologie und Chirurgie der Gallenwege. Leipzig: Vogel, 1890.
2. Bakes J. Die Choledochopapilloskopie nebst Bemerkungen uber Hepaticusdrainage und Dilatation der Papille. Arch Klin Chir 126:473, 1926.
3. McIver MA. An instrument for visualizing the interior of the common duct at operation. Surgery 9:112, 1941.
4. Wildegans H. Endoskopie der tiefen Gallenwege. Langenbecks Arch Klin Chir 276:652, 1953.
5. Shore JM, Morgenstern L, Berci G. An improved rigid choledochoscope. Am J Surg 122:567, 1971.
6. Berci G, Shore JM, Morgenstern L, Hamlin JA. Choledochoscopy and operative fluorocholangiography in the prevention of retained stones. World J Surg 2:411–427, 1978.
7. Phillips E, Berci G, Carroll B, et al. The importance of intraoperative cholangiography during laparoscopic cholecystectomy. Am Surg 55:267–272, 1989.
8. Sackier JM, Berci G, Phillips E, Carroll B, Shapiro S, Paz-Partlow M. The role of cholangiography in laparoscopic cholecystectomy. Arch Surg 126:1021–1026, 1991.
9. Berci G. Intraoperative and postoperative biliary endoscopy (choledochoscopy). Endoscopy 21:299–384, 1989.
10. Cotton PB, Lehman G, Vennes J, et al. Endoscopic sphincterotomy, complications and their management: an attempt at consensus. Gastrointest Endosc 37:383–393, 1991.
11. Morgenstern L, Wong L, Berci G. 1200 open cholecystectomies before the laparoscopic era: a standard for comparison. Arch Surg 127:400–403, 1992.

19

Small Bowel Enteroscopy and Intraoperative Endoscopy

Talmadge A. Bowden, Jr.

It has been more than 20 years since the first published reports on small bowel endoscopy appeared in the literature.[1, 2] Since 1972, vigorous efforts by investigators in Japan and Europe have produced three types of enteroscopic techniques, none of which has been entirely satisfactory. In addition, a variety of enteroscopes have been developed, tested, and discarded,[3] leaving the day-to-day diagnostic evaluation of the small bowel to barium contrast studies, isotope scans, and arteriography, tests whose limitations are also well known and documented.[4–7]

In spite of the frustrations experienced by enteroscopists, the drive to develop a practical and reliable instrument and technique has continued, producing some measurable progress over the past 5 years, but even with these recent advances, enteroscopy must still be considered an emerging technology.

The anatomy of the small bowel does not lend itself well to endoscopic examination because the 2- to 3-m length of small intestine from the ligament of Treitz to the terminal ileum is attached by its mesentery to the superior mesenteric artery, which measures only 14 to 15 cm in length. This results in a coiling effect, which combined with the freedom of movement of the small intestine restricts passage of any type of enteroscope. This chapter updates and positions current enteroscopic methods and endoscopes and reviews the most consistent method of examining the small intestine—intraoperative endoscopy.

ENTEROSCOPY

Enteroscopy has developed along three main lines:[7]

1. Rope-way endoscopy, which is advancement of an endoscope through the small bowel over a previously passed "string." This method requires a two-channel enteroscope and, unfortunately, is quite painful and must be performed under general anesthesia. The technique has received little attention and has essentially been abandoned and will not be discussed here in any further detail.

2. Push-type enteroscopy, which requires the peroral insertion of a long endoscope into the proximal small bowel.

3. Sonde-type enteroscopy, which uses a long, thin endoscope that is propelled through the intestine by natural peristalsis enhanced at times by pharmacologic stimulation. All of these methods have distinct advantages and disadvantages.

Push Enteroscopy

This is by far the most common method of enteroscopy practiced routinely by most endoscopists.[7, 8] Push enteroscopes have recently been developed and are commercially available. The Olympus Corporation, New Hyde Park, NY, currently has a designated push enteroscope (SIF-10) with an outer diameter of 11.3 mm, a biopsy channel of 2.8 mm, and a shaft length of

214

167 cm. The current market price is about $17,000. In general, this enteroscope does not offer significant advantages over the more commonly used standard pediatric or adult colonoscopes. The smaller diameter of the insertion tube on the pediatric endoscope does make its passage somewhat easier than that of the adult colonoscope. The primary limitation to push enteroscopy is the curved anatomy of the stomach and duodenum. The opposing curves of the stomach and duodenum dissipate the propelling force transmitted to the instrument shaft and usually result in a large loop forming in the stomach. Using a push-pull hooking technique and applying the liberal use of fluoroscopy, an adult or pediatric colonoscope can usually be passed into the proximal jejunum for a distance of approximately 2 ft beyond the ligament of Treitz. In an effort to extend the reach of the enteroscopic examination, the Olympus Corporation has recently developed a prototype instrument (SIF-10L) that uses an overtube back-loaded onto the shaft of the orally passed endoscope. Using standard push methods, the endoscope tip is advanced into the proximal jejunum. At this point, the overtube is advanced into the esophagus and stomach to the second portion of the duodenum. The endoscope, thus stiffened, limits gastric and duodenal looping of the instrument as it is advanced. Experience with this new instrument indicates that the enteroscope can be advanced up to 6 or 7 ft beyond the ligament of Treitz, resulting in an examination of essentially the entire jejunum.[9, 10]

The ability to pass this instrument deeper into the small intestine does have some disadvantages. Because of the long working length of the instrument (200 cm), two operators are required to insert the enteroscope, one to control the tip and the other to advance the instrument. The insertion of the overtube can result in significant pain, so heavy sedation is at times necessary. Because of the extended length of the instrument, biopsy forceps have been reported to fail to open at maximum insertion depths. Procedure times are not excessive and have been reported to range between 12 and 34 minutes. Some complications have been reported. They have primarily been due to the insertion of the overtube, with trauma to the ampulla of Vater and subsequent pancreatitis and a Mallory-Weiss tear. This instrument, as with other previously developed enteroscopes, is still in a clinical testing stage and its safety profile has not been defined.

Push enteroscopy has a broad range of indications, but the most common one is the evaluation of the patient with gastrointestinal bleeding of obscure causes.[11] Experience suggests that the examination has a significant yield in this group of difficult cases. In one series, a source was found for the bleeding in more than 40% of the patients examined. The most common cause of this bleeding has been reported as arteriovenous malformations. Furthermore, push enteroscopy offers the opportunity not only to localize these areas but also to treat them with bipolar electrocautery. Other uses for push enteroscopy have been small bowel biopsy and polypectomy and the confirmation or exclusion of abnormalities identified on x-ray studies. Additional reported uses have been the placement of enteric feeding tubes, enteroclysis, and cholangiography in patients with hepaticojejunostomies.[12]

An additional variation of push enteroscopy is the retrograde examination of the terminal ileum during colonoscopy. With some practice and experience and the use of fluoroscopy in the early part of the learning curve, coupled with a colonoscope free of loops and twists, the ileocecal valve can frequently be intubated and up to 50 cm of ileum examined. Retrograde ileoscopy requires several steps for a successful examination:

1. The ileocecal valve must be identified,
2. The endoscope must be passed beyond the valve into the bottom of the cecum,
3. The endoscope tip is flexed while the operator attempts to imbed it against the valve to pull the valve open,
4. Gentle air insufflation is performed at this point coupled with forward and medial insertion,
5. Once in the ileum, the endoscope is advanced with hook and pull maneuvers.

Excessive insufflation is to be avoided because it can result in significant patient discomfort. Retrograde enteroscopy can be useful in diagnosing Crohn's disease, tuberculosis, and small bowel lymphoma.[7] It also seems prudent that when evaluating a patient for bleeding of obscure cause with colonoscopy, retrograde enteroscopy also be performed.

Sonde Enteroscopy

The development of the sonde enteroscope has received the most attention by instrument makers over the past years, with at least six prototypes being developed and discarded.[7] The word sonde is derived from French roots and literally means "bend." These types of instruments all have in common a balloon at the end of the enteroscope that acts as a bolus upon which peristalsis advances the instrument through the small bowel. Once full insertion is verified by x-ray studies, the endoscopic examination is performed during withdrawal of the enteroscope. All sonde instruments have been limited in their inability to deflect the tip, and the small diameter eliminates the possibility for a biopsy channel. Currently, the commercially available sonde enteroscope marketed by the Olympus Corporation is the SIF-SW (small intestinal fiberscope-Sonde, wide).[11, 13] This instrument is 5 mm in diameter and has a working length of 2560 mm. The forward angle of view is 120°. This instrument has many of the limitations of its predecessors in that procedure times can be quite lengthy, ranging from 6 to 8 hours, and visualization is not complete because of the lack of tip deflection. In addition, therapeutic capability is not available because of the lack of a biopsy channel.

Because the perfect enteroscope has yet to be developed, several investigators have recently reported on a variety of concepts and techniques. Gostout and associates[14] have suggested a team approach to small bowel enteroscopy that will serve to shorten position time as well as examination time. This approach clearly requires a well-trained and motivated nursing staff. In addition, Gostout and coworkers have also suggested guidewire passage to facilitate the advancement of the enteroscope. Dabezies and associates[15] have been investigating video enteroscopy. The advantages to the application of video technology to enteroscopy certainly apply in this area, as in others, in that instruments can be longer, more flexible, and more resilient. The limiting factor at this point is chip size, which demands a larger instrument with the subsequent necessity for oral rather than transnasal passage. The ability to deflect the tip has frustrated all investigators and developers to date. The addition of cables for this feature requires that the instrument be larger, heavier, and stiffer. This, of course, defeats the advantages of patient comfort and requires more sedation for the examination. Sonde enteroscopy is currently practiced by only a few endoscopists. Available data do, however, suggest that the examination using current instruments is safe and somewhat effective. The primary usefulness of the instrument is in patients with bleeding of obscure cause; when used in this context in these highly selected patients, a diagnosis can be expected in approximately one quarter to one third of patients. Serious complications have not been reported, but the procedure is limited by the time required to complete the examination, patient discomfort, lack

of tip control, incomplete mucosal examination, lack of a therapeutic channel, and inability to mark lesions discovered during the examination.

One area of enteroscopy that has not been clearly addressed is the financial considerations of the examination. Push enteroscopy using a colonoscope, either pediatric or adult in a standard unit, will not have many other significant cost considerations. However, enteroscopy using the specialized endoscopes with fluoroscopy can be expected to result in greater cost. Specialty enteroscopes of either the push or sonde type can be expected to range between $14,000 and $22,000. Significant time is required to complete sonde enteroscopy, and additional personnel are required. At present, Medicare and some insurers reimburse for small bowel endoscopy. The exact facility and professional fees have not been consistently defined.

Enteroscopy has been receiving more and more attention over the last few years; however, its clinical usefulness has still not been established, and some physicians doubt its efficacy.[16] One of the stated disadvantages of enteroscopy, particularly of the sonde type, is the fact that only a diagnosis can be made. This, however, is not entirely bad because it does provide a reason for a patient's symptoms, and even though it may not specifically localize a site for surgery, it does provide information and a "road map" for the surgical team.

INTRAOPERATIVE ENDOSCOPY

A wide spectrum of conditions exist in which intraoperative endoscopy has been reported to be useful.[17–22] The procedure has the ability not only to enhance and refine information previously obtained but also to discover a pathologic condition unknown prior to exploration. The method for gastrointestinal panendoscopy has been well described,[17] but since the technique for small bowel intraoperative endoscopy is somewhat tricky, it probably deserves retelling. For most examinations, an adult colonoscope is the instrument of choice because of its length. In many instances, the narrower pediatric colonoscope will suffice. If available, a sonde enteroscope would certainly be the less traumatic instrument to use because of its flexibility and narrow diameter, but tip deflection would not be possible. If the surgeon is not an endoscopist, certainly preoperative consultation and review of the case and proposed procedure with a skilled endoscopist is appropriate. The anesthesiologist should also be consulted because it will be necessary to position the equipment to the left of the patient, and the passage of the endoscope may interfere with previously placed endotracheal tubes, nasogastric tubes, and esophageal stethoscopes.

It is advantageous to have a nasogastric tube in place prior to passage of the colonoscope. This tube serves two purposes: it acts as a guide to proper insertion of the endoscope to the side of the endotracheal tube and prevents overdistention of the stomach with the potential for tearing the gastric wall or short gastric vessels during the examination. It is easier to insert the endoscope into the duodenum before the abdomen is opened and the tamponade effect of the abdominal wall on the stomach is lost. Once the abdominal cavity is entered, the surgeon performs a thorough exploration. In some conditions, such as small bowel cancers or lymphomas, the diagnosis can be made and the pathologic site localized at this point, and intraoperative endoscopy will not be necessary. The advancement of the endoscope to the cecum requires several pairs of hands. It is quite necessary that a mobile small bowel and mesentery be present for easy passage of the endoscope through the intestinal tract. All adhesions should be lysed.

Throughout the passage of the endoscope to the terminal ileum, two loops will tend to form, one along the greater curvature of the stomach and the second along the greater curvature of the duodenum. To minimize this effect and to allow some straightening of the endoscope, an assistant places the right hand on the stomach and the left hand on the duodenum to keep the instrument shaft as straight as possible. Passage of the instrument beneath the mesenteric vessels in the horizontal portion of the duodenum can be an area of potential iatrogenic mucosal trauma. It must be emphasized that passage through this area is performed with great care and under direct vision. Once the endoscope has passed beyond the ligament of Treitz, the surgeon grasps the tip of the endoscope and, in concert with the endoscopist who gently pushes the instrument, the surgeon pulls the tip forward into the small bowel. After advancement is accomplished for a distance of 2 to 3 ft into the small bowel, the proximal intestine is pleated onto the instrument shaft. This pleating will occur throughout the procedure as more and more instrument is passed into the distal intestine. Advancement through the small bowel is always performed under *direct vision*. This is necessary because small areas of mucosal trauma may occur. Lesions that are detected during this phase are marked with a silk suture

through the serosa of the bowel only. Full-thickness passage of suture material is to be avoided. As the instrument is advanced, the small bowel will begin to coil onto the shaft, and large loops will form. Excessive tension on the mesentery is to be avoided, and it should be checked frequently. With a standard colonoscope, the cecum should be reached in most examinations. Occasionally, for a variety of reasons the distal ileum cannot be reached, and examination of this area of the intestine must be performed in a retrograde fashion by passing the endoscope through the colon.

Once the cecum is reached, the operating room lights are dimmed or turned off and, using the technique of transillumination from the endoscope light, the bowel wall can be clearly outlined. This technique delineates the blood vessels in the bowel wall, and the smallest of vascular formations can be identified. The small bowel is examined in 10-cm segments by insufflating the bowel with air, inspecting with transillumination, and marking lesions as indicated. Air is then removed and an assistant, using the index and middle fingers in a scissoring manner, compresses the intestine to avoid distention of the distal bowel as the endoscope is removed. Occasionally, a suction artifact can result in a submucosal hematoma, which can mimic a vascular lesion. When this occurs, the dilemma can be resolved by using reverse transillumination, a technique that is performed by turning off the endoscope light and focusing a bright operating room light on the surface of the bowel. Using the magnification of the endoscope, the characteristic vascular network of an ectasia can be clearly distinguished from the solid submucosal hemorrhage. When the examination is completed, the endoscope is removed, and the surgical excision is dictated by the intraoperative findings. If only a few lesions are found, simple ellipse is appropriate. When lesions are grouped, limited resection is done. If lesions are multiple, they can be oversewn from the outside using endoscopic guidance or a combination of endoscopic cautery and oversewing.

Intraoperative endoscopy has been used for a wide variety of conditions, and the literature is replete with case reports and small series experiences. The widest use of intraoperative endoscopy has been in the management of occult and gastrointestinal bleeding.[18, 20] With the increased use of nonoperative enteroscopy, lesions are being discovered in the small bowel with increasing frequency. Since therapeutic potential cannot be realized at present with sonde enteroscopes, intraoperative endoscopy offers this choice. Intraoperative endoscopy will not be necessary on a frequent basis. Using standard investigative techniques of gastroscopy and colonoscopy with angiography, gastrointestinal bleeding sites can be identified in at least 95% of patients. Only a small number of patients (1 to 5%), bleed from the small intestine; however, when a small bowel source is suspected and other areas have been eliminated by standard testing, intraoperative endoscopy offers the only consistent method of specific localization and treatment of such lesions. In addition, the rest of the gastrointestinal tract can be completely cleared of other potential lesions with this technique. Other uses of intraoperative enteroscopy have been reported,[23] with treatment strategies for Peutz-Jeghers disease and other polyposis syndromes being suggested.

Intraoperative endoscopy is still the final determination on small bowel pathologic conditions because it offers a complete view of the mucosal surface for the endoscopist and a transilluminated and surface view for the surgeon. Intraoperative endoscopy, however, is not perfect, and some vascular ectasia has been missed with the technique.[24]

CONCLUSION

Enteroscopy has made significant advances in the past few years but remains a difficult, time-consuming process with instruments that have frustrating limitations. Investigation in the area of enteroscopy continues, and it is anticipated that technology will respond to the limitations that exist in instrumentation. Until that time, push enteroscopy, using readily available instruments will continue to be the most common method for investigating the proximal small bowel. Enteroscopy using expensive instruments is probably best performed by groups interested in this process or in medical centers. Intraoperative endoscopy continues to be the only consistent method of examining the small bowel, and perhaps an intraoperative enteroscope with the flexibility and diameter of the traditional enteroscopes will be developed.

Acknowledgment

The author would like to recognize Mary Last for her assistance and support in the preparation of this manuscript.

References

1. Classen M, Fruhmorgen P, Koch H, et al. Enteroskopie-fiberendoskopie von jejunum und ileum. Dtsch Med Wochenschr 11:401–411, 1972.
2. Deyhle P, Jenny S, Fumagnalli J, et al. Endoscopy of the whole small intestine. Endoscopy 4:155–157, 1972.
3. Tada M, Akasaka Y, Misaki F, et al. Clinical evaluation of a sonde-type small intestine fiberscope. Endoscopy 8:33–38, 1977.
4. Maglinte DD, Hall R, Miller RE, et al. Detection of surgical lesions of the small bowel by enteroclysis. Am J Surg 147:225–228, 1978.
5. Nolan DJ: Radiology of the small intestine. In: Nelson RL, Nyhus LM, eds. Surgery of the small intestine. Norwalk, CT, Appleton & Lange, 1987:59–83.
6. Treves S, Grand RJ, Eraklis AJ. Pentagastrin stimulation of technetium-99m uptake by ectopic gastric mucosa in a Meckel's diverticulum. Radiology 128:711–712, 1978.
7. Bowden TA. Endoscopy of the small intestine. Surg Clin North Am 69:1237–1247, 1989.
8. Parker HW, Agayoff JD. Enteroscopy and small bowel biopsy utilizing a peroral colonoscope. Gastrointest Endosc 29:139–140, 1983.
9. Barkin JS, Reiner DK, Lewis BS, et al. Diagnostic and therapeutic jejunoscopy with the SIF-10L enteroscope: longer is really better (abstract). Gastrointest Endosc 36:214, 1990.
10. Shimizu S, Tada M, Kawai K. Development of a new insertion technique in push-type enteroscopy. Am J Gastroenterol 82:844–847, 1987.
11. Lewis BS, Waye JD. Chronic gastrointestinal bleeding of obscure origin: role of small bowel enteroscopy. Gastroenterology 94:1117–1120, 1988.
12. Gostout CJ, Bender CE. Cholangiopancreatography, sphincterotomy, and common duct stone removal via Roux-en-Y limb enteroscopy. Gastroenterology 95:156–163, 1988.
13. Tada M, Shimizu S, Kawai K. A new transnasal sonde-type fiberscope (SSIF VII) as a pan-enteroscope. Endoscopy 18:121–124, 1986.
14. Gostout C, Schroeder K, Burton D. Small bowel enteroscopy: an early experience in gastrointestinal bleeding of unknown origin. Gastrointest Endosc 37:5–8, 1991.
15. Dabezies M, Fisher R, Krevsky B. Video small bowel enteroscopy: early experience with a prototype instrument. Gastrointest Endosc 37:60–62, 1991.
16. Ament M. A large investment for small intestinal endoscopy (editorial). Gastrointest Endosc 29:59–60, 1983.
17. Bowden TA. Intraoperative endoscopy of the gastrointestinal tract. In: Dent T, Strodel W, Turcotte J, eds. Surgical endoscopy. Chicago: Year Book Medical, 1985:167.
18. Bowden TA. Intraoperative endoscopy of the gastrointestinal tract: clinical necessity or lack of preoperative preparation? World J Surg 13:186–189, 1989.
19. Bowden TA. Intraoperative gastrointestinal endoscopy. In: Cameron J, ed. Current surgical therapy. Philadelphia, BC Decker, 1989:364–366.
20. Bowden TA, Hooks VH, Mansberger AR. Intraoperative gastrointestinal endoscopy in the management of occult gastrointestinal bleeding. South Med J 72:1532–1534, 1979.
21. Bowden TA, Hooks VH, Mansberger AR. Intraoperative gastrointestinal endoscopy. Ann Surg 191:680–687, 1980.
22. Bowden TA, Hooks VH, Teeslink CR, et al. Occult gastrointestinal bleeding: locating the cause. Am Surg 46:80–87, 1980.
23. Mathus-Vliegan E, Tytgat G. Intraoperative endoscopy: technique, indications and results. Gastrointest Endosc 32:381–384, 1986.
24. Lewis B, Wenger J, Waye J. Intra-operative endoscopy versus SBE, are the findings comparable? (abstract) Gastrointest Endosc 36:218, 1990.

20

Technique of Diagnostic Colonoscopy

Kenneth A. Forde

The successful passage of a thin, flexible tube (an endoscope) through a tortuous, contracting organ that has a moist surface, often contains fluid, and is to some extent fixed (the colon) is essentially an art. Although much of it can be articulated and some of it can be standardized, it remains to a large extent a matter of style. Each author therefore customarily expounds on the particular technique he or she has mastered and found effective.[1-3] This author will not alter that tradition.

The elements necessary for successful colonoscopy include (1) adequate preparation of the patient, both psychologic and mechanical; (2) adequate preparation of the endoscopist, which includes knowledge of the instrumentation, knowledge of colonic anatomy (including postoperative changes) and pathology, and the limitations and hazards of the procedure itself; (3) mastery of the principles and techniques of insertion as well as examination; and (4) use of the services of a well-trained and alert gastrointestinal endoscopic assistant.

PATIENT PREPARATION

Anything that decreases the reflex excitability of the patient makes the procedure more tolerable, lessens the amount of analgesic and sedative medication needed, and often facilitates the examination for the endoscopist as well. This is why "informed consent" involves not only enunciation of potential hazards but also some simple description of the technique, explanation of possible periodic discomfort, discussion of the importance of and technique of preparation,

and reassurance that the morbidity of the procedure is indeed low and that the examiner is prepared to provide prompt management of adverse sequelae. The patient should understand that there is time following the endoscopic procedure to discuss and decide upon open surgical intervention should it be necessary. This author has found it extremely useful to air these concerns before the procedure is initiated. It is also important to discover if the patient has a history of unusual bleeding after injury, is taking drugs that might modify platelet function (therefore requiring their discontinuation if possible several days before the procedure), and whether antibiotics are needed to protect diseased cardiac valves or indwelling prosthetic materials. In this regard, this author essentially follows the guidelines of the American Heart Association.[4]

Excellent mechanical bowel preparation is absolutely necessary if an efficient, safe, and informative colonoscopic examination is to be achieved. If the mucosa is not well visualized, the diagnosis may be inaccurate or impossible, and instrumental damage may go unrecognized. Furthermore, a complication such as perforation would have increased morbidity if the fecal content in the bowel lumen is significant. Except in the presence of acute bleeding, active inflammation, suspected ischemia, or a recently created anastomosis, vigorous and thorough mechanical preparation is employed by most colonoscopists. There are several forms of mechanical preparation possible, but the polyethylene glycol electrolyte lavage solutions (this author's preference) enjoy the greatest popularity at present. Other forms of preparation that are sometimes employed involve the combination of a saline cathartic (usually sodium phosphate or magnesium citrate) and enemas or colonic lavages. With the latter, there must be more concern about electrolyte imbalance, especially in patients who take diuretic medications chronically. In addition, the preparation time is usually longer (2 to 2.5 days). Some postgastrectomy patients experience symptoms of dumping syndrome after saline cathartic administration.

PREPARATION OF THE ENDOSCOPIST

The endoscopist should be qualified to perform the procedure as enunciated by the guidelines of several organizations concerned with the performance of endoscopy.[5, 6] If the patient undergoing endoscopy has had a barium enema examination, it is useful for the endoscopist to review the results. It is often helpful in predicting anatomic variations or potential difficulty in insertion as well as in localization of lesions. The colonoscopist should also have received training in the use of fluoroscopic and electrocautery equipment, as they will be necessary at times in diagnostic examination. Equipment for resuscitation should be available, as should staff members who are qualified to perform cardiopulmonary resuscitation.

TECHNIQUE OF INSERTION

One of the concepts the endoscopist must understand from the outset is that the examiner is initially attempting to reach the highest level of insertion (usually the cecum) as expeditiously as possible, with careful inspection planned for the withdrawal phase of the examination. An exception is when one is looking for vascular ectasias (areas of angiodysplasia, arteriovenous malformations), which are most commonly found in the cecum and ascending colon. In such cases, the colonoscopist is especially on the lookout in the insertion phase when one is certain that the area visualized has not been previously traumatized, because submucosal hemorrhage from instrumental contusion or suction can occasionally cause confusion in recognizing these tiny lesions. Of course one always maintains an alert posture on insertion and does not ignore lesions of significance when encountered, noting at least their location. Hints that lesions may be present should not be ignored. For example, a trail of bloody mucus (what we

have called the "herald sign") suggests that there must be some mucosal lesion or disruption ahead.

Another concept to be grasped is that one places the instrument in positions that allow the bowel to be pleated or accordioned over it rather than simply pushing the instrument into the colon. One should try to make a small portion of the instrument go a long distance—in other words, with more than one-to-one movement. This is why to-and-fro movement, jiggling, or shaking the instrument shaft (also called dithering) can be so effective.

Still another caveat is to know where the lumen is at all times. This not only will assure greater efficiency in insertion but also will decrease the likelihood of instrumental impingement on the bowel wall, with consequent bowing of the bowel as more of the instrument is inserted. During insertion, it is more efficient if the bowel is not widely dilated, as from over-insufflation. Telescoping is more feasible if the colonic mucosa can cling to the instrument, so to speak. One should always leave a little distance between the instrument tip and the open lumen ahead. With a "red-out" (instrument tip against the mucosa), no progress is possible. One should also recognize paradoxical movement and use it to advantage. Paradoxical movement occurs when a loop is being formed or reduced. If the examiner cannot see where the instrument is going, it is important to withdraw it, identify the lumen, and start over. One should resist the temptation to "hold on to conquered territory." If a certain point in the colon was previously reached, the chances are overwhelming that it will be reached again.

These and other caveats help to avoid dangerous and painful stretching of the bowel wall or mesentery, as well as the creation of loops that prevent the force of insertion from being transmitted to the tip of the instrument. Pain, resistance to movement, and blanching of the mucosa are danger signs to be avoided. When these symptoms or signs are encountered, one should change the maneuver or abandon the procedure.

Modern colonoscopes are constructed in such a fashion that the right hand is necessary only to manipulate the body or shaft of the instrument by grasping it firmly but not too tightly, being sensitive to the need for torque (twisting in any direction) as an aid in directing the instrument tip, often complementing the left-to-right deflection. Sometimes it is necessary for the examiner's right hand to be taken off the instrument shaft—for example, to insert or manipulate an accessory instrument. At such times, an assistant's hand should replace that of the endoscopist on the instrument shaft. The left hand is used to grasp the head with the controls, mainly in the palm and fourth and fifth fingers fully and the middle finger slightly in such a fashion that the index and middle fingers can at all times easily reach the suction (proximal) button and the air-water (distal) injection button, respectively (Fig. 20–1). The left thumb is used only to rotate the wheels, which results in up-and-down and left-to-right deflection. Although the beginner tends to think of and use these knobs separately, it is more efficient to learn to use them together so that an almost rotatory motion is accomplished using the left thumb. In fact, the left thumb and right hand, through the integrated simultaneous combination of tip deflection with the left hand and rotation (torquing), insertion, and withdrawal with the right hand, allow for efficient insertion and withdrawal of the instrument throughout the procedure. This is why this author prefers to insert the instrument with both dial controls in the unlocked position.

Before beginning a diagnostic procedure, it is necessary to ensure that the instrument to be used is in working order; that air, water, and

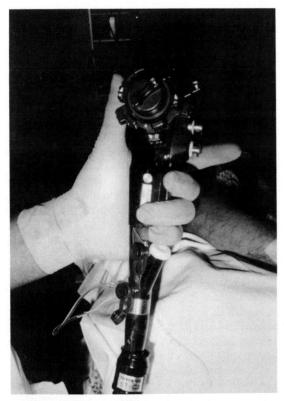

Figure 20–1. Position of the left hand and fingers holding the colonoscope.

suction channels are operating properly; and that biopsy forceps, cytology brush, snare, and cautery are available. If fluoroscopy is available, we customarily place an external splinting device on the colonoscope in case it is needed during the examination, especially with some of the older, stiffer instruments.

If a patient needs antibiotics around the time of the procedure, they are customarily administered intravenously in the holding or recovery area 20 to 30 minutes before initiating the examination. If an abdominal wall (including inguinal) hernia is present, it is noted and at the conclusion of the procedure its continuing reducibility is confirmed. We begin the procedure by placing the patient in the left lateral recumbent position, unless one is inserting the instrument through a colostomy stoma, in which case the patient remains supine. Monitoring devices (sphygmomanometer, pulse oximeter) are attached, and a small needle is inserted in an upper extremity vein through which medication (usually meperidine and midazolam) is administered. This author leaves the needle in place so that further medication (analgesic, sedative, or antispasmodic agents) may be given during the procedure, if necessary, and as a conduit for the naloxone administered at the conclusion of the examination to counteract the effect of the meperidine. If this author is examining a patient in whom areas of angiodysplasia are suspected but are not readily observed, the naloxone is administered before the instrument leaves the ascending colon because it is thought by some that meperidine may prevent visualization of these tiny lesions.

Although the endoscopist's assistant has many roles in the endoscopy suite, his or her role in certain specific activities is essential for the most efficient conduct of the examination. For example, whenever the endoscopist removes the right hand from the instrument shaft (as for the insertion of snares and other accessory instruments), the assistant should automatically place a hand on the shaft to prevent the instrument from slipping out of the colon. If the external splinting device is used, the assistant must keep it in position at the anus to prevent possible perforation if the device is accidentally inserted further as the colonoscope is advanced. If abdominal pressure is needed during intubation, it is usually the assistant who performs this function.

The examination is begun by inspection of the perianal region for fissures, fistulas, hemorrhoids, condylomas, and rare neoplasms such as melanoma and anal gland and squamous carcinomas. The lubricated, gloved right index finger is gently inserted into the rectum, and a rectal examination (including the posterior prostate in older men) is carefully performed. The endoscopist may unfortunately be the only individual performing routine rectal examination on the patient and should not neglect the opportunity for discovering important local pathologic conditions.

Leaving the right index finger in the rectum and using the left hand, the operator places the lubricated instrument tip perpendicular to the right index finger, and using the right thumb, gently inserts the instrument tip as the right index finger is withdrawn (Fig. 20–2). The operator then takes the head of the instrument in the left hand (making sure that the dial controls are in the unlocked position) and holds the instrument shaft with the right hand, the instrument being draped on the examining table between the examiner and the patient's right thigh. This simple maneuver prevents the weight of the portion of the instrument that is outside the body from producing too much countertraction, which may induce the instrument to slip out of the colon.

Once in the rectum, a small amount of air insufflation is necessary to visualize the direction of the lumen, as well as to adequately examine the entire circumference of the rectum because its lumen is usually quite large compared with other regions of the colon. From this point on, the strategy is to avoid creating a loop in the sigmoid colon by keeping it as straight as possible from the beginning of the examination. If the instrument were simply inserted following the course of the visualized lumen, one would be led to the examiner's left (the patient's right side), and a so-called alpha (α)-loop might be created; I try to avoid this by purposefully

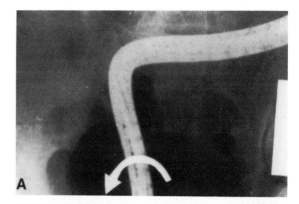

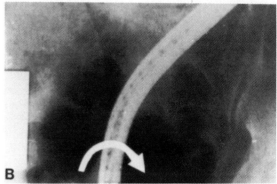

Figure 20–3. (A, B) Torquing the instrument to prevent formation of a sigmoid loop.

turning the instrument shaft to the right, using tip deflection with the left thumb to permit visualization of the lumen (Fig. 20–3). For a couple of minutes this may seem awkward to the beginner, but it is well worth it if looping of the sigmoid colon is thus avoided. Whenever possible, we attempt jiggling the instrument (shaking it in place with negligible pushing) and perform to-and-fro insertion and withdrawal motions, allowing telescoping of the bowel over the instrument.

The sigmoid colon (Fig. 20–4A) is of variable length but is often longer than commonly known to the nonendoscopist. Consequently, the first truly acute angle encountered by the fledgling endoscopist (and embarrassingly by experienced endoscopists who do not employ fluoroscopy or follow the locations of lesions to the operating room) is often thought to be the splenic flexure. It usually is not, but rather is the sigmoid colon–descending colon junction after a long sigmoid colon has been traversed. It is important to recognize this fact so that subsequent maneuvers are more logical and effective.

If the distal descending colon has been reached with the sigmoid colon in a relatively straight configuration, insertion is continued, still torquing the shaft to the right as the de-

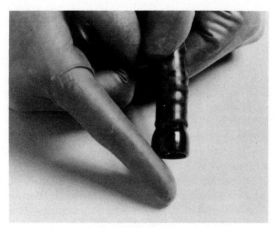

Figure 20–2. Insertion of the instrument tip.

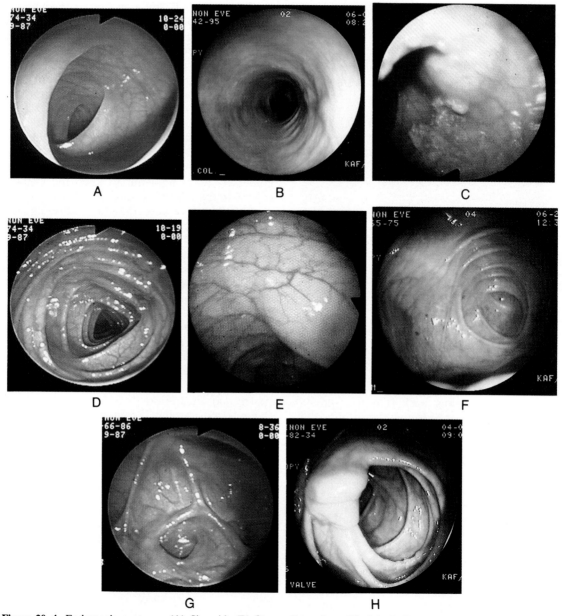

Figure 20–4. Endoscopic anatomy. **(A)** Sigmoid. **(B)** Descending colon. **(C)** Splenic flexure. **(D)** Transverse colon. **(E)** Hepatic flexure. **(F)** Ascending colon. **(G)** Appendiceal orifice. **(H)** Ileocecal valve.

scending colon is intubated. If, however, the sigmoid colon has not been maintained in a straight position, further attempts at advancing the instrument into the descending colon will be thwarted through either resistance to passage or less than one-to-one movement of the instrument tip and patient discomfort from bowing of the sigmoid colon and stretching of its wall and mesentery (Fig. 20–5). Maneuvering at this point must be changed or discontinued lest the result be disruption of the apex of the sigmoid colon or a tear of the mesentery with consequent

internal bleeding (which may not be apparent until its consequences appear sometime after the procedure has been concluded). If the examiner recognizes the formation of this loop, the appropriate first maneuver is to withdraw the instrument, torquing it in a clockwise direction; advancement may then be possible (see Fig. 20–3B).

Sometimes a more complex loop, the α-loop, is formed, and is often not reducible by withdrawal and clockwise rotation when the instrument tip is in the descending colon. In fact, the

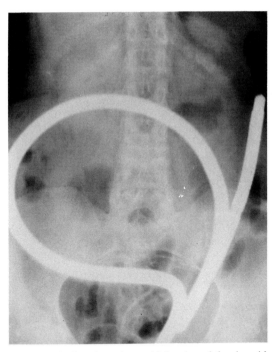

Figure 20–5. Creating a loop with bowing of the sigmoid.

instrument often slips back into the sigmoid colon, or one keeps re-forming the α-loop. This type of loop is most easily reduced without losing ground if the examiner can reach the splenic flexure (if the patient is tolerating the loop without discomfort) and hook the tip around the medial aspect of the splenic flexure by acute tip deflection, and then by withdrawal and counterclockwise or clockwise rotation one can reduce the α-loop and thus straighten the sigmoid colon. Having done this, it may be possible to achieve further intubation and progress into the transverse colon. At times, however, attempting further insertion results in reformation of the loop. To remedy this one can reduce the loop and have an assistant apply abdominal pressure (often from the epigastrium and sometimes from the right, down to the pelvis) to keep the loop from re-forming. This is an important concept because this author thinks it is potentially dangerous for the assistant to actually attempt reduction of the loop of bowel with the instrument in it. If fluoroscopy is available, one first hooks the tip of the colonoscope around the splenic flexure, locking or holding the dial controls firmly in place. It is usually possible to reduce the loop and then slide the well-lubricated external splinting device over the instrument under fluoroscopic guidance up to the proximal descending colon (but not to the flexure for fear of putting too

much tension on the lienocolic attachments) (Fig. 20–6). This author usually inserts the splinting device with a constant rotatory motion in the same direction, thus minimizing the possibility of laceration and lifting up of a flap of intestinal mucosa. If the device does not slide easily or the patient experiences discomfort, its use should be discontinued. If the mucosa appears inflamed and friable, if active bleeding is present, or if fluoroscopy is not available, it is dangerous to use the external splinting device. It should never be used without fluoroscopic guidance. It is important to keep the sigmoid colon straight during insertion of the splinting device and to be sure that the entire sigmoid colon has indeed been straightened and splinted. Otherwise, one could be wedging the device against the bowel wall unknowingly at a point of angulation in the sigmoid colon or at the sigmoid colon–descending colon junction, with the potential for perforation.

Among the problems most commonly encountered in attempting sigmoid colon intubation are spasm and diverticulosis, often in conjunction. It is tempting when spasm is first encountered to overinsufflate with air. This is an error because it may only produce further spasm and frustration. It is best to wait a few seconds, positioning the instrument tip in the center of the lumen ready to proceed when the bowel relaxes. Diverticulosis, although it may be universal, is most commonly encountered in the sigmoid colon, where the bowel may also be less pliable, more thick-walled, more angulated, and more fixed, which are all possibly related to bouts of previous inflammation or prolonged spasm. One has to be able to differ-

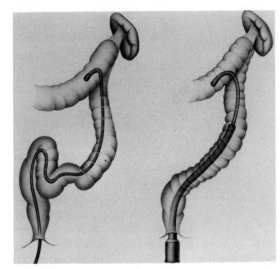

Figure 20–6. Hooking the splenic flexure and straightening and splinting the sigmoid.

entiate the ostium of a diverticulum from the lumen, and some diverticula are so wide-mouthed or so long that they may simulate the colonic lumen. Before advancing the instrument, it is important to look ahead and around, gaining some perspective on "the lay of the land." The lumen is usually at a 90° angle from any diverticular orifice, but the colon may then have an acute turn or spiral that changes the configuration, almost from endoscopic frame to endoscopic frame (Fig. 20–7). Occasionally it is possible to jiggle the instrument, allowing the tip to find the lumen, but diverticular-laden bowel is often too stiff to permit this. One usually recognizes when the descending colon is reached by its open "tunnel view," which it assumes because it is fixed along the white line of Toldt (Fig. 20–4B). Sometimes, however, one is confused about location because the interhaustral septa of the descending colon may be so thickened in extensive diverticular disease that the bowel takes on the appearance of the transverse colon in this region.

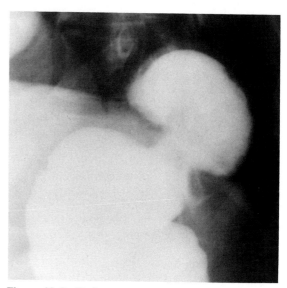

Figure 20–8. Barium enema splenic flexure herniation through the diaphragm with obstruction on retrograde filling.

The splenic flexure is sometimes clearly identifiable by a bluish globular viscus depressing the bowel (Fig. 20–4C). The endoscope usually slides around the normal splenic flexure quite easily, but if there is difficulty, especially in a patient with previous operation or injury, one should be concerned about fixation at this point making the spleen and colon more vulnerable to injury. On one occasion in this author's experience, we resorted to a barium study when there was failure to progress easily beyond this point. This study demonstrated the presence of a diaphragmatic hernia–containing colon (Fig. 20–8).

Sometimes the angle of the bowel at the splenic flexure is so acute that the lumen of the distal transverse colon is not easily visualized or entered. With a small loop in the splenic flexure, it is often easier to intubate the transverse colon, but a loop that is too large may produce so much elevation that the diaphragm is impinged on, causing shoulder discomfort. Sometimes gentle to-and-fro motion will allow the tip to enter the transverse colon, but the examiner should not withdraw the endoscope too vigorously with a fixed loop at this location for fear of damaging the spleen.

Another maneuver that sometimes results in easier intubation of the transverse colon is placing the patient in the supine position when the splenic flexure is reached. Only after the distal transverse colon has been definitely entered does the examiner cease concentration on the clockwise torque that was used to maintain the straight sigmoid colon configuration.

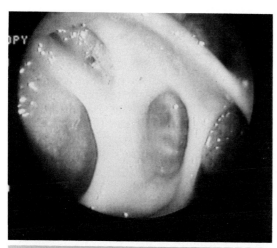

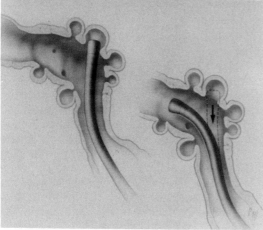

Figure 20–7. Finding the lumen with extensive diverticulosis.

The transverse colon can usually be identified by its triangular so-called cathedral ceiling appearance resulting from its suspension by the three teniae coli (Fig. 20–4D). Seeing the transmitted cardiac apical impulse helps identify the left transverse colon, as does the initial appearance of the adjacent broad bluish green background shadow of the left lobe of the liver.

Since the transverse colon is usually on a long mesentery and is not as fixed as the rest of the colon, it is easier to intubate if the examiner resists the temptation to insert a large segment of the instrument. The midtransverse colon often dips into the pelvis (Fig. 20–9) and may lead the tip of the colonoscope into this area, producing so much looping that attempts at advancement become ineffective. This is why transillumination in the right lower quadrant may indicate that the mid–transverse colon has been reached, and not the cecum, as the novice may think. I have found that by keeping the instrument in midposition, using to-and-fro and jiggling motions, the examiner can progress rapidly through the "gothic straits" (a term for the transverse colon) until the hepatic flexure is reached. If one remembers to keep the proximal

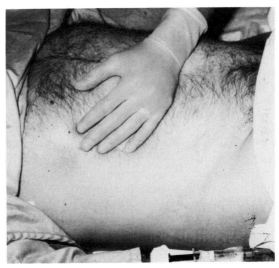

Figure 20–10. The assistant's hand is applying pressure to the transverse colon loop.

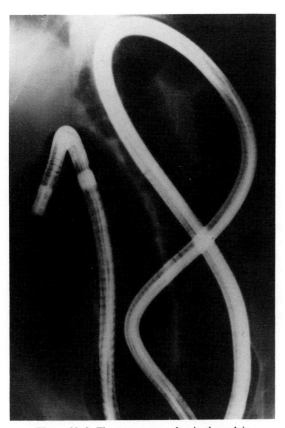

Figure 20–9. The transverse colon in the pelvis.

transverse colon deflated and deflects the tip of the instrument so that it is pointed in the direction of the patient's head, on slight withdrawal the transverse colon may be shortened by reduction of its loop, thus making insertion into the distal ascending colon easier.

At times the hepatic flexure is fixed because of a previous right upper quadrant operation. Sometimes it is necessary for the assistant to hold up the transverse colon for the distal ascending colon to be intubated (Fig. 20–10).

The hepatic flexure may represent a significant challenge, even for the experienced endoscopist. If the patient has undergone a previous right upper quadrant surgical procedure, there may be fixation and less maneuverability of the flexure, which is often a series of loops and may be quite redundant. One of the traps in endoscopic localization is that with angulation and spiraling at the hepatic flexure, the endoscopic appearance of the confluence of the teniae may be simulated (what has often been dubbed "the fool's cecum"), but of course there is no ileocecal valve!

Sometimes with a very redundant transverse colon, one makes a complete circle with the endoscope in the bowel, forming a so-called gamma (γ)-loop. If this is well tolerated by the patient and if there is length remaining in the instrument, it is actually easier to continue passage into the ascending colon and to the cecum (Fig. 20–11). The major problem occurs on withdrawal. As one reduces the γ-loop, much of the reduction will be done blindly, and the colon in this area will not be well examined. Ideally, then, with withdrawal and rotation, the

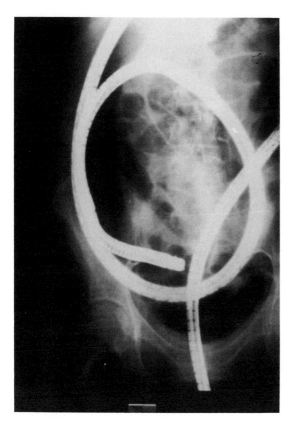

Figure 20–11. There is a gamma loop in the transverse colon, but cecal intubation is possible.

examiner should try to reduce and then straighten the transverse colon, allowing more efficient advancement into the proximal ascending colon or, if one has reached the cecum in the γ configuration, the transverse colon should be straightened (optimally with fluoroscopy) before the instrument is withdrawn from the ascending colon. The most important element in rounding the hepatic flexure is a deflated, straightened transverse colon in a patient who has not undergone a previous right upper quadrant operation.

Identification of the hepatic flexure by the overlying hepatic shadow may be very misleading in that the hepatic shadow may be cast from the distal transverse colon all the way up to the middle of the ascending colon. Rarely, one fortuitously encounters a globular bluish green shadow (the gallbladder) projecting from a broader, flat shadow of similar hue (the liver), and only then can one identify the hepatic flexure with absolute certainty (Fig. 20–4E). As one progresses, to the ascending colon, however, the folds are endoscopically of lower profile (Fig. 20–4F). If the ascending colon is not fixed (as from previous information or opera-

tion), one can often collapse it onto the tip of the instrument with gentle suction once the endoscope has rounded the corner into the distal ascending colon. Sometimes it is necessary to place the patient in the prone position to advance the instrument into the ascending colon. An assistant may also position the cecum with pressure in the right side of the groin or the middle or even left side of the lower abdomen (depending on the cecal position in the individual patient) to allow total colonoscopy.

It is important to be able to confirm total intubation of the colon by observing the confluence of the teniae coli and the appendiceal orifice, but the ileocecal valve must also be visualized (Fig. 20–4G). The appearance of the valve as observed by the endoscopist is varied and is rarely seen en face without special manipulation but is always identified as a submucosal mound. With the very significant amount of adipose tissue present, the yellowish appearance will sometimes overcome the normal pink hue of the mucosa (Fig. 20–4H). The endoscopist must always remember that a varying amount of cecum may lie proximal to the ileocecal valve and, like the radiologist, he or she has to be concerned about missing a cecal lesion if the cecum is not entirely visualized. Pressure on the abdominal wall to indent the bowel at the tip of the instrument or noting light transmitted through the abdominal wall may occur in the right lower quadrant if the tip of the instrument is in bowel that at that moment is in the right lower quadrant, but the possibilities of anatomic location range from sigmoid colon (sic) to transverse colon to cecum. Only the aforementioned internal landmarks or seeing the tip of the instrument at the end of the air column on fluoroscopy are infallible in confirming total colonic intubation.

WITHDRAWAL AND INSPECTION

Having reached the cecum, redundant endoscope is withdrawn to keep the bowel as straight as possible. If fluoroscopy is used, at this point, the configuration of the endoscope in the bowel should resemble a question mark or the numeral 7. I customarily withdraw the splinting device back toward the control section of the instrument shaft if or when there is enough remaining endoscope outside the body. The definitive examination is now undertaken, releasing the bowel from the instrument in the manner in which one lets a kite ascend. As the bowel wall moves away, it is examined carefully. With the wide angles of view now possible, it is easier to visualize most of the mucosa without much tip deflection. However, there are still potential blind spots for even the most expert and alert endoscopist. They occur at sharp angles, of which the most common are the medial aspect of the distal ascending colon at the hepatic flexure, the medial aspect of the distal transverse colon at the splenic flexure, and the medial aspect of the distal descending colon at the junction of the sigmoid colon and descending colon. The process of withdrawing the instrument has to be relatively slow and deliberate, anticipating when pleated bowel is about to slip away and keeping up with it, having the "endoscopic conscience" to reintubate an area not seen well, to irrigate away debris, and to aspirate fecal fluid to visualize the entire mucosal surface. It is on withdrawal through a tortuous sigmoid colon (a more frequent site of pathology than the ascending colon) that the challenge is greatest and coordination of tip deflection and shaft rotation at times becomes as challenging as the process of insertion. As an area of bowel is examined, it is deflated by suction to improve the patient's comfort. When the rectum is reached, it is frequently necessary to deflect the tip acutely, retroflexing the instrument to visualize the distal anorectum, otherwise, small, low-profile lesions may be overlooked (Fig. 20–12).

Despite the use of monitoring devices, as is customary at present, throughout the course of the examination, this author relies on the assistant's observation of the patient for discomfort,

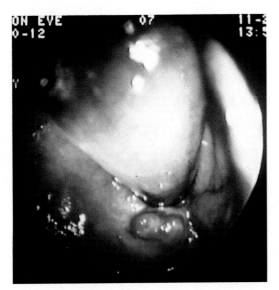

Figure 20–12. The endoscope tip is retroflexed in rectum.

degree of responsiveness, adequate respiratory exchange, clamminess, and abdominal distention. At the conclusion of the procedure (or earlier, if it is thought necessary), naloxone is administered and it is verified that hernias, if present, are still reducible.

There are certain conditions in individuals who present for diagnostic examination that require further discussion.

Colostomy

In the patient with a terminal colostomy, digital examination before initiation of the procedure is still important to assess whether significant stricture exists that might need dilation or skin release and whether or not there is subcutaneous herniation of bowel in which the endoscope may be trapped. One can usually be more liberal with air insufflation in the ostomate. In fact, it is sometimes necessary to insufflate almost throughout the procedure to achieve visualization because air will escape around the instrument at the colostomy site when the sphincter is not present.

Strictures

Colonoscopic evaluation of an area of stricture has its own hazards and limitations. If the area of narrowing has been discovered at endoscopy and is in a patient with a history of inflammatory bowel disease, there must be greater concern about overinsufflation. In the examination of any patient with a stricture, one may inadvertently overdistend the more proximal bowel, resulting in a risk of perforation (Fig. 20–13).

If the stricture cannot be traversed, one cannot rule out malignancy above the instrument tip, even with normal cytologic features through the stricture. However, at times, despite normal biopsy results, a cytology brush passed beyond the instrument tip into the area of stricture may yield malignant cells (Fig. 20–14).[7, 8] Sometimes the specimen is adequate for the pathologist to make a definitive diagnosis of carcinoma. The endoscopist should not be surprised at this combination (normal biopsy results and abnormal cytologic features) because the mucosa at the presenting distal end of the stenotic colon cancer is often normal bowel wall that is edematous because of pressure from the proximal mass. With an area of stricture, there may be more tendency toward looping of the distal bowel, which also increases the risk of perforation at

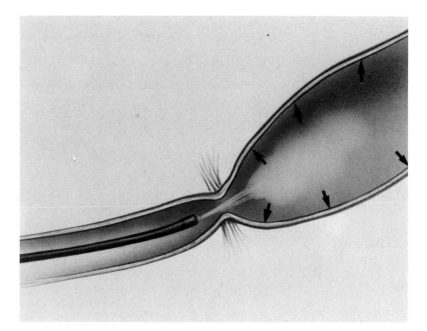

Figure 20–13. Overinsufflation of the bowel proximal to a stricture.

the site of the stricture or distal to it (Fig. 20–15). At an area of stricture, the bowel may be externally fixed because of inflammation or tumor extension, and overzealous manipulation may cause disruption at this site, with bowel perforation (Fig. 20–16). If a distal colon tumor is producing some stenosis but does not totally obstruct the progress of the endoscope, the examiner has to decide whether or not to attempt more proximal intubation in the indicated search—for example, for a synchronous neoplasm. Fixation, as previously mentioned, is a concern, as is overdistention of the noninvolved, and therefore more distensible-appearing, portion of the lumen (Fig. 20–17). Unless the area of narrowing is trivial, total endoscopy in most

circumstances should probably be deferred. Although all strictures should be sampled cytologically when feasible (with areas of angulation or fixation, the cytology brush may not be steerable into the lumen), it must be recalled that too early brushing of an anastomotic site may be misleading because one may harvest suspicious or atypical cells from granulation tissue.

Bleeding

Occasionally, it is necessary to perform diagnostic colonoscopy in the management of a patient with acute bleeding from the anus.[9] It is sometimes called for when the patient is not

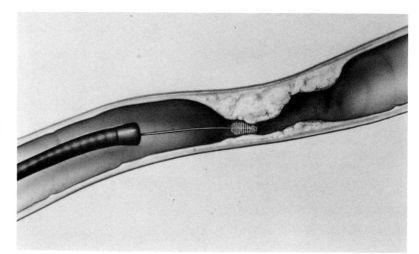

Figure 20–14. Cytologic sampling through a stricture.

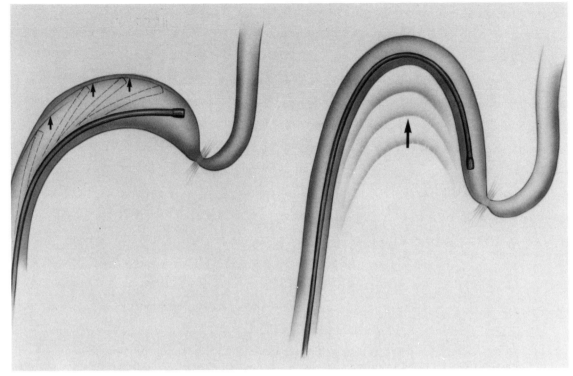

Figure 20–15. Bowing distal to the stricture.

bleeding rapidly enough for angiography to be revealing, when a nuclear scan may be abnormal but not localizing, or in a patient who continues to require blood volume replacement and the possibility of blind exploration exists. These patients are usually desperately ill and often in shock and require resuscitation and monitoring.

They may need to undergo colonoscopy in the intensive care unit or operating room. Preparation of the bowel under these circumstances is not usually possible and, fortunately, blood is such an excellent cathartic that if the patient is bleeding actively enough there will not be a need for preparation. The greatest discourage-

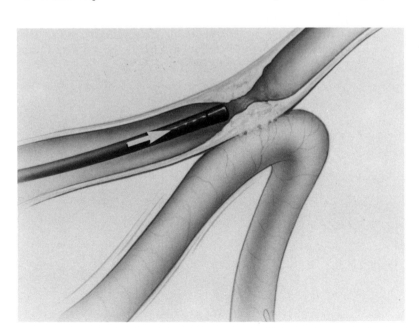

Figure 20–16. Fixation in the presence of a stenotic lesion.

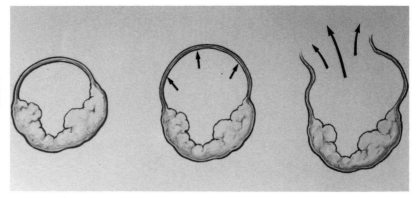

Figure 20–17. Mechanism of disruption, with overdistension in the presence of a near-circumferential lesion.

ment for the endoscopist who has had limited experience with examination of the actively bleeding patient is that there is often clotted blood in the rectum, which makes initiation of the examination frustrating. I routinely wash out the rectum before initiating the examination. Colonoscopy under these circumstances is innately more hazardous and should not, in my opinion, be attempted without previous significant experience in routine diagnostic colonoscopy. The patient, if possible, as well as the family and referring physician, should be made aware of the greater potential for complications and that a nonbleeding but low profile or submucosal condition could be overlooked in the presence of acute massive bleeding. In fact, we recommend that all patients examined acutely for bleeding undergo a follow-up elective diagnostic colonoscopy. During bleeding, diagnostic colonoscopy is often done with only small amounts of analgesia or sedation because of the

already unstable condition of the patient. It is important to have an adequate irrigating device (preferably of the jet variety) (Fig. 20–18) because a blood clot should be fragmented or dispersed rather than aspirated (Fig. 20–19). It is sometimes necessary to alter the patient's position so that the blood can collect in the dependent portion of the bowel lumen, and the instrument is then passed in the space above it. The findings at emergency colonoscopy for bleeding must be carefully and strictly interpreted.[11] If one cannot identify the lumen, the examination should be terminated. If bleeding has ceased and there is a tenacious blood clot present, the procedure will rarely be possible, and even if it is, the cause of bleeding will be inconclusive. Even if a bleeding source is found, colonoscopic localization may be difficult without fluoroscopy. Sometimes it is feasible or necessary to examine such patients intraoperatively.

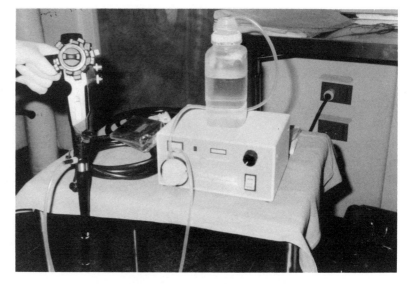

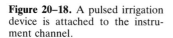

Figure 20–18. A pulsed irrigation device is attached to the instrument channel.

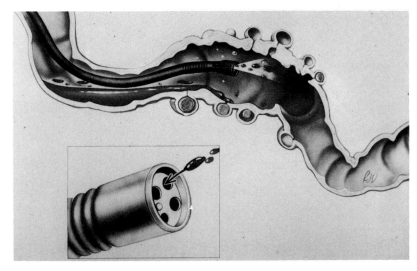

Figure 20–19. Colonoscopy during acute bleeding.

INTRAOPERATIVE DIAGNOSTIC COLONOSCOPY

Emergent Intraoperative Colonoscopy for Bleeding

Although colonoscopy without celiotomy is logistically easier and more desirable for patient management, there are uncommon situations in

which it becomes necessary to examine the acutely bleeding patient at the time of abdominal exploration but before the bowel is entered or resected. Under these circumstances the surgeon should place an occlusive intestinal clamp across the terminal ileum as early as possible and thread the colonoscope carefully up to the cecum, being sure that the bowel is adequately pleated over the instrument, especially in the sigmoid region where it will more commonly be bowed up without the presence of the tampon-

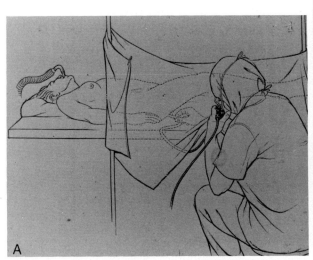

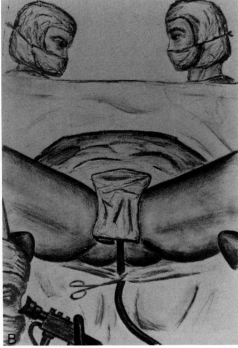

Figure 20–20. (A) Position and draping for intraoperative colonoscopy. (From Forde KA, Intraoperative colonoscopy. In: Hunt RH, Waye JD, eds. London: Chapman & Hall, 1981:192.) **(B)** Alternative position for intraoperative colonoscopy.

ade of the intact abdominal wall. All the endoscopist should do during this maneuver is ensure patency of the lumen of the instrument with the constant flow of water through the biopsy channel. When the cecum has been reached, the examination is begun, with irrigation being carried out as the endoscope is withdrawn. If a bleeding site is identified, the surgeon palpates the tip of the instrument and places a seromuscular suture to mark the area. Before the instrument is completely withdrawn, attempts should be made to decompress the bowel as much as possible, certainly before removing the occlusive clamp from the distal ileum.

Nonurgent Intraoperative Colonoscopy

At present, colonoscopy is occasionally required for diagnosis intraoperatively for three main indications: (1) enigmatic but nonacute gastrointestinal bleeding of significance, (2) location of the site of a previously removed malignant polyp when it has been decided that resection is necessary, and (3) when preoperative colonoscopy is not possible.

As part of the evaluation of chronic or recurrent enigmatic but significant gastrointestinal bleeding, intraoperative colonoscopy has been undertaken with significant success in this small but difficult group of patients. When intraoperative colonoscopy is planned either emergently or nonemergently, the patient is positioned before celiotomy so that the endoscopist will later be able to perform the examination without contaminating the operative field. Some exam-

iners prefer to place the patient's legs in stirrups, whereas others (this author included) prefer to elevate the thighs on pillows and approach the examination later from the patient's right side (Fig. 20–20). The colonoscope needs only the usual cleaning and disinfection; it does not need sterilization because it will not be in the operative field. This author customarily verifies that suction and irrigation are available and in working order and then inserts the instrument a few centimeters into the rectum, placing it carefully under the operating table until positioning, skin preparation, and other preliminary procedures are accomplished. After the abdomen has been opened and the surgeon has placed an occlusive clamp on the terminal ileum, the endoscopist takes up a position below or outside the sterile drapery or screening and proceeds with the examination. With video endoscopy, the examiner may easily stand as during routine colonoscopy or may sit if preferred (Fig. 20–21). Members of the surgical team may also view the endoscopic image, but it is important for the surgeon to aid in the passage of the instrument, especially by keeping the sigmoid colon from bowing up out of the pelvis and, at times, keeping the bowel in a relatively straight position so that the lumen may be more easily negotiated. Transillumination may be necessary to identify submucosal vascular lesions, and these lesions, as well as polypectomy sites (Fig. 20–22), may be marked by the surgeon with seromuscular sutures for identification. Sometimes the surgeon has to divide adhesive bands or "take down" (separate) the sigmoid colon from its lateral attachments to facilitate intubation. If one is searching for a polypectomy site

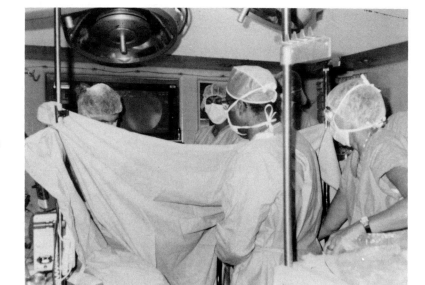

Figure 20–21. Intraoperative video colonoscopy in progress.

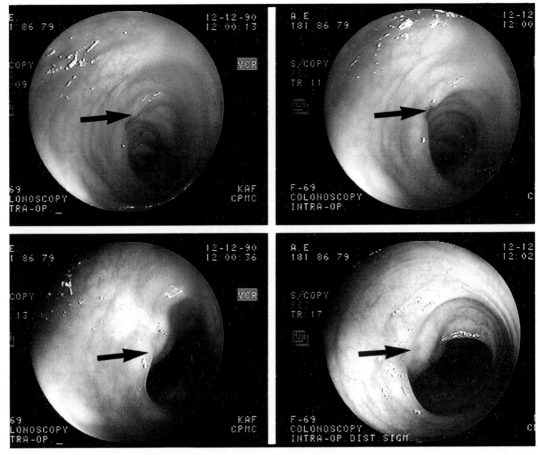

Figure 20–22. Polypectomy site identified by intraoperative colonoscopy.

(most often in the sigmoid colon), and therefore total colonoscopy is not the goal, the occlusive clamp may be placed more distally—for example, on the transverse colon. However, the surgeon should watch carefully for the escape of air into the proximal bowel and, in fact, at the conclusion of the procedure should be sure that the colon is adequately decompressed before the instrument is withdrawn from the rectum.

With adequate preparation of both patient and examiner, a good background knowledge of normal and postoperative anatomy and of the pathologic states that may affect the colon, the technical aspects of colonoscopic intubation are possible to master and should result in minimal morbidity.

References

1. Waye JD. Colonoscopy intubation techniques without fluoroscopy. In: Hunt RH, Waye JD, eds. Colonoscopy techniques, clinical practice and color atlas. Chicago: Year Book Medical Publishers, 1981:147–178.
2. Sugawa C, Schuman BM. Primer of gastrointestinal fiberoptic endoscopy. Boston: Little, Brown, 1981:99–131.
3. Shinya HS. Colonoscopy. New York: Igaku-Shoin Medical Publishers, 1982:48–76.
4. Dajani AS, Bisno AL, Chung KJ, et al. Prevention of bacterial endocarditis. Recommendations by the American Heart Association. JAMA 264:2912–2922, 1990.
5. Society of American Gastrointestinal Endoscopic Surgeons. Granting of privileges for gastrointestinal endoscopy by surgeons. Los Angeles: Publication 0011. 1992.
6. American Society for Gastrointestinal Endoscopy. Principles of training in gastrointestinal endoscopy. Manchester, MA: 1992.
7. Forde KA, Treat MR. Colonoscopy in the evaluation of strictures. Dis Colon Rectum 28:699–701, 1985.
8. Jeevanandam V, Treat MR, Forde KA. A comparison of direct brush cytology and biopsy in the diagnosis of colorectal cancer. Gastrointest Endosc 33:370–371, 1987.
9. Schuman BM: Vision for the blind colectomy (editorial). Gastrointest Endosc 27:238–239, 1981.
10. Forde KA: Bleeding from the small intestine and colon. In: Madden RE, ed. Problems in general surgery. Philadelphia: JB Lippincott, 1987:4:363–372.

21

Therapeutic Colonoscopy
Polypectomy, Management of Bleeding, and Decompressive Techniques

William I. Wolff and Hiromi Shinya

HISTORY

In the early 1970s, diagnostic and therapeutic colonoscopy was at about the stage that laparoscopic surgery was a few years before—a promising but untested procedure. There were certain notable differences, however. Video cameras were not yet invented. The techniques were either self-taught or required peeking through an observer scope attached to the eyepiece of the colonoscope. (Imagine the situation in the early days at the Beth Israel Medical Center with 15 visitors or more standing around and "trying to get a look").[1] There were many who claimed the procedure was unnecessary, uninformative, and dangerous.[2-4] Our early reports were turned down by all the radiology journals.[5] We did not know ourselves whether complete colonoscopy and polypectomy were akin to landing a plane on a naval carrier in a heavy sea—something that could be accomplished safely but only by a highly skilled few. There were no courses to be taken and we never thought of trying it out on pigs.

Then again, as Ogden Nash once commented, "Progress may have been all right once, but it went on too long."

MEDICATION AND MONITORING

Premedication of the patient for therapeutic endoscopic procedures is similar in most respects to that used for diagnostic colonoscopy. However, the procedure may last longer, requiring intraoperative supplementation of medication and the need for a higher degree of patient cooperation, necessitating larger dosages.

The selection of drugs and dosages must be tailored to any given patient. For sedation, we generally employ diazepam (Valium) or midazolam (Versed) administered slowly by the intravenous route in appropriate doses.

These agents are generally preceded by meperidine (Demerol) administered intravenously through the same needle in doses of 25 to 100 mg. This is readily reversed, if necessary, by naloxone (Narcan) given in doses of 0.4 mg intravenously or intramuscularly, which may be safely repeated, if necessary, every 4 to 6 minutes. (Naloxone is contraindicated in any patient who is participating in a methadone maintenance program.)

Great care must be taken to avoid cardiac or respiratory depression, particularly in cardiac patients and older individuals. Equipment is currently available for finger monitoring of patients to provide continuous recording of blood pressure, pulse rate, and blood oxygen saturation during the procedure. Although not required in the majority of patients, this type of monitoring can prove useful in selected cases, and pulse oximetry is becoming a standard for care.

Ordinary traditional sigmoidoscopy, and both diagnostic and therapeutic colonoscopy, can be associated with a transient bacteremia. Hence, prophylactic antimicrobial therapy has been recommended for individuals at high risk for the development of endocarditis, including those with intravascular foreign bodies such as prosthetic heart valves, pacemakers, and the like; valvular disorders, including mitral valve prolapse; rheumatic heart disease; septal defects; and other congenital anomalies. In this regard, the recommendations of the American Heart Association are suggested.[6]

GENERAL COMPLICATIONS OF COLONOSCOPY

Complications associated with therapeutic colonoscopy are related to the endoscopic undertaking in general, as well as additional complications related to the special procedure under consideration. The latter will be considered separately.

General complications include the following: (1) cardiopulmonary complications, (2) phlebitis, (3) perforation, (4) hemorrhage, (5) vasovagal reactions, and (6) postcolonoscopy distention.

Cardiopulmonary Complications

Patients with known cardiopulmonary disease are at special risk from any form of endoscopy (see "Medication and Monitoring"). Individuals in this category are particularly prone to oversedation. The bowel preparation process must be carried out with special attention to avoiding hypovolemia or water intoxication, conditions that may lead to myocardial infarction and heart failure.

Hypoxia may result from oversedation or pulmonary ventilatory restriction secondary to mechanical overdistention of the bowel if air insufflation is excessive, particularly in the difficult case.

Oversedation is avoided by (1) careful assessment with regard to appropriate drug selection and dosage and (2) slow and cautious intravenous drug injection. Added monitoring measures already alluded to, and the ready availability of resuscitation equipment, together with properly trained personnel, constitute important factors in caring for the high-risk patient.

Phlebitis

Thrombophlebitis, usually at the site of intravenous injection, occurs not infrequently (0.5% to 10% of cases).[7] Selection of a larger vein for injection, when available, and flushing of the vein with 5 to 10 mL of normal saline immediately after injection may reduce the incidence of this complication. In any event, serious aftereffects are rare.

Perforation

Perforation is a hazard of the endoscopic process in general and of the special therapeutic procedure embarked upon in particular. Inexperience is a common denominator, but perforations can and do occur even in the best hands, albeit rarely. When we initially undertook colonoscopy in 1969, we recognized the possibility of perforation as an important risk and therefore deliberately refrained from reporting on this new procedure—at the risk of losing priority—until we had completed more than 200 cases without any complication whatsoever.[7, 8] We firmly believe that this enabled colonoscopy to develop and spread without the stigma of potentially being a highly dangerous procedure. In addition, this emphasized the fact that any complications involved should properly be attributable to shortcomings of the individual attempting it rather than to the method itself.[4]

During instrument introduction and in diagnostic colonoscopy, perforation is usually the result of overvigorous insertion of the instrument or unfamiliarity with the colonic anatomy. Sometimes the orifice of a large diverticulum can be mistaken for the lumen.

Inexperienced endoscopists, who should avoid therapeutic procedures for the most part, are better off using smaller doses of premedication so that patient discomfort can be monitored carefully. Resistance to advancement of the instrument is a warning sign, and its cause may sometimes be ascertained through the adjunctive use of fluoroscopy. The latter also facilitates recognition of marked bowing of the scope or looping of a colonic segment. Advancement of a colonoscope against resistance should never be attempted, even if the colonic lumen can be seen.

Excessive rotational motion may also result in perforation by tearing the bowel wall. Such incidents occur most commonly in the sigmoid colon or at the splenic flexure. The key to successful and safe introduction of the instrument is the ability to visualize the colonic lumen at all times without stretching its wall. Gentleness is the watchword.

Luminal narrowings such as those resulting from tumor, fibrosis secondary to recurrent episodes of diverticulitis, strictures, anastomotic rings, and the like may limit advancement of the instrument and require careful assessment before any attempts at pushing the instrument through are made. Retreat is more commonly a manifestation of wisdom than of timidity and is usually a judicious maneuver.

Perforations resulting from specific therapeutic procedures will be discussed later.

Hemorrhage. Hemorrhage during instrument insertion or diagnostic colonoscopy is almost always extrinsic to the colonic lumen, generally resulting from tearing of the mesentery or colonic ligaments by vigorously pushing, twisting, or pulling the instrument.

Splenic rupture may occur when excessive tension is placed on the splenic flexure of the colon, either while advancing the colonoscope or while straightening the splenic flexure of the colon.

Vasovagal Reaction. So-called vasovagal reactions are manifested by the patient's experiencing cold clammy skin, diaphoresis, bradycardia, and hypotension. Presumed causes include overstretching of the mesentery and other colonic attachments. The patient usually complains of abdominal pain before the onset of a vasovagal reaction. By avoiding maneuvers causing pain, the reaction can usually be prevented.

When the reaction does occur, the endoscopist should terminate the procedure promptly and withdraw the instrument, aspirating whatever air is present during the withdrawal. The patient's legs should be elevated and efforts directed at restoring blood pressure and pulse rate, lest cardiac ischemia result in myocardial infarction. If meperidine or similar analgesia was given as premedication, drug reversal through the administration of 0.4 mg naloxone intravenously, in repeated doses if necessary, to a total of 10 mg is suggested.

Continual sweating and hypotension should be addressed by additional intravenous fluids and oxygen administration by face mask.

Postcolonoscopy Distention. The so-called postcolonoscopy distention syndrome is characterized by an uncomfortable, painful, or distended abdomen following the procedure. It is commonly seen after a prolonged or difficult procedure or when the endoscopist is inexperienced. It is a consequence of excessive insufflation of air, which can force the ileocecal valve to become incompetent and extend air filling well up into the small intestine. If the operator fails to reach the cecum after a prolonged attempt, overdistention can be avoided by having the right side of the abdomen gently compressed by an assistant while insufflated air is aspirated.

Prolonged abdominal distention and pain after any endoscopic procedure may be confused with bowel perforation: proper diagnosis may be made either with the help of fluoroscopy or anteroposterior radiographs with the patient appropriately positioned. When findings signifying overt perforation are lacking, distress may be alleviated by spontaneous evacuation of air, sometimes abetted by the insertion of a rectal tube and sometimes by reinsertion of the colonoscope.

COLONOSCOPIC POLYPECTOMY

Background

Endoscopic removal of colorectal polyps by retrograde colonoscopic means, first performed at the Beth Israel Medical Center in New York in September 1969,[2] is regarded as a landmark in the management of colorectal tumors.[10] Moore called it a "quantum advance in abdominal surgery"[11] and Dunphy labeled the approach "a major contribution to abdominal surgery"[12] when a report was presented before the American Surgical Society at its annual meeting in 1973.[13] Earlier reports on the subject had previously been presented before the New York Surgical Society in February 1970, at the American Society for Gastrointestinal Endoscopy in May 1972, and before the American College of Surgeons in October 1972.[14]

After an article appeared in the *New England Journal of Medicine* the same year,[10] the journal's eminent editor, Franz J. Ingelfinger, was prompted to make a most convincing observation on the then highly controversial subject of the malignant potential of colonic polyps, stating, "...there is no more controversy; it has petered out. Why? Because the development of fiberoptic colonoscopes has made it possible to remove polyps safely, at reasonable expense and with only moderate trouble, from almost any part of the colon without necessitating laparotomy. This technical development has made the controversy concerning the malignant potential of colonic polyps academic..."[15]

This commentary was based on the historical fact that only polyps reachable through traditional rigid sigmoidoscopy had, in the past, lent themselves to recognition, identification as such by biopsy and, sometimes, endoscopic removal. The limitations of this body of evidence were well appreciated. At that time, contrast enema was the only alternative method of diagnosing (with varying degrees of sensitivity and specificity) lesions higher than the 18- to 25-cm insertion level attainable with the rigid sigmoidoscope.

The contrast enema study, whether direct or using the Mälmo (air contrast) technique, not infrequently missed existing polyps, as subsequent comparisons of endoscopic and radiologic methods of examination clearly proved.[5] As often as not, radiologic assessment alone posed the perplexing problem of whether the filling defect revealed by the study represented a malignant process, and, then, what to do if the exact nature of the process was not amenable to radiologic determination. Only mobile filling defects or those in which a stalk was visualized could really be labeled polyps, and even when so categorized, the issue of malignant change remained unresolved. Colonoscopy provided an answer to the dilemma.

At present, endoscopic polypectomy is practiced throughout the world, being performed in hospitals, free-standing medical units, and physicians' offices by individuals of widely disparate training and backgrounds with, by and large, satisfactory results. At its onset, polyp removal at colonoscopy was regarded as a perquisite of surgeons and was later on enthusiastically promoted by colorectal surgeons. Now it is widely performed by hundreds of endoscopically trained gastroenterologists as well.

There is no question, however, that at present colonoscopic polyp removal should be attempted only by individuals with extensive experience in diagnostic colonoscopy. Also called for is an acceptable level of familiarity with the gross presentation of bowel pathology[16, 17] and a working knowledge of electrocautery or laser equipment, or both.

Problems with respect to the qualifications of individuals to perform polypectomy remain paramount, however, and institutions and professional groups must refer to published material[18] and guidelines such as those put out by societies such as The American Society for Gastrointestinal Endoscopy, The Society of American Gastrointestinal Endoscopic Surgeons, The Society for Surgery of the Alimentary Tract, and others in the United States as well as similar organizations abroad.

The further management of the patient whose polyp has been removed and analyzed by a competent pathologist is still a matter of conflicting opinion.[19] This subject will be dealt with later on in this chapter. There is consensus, however, regarding the need for a meticulous search for a synchronous mature colorectal cancer whenever a polyp is discovered. This is irrespective of the histopathologic features of neoplastic polyps. The value of, need for, and

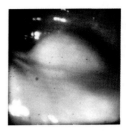

Figure 21–1. Endoscopic view of a small (0.5 cm) polyp.

appropriate timing of subsequent checkup diagnostic colonoscopy for early detection of additional polyps or new cancers have not been definitively clarified, however, and remain matters of increasing concern in terms of appropriate patient care versus the cost–benefit ratio.

Small or diminutive polyps are receiving increasing attention based on the concerns indicated previously for polyps in general. They may not be as harmless as once regarded. Also, it has been suggested that they may represent sentinel indicators of coexisting or impending bowel pathology (Fig. 21–1).[20–24]

General Principles

Removal of colorectal polyps by the endoscopic route is the most frequently employed, and possibly the most fruitful, therapeutic application of colonoscopy.

If a colorectal polyp is discovered by contrast enema, the correctness of the diagnosis can be verified only by endoscopic examination because appropriate treatment depends on the nature of the local pathology (incorrect radiologic diagnoses are not unheard of) and the presence or lack of other bowel pathology.

If we define a polyp as any abnormal protrusion into the bowel lumen from the wall, a whole list of possibilities must be considered (Table 21–1). As noted, included are local inflammatory lesions, small cancers, nonneoplastic tumors such as hamartomas or lipomas, anatomic variants, and even artifacts.

Endoscopy generally allows a more precise diagnosis in most instances. If the lesion proves to be a neoplastic polyp, it can be assessed in terms of (1) its gross morphologic features and probable histopathologic features, (2) its size and configuration, and (3) the presence or lack of an associated additional abnormality or disease process. If gross observation is not sufficiently adequate, appropriate biopsy specimens can and should be obtained, unless the specimen itself can be readily removed. However, for

Table 21–1. CLASSIFICATION OF POLYPS OF THE COLON AND RECTUM

I. Nonneoplastic
  A. Inflammatory
    1. Inflammatory polyp
    2. Pseudopolyposis
    3. Colitis cystica profunda
    4. Lymphoid polyps and polyposis
  B. Growth Anomalies
    1. Juvenile (retention)
    2. Generalized juvenile polyposis
    3. Peutz-Jegher polyposis
  C. Hyperplastic
    1. Hyperplastic (metaplastic)
II. Neoplastic
  A. Carcinoid
  B. Leiomyoma
  C. Lipoma
  D. Neurofibroma
  E. Metastatic Carcinoma, Leukemia, and so on
  F. Adenoma
    1. Tubular adenoma (adenomatous polyp)
    2. Villotubular adenoma
    3. Villous adenoma
  G. Polypoid Carcinoma

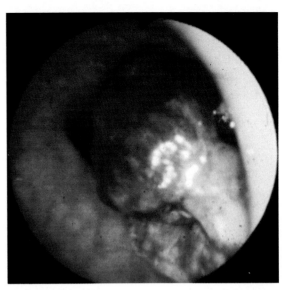

Figure 21–2. Endoscopic view of a polypoid carcinoma with stalk.

certain intramural lesions such as lipomas, leimyomas, carcinoids, vascular malformations, and the like, biopsy is better avoided, and endoscopic removal should not be attempted.

The major significance of colorectal polyps is related to cancer: is the lesion in question a polypoid carcinoma (Fig. 21–2), is it a "malignant polyp," or is it a polyp that may, with time, become malignant? The once celebrated controversy in regard to polyp malignancy relates to the neoplastic variety otherwise known as adenomas. These, and hyperplastic polyps, numerically constitute the vast majority of lesions considered under the rubric polyps. Terminology tends to be somewhat confusing. Table 21–2 provides a breakdown on the subject. Table 21–3 relates currently favored terminology, along with terms used in the past, which are apt to cause confusion.

Large bowel cancer is a disease treated by surgery that is on the increase in the United States and that if diagnosed at an early stage can be cured (Fig. 21–3). Until colonoscopy came upon the scene, salvage rates were at a standstill. It is hoped that by removing polyps, cancer can be attacked at an earlier stage or prevented.[25, 26]

Current thinking on the subject embraces the concept that in certain neoplastic polyps, the polyp epithelium undergoes progressive dysplasia of increasing severity. Finally, a localized, nonpenetrating but *full-blown cancer* forms, known as *carcinoma in situ*. When and if this

process goes on to penetrate the lamina propria, it becomes a clinically important true or *invasive* cancer (Fig. 21–4). This cytologic sequence, of course, has never been documented except indirectly, but it is supported by a compelling body of evidence. Once the lamina propria has been broached, the cancer cells may enter the blood stream or lymphatics, or both, and metastasize (Fig. 21–5) or they may continue to invade the large bowel wall beyond the submucosal layer, or both. Cancers that do not penetrate the lamina propria (carcinoma in situ) are also referred to in some reports as intramucosal cancer, focal carcinoma, and superficial cancer, terms that only serve to confuse the clinician. To repeat, these last are not true cancers in a clinical sense and should not be regarded or reported as such.

Whether epithelial *hyperplasia* rather than *dysplasia* plays a role in the sequence alluded

Table 21–2. BREAKDOWN OF POLYP TERMINOLOGY

Nonneoplastic	Neoplastic
Hyperplastic	Carcinoid
Hyperplastic (metaplastic)	Leiomyoma
	Lipoma
Inflammatory	Neurofibroma
Inflammatory polyp	Metastatic carcinoma,
Pseudopolyp	Leukemia, and so on
Colitis cystica profunda	Adenoma
Lymphoid polyps	Tubular (adenomatous
	polyp)
Growth Anomalies	Villotubular adenoma
Juvenile (retention)	Villous adenoma
Peutz-Jegher polyposis	Polypoid carcinoma

Table 21–3. CURRENT AND PAST POLYP TERMINOLOGY

Current Terminology	Old Terminology
Nonneoplastic	*Nonneoplastic*
Juvenile polyp	Retention polyp
Hyperplastic polyp	Metaplastic polyp
Neoplastic	*Neoplastic*
Tubular adenoma	Adenomatous polyp
Villous adenoma	Papillary polyp
Villotubular adenoma	Villoglandular polyp
Polypoid carcinoma	Malignant polyp

to is uncertain but, in general, hyperplastic polyps are benign lesions with no propensity for malignant change.[27]

The evidence that certain specimens of these *neoplastic* polyps have a significant propensity for malignant degeneration is very strong. Many students of the subject believe that most, if not all, colon cancers have a polyp precursor and that polyp removal can either prevent colon cancer or allow its mastery at an early and prognostically favorable stage. The tendency for malignant change in polyps is related to (1) histologic features, (2) polyp size and location, and (3) total number—whether they occur synchronously or metachronously.

The fact of the matter, however, is that *the majority of colorectal polyps are benign* and without malignant potential.

Contraindications and Restrictions

Contraindications to polyp removal are both absolute and relative. Not the least of consid-

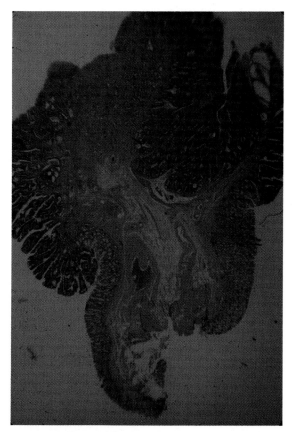

Figure 21–4. Photomicrograph of a pedunculated polyp with invasive carcinoma in the head.

erations should be the skill and experience of the endoscopist in a given situation. Removal of a small pedunculated polyp on a long stalk in the rectosigmoid colon is not equivalent to removing a large, broad-based or sessile lesion in the thin-walled cecal area.

Certainly, the general condition of the patient must be a known quantity, as must the lack of hemorrhagic diathesis, as elicited by a careful history taking, review of current medications and, if needed, appropriate laboratory studies.

The presence of significant associated inflammatory disease may be a deterrent to polyp removal.

Bowel preparation must be more than adequate so that the entire circumference of the adjacent bowel wall is clearly within the field of view. Also, unimpeded access to the segment of colon containing the polyp is called for should there be any bleeding from the polypectomy stump.

The availability of backup support should also be a consideration. Difficult polyps—rendered so by size, configuration, location, or number (Fig. 21–6)—are sometimes best managed in an institutional setting as opposed to an office, so

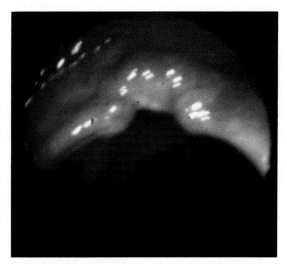

Figure 21–3. Endoscopic view of an early carcinoma with ulceration.

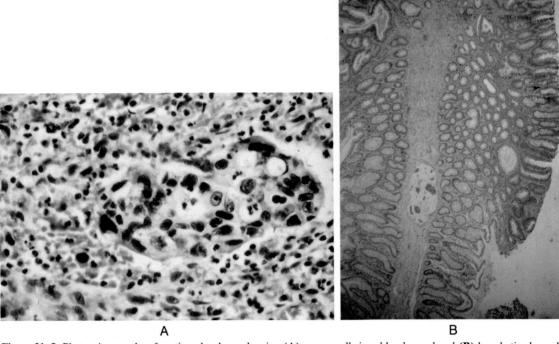

Figure 21–5. Photomicrographs of sectioned polyps, showing **(A)** cancer cells in a blood vessel and **(B)** lymphatic channels of a stalk.

that the means are readily available for prolonged monitoring, radiologic studies, or blood transfusion. Certainly, advanced age, cardiac or pulmonary problems, associated pregnancy, brittle diabetes, and similar problems call for maximal prophylactic safety measures.

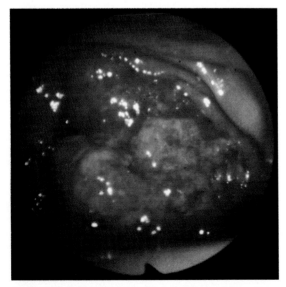

Figure 21–6. Endoscopic view of a large polyp almost completely blocking the lumen.

Biopsy and Cytologic Studies

Whether or not biopsy should be done prior to endoscopic polypectomy depends on a number of considerations. Obviously, if there is an adjacent overt cancer that will have to be removed surgically, and the anticipated extent of resection will include the polyp, biopsy is unnecessary and probably contraindicated. If, conversely, a synchronously occurring separate cancer is noted at a distance, polyp removal and pathologic assessment may contribute materially to the need for and extent of further surgical bowel removal at the time of laparotomy. If polyp size or configuration is such that complete endoscopic removal is unlikely at the time, or at a single sitting, strategically taken biopsy specimens may prove most helpful in total management.

When a number of polyps are encountered, biopsy of those polyps not contemplated for immediate removal can prove to be a prudent measure.

Small lesions can be completely excised with several bites of the biopsy forceps. Large lesions should be sampled wherever gross anatomic distortions are noted (Fig. 21–7) or at central and marginal zones, or both. This can assure specimens from normal surrounding tissues,

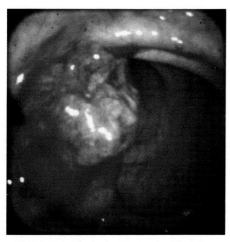

Figure 21–7. Endoscopic view of an adenomatous polyp, showing grossly invasive cancer in the head.

with additional deep bites taken from obviously diseased areas.

Biopsies can be useful in inflammatory diseases and will sometimes reveal parasites when previous stool studies have been uninformative.

Lesions such as lipomas and certain others, such as vascular malformations, need not or should not be biopsied.

A variety of biopsy forceps are available, and operators should attain a familiarity with them. We prefer the use of cold biopsy forceps without coagulation. In our experience, the amount of ensuing bleeding is minimal and of little consequence. Mere fulguration, recommended by some investigators, has the disadvantage of not providing a histologic diagnosis, as well as the added risk of bowel perforation.

Biopsy specimens are taken by introducing the biopsy forceps so that it protrudes 1 to 2 cm beyond the instrument tip and then advancing the tip without moving the forceps in most instances. Specimens are immediately placed in formalin after being pulled back through the biopsy channel. To avoid crushing and distortion of larger specimens, the entire instrument should be removed, with the forceps tip slightly protruding, the specimen should be released into the formalin jar before the forceps is removed.

Snare-Cautery Devices

There are a variety of snare-cautery devices that should be studied by the endoscopist, and a working familiarity should be acquired for those used. Basically, however, there are only two types.

The simplest is a strand of braided wire folded back on itself and threaded through polytetrafluoroethylene (Teflon) tubing.[17] This arrangement, devised by Shinya in 1969, is still employed by him and his associates today, and more than 30,000 polyps have been removed with this device, with eminently successful results. Its employment is greatly enhanced when a knowledgeable assistant is available to form the loop within the bowel lumen as viewed through an observer scope or on a video screen. Electrocautery is applied by electrodes fixed to the tail portions. The operator is responsible for the strength and duration of the electrical impulse once the snare is positioned and tightened to his or her satisfaction. The loop is readily loosened and reapplied as desired. When the operation is complete, the wire loop is withdrawn. When circumstances dictate, the loop can be used to grasp the polyp and hold it against the tip of the endoscope as the instrument is withdrawn. Under other conditions, the operator holds the transected polyp or polyp segment to the tip of the endoscope by the application of suction.

The commercial type of snare wire is manipulated and rotated by use of a variety of types of handles that remain outside the body once the snare device is inserted through the appropriate instrument channel. The size and shape of the loop are not readily adjustable. There have been reports of difficulties encountered in removing the wire, which is a real problem when the polyp encircled is not transected (see "Postpolypectomy Complications").

The advantages of the commercial snare are that it can be used more easily by a gastrointestinal assistant with minimal training and that it is quite satisfactory for small polyps. Moreover, commercial snares are now available in many sizes and shapes and wire thicknesses for particular situations. This means, of course, that a sizable inventory must be on hand to deal with various potential problems. Therefore, commercial snares tend to be less cost-effective.

Electrocautery

The chief applications of electrocautery in colonoscopy are polyp removal and treatment of bleeding sites. Electrocautery devices are familiar to most surgeons, and the most important aspect of their use is that the operator be familiar with the particular device being used. The method involves the passage of an electric current of sufficient voltage, density, and duration to produce tissue necrosis. Most units have designated *cutting* modes or *coagulation* modes, or a blend of both. Units commonly employed are *monopolar* or *bipolar*. The former involves a single electrode and a larger indifferent grounding plate. The latter uses two small electrodes at the tip of the instrument across which a current flows. Grounding is not required. Use of the monopolar modality calls for special safeguards in patients who have cardiac pacemakers.

A fairly recent innovation in bipolar electrodes is the *BICAP probe* (ACMI, Stamford, CT) in which there is a sheathed, rounded multichannel probe containing a central opening through which fluid may be perfused continuously or in jets. The probe is inserted through the biopsy channel of the colonoscope. It has been used to control bleeding sites in both the upper and lower gastrointestinal tract.

Use of the electrocautery technique is described in "Technique of Polypectomy" and "Vascular Malformations." The cutting current is never used for polyp removal, but some endoscopists employ a combination of cutting and coagulation (blend). The electrocautery equipment, including connections, grounding plate, and current, should be checked and calibrated each day.

Snare wires are usually insulated by an appropriate sheath, but the operator should wear rubber gloves, particularly with the open wire loop technique.

Gas explosion is not a concern in the properly prepared bowel as demonstrated by us early on[28] and by many others since.

The *hot biopsy* forceps allows a small biopsy specimen to be taken at the same time the surrounding tissue is electrocoagulated. The need for a specimen that can be studied histologically and the difficulty in retrieving tiny polyps endoscopically resected have led to wider acceptance of the hot biopsy forceps. Although generally regarded as extremely safe, there is evidence that, in certain colons at least, there is appreciable risk of hemorrhage or perforation.[29] Williams, long an advocate of the technique, points out how these dangers may be minimized.[30]

The *heater probe* (Olympus HPU, Olympus Corp., Lake Success, NY) is an electric thermal coagulation device with irrigating channels.

Lasers

Laser application to the gut via the endoscope is now a widely used technique. Undertaken early on at our institution by Waitman and associates,[31, 32] it has been employed successfully

in the treatment of a variety of hemorrhagic lesions and obstructing neoplasms. In the latter situation, the goal is generally palliative alleviation of the obstruction. Laser usage, in both the upper and lower gastrointestinal tract, usually requires large-diameter, multichannel endoscopes so that lavage and suction may be performed simultaneously. Lavage is accomplished with fluid or carbon dioxide gas.

Commonly, two forms of laser energy have been tried in these photocoagulation procedures, namely, the argon laser and the neodymium-doped yttrium-aluminum-garnet (Nd:YAG) laser. The latter is preferred by many for treating vascular lesions because of greater hemostatic efficiency. In either instance, a satisfactory outcome more often than not requires two or more endoscopic sessions 2 to 4 days, or longer, apart. In the case of obstructing tumors, numerous repeat procedures are needed at intervals of weeks or months for recurrent obstruction, if the patient survives that long.

In our unit, Ghazi has treated large, broad-based sessile colonic polyps with the Nd:YAG laser, either alone or in combination with endoscopic snare polypectomy, with a reasonable degree of success in these notoriously difficult cases.[33]

As with other gastrointestinal tract cancer, laser therapy is rarely undertaken in colorectal cancer as a curative procedure or as the primary mode of management. Its major indications are to relieve obstruction or control bleeding but not to alleviate pain. Before accepting a patient for laser therapy, the endoscopist should have as much information as possible in terms of the patient's general condition, the nature and extent of the tumor, and the local tumor pathology. The last requires a contrast enema study, imaging studies, and diagnostic endoscopy, including, when feasible, endoscopic ultrasonography. As noted, repetitive sessions are commonly needed. This fact, plus the rigorous bowel preparation regimen required, must be weighed in the balance when making a decision regarding the choice of therapy.

Complication rates are significant; however, when compared with those associated with alternative methods of management, they are acceptable.[34, 35]

Selected small rectal cancers (defined as less than 3 cm in length and less than one third of the bowel circumference) have been ablated using endoscopic laser therapy as the primary modality, with fair success.[36]

Advances in instrument design and new laser forms currently being tried may well change the picture in the next few years.

Technique of Polypectomy

Polyp removal via the colonoscope should be attempted only by those with broad experience in using the colonoscope and its accessories. The polyp must be visualized clearly, its size and configuration assessed, and a decision made as to whether it should be biopsied, electrocoagulated, removed entirely or piecemeal, or left alone. It is best to only biopsy frank carcinomas, with no attempt at complete removal. Sometimes, a polypoid carcinoma can be fully resected through the endoscope.

Diminutive Polyps. Small polyps, 5 mm in diameter or less, may be completely excised with several bites of the biopsy forceps and the base coagulated. Alternatively, the hot biopsy forceps can be employed to remove the polyp completely with coagulation.

Small Sessile Polyps. Small sessile polyps can be removed by the standard snare-cautery technique. The snare must be positioned carefully at the base and gently tightened and the polyp lightly tented toward the lumen, at which point the coagulation current is applied.

In applying the snare wire to small lesions, great care must be exercised to avoid including normal colonic mucosa in the snare loop. This state of affairs should be suspected when there is more resistance than usual in transecting the tissue than when coagulating through a polyp. It should be regarded as a warning sign and the snare loop immediately released. The area of coagulation must then be carefully examined. This occurrence can generally be avoided if the mucosa is tented first and the polyp oscillated to-and-fro.

Polyps with Long Stalks. For polyps with long stalks, the snare should be placed so that at least 1 cm of stalk remains when the polyp is removed. This avoids the possibility of perforation, and if bleeding occurs from the transected stalk, it can readily be resnared to achieve hemostasis (Fig. 21–8).[17]

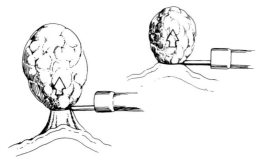

Figure 21–8. Proper level for snare cautery transection of polyps.

POLYPECTOMY TECHNIQUE
Short and heavy stalk

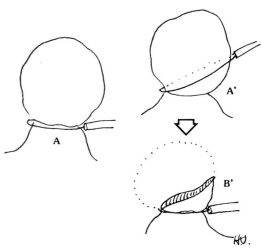

Figure 21–9. Polypectomy technique for a short or heavy stalk.

Polyps with Short Stalks. When the stalk is short, the snare should be placed as close as possible to the body of the polyp. This can be accomplished by not tightening the loop completely once the polyp is lassoed. This allows the snare to be placed close to the neck of the polyp before finally tightening and constricting the tissue (Fig. 21–9).

Some operators advocate tightening the noose to the point of complete strangulation before applying electric current. We regard this maneuver as both unnecessary and dangerous: premature transection of the stalk by strangulation before the current is applied can lead to hemorrhage and loss of visualization. Moreover, prolonged strangulation can bring about a spasm of the colonic musculature, with loss of clear visualization of the endoscopic field.

A word of caution is in order with respect to tightening the snare loop: this should not be done until the loop is in the correct position. However, once tightening on the head of the polyp has begun, the snare loop should not be released or repositioned lest the partially sectioned area start bleeding and obscure the field. It is preferable to complete the transection with cautery and then reapply the snare to cut off the remainder of the polyp.

Large Polyps. Large polyps with a broad base are best removed in sections until the head is reduced adequately to reveal its base. If there is a pedicle, it can be appreciated by oscillating the polyp head in various directions. One must avoid pulling the polyp lest the mucosa to which it is attached be stretched and coagulated. If this goes unnoticed, late perforation may ensue.

POLYPECTOMY TECHNIQUE
Large and wide based

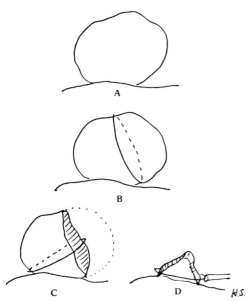

Figure 21–10. Piecemeal removal of a large, broad-based polyp.

Large, broad-based polyps are subject to the risk of transecting at a level too close to the bowel wall. Coagulation may be prolonged before complete transection occurs, and necrosis of the colonic wall may ensue. Such polyps should be removed piecemeal or segmentally, at several sittings if necessary (Fig. 21–10).

Large Sessile Polyps. These polyps, particularly those 2 cm in diameter or greater, are subject to the limitations just described. Partial removal, if feasible, or taking extensive biopsy specimens, or both, should be considered so that a decision may be reached to either attempt endoscopic removal or resort to laparotomy.

Large villous adenomas can remain benign for many years but have the greatest propensity for malignant change. When benign, segmental removal can be carried out by obliquely placed cuts, at sequential sittings if necessary.

The endoscopic presentation of large sessile polyps is the single most important variable in arriving at a decision about whether or not to attempt endoscopic removal. Soft, smooth, velvety lesions are apt to be benign, whereas hard, granular, ulcerated lesions have a good chance of being malignant. Polyps larger than 3 cm in diameter or those with gross appearance suggesting malignant change are preferably treated by bowel resection when the patient's condition permits (Fig. 21–11). Otherwise endoscopic resection may be attempted with great caution exercised at all times. Even then the risks are appreciable.

Specimen Retrieval. Specimens are best retrieved, as noted, by applying suction when the head of the polyp is up against the tip of the instrument. If the specimen is lost, it can often be retrieved by passing the endoscope beyond the polypectomy site and instilling 1000 to 2000 mL water or normal saline through the instrument. The patient then usually passes the specimen along with the fluid into a bedpan after the colonoscope is withdrawn, aspirating air en route.

Multiple Polyps. When multiple polyps are encountered, the number that can be removed at a single sitting depends on the experience and dexterity of the operator, on the size of the polyps and their configuration, on the total number present, and on their location.

Usually the endoscope is introduced all the way to the cecum to evaluate the situation, and a decision is then made. If many polyps are

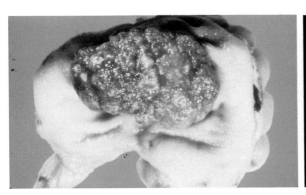

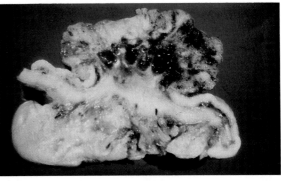

A   B

Figure 21–11. (A, B) Photographs of a large (benign) villous adenoma, which is best removed by colectomy.

encountered, removal from the same colonic segment at a given sitting is advised so that if postoperative complications occur, the area of involvement can be accurately located. The remaining polyps are saved for one or more additional sessions.

As mentioned, polypectomy is usually performed on withdrawal after luminal inspection up to the cecum. However, small polyps may be managed on the way in, lest they be difficult to locate on the way out.

Use of the Splinting Device. Retrieval of multiple specimens from the transverse or ascending colon can be a tedious and, occasionally, troublesome undertaking. In such cases, the long colonoscope must first be inserted with the splinting device. Once in place, the long instrument can be withdrawn and a shorter scope introduced through the splinting tube. The latter then passes readily into the transverse or ascending colon, and the polyps are resected and retrieved fairly easily. Of course, any polyps having an appearance indicative or suggestive of malignant change should be removed first.

Management of Malignant Polyps

The management of malignant polyps of the large bowel continues to be a subject of some controversy but with large areas of general agreement. Basic to any meaningful discussion is a clear understanding as to what constitutes a malignant polyp in a clinical sense. The literature contains numerous reports in which the same or similar terms are applied to what we now recognize as clearly different entities. Conversely, a variety of names are used for essentially the same lesions. A clear understanding of nomenclature is obviously mandatory.

Of crucial concern is the definition of what constitutes malignant change in a polyp. Certain gross features are suggestive when the polyp is viewed endoscopically—for example, areas of fixation to the bowel wall. It is only microscopic examination, however, that provides the answer through specimens obtained either by biopsy or polyp removal. Normal biopsy results alone are not dependable, as they may not be representative of the entire lesion.

A critical distinction must be made between *invasive* and *noninvasive cancer.* Invasion is, by accepted definition, penetration of the lamina muscularis mucosae (Fig. 21–12). Nonpenetrating cancer is carcinoma in situ. This is a true histologic cancer but is not clinically significant. Carcinoma in situ may be a stage of cancer that

occurs earlier than invasive cancer, but this progression has never actually been demonstrated, for a polyp once removed cannot "further testify against itself." It goes without saying that determining whether invasion is present requires removal of the entire polyp and sectioning, with appropriate orientation by the pathologist. Even then there are occasional instances when the findings are equivocal.

Using the terminology we prefer (see Table 21–3), Tables 21–4 through 21–6 analyze some 26,630 polyps removed endoscopically. Table 21–7 analyzes a later series of 15,416 polyps. The relative frequency, histologic analysis, and incidence of malignant changes are demonstrated. It should be emphasized that these numbers apply only to polyps lending themselves to endoscopic resection. Many villous adenomas, for example, are too large for this procedure to be done safely. In general, malignant changes occur in 3% to 5% of tubular adenomas, in 8% to 12% of villotubular adenomas, and in 30% to 40% of villous adenomas.

It is quite clear that as far as the individual polyp is concerned, the histologic pattern has an important bearing on the chance of malignant change. In addition, because of the relative frequency of occurrence among the three types of adenoma, it is equally clear that as far as colon cancer is concerned, the tubular adenoma plays an important role because its relatively low propensity for malignant alteration is counterbalanced by its higher rate of occurrence. It is also quite apparent, however, that *the vast*

Table 21–4. POLYPS REMOVED ENDOSCOPICALLY

1969–1978 (Total 7000 Polyps)		1969–1986 (Total 19,630 Polyps)	
Nonneoplastic		*Nonneoplastic*	
1173 (17%) **Total**		4139 (21%) **Total**	
		Hyperplastic	2256
		Inflammatory	793
		Juvenile	747
		Hamartomas	343
		Submucosal	
		Lipomas	28
		Leiomyomas	12
		Lymphoid	19
		Carcinoids	5
		Hodgkin's disease	1
Neoplastic		*Neoplastic*	
5827 (83%) **Total**		15,416 (79%) **Total**	
Adenomas	5786	Adenomas	15,289
Polypoid carcinoma	41	Polypoid carcinoma	41

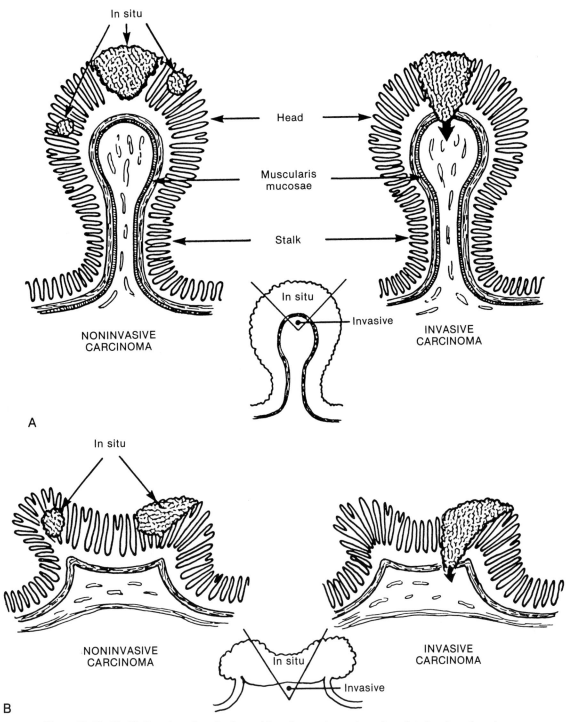

Figure 21–12. (A, B) Drawings show in situ and invasive carcinoma in pedunculated and sessile polyps.

Table 21–5. HISTOLOGIC ANALYSIS OF ADENOMAS

	No.	%
Tubular adenomas	3725	64.3
Villotubular adenomas	1542	26.7
Villous adenomas	519	9.0
TOTAL	5786	100

majority of adenomas do not progress to carcinoma.

It has long been recognized that the incidence of malignant change is related not only to histopathology but also to polyp size. This holds true for all forms of adenomatous polyps, whether tubular or villous. Figure 21–13 shows an analysis of our data relating the presence of invasive cancer to polyp size as well as the histologic format. It is worthy of note that invasive cancer is present even in very small neoplastic polyps of various categories. When polyps are analyzed for carcinoma in situ, a very similar pattern emerges.

Colonoscopic polypectomy is, therefore, either prophylactic or therapeutic in terms of cancer. When the histologic section shows the presence of invasive cancer, the further management of the patient comes into question. This consideration applies to approximately 5% to 10% of neoplastic polyps removed endoscopically. Some researchers believe all patients should have colonic resection if their condition permits.[37–49] However, most investigators with vast experience, including ourselves, hold that this is unnecessary in many instances, particularly in pedunculated polyps with the cancer confined to the head. The problem is more acute in sessile or broad-based polyps and clearly does not apply at all when incomplete removal is a possibility.

As long ago as 1975, we offered the following guidelines for early surgical intervention: (1) the presence of cancerous invasion at or close to the plane of resection, (2) a high histologic grade

Table 21–6. MALIGNANT CHANGE IN ADENOMAS

	No.	% With Carcinoma In Situ	% With Invasive Carcinoma
Tubular adenomas	3725	12	3
Villotubular adenomas	1542	11	8
Villous adenomas	519	15	10
TOTAL	5786	12	5

Table 21–7. COLONOSCOPIC POLYPECTOMY: INCIDENCE OF "MALIGNANT" POLYPS (15,416 NEOPLASTIC POLYPS EXCISED SEPTEMBER 1969–DECEMBER 1986)

	No.	%
Benign	11,603	75
Dysplasia	1,598	10
Carcinoma in situ	1,548	10
"Malignant" polyps	667	5
Adenoma with invasive carcinoma	540	4
Polypoid carcinoma	127	1

of malignancy, (3) the finding of cancer cells in the lymphatics, (4) the presence of polypoid carcinomas (in which the entire polyp is cancerous), and (5) the uncertainty of complete removal.[43] These criteria have largely been accepted and promulgated. Haggitt and colleagues studied the problem in detail and offered criteria based on "levels," but it should be noted that 35% of their patients were never subjected to endoscopic polypectomy, surgical resection being the primary procedure.[50]

In a recent report before the Society of American Gastrointestinal Endoscopic Surgeons, we presented additional follow-up data but pointed out that the issue still lacks definitive resolution. We offered what we currently regard as significant determinants (Table 21–8) and suggested a data sheet whereby uniform and comprehensive factors might be recorded at the time of polypectomy (Table 21–9).[19] It is apparent that the final word has yet to be spoken.

Recently, attention has been directed at small (up to 10 mm) or diminutive (up to 5 mm) polyps.[20–23] Once thought to be mostly hyperplastic polyps, accumulated evidence shows that 30% to 80% of these lesions are neoplastic in nature.[20–23, 51, 52] In addition, although the incidence of malignancy is low (0.1% to 3.2%), it is the current consensus that all small or diminutive polyps should be removed when encountered.

Table 21–8. SIGNIFICANT DETERMINANTS RELATING TO DECISION-MAKING FOR SURGERY AFTER ENDOSCOPIC REMOVAL OF MALIGNANT COLONIC POLYPS

1. Tumor at or close to plane of resection
2. Extensive polyp involvement by cancer
3. Piecemeal (*i.e.*, ? complete) resection
4. Villous adenoma
5. Locally recurrent tumor
6. Highly undifferentiated cancer
7. Lymphatic or vascular invasion
8. Polypoid carcinoma
9. Physician's, surgeon's, or patient's decision

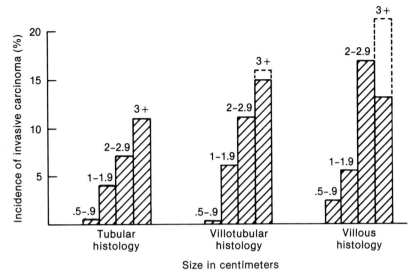

Figure 21–13. The graph shows the incidence of invasive cancer based on polyp size (numbers in centimeters above the bars) and histology. (From Shinya N. Colonoscopy: diagnosis and treatment of colonic diseases. New York, Tokyo: Igaku-Shoin, 1982.)

Polypectomy Complications

The complications associated with endoscopic polypectomy are (1) those common to the endoscopic procedure itself and (2) those peculiar to polyp removal. The former have already been covered.

Complications arising from polypectomy are related to several factors, chief among which are the skill and experience of the operator; the size, configuration, and location of the polyp; the adequacy of bowel preparation; the technique employed; and the reliability of the equipment employed. In experienced hands, the incidence should not exceed 1%. In our own hands, it has been less than 0.01% (Table 21–10).

The specific complications encountered include (1) bleeding, (2) perforation, (3) transmural burns, (4) snare entrapment, and (5) ensnared bowel.

Postpolypectomy Hemorrhage. Bleeding is the most frequent complication encountered, representing about 50% of the difficulties. It can vary from a slow ooze to brisk hemorrhage requiring blood transfusion, and it may be immediate or delayed. High on the list of preventive measures is a careful history for any bleeding diathesis or for the use of certain medications, notably aspirin. Salicylates should be discontinued at least 10 days prior to the contemplated procedure. Patients receiving anticoagulant therapy should discontinue the medication at least 5 days in advance of the procedure. Bleeding and coagulation times must be checked within 8 hours of the event.

Table 21–9. POLYPECTOMY DATA SHEET (BETH ISRAEL MEDICAL CENTER)

Number of Lesions:										Endoscopist:					
Anatomic Location	**Nature of Lesions**				**Size (cm)**	**Clinical Features (Gross)**						**Procedure**			
	Pedunculated		*Sessile*												
Distance (cm)	*Long stalk*	*Short stalk*	*Wide-base sessile*	*Narrow-base sessile*		*Lobulated*	*Ulcerated*	*Villous*	*Polypoid*	*Flat*	*Partial circumference*	*Excision complete*	*Excision incomplete*	*Biopsy only*	*Complete piecemeal*	*Coagulation*
1. ___ ( )	☐	☐	☐	☐	———	☐	☐	☐	☐	☐	☐	☐	☐	☐	☐
2. ___ ( )	☐	☐	☐	☐	———	☐	☐	☐	☐	☐	☐	☐	☐	☐	☐
3. ___ ( )	☐	☐	☐	☐	———	☐	☐	☐	☐	☐	☐	☐	☐	☐	☐
4. ___ ( )	☐	☐	☐	☐	———	☐	☐	☐	☐	☐	☐	☐	☐	☐	☐
5. ___ ( )	☐	☐	☐	☐	———	☐	☐	☐	☐	☐	☐	☐	☐	☐	☐

Table 21–10. COMPLICATIONS OF DIAGNOSTIC AND THERAPEUTIC COLONOSCOPY 60,305 PROCEDURES PERFORMED (JULY 1969–DECEMBER 1986)

	Diagnostic	Therapeutic
Perforation	0	2
Hemorrhage	0	32
Death	0	0
Other	3 (vasovagal reaction)	1 (fever)

Postpolypectomy Perforation. This is the result of a transmural burn. It may be recognized immediately or after a number of hours, or its recognition may be delayed. Classically, an immediate significant perforation will be manifested by abdominal pain, fever, leukocytosis, abdominal tenderness with rebound tenderness, and the appearance of intra- or retroperitoneal air or air under the diaphragm seen on x-ray film with the patient upright or on an anteroposterior view with the patient in a lateral recumbent position. At the other extreme is the "silent" perforation that is unassociated with symptoms or signs and is discovered only on an incidental radiologic study performed after the procedures.[53, 54]

Postpolypectomy Transmural Burns. These are related to both technique and the equipment used. They are encountered with greatest frequency when the configuration of the polyp is sessile and in the polyp with a short, wide stalk. These burns occur when the removal of pedunculated polyps is accompanied by the snare being placed too close to the attachment of the polyp to the bowel wall, which can happen when the polyp is not entirely free and its body rests against adjacent bowel wall.

Snare Entrapment. As previously noted, problems are sometimes encountered in attempting to withdraw the snare wire when a commercial type of unit is used. A number of solutions have been offered when the polyp is incompletely transected, including (1) leaving the wire in place in the colon for several days, during which time the polyp may slough off and release it, (2) leaving the wire in place and again attempting to remove it using the homemade snare described previously (best attempted by a more experienced endoscopist), and (3) resorting to laparotomy.

This problem is not seen with the homemade snare device, as pulling one end will bring the whole wire through after the polytetrafluoroethylene tubing ensheathing it is withdrawn.

Entrapment generally results when there is too much tissue in the snare, the electrocautery unit is set wrong, or there is a mechanical misarrangement. Aggressive attempts at resection using a strong coagulation or cutting current can bring about bowel perforation and should be avoided.

Ensnared Bowel. Careless employment of the snare wire loop or applying it with an inadequate or incomplete view of the area can result in inadvertent incorporation of adjacent bowel wall during polypectomy. This can cause a transmural burn and perforation. As previously noted, the need for excessive amounts of current when transecting may provide a clue to this possibility.

VOLVULUS

Colonoscopy has been shown to be of value in the management of large bowel distention, both mechanical and adynamic in origin. Classically, volvulus of the colon was treated surgically, particularly if bowel viability is threatened or if distention is excessive.[55] Sigmoidoscopy was sometimes employed. Ghazi and colleagues were the first to describe the application of the fiberoptic colonoscope to treat a case of sigmoid volvulus. They pointed out the advantages offered over traditional rigid sigmoidoscopic methods.[56] Careful scrutiny of the wall during endoscopic decompression is deemed imperative lest ischemic and gangrenous changes that are already present be overlooked. If these changes are present, of course immediate operative intervention is called for.

Endoscopic management of this condition has been reported by a number of groups, notably Brothers and colleagues,[57] Ballantyne and colleagues,[55] and Geer and associates.[58]

Because recurrent volvulus is not uncommon after endoscopic decompression, leaving an indwelling catheter inserted through a colonoscopic overtube has been suggested.[59]

PSEUDOOBSTRUCTION AND OGILVIE'S SYNDROME

Disturbances of bowel motility associated with moderate to severe obstructive phenomena have been described, both on a chronic and acute basis. One form, described by Ogilvie in 1948,[60] has been perpetuated using his name and is called Ogilvie's syndrome.

We have encountered this condition in a number of clinical circumstances (in idiopathic conditions,[61, 62] in obstetric and gynecologic conditions,[63] associated with methadone maintenance therapy[64, 65]) and have indicated the potential value of colonoscopy in the management of these cases. It is currently regarded as a safe and effective diagnostic and therapeutic tool by Strodel and Eckhauser.[66] Gosche and associates[67] regard it as the treatment of choice, as do Dent and colleagues.[68] Complications can and do occur (3% in Dent's collected series) but, as these authors point out, they should be minimal if the colonoscopist is experienced and careful.

Despite its initial wide acceptance, however, there are some investigators who are less enthusiastic. Sloyer and coworkers[69] reported 25 cases successfully managed without colonoscopic decompression, an approach endorsed by Surawicz,[70] whose experience has led to "less dramatic" results with endoscopic efforts.

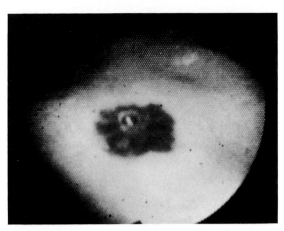

Figure 21–14. Endoscopic view of an arteriovenous malformation in the cecum.

VASCULAR MALFORMATIONS

Vascular malformations, which are referred to in various ways as shown in Table 21–11, are being observed with increasing frequency as expertise in colonoscopy becomes more widespread. They are now recognized as an important causative mechanism for overt or occult lower bowel bleeding.

These vascular lesions have been studied extensively by Boley and Brandt[71] whose reports are worthy of perusal. Their more than coincidental association with aortic stenosis has been discussed by Greenstein and associates.[72]

Although colonoscopic recognition and localization of the various vascular malformations and estimation of their role in bleeding phenomena were the early contributions of complete large bowel endoscopy, current advances in technology and skill have led to methods of definitive management by this route. Endoscopic electrocoagulation and laser ablation are being employed by more experienced and skilled endoscopists with increasing frequency and success. The various modalities reported include monopolar electrocoagulation, bipolar

Table 21–11. VARIOUS TERMS FOR VASCULAR MALFORMATIONS

Angiodysplasia	Arteriovenous fistula
Vascular ectasia	Arteriovenous anastomosis
Arteriovenous malformation	Hemangioma
	Arteriovenous shunt
Angioma	Angiectasia
Telangiectasia	

electrocoagulation, heater probes, argon laser, Nd:Yag laser, and endoscopic sclerosis.[73–77]

Early on in the era of colonoscopy, we reported a number of cases of recurrent serious gastrointestinal tract bleeding episodes, the source of which had eluded the most exhaustive diagnostic workup then available (Fig. 21–14). In each instance, an arteriovenous malformation in the colonic mucosa was discovered, only by colonoscopy.[78] Such disclosures are now routine because complete colonoscopy is the rule.

When discovered, the majority of symptomatic vascular anomalies can be managed endoscopically. Surgical intervention with resection is reserved for cases in which the bleeding cannot be controlled or endoscopic ablation is either unsuccessful or ill-advised. Such decisions are based on local manifestations, such as large size or multiplicity. Even then it has been stated that up to 20% of patients can expect to have rebleeding episodes.[71]

Management of these vascular lesions is by electrocoagulation or photocoagulation. At our institution, Waitman and colleagues[79] reported on successful control without complication in more than 250 patients with arteriovenous malformations of the gastrointestinal tract using argon laser photocoagulation. They have switched to the neodymium:YAG laser as the preferred modality, and their more recent report provides an excellent analysis of the subject.[80] Others concur.[77]

Apparently the choice of photocoagulation or electrocoagulation is a matter of personal preference, augmented by experience. We have encountered no problems in a fairly large number of patients treated by carefully calibrated and applied electrocoagulation. Howard and colleagues,[74] in 1982, reported 26 patients so managed, with one delayed perforation. Brandt and Rogers,[81] in 1988, stated that all methods give the same results. Trudel and associates,[73] in 1988, reported 78 patients managed by electrocoagulation without morbidity or mortality. Danesh and associates[82] had a similar favorable experience and strongly advocate a gentle, cautious approach with repeated sessions rather than "undue local heating in one."

General experience has been that rebleeding is more often than not from new or missed lesions as opposed to inadequate treatment.

Laser photocoagulation is not without its complications, notably perforation or bleeding, but they should be infrequent when it is employed by those familiar with the technique and equipment. The long-term results are usually good, but rebleeding does occur, from both treated and other sites. As noted by Rutgeerts and colleagues,[77] "more important for the outcome, however, is the number of lesions. The more numerous the lesions the less efficacious laser photocoagulation is in decreasing the rate of bleeding."

An interesting question has been posed as to whether an incidentally encountered vascular ectasia should be biopsied or treated. Our inclination, concurred in by Brandt and Rogers,[81] is to leave it alone. Rogers, however, in his discussion of Brandt's article[83] expresses the opposite viewpoint.

BLEEDING

Acute Bleeding

Colonoscopy can be performed during the active phase of a lower gastrointestinal bleeding episode as long as the patient is hemodynamically stable. Blood acts somewhat as a cathartic so that the colon can be examined with varying degrees of success. Sometimes, although the exact nature of the pathology cannot be determined, the *location* of the bleeding can be ascertained. This is helpful when surgical intervention is contemplated.

Chronic Bleeding

Colonoscopy is the best tool for diagnosing the cause of lower gastrointestinal bleeding. As long as the bowel preparation is adequate, a colonic bleeding site may generally be found. Angiodysplasias or arteriovenous malformations frequently occur in the cecum. They may or may not be actively bleeding at the time of diagnosis (see earlier discussion).

Although much has been published on the subject of endoscopic management of acute and chronic *upper* gastrointestinal tract bleeding, there is considerably less information with respect to the lower bowel. At first it was thought that retrograde colonoscopy had little to offer— and possibly was excessively risky—for the patient with acute, active bleeding from the lower bowel. The accomplishment of appropriate bowel cleansing and visualization was deemed unlikely. Forde and Treat[84] approached the problem aggressively and suggested that the rate of bleeding is the central issue. They proposed division of patients into the following three major groups to determine clinical response: (1) acute bleeding, (2) recent major bleeding, and (3) chronic minor and occult bleeding. The latter two groups have been adequately discussed previously, and the invaluable contributions made by colonoscopy are now widely recognized,[84-86] in terms of both lesion identification and therapy. In evaluating reports on the subject, it is wise to ascertain just what is referred to when the term emergency colonoscopy is used. Patients who have experienced a recent major episode of gastrointestinal bleeding that has stopped are very likely to have colonoscopy recommended. Such examinations can, and frequently are, very fruitful but, as Forde points out, these individuals are not undergoing emergency colonoscopy. Also, he notes, they often require more vigorous and prolonged preparation than do routine cases and urges that this be carried out whenever feasible.

The acute bleeding problems posing the greatest difficulty are those in which the bleeding is active and vigorous and associated with volume depletion requiring transfusion, prompt diagnosis, and therapy if survival is to be achieved. Assuming that an upper gastrointestinal tract source has been ruled out by appropriate diagnostic measures, rigid or flexible sigmoidoscopy is in order to eliminate the possibility of a low-lying source.[87-89] In such cases, the traditional rigid scope has many advantages, as the flexible instrument requires adequate mechanical cleansing of the rectum.

If these measures fail to resolve the clinical problem, the diagnostic and therapeutic options include radionuclide scanning, selective mesenteric angiography, and colonoscopy. If the former have been tried and transcatheter instillations of vasoconstrictors or emboli, or both, have proved inadequate, true emergency colonoscopy appears to be a procedure of last resort. At this stage, patients are usually critically ill and possibly in shock—far from ideal candidates for the procedure. Laxatives and colonic lavage are dangerous, but rectal irrigation with saline or tap water is necessary to remove blood clots. Examination is usually difficult because anatomic landmarks may be obscured by blood. When clots are encountered, they must be dispersed by jets of saline, and observation of the field of vision by gravitational puddling of fluid blood can sometimes be helped by changing the patient's position. Overdistention of the bowel by instillation of air or fluid must be avoided. Initial efforts must be directed at maximal insertion, with more careful examination of the bowel wall being done on withdrawal.

If a demonstrated or possible source of the bleeding is found, its precise localization within the colon is more easily identified if the procedure has been done with fluoroscopic monitoring.

The course to follow when the bleeding source is found depends on the nature of the lesion. At the very least, the procedure localizes the segment of bowel involved so that if laparotomy is required the surgeon's job is made that much easier.

The endoscopist must at all times proceed cautiously but with dispatch. An unduly long examination may permit excessive further deterioration of the patient's condition.

References

1. Wolff WI, Shinya H. Modern endoscopy of the alimentary tract. In: Ravitch M, Steichen F. Current problems in surgery. Chicago: Year Book Medical Publishers, 1974.
2. Wolff WI. Colonoscopy. History and development. Am J Gastroenterol 84:1017–1025, 1989.
3. Turell R, Marshak RH. Coloscopy with some reference to polypoid lesions. NY State J Med 72:2615, 1972.
4. Wolff WI. Colonoscopy and endoscopic polypectomy (editorial). NY State J Med 73:641–642, 1973.
5. Wolff WI, Shinya H, Geffen A, et al. Comparison of colonoscopy and the contrast enema in five hundred patients with colorectal disease. Am J Surg 129:181–186, 1975.
6. American Heart Association. Prevention of bacterial endocarditis. JAMA 264(22):2919–2922, 1990.
7. Langdon DC, Harlon JR, Bailey RI. Thrombophlebitis with diazepam used intravenously. JAMA 223:184–185, 1973.
8. Wolff WI, Shinya H. Colonofiberoscopy. JAMA 217:1509–1512, 1971.
9. Wolff WI, Shinya H, Geffen A, et al. Colonofiberoscopy. Am J Surg 123:180–184, 1972.
10. Wolff WI, Shinya H. Polypectomy via the fiberoptic colonoscope. N Engl J Med 288:329–332, 1973.
11. Moore FD. Discussion of Colonic Polyps by Wolff WI, Shinya H. Ann Surg 178:376, 1973.
12. Dunphy JE. Discussion of Colonic Polyps by Wolff WI, Shinya H. Ann Surg 178:377, 1973.
13. Wolff WI, Shinya H. A new approach to colonic polyps. Ann Surg 178:367–376, 1973.
14. Wolff WI, Shinya H. Colonfiberoscopic management of colonic polyps. Dis Colon Rectum 16:87–93, 1973.
15. Ingelfinger FJ. Malignant potential of colonic polyps. In: Ingelfinger FJ, Relman AS, Finland M, et al, eds. Controversy in internal medicine. II. Philadelphia: WB Saunders, 1974.
16. Hunt RH, Waye JD. Colonoscopy: Technique, clinical practice and colour atlas. London: Chapman and Hall, 1981.
17. Shinya H. Colonoscopy: diagnosis and treatment of colonic diseases. New York, Tokyo: Igaku-Shoin, 1982.
18. Wolff WI. Hospital privileges for gastrointestinal endoscopy. Bull Am Coll Surg 66(11):17–20, 1981.
19. Wolff WI, Shinya H, Cwern H, et al. Cancerous colonic polyps. "Hands on" or "hands off." Am Surg 56:148–152, 1990.
20. Cosgrove JM, Wolff WI, Tenenbaum N, et al. An appraisal of small and diminutive colonic polyps. Surg Endosc 5:143–145, 1991.
21. Achkar E, Carey W. Small polyps found during sigmoidoscopy in asymptomatic patients. Ann Intern Med 109:880–883, 1988.
22. Tripp MR, Morgan TR, Sampliner RE, et al. Synchronous neoplasms in patients with diminutive colorectal adenomas. Cancer 60:1599–1603, 1987.
23. Urbanski SJ, Haber G, Kartan P, et al. Small colonic adenomas with adenocarcinoma: a retrospective analysis. Dis Colon Rectum 31:58–61, 1988.
24. Ways JD, Lewis BS, Frankel A, et al. Small colon polyps. Am J Gastroenterol 83:120–122, 1988.
25. Wolff WI, Shinya H. Earlier diagnosis of cancer of the colon through colonic endoscopy (colonoscopy). Cancer 34:912–931, 1974.
26. Wolff WI, Shinya H. The impact of colonoscopy on the problem of colorectal cancer. In: Ariel IM, ed. Progress in clinical cancer. New York: Grune & Stratton, 1978:VII:51–69.
27. Jass J. Nature and clinical significance of colorectal hyperplastic polyp. Semin Colon Rectal Surg 2:246–252, 1991.
28. Ragins H, Shinya H, Wolff WI. The explosive potential of colonic gas during colonoscopic electrosurgical polypectomy. Surg Gynecol Obstet 138:554–556, 1974.
29. Dyer WS, Quigley EMM, Noel SM, et al. Major colonic hemorrhage following electrocoagulating (hot) biopsy of diminutive colonic polyps. Gastrointest Endosc 37:361–362, 1991.
30. Williams CB. Small polyps: the virtue and dangers of hot biopsy (editorial). Gastrointest Endosc 37:94–95, 1991.
31. Waitman AM, Grant DZ, Chateau F. Endoscopic laser photocoagulation of bleeding gastrointestinal telangiectasia (abstract). Gastrointest Endosc 27:139–140, 1981.
32. Waitman AM, Grant DZ, Chateau F. Endoscopic management of vascular abnormalities. In: Silvis SE, ed. Therapeutic gastrointestinal endoscopy. New York, Tokyo: Igaku-Shoin, 1985.
33. Ghazi A, Ferstenberg H, Shinya H. Endoscopic gastroduodenal polypectomy. Ann Surg 200:175–180, 1984.
34. Mathur-Vliegen EMH, Tygat GNJ. Laser ablation and palliation in colorectal malignancy—results of a multicenter inquiry. Gastrointest Endosc 32:393–399, 1986.
35. Mellow MH. Endoscopic therapy of colorectal neoplasms. Gastrointest Endosc Clin North Am 2:543–552, 1992.
36. Brunetaud JM, Maunoury V, Cochelard D, et al. Laser palliation for rectosigmoid cancers. Int J Colorectal Dis 4:6–8, 1989.
37. Webb WA, McDaniel L, Jones L. Experience with 1000

colonoscopic polypectomies. Ann Surg 201:626–632, 1985.

38. Colacchio TA, Forde KA, Scantlebury VP. Endoscopic polypectomy: inadequate treatment for invasive colorectal carcinoma. Ann Surg 194:704–770, 1981.

39. Waye JD. An approach to malignant polyps. Gastrointest Endosc 30:310–311, 1984.

40. Wilcox GM, Colaccio TA. Reply to selected summary: is polypectomy alone adequate for carcinoma in-situ? Gastroenterology 83:716–717, 1982.

41. Lockhard Mummery HE, Dukes CE. The surgical treatment of malignant rectal polyps. Lancet 2:751–755, 1952.

42. Carden ABG, Morson BC. Recurrence of the local excision of malignant polyps of the rectum. Proc R Soc Med 57:1–3, 1964.

43. Wolff WI, Shinya H. Definitive treatment of "malignant polyps" of the colon. Ann Surg 182:516–525, 1975.

44. Christie JP. Malignant colon polyps—cure by colonoscopy or colectomy? Am J Gastroenterol 79:543–547, 1984.

45. Coutsoftides T, Sivak MV Jr, Benjamin JP. Colonoscopy and the management of polyps containing invasive carcinoma. Ann Surg 188:638–641, 1978.

46. Langer JC, Cohen Z, Taylor BR, et al. Management of patients with polyps containing malignancy removed by colonoscopic polypectomy. Dis Colon Rectum 27:6–9, 1984.

47. Lipper S, Kahn LB, Ackerman IV. The significance of microscopic invasive cancer in endoscopically removed polyps of the large bowel: a clinicopathologic study of 51 cases. Cancer 52:1691–1699, 1983.

48. Nivatvongs S, Goldberg SM. Management of patients who have polyps containing invasive carcinoma removed via colonoscope. Dis Colon Rectum 21:8–11, 1978.

49. Morson BC, Whiteway JE, Jones FA, et al. Histopathology and prognosis of malignant colorectal polyps treated by endoscopic polypectomy. Gut 25:437–444, 1984.

50. Haggitt RC, Glotzbach RE, Soffer EE, et al. Prognostic factors in colorectal carcinomas arising in adenomas: implications for lesions removed by endoscopic polypectomy. Gastroenterology 89:328–336, 1985.

51. Church JM, Fazio VW, Jones IT. Small colorectal polyps. Dis Colon Rectum 31:50–53, 1988.

52. Feczko PJ, Bernstein MA, Holpert R, et al. Small colonic polyps. Radiology 152:301–303, 1984.

53. Overhall BF, Hargrove RJ, Ferris RK, et al. Colonoscopic polypectomy: silent perforation. Gastroenterology 20:112–113, 1976.

54. Nivatvongs S. Complications in colonoscopic polypectomy. Am Surg 54:61–63, 1988.

55. Ballantyne GH, Brandner MD, Beart RW. Volvulus of the colon. 202:83–92, 1985.

56. Ghazi A, Shinya H, Wolff WI. Treatment of volvulus of the colon by colonoscopy. Ann Surg 183:263–265, 1976.

57. Brothers TE, Strodel WE, Eckhauser FE. Endoscopy in colonic volvulus. Ann Surg 206:1–4, 1987.

58. Geer DA, Arnaud G, Beitler A, et al. Colonic volvulus. The Army Medical Center experience 1983–1987. Am Surg 57:295–300, 1991.

59. Dabezies MA, Krevsky B, Kolenda B. An overtube for decompression of sigmoid volvulus. Gastrointest Endosc 34:6:491, 1988.

60. Ogilvie A. Large intestine colic due to sympathetic deprivation. A new clinical syndrome. Br Med J 2:671–673, 1948.

61. Spira IA, Rodriques R, Wolff WI. Pseudo-obstruction of the colon. Am J Gastroenterol 65:397–408, 1976.

62. Spira IA, Wolff WI. Gangrene and spontaneous perforation of the cecum as a complication of pseudo-obstruction of the colon. Dis Colon Rectum 19:557–562, 1976.

63. Spira IA, Wolff WI. Colonic pseudo-obstruction following termination of pregnancy and uterine operation. Am J Obstet Gynecol 126:7–12, 1976.

64. Spira IA, Rubenstein R, Wolff WI, et al. Fecal impaction following methadone ingestion simulating acute intestinal obstruction. Ann Surg 181:15–19, 1975.

65. Rubenstein R, Spira IA, Wolff WI. Management of surgical problems in patients on methadone maintenance—analysis of 100 cases. Am J Surg 131:566–569, 1976.

66. Strodel WE, Eckhauser FW. Therapeutic and diagnostic colonoscopy in non-obstructive colonic dilatation. Ann Surg 197:416–421, 1983.

67. Gosche JR, Sharpe JN, Larson GM. Colonoscopic decompression for pseudo-obstruction of the colon. Am Surg 55:111–115, 1989.

68. Dent TL, Kukora JS, Strodel WE. Colonoscopic decompression: treatment of choice for acute pseudo-obstruction of the colon (Ogilvie's syndrome). In: Dent TL, Strodel WE, Turcotte JG, et al., eds. Surgical endoscopy. Chicago: Year Book Medical Publishers, 1985.

69. Sloyer AF, Panella VS, Demas BE, et al. Ogilvie's syndrome: successful management without endoscopy. Dig Dis Sci 33:1391–1396, 1988.

70. Surawicz CM. Ogilvie's syndrome (acute colonic pseudo-obstruction). In: Gitnick G, ed. Current gastroenterology. Vol 10. Chicago: Year Book Medical Publishers, 1990.

71. Boley SJ, Brandt LJ. Vascular ectasias of the colon. Dig Dis Sci 31(Suppl):265–425, 1986.

72. Greenstein RJ, McElhinney AJ, Reuben D, et al. Colonic vascular ectasias and aortic stenosis: coincidence or causal relationship? Am J Surg 151:347–351, 1986.

73. Trudel JL, Fazio VW, Sivak MV. Colonoscopic diagnosis and treatment of arteriovenous malformations in chronic lower gastrointestinal bleeding. Dis Colon Rectum 31:107–110, 1988.

74. Howard DM, Buchanan JD, Hunt RH. Angiodysplasia of the colon. Experience of 26 cases. Lancet 2:16–19, 1982.

75. Rogers BHG, Adler F. Hemangiomas of the cecum. Colonoscopic diagnosis and therapy. Gastroenterology 71:1079–1082, 1976.

76. Tedesco FJ, Griffin JW Jr, Klein AG. Vascular ectasia of the colon: clinical, colonoscopic and radiographic features. J Clin Gastroenterol 2:233–238, 1980.

77. Rutgeerts P, Van Grompel F, Geboes K, et al. Long term results of treatment of vascular malformations of the gastrointestinal tract by neodymium:YAG laser photocoagulation. Gut 26:586–593, 1985.

78. Wolff WI, Grossman MB, Shinya H. Angiodysplasia of the colon: diagnosis and treatment. Gastroenterology 72:329–333, 1977.

79. Waitman AM, Grant DZ, Chateau F. Endoscopic management of vascular abnormalities. In: Silvis SE, ed. Therapeutic gastrointestinal endoscopy. New York, Tokyo: Igaku-Shoin, 1985.

80. Grant DZ, Scherl EJ, Waitman AM, et al. Laser therapy of vascular abnormalities. In: Silvis SE, ed. Therapeutic gastrointestinal endoscopy. 2nd ed. New York, Tokyo: Igaku-Shoin, 1990.

81. Brandt LJ, Rogers BHG. A cecal angiodysplastic lesion is discovered during diagnostic colonoscopy performed for iron-deficiency anemia associated with stool positive

for occult blood. What therapy would you recommend? Am J Gastroenterol 83:710–711, 1988.

82. Danesh BJZ, Spiliadis C, Williams CB, et al. Angiodysplasia—an uncommon cause of colonic bleeding. Int J Colorectal Dis 2:218–222, 1987.

83. Rogers BHG. Discussion of article by Brandt LG, Rogers BHG. Am J Gastroenterol 83:710–711, 1988.

84. Forde KA, Treat MR. Colonoscopy for lower gastrointestinal tract bleeding. In: Dent TL, Strodel WE, Turcotte JG, Harper ML, eds. Surgical Endoscopy. Chicago: Year Book Medical Publishers, 1985:261–274.

85. Tedesco FJ, Waye JD, Raskin JB, et al. Colonoscopic evaluation of rectal bleeding: a study of 304 patients. Ann Intern Med 89:907–990, 1978.

86. Teague RH, Thornton JR, Manning AP, et al. Colonoscopy for investigations of unexplained rectal bleeding. Lancet 1:1350–1351, 1978.

87. Orecchia PM, Hensley EK, Donald PT. Localization of lower gastrointestinal hemorrhage. Arch Surg 120:621–625, 1985.

88. Noer RJ. Hemorrhage as a complication of diverticulitis. Ann Surg 141:674–677, 1955.

89. Knight CD. Massive hemorrhage from diverticular disease of the colon. Surgery 42:853–856, 1957.

22

Colonoscopy in the Diagnosis and Treatment of Colorectal Malignancy

Theodore R. Schrock

Cancer of the colon and rectum is a serious problem throughout the world. It is the second most common cause of death from malignant disease in many developed countries.[1] In the United States, approximately 150,000 new cases of colorectal cancer are diagnosed and about 60,000 deaths occur from this disease annually.[2] Colorectal cancer is responsible for 20,000 deaths each year in Britain.[3]

Colonoscopy has established a prominent place in the diagnosis and treatment of colorectal malignancy since its introduction 25 years ago.[4] Colonoscopy is used to screen patients at high risk of the development of colorectal cancer. Benign neoplastic polyps, believed to be the precursors of most cancers of the large bowel, are detected and removed by colonoscopy. Colonoscopic polypectomy is sufficient treatment for some malignant polyps. In most instances, symptoms of cancer are investigated initially by colonoscopy. Known or suspected malignancy is evaluated by colonoscopy to inspect the lesion directly, biopsy the tumor, and search for synchronous neoplasms. Colonoscopic methods can assist in the palliation of some unresectable cancers of the distal bowel. Colonoscopy is an essential feature in the follow-up of patients after excision of benign or malignant neoplasms. The role of colonoscopy in contemporary management of colorectal cancer is discussed in this chapter.

SCREENING OF PERSONS AT AVERAGE RISK

There are two basic approaches to earlier detection of large bowel cancer: (1) education about symptoms and signs of cancer in the hope that both patients and physicians will act more quickly to detect the disease and (2) screening of asymptomatic persons.[5] The value of early diagnosis in symptomatic patients is beyond dispute, but the usefulness of screening asymptomatic persons remains unproved.[5-9]

General Principles of Screening

Screening is the search for disease by testing large populations of asymptomatic individuals.[5, 10] *Case finding* is the diagnosis of disease at an early stage in patients who consult a physician, whether or not these patients are symptomatic.[10] In screening, the health care system seeks out individuals with the disease, and in case finding patients take the initiative.[5] Cancer *surveillance* is a form of screening in which an at-risk population (*e.g.*, patients with ulcerative colitis [UC]) is investigated on a regular schedule to prevent or detect the onset of malignancy.[11]

Criteria for screening programs for any disease have been defined.[12] The natural history of the condition must be known, there must be a

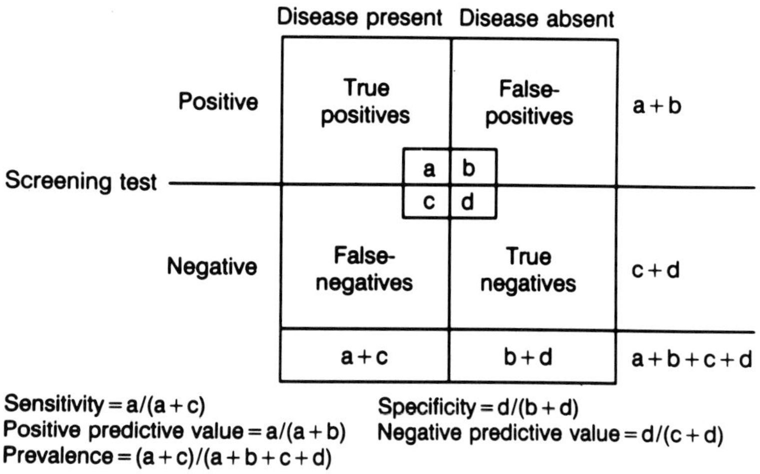

Figure 22-1. Evaluation of screening tests. (From McGill DB, Ahlquist DA. Screening for colorectal disease. In: Phillips SF, Pemberton JH, Shorter RG, eds. The large intestine: Physiology, pathophysiology, and disease. New York: Raven Press, 1991:336.)

	Disease present	Disease absent	
Positive	True positives	False-positives	a + b
Screening test	a	b	
	c	d	
Negative	False-negatives	True negatives	c + d
	a + c	b + d	a + b + c + d

Sensitivity = a/(a + c)   Specificity = d/(b + d)
Positive predictive value = a/(a + b)   Negative predictive value = d/(c + d)
Prevalence = (a + c)/(a + b + c + d)

recognizable latent stage, acceptable tests with high specificity and sensitivity must be available, treatment should be generally accepted, and early diagnosis and treatment should improve the prognosis.[13]

Results of screening studies are expressed in a variety of statistics as shown in Figure 22-1.[9] The positive predictive value is most useful to the clinician.[14] It gives a direct indication of the odds that the abnormal test result is due to the disease in question.

A number of biases can confuse the interpretation of cancer screening studies.[15] In general, these biases make a screening test appear more effective than it actually is.[15] *Lead time bias* is the result of earlier detection of a disease that does not translate to improved survival. Patients who have been screened may appear to live longer than individuals who have not just because the interval from detection to death is longer, yet the two groups still die at the same point. *Length time bias* arises because a screening test is more likely to detect slowly growing tumors that are prevalent in a population for long periods. Slowly growing tumors in general are less aggressive and have more favorable outcomes. *Overdetection bias* is detection of very early lesions that might not progress to invasive cancer if left alone. Inclusion of such lesions may make it appear that the screened population is better off than the general population. *Volunteer bias* makes a test appear more or less effective, depending on the characteristics of the individuals who volunteer for the screening program.[15]

Screening for Colorectal Cancer

Colorectal cancer meets most of the criteria for screening. The natural history is well estab-

lished. Polyps are precursors of malignancy. Carcinoma has a latent stage; it becomes symptomatic relatively late, often when the tumor has spread beyond the bowel wall.[1] Surgical resection is the standard treatment, and survival following resection is directly related to the degree of spread at the time of operation.[1, 5] What remains at issue is the adequacy of current screening tests and the uncertainty that mortality rates will be lowered as a result of the wide application of these tests.

The adenoma-carcinoma sequence is an important constituent in arguments for the value of screening programs.[16] If most cancers arise in adenomas, detection and removal of benign neoplasms by screening is cancer prevention.[1, 16, 17] The consensus has been and remains that most carcinomas of the large bowel, perhaps 90% or so, develop within adenomas.[18–21] Basic science support of this sequence comes from a recent report that a human colonic adenoma cell line has been changed from the premalignant state to its malignant counterpart by exposure to a carcinogen (N-methyl-N'-nitro-N-nitrosoguanidine) in vitro.[22]

What percentage of carcinomas, if any, arise de novo remains unclear.[3, 23, 24] Claims that "at least 80%" of cancers arise de novo may be valid in Japan and other low-risk areas but seem unlikely for Western populations.[25, 26] The finding of polypoid carcinomas as small as 2 to 7 mm demonstrates that there may not be an endoscopically identifiable benign phase in every case, nor is there always a long phase of development to cancer.[19]

Methods of Screening

The American Cancer Society has issued guidelines for screening of asymptomatic persons at average risk of acquiring colorectal cancer. The following program is recommended: (1) from age 40 to 50 years, an annual digital rectal examination and fecal occult blood test (FOBT); (2) from age 50 years, sigmoidoscopy, preferably flexible, every 3 to 5 years after two normal annual examinations.[5, 6, 15, 27, 28] The National Cancer Institute and other groups have supported these recommendations, but dissenting views are plentiful. These screening tests are now discussed.

Fecal Occult Blood Test

The FOBT is the most important element in large scale studies of screening of persons at average risk. Of course, the FOBT is used also by individual clinicians in case finding.

The most common test for fecal occult blood employs guaiac-impregnated slides (Hemoccult, SmithKline Diagnostics, Inc., San Jose, CA). Positive test results are found in 2% to 6% of participants in screening programs. Colorectal cancer is detected in 5% to 10%, and adenomas are found in 10% to 43% of individuals with positive test results in these circumstances.[29–31] The false-positive rate in large screening studies varies from 3% to 5%.[5, 32, 33] Overall, the positive predictive value for invasive cancer is 11% to 24%, and for adenomas it is 36% to 41%.[34, 35] In one trial, overall positive predictivity was lower than that reported by others, and it increased with age from 1.6% for individuals younger than 60 years to 3.6% for those older than 70 years.[36]

The insensitivity of the FOBT for cancer represents the major obstacle to screening efficacy.[37] In one study, the sensitivity for neoplasia was 21% (false-negative rate of 79%).[34] In general, however, the false-negative rate is about 30% to 40%.[5, 32, 33] False-negative test results reflect inadequate sampling in some patients, but in many cases the test result is negative because the neoplasm does not shed enough blood to be detected.[38] Generally, carcinomas must ulcerate before they bleed. Small polypoid adenomas (less than 1 cm) are unlikely to bleed, and even polyps as large as 2 cm do not bleed in every instance.[37, 39, 40] Detection of small adenomas by the FOBT is almost certainly serendipity.[41] The Hemoccult test is significantly more sensitive for carcinoma of the sigmoid and descending colon (81%) than for rectal cancer (45%) or ascending colon cancer (47%).[42, 43]

Rehydrating Hemoccult slides changes the findings.[44] In a representative study, positivity rose from 2.4% to 9.8% and sensitivity increased from 81% to 92% with rehydration, but specificity decreased from 98% to 90%, and positive predictivity dropped from 5.6% to 2.2%.[36] Selection of a method of processing the FOBT requires a compromise between sensitivity and specificity.[35]

HemoQuant (SmithKline Beecham Clinical Laboratories, Van Nuys, CA) is a quantitative assay of fecal hemoglobin by fluorimetry of porphyrins derived from heme in the assay reaction or during intestinal transit.[45] Another method of testing for occult blood is immunologic determination of fecal hemoglobin and transferrin levels.[46] It remains to be seen whether these more complex and expensive tests are sufficiently advantageous to replace the Hemoccult test.[38]

There is only suggestive evidence that mass screening for fecal occult blood in patients at average risk of acquiring colorectal cancer achieves the goal of reducing mortality from this disease.[36, 47–49] Cancers detected in screened populations routinely are less advanced than those detected in control groups. In one study of more than 107,000 asymptomatic individuals, 52% of cancers detected were Dukes' stage A compared with 10.6% that were Dukes' stage A in the control group.[29] However, the biases discussed earlier may have influenced these findings. The results of prospective controlled trials that should answer the central question are anticipated in a few years. In the practice setting, the FOBT alone is an uncommon manner of colorectal cancer detection; most cancers present with symptoms.[50]

The possible presence of colorectal cancer in a person with a positive FOBT is the greatest concern.[51] It is also true that abnormal blood in stool usually reflects other, often trivial, pathologic findings.[37] Occult fecal blood requires evaluation by history, physical examination, laboratory studies, and anoscopy.[52] Rigid proctosigmoidoscopy helps detect anorectal disease, but it has limited value in patients with occult bleeding.[42] The entire colon must be examined by a combination of flexible sigmoidoscopy and double-contrast barium enema or by colonoscopy.[53] Surprisingly, 35% of individuals with positive FOBT results in one study had an inadequate diagnostic workup limited to a repeat FOBT or sigmoidoscopy, or both.[48] Comparison of strategies to evaluate a patient with a positive FOBT result is detailed in Table 22–1. Further discussion of these diagnostic techniques follows.

Table 22–1. PERFORMANCE OF SEVEN DIAGNOSTIC STRATEGIES FOR SCREENEES WITH A POSITIVE FECAL OCCULT BLOOD TEST

| Strategy | Strategy Sensitivity | | | | Net Benefits and Costs* | | | | Cost-effectiveness Ratio | |
	Localized Ca	Disseminated Ca	Polyps >0.5 cm	Strategy Specificity	Fatal Ca Prevented	Major Morbidity	Minor Morbidity	Cost	Per Fatality Prevented	Per Life-year Saved
RSIG	0.20	0.20	0.10	0.98	0.70	0.10	0.36	$ 81,333	$116,190	$13,832
FSIG	0.50	0.50	0.50	0.98	1.75	0.62	1.82	$168,607	$ 96,347	$11,470
BE	0.80	1.0	0.60	0.95	2.82	0.35	2.16	$211,040	$ 74,837	$ 9,385
RSIG + BE	0.84	1.0	0.64	0.93	2.94	0.41	2.31	$237,177	$ 80,671	$ 9,604
FSIG + BE	0.90	1.0	0.80	0.93	3.15	0.81	2.89	$287,580	$ 91,294	$10,868
CO	0.95	1.0	0.90	1.0	3.32	1.03	3.68	$281,697	$ 84,720	$10,086
CO + BE	0.99	1.0	0.96	1.0	3.46	1.03	3.68	$354,853	$102,410	$12,192

From Barry MJ, Mulley AG, Richter JM. Effect of workup strategy on the cost-effectiveness of fecal occult blood screening for colorectal cancer. Gastroenterology 93:301–310, 1987.
*Per 10,000 screened.
BE = barium enema; Ca = carcinoma; CO = colonoscopy; FSIG = flexible sigmoidoscopy; RSIG = rigid sigmoidoscopy.

Proctosigmoidoscopy

Proctosigmoidoscopy is described in detail in Chapter 23. Rigid sigmoidoscopy was the screening procedure used in the landmark study that found that no patient acquired rectal cancer within 7 years of normal sigmoidoscopic examination.[54] Today, flexible proctosigmoidoscopy is preferred over rigid proctosigmoidoscopy because it examines two to three times more bowel length and detects two to six times the number of lesions.[55, 56] Flexible sigmoidoscopy has a sensitivity for neoplasms of the distal colon and rectum of nearly 94%, and the positive predictive value in this location is 100%.[34]

Until 25 years ago, nearly 50% of large bowel tumors occurred in the distal colon or rectum.[15] Since then, a shift to the right of cancer distribution has been reported by many groups.[57, 58] An occasional dissenting view appears.[59] Currently, the most proximal and distal 20 to 25-cm segments of the large bowel each harbor about 25% of the cancers.[58] The practical implication is that flexible proctosigmoidoscopy is better than rigid sigmoidoscopy for screening, but the data also support an opinion that screening should evaluate the entire colon and rectum.[58] Fully 50% of colonic cancers that are too far proximal to be seen with the rigid sigmoidoscope are also too high to be reached with the flexible one. Flexible proctosigmoidoscopy alone clearly is inadequate to evaluate patients with a positive FOBT result.[52, 53]

Studies of screening sigmoidoscopy to detect cancer in individuals with negative FOBT results who are at average risk of acquiring colorectal cancer have reached equivocal conclusions, in part because most of the data are uncon-

trolled.[15, 60] In a representative study, flexible sigmoidoscopy with a 60-cm scope was performed in 412 asymptomatic veterans.[61] A total of 132 polyps were detected in 93 subjects (22.6%), and four invasive carcinomas were found (4.3%). The cost of detecting each potentially curable carcinoma was $47,174.[61]

Carcinomas detected by screening flexible proctosigmoidoscopy typically are in an early stage, but it is unclear whether screening improves survival.[61] Two recent retrospective case control studies concluded that the risk of death from colorectal cancer was reduced among individuals who had a single screening sigmoidoscopic examination compared with the risk for those who never had one.[62, 63] The risk of death from distal cancers was markedly reduced for 10 years after a single examination; fatal colon cancer above the reach of the sigmoidoscope did not show this difference.[62] The specificity of the negative association for cancer within the reach of the sigmoidoscope is consistent with a true efficacy of screening.[62] Despite these encouraging results, a properly conducted randomized trial with colorectal cancer mortality as an outcome is needed to provide a definitive answer.[15]

Proctosigmoidoscopy and Barium Enema

A combination of proctosigmoidoscopy to examine the distal colon and rectum and barium enema to study the proximal bowel can be used to evaluate patients with positive FOBT results.[64–68] This approach is not recommended for individuals with negative FOBT results who are at average risk of acquiring colorectal cancer.

Barium enema has a good record of accuracy in the detection of malignant lesions.[65, 69] Review of 19 English language radiologic publications between 1980 and 1989 showed that 15 of 19 investigations had a radiologic sensitivity of 90% to 100% for detection of colorectal cancer, with a median sensitivity of 94%.[69] Detection of benign neoplasms, especially small ones, is not as reliable. Barium enema is 80% to 95% sensitive for detection of polyps greater than or equal to 1 cm and 50% to 85% sensitive for detection of polypoid lesions less than or equal to 1 cm.[69]

In one study, double-contrast barium enema and flexible sigmoidoscopy were used to assess 530 patients with positive FOBT results. An adenoma greater than or equal to 1 cm was found in 13.4% of cases, and a carcinoma was diagnosed in 4.9% of cases overall.[70] The sensitivity for neoplasms greater than or equal to 1 cm at the primary assessment was 72% for double-contrast barium enema and 86% for sigmoidoscopy; the sensitivity for the combined methods was 94%, and the specificity was 99%.[70] Colonoscopy was performed in very few of these patients.

A drawback to double-contrast barium enema is the number of false-positive findings of diminutive polyps.[70] In one study, about 13% of all sizes of polyps seen on barium enema were artifacts, and 28% of presumed adenomas less than or equal to 1 cm in diameter were false positives.[70]

Colonoscopy

The technique of diagnostic colonoscopy is described in Chapter 21. Colonoscopy permits direct inspection of the entire colonic mucosa in more than 90% of patients.[71, 72] Perhaps 30% of colonoscopies are technically difficult, but a claim that attempted complete colonoscopy routinely fails to reach the cecum in 25% of patients does not mesh with actual experience.[69]

The ability of colonoscopy to detect large colorectal polyps ($\geq$1 cm) was studied in a blinded trial featuring tandem colonoscopy. The rate of missed lesions was less than 5% during the index colonoscopic examination in the well-prepared colon.[73] In a study of specimens of colon resected for cancer, the findings on preoperative colonoscopy agreed with the pathology report 96% of the time in patients with synchronous polyps greater than or equal to 1 cm.[74] When polyps of all sizes were included, with many less than 5 mm, colonoscopy agreed with the pathology report in 89% of cases.[74] Small lesions are the major source of error; the

endoscopist misses at least 20% to 30% of polyps 2 to 5 mm in diameter.[75] There is no doubt that colonoscopy can miss large lesions too, especially in flexures.

Colonoscopy rather than proctosigmoidoscopy is required when all of the colon must be inspected. In one study, flexible sigmoidoscopy was performed in asymptomatic men older than 50 years of age, followed immediately by colonoscopy regardless of the sigmoidoscopic result.[76] Polyps were found in proximal colonic segments in 20% of patients who had no adenomas on sigmoidoscopy.[76] The majority of proximal neoplasms were small ($\leq$1 cm) tubular adenomas, and it remains to be determined whether small proximal adenomas are worth finding.[76] In another study, the 130-cm colonoscope was substituted for the flexible sigmoidoscope for screening, using the usual sigmoidoscopy enema routine for preparation.[77] There was no advantage to using the colonoscope in this way.[77]

Many studies have compared colonoscopy with a combination of flexible proctosigmoidoscopy and air-contrast barium enema for the evaluation of patients with positive FOBT results.[53, 68, 78] Some of these studies lack proper controls to support their conclusions. For example, colonoscopy by experts was contrasted with radiographic studies of uneven quality, and as a result, 30% to 40% of significant lesions found at colonoscopy had been missed by barium enema.[79] In another study, patients preferred colonoscopy over barium enema, but patients were sedated for colonoscopy and not for the x-ray studies.[80] An article from the radiology literature collected 18 cases of colonic neoplasm 2 to 8 cm in diameter from six institutions; all lesions were missed by colonoscopy and were seen on barium enema, with the implication that gross diagnostic errors are common during colonoscopy.[81] Another radiologist claimed that approximately 10% to 20% of colorectal lesions detected on barium enema are missed by colonoscopy, mostly because of failure to examine the ascending colon; there was no information on the size and histologic diagnosis of these radiographic findings.[69]

The bulk of objective evidence is persuasive that colonoscopy has a higher sensitivity for tumors greater than or equal to 5 mm when compared with a combination of flexible sigmoidoscopy and double-contrast barium enema.[27, 53, 75, 82–84] A prospective study of patients with polyps discovered during fiberoptic sigmoidoscopy compared the accuracy of barium enema performed by experienced radiologists to colonoscopy performed by experienced gastroenterologists who were blinded to the radiographic findings.[84] Synchronous proximal polyps larger than 0.5 cm in diameter were found by colonoscopy in 40% of 114 patients, but the sensitivity of double-contrast barium enema in detecting these lesions was only 26%.[84] Another study directly compared colonoscopy and air-contrast barium enema by using both procedures in patients with distal polyps; specificity was 91% for endoscopy and 72% for barium enema in detection of lesions greater than or equal to 7 mm in diameter.[75]

Cost considerations are important in designing a mass screening program, and no doubt colonoscopy for individuals with a positive FOBT result is more costly, at least initially, than alternative strategies.[53, 68, 78] Conversely, the higher initial cost of colonoscopy may be offset by its greater sensitivity and its capacity for biopsy and treatment.[85] In one study, colonoscopy as the first test had a cost of $2139/treatable lesion compared with a cost of $2895 for a combination of proctoscopy and barium enema.[85] Another study calculated the cost/fatality prevented by FOBT screening; the authors concluded that the cost was lower if patients with positive FOBT results were evaluated by colonoscopy rather than by a combination of flexible sigmoidoscopy and barium enema (see Table 22–1).[53]

There are additional arguments for total colonoscopy as the initial choice in most patients who have positive FOBT results. If a double-contrast barium enema shows no lesion in a patient with occult fecal blood, most clinicians feel compelled to perform colonoscopy anyway.[52] (A minority opinion is that the residual risk to patients who have positive FOBT results but do not have a familial trait may be low enough that the dangers of colonoscopy could outweigh the potential benefits.)[86] Further, if a lesion is seen on flexible sigmoidoscopy or barium enema, colonoscopy is needed to biopsy or remove the lesion and to look for synchronous lesions.[4, 27, 87, 88] Finally, lesions seen on barium enema, even if genuine, may or may not be the source of occult bleeding, and colonoscopy may help make this determination.

Rather than screen with an indirect test (FOBT) or a limited test (proctosigmoidoscopy), one could argue for total colonic evaluation of individuals at average risk by colonoscopy or barium enema regardless of FOBT status.[33, 69, 89–91] In the opinion of one authority, there is fairly good evidence that examination of the entire large intestine every 5 to 10 years in individuals aged 50 to 70 years would reduce the mortality rate of colorectal cancer.[90] Neither colonoscopy nor barium enema is generally thought of as a screening method because both involve discomfort and carry some risk, but if one really wanted to reduce colorectal cancer's toll, this would be one way to do it.[90] Colonoscopy is the more effective of the two methods, but it is more expensive.[90]

Several investigations of colonoscopy to screen persons at average risk of acquiring colorectal cancer have been reported. One study of asymptomatic men older than 50 years disclosed adenomas (most of them small) in 41% of cases and invasive cancer arising in adenomas in 1.7% of cases.[89] Another group found adenomatous polyps in 41% of 105 healthy men older than 50 years with negative FOBT results who underwent full colonoscopy.[91] The authors of both studies expressed a view that colonoscopy may be a better screening test than the FOBT. In another prospective study in which the FOBT missed 65% of the polyps and 40% of the carcinomas, the authors recommended that colonoscopy become the screening test of choice for colorectal cancer.[33]

The cost-effectiveness of two strategies of screening for colon cancer have been compared.[92] The first strategy included yearly FOBTs and sigmoidoscopy starting at age 50 years. Positive FOBT results were followed by colonoscopy. If FOBT results were negative and if adenomatous polyps were seen by flexible sigmoidoscopy, colonoscopy was performed; if sigmoidoscopy revealed no polyps, sigmoidoscopy was repeated 1 year later and every 3 to 5 years thereafter.[92] The second strategy was screening with colonoscopy. If colonoscopy was normal, the examination was not repeated. If adenomatous polyps were found, follow-up colonoscopy was performed every 3 to 5 years.[92] Cost analysis was performed by making a number of crucial assumptions. The 10-year cost of screening with sigmoidoscopy averaged about $1700, compared with $2500 for colonoscopy. The cost of identifying one patient with an adenomatous polyp was $8766 with sigmoidoscopy and $5988 with colonoscopy.[92] The calculated cost of preventing one death from colon cancer was $444,133 with sigmoidoscopy versus $347,214 with colonoscopy. The authors concluded that (1) colon cancer prevention with current screening methods is very expensive and (2) screening with sigmoidoscopy and FOBT may not be cost-effective compared with screening with colonoscopy.

Despite studies like those cited, the majority of fact and opinion does not support the use of colonoscopy for initial screening of asymptomatic persons at average risk of acquiring colorectal cancer.[1, 93, 94] Compared with the FOBT and flexible proctosigmoidoscopy, colonoscopy places greater demands on the patient, a more extensive bowel preparation is needed, sedation usually is required, there are more complications, and the initial cost is higher.[1] By consensus, at present screening colonoscopy should be reserved for individuals with positive FOBT results or those at high risk of colorectal neoplasia.[1, 93, 94] Barium enema likewise has little support as a screening test in persons at average risk.[69]

Other Studies

Upper Gastrointestinal Endoscopy. Esophagogastroduodenoscopy (EGD) is listed among screening tests for colorectal cancer only because it plays a controversial role in the evaluation of patients who have positive FOBT results.[5] In one prospective study, EGD and colonoscopy were performed in 100 patients with occult fecal blood or iron deficiency anemia or both.[95] Colonoscopy yielded a possible source of bleeding in 26% of patients, EGD was abnormal in 36% of patients, and one or the other was abnormal in 53% of patients.[95] Colonoscopy resulted in a higher cancer detection rate, yet EGD detected the origin of occult bleeding in 68% of patients in whom the source was found, and EGD resulted in a change of therapy in 30% of all 100 patients.[95] Interpretation of this study is confounded by the inclusion of anemic patients.

When cost is a consideration and the goal of screening is to reduce the mortality rate of colorectal cancer, patients with a positive FOBT result and no symptoms referable to the upper gastrointestinal tract should have colonoscopy first.[5] If colonoscopy is normal, it probably is unnecessary to investigate further.[5, 95] If fecal occult blood is found on repeat testing, another colonoscopy is called for, and EGD should be performed for persistent occult bleeding. Enteroscopy is performed alone or as part of an abdominal operation in some patients with chronic occult bleeding (see Chap. 19).

Carcinoembryonic Antigen and Other Markers. Carcinoembryonic antigen (CEA) and other tumor markers have severe limitations as screening tools for the early diagnosis of colorectal cancer, and none has proved useful to date.[14]

Conclusions

Screening for colorectal cancer in persons at average risk remains controversial because there is no proof yet that mortality rates can be reduced by these efforts.[5–7, 29] Retrospective case control studies of screening proctosigmoidoscopy are encouraging but not conclusive.[62, 63] The available evidence suggests that screening the population with the FOBT results in a greater yield of tumors that are localized to the bowel wall at the time of diagnosis and treatment.[35] These tumors have favorable features, and it is logical to believe that the prognosis will be better than in patients who are symptomatic at the time of diagnosis.[35] Because of potential biases, however, the mortality results of controlled trials must be awaited before it is clear whether screening has real value.[35] Currently, four randomized clinical trials of FOBT are under way.[96]

Analysis of a mathematical model indicates that an annual FOBT for screening persons older than age 40 years who are at average risk of acquiring colorectal cancer may reduce mortality from this disease by about one-third.[97] Either colonoscopy or barium enema may reduce mortality by about 85%, and a 3- to 5-year frequency of endoscopy or barium enema preserves 70% to 90% of the effectiveness of performing these procedures annually. Beginning screening at age 50 years reduces effectiveness by 5% to 10%.[97] Decisions made in devising such mathematical models for evaluation of a medical procedure may cause the value assigned to a test to vary by a factor of up to 10.[90]

Hope persists that with a disease so common, an intervention that improves survival by only a small percentage can save a significant number of lives.[35] In case finding, the patient may be directed promptly to a thorough and expensive procedure such as colonoscopy. In contrast, for screening to be cost-effective, it should begin with a test that is predictive, inexpensive, and acceptable in terms of risk and comfort.[5] Thus, colonoscopy is of little use at present in screening of persons at average risk.

SCREENING AND SURVEILLANCE OF PERSONS AT HIGH RISK FOR COLORECTAL CANCER

The presence of a colorectal neoplasm now or in the past is the most common factor placing a person at high risk for the development of cancer of the large bowel.[5] Only about 15% of patients who acquire colorectal cancer have discernible high-risk features other than sporadic adenomas, and the great majority of these persons have a history of colorectal cancer in first-degree relatives.[5] Inflammatory bowel disease and ureterosigmoidostomy also predispose to colorectal cancer. Earlier and more complete examination is appropriate for individuals at high risk, and colonoscopy is an important part of this effort.

Presence of Colorectal Neoplasms

The presence of one or more benign or malignant epithelial neoplasms in the colon or rectum requires a search for synchronous lesions.[4, 98–100] Most frequently, the index lesion is detected by proctosigmoidoscopy, but regardless of how the initial neoplasm comes to light, the entire colon and rectum should be evaluated, and synchronous polyps should be removed if possible.[101] The gross appearance of distal lesions is unreliable, and a correct diagnosis can be made only by biopsy.[102] The controversial implications of hyperplastic polyps in the distal bowel are discussed in Chapter 7.

Colonoscopy following the detection of adenomatous index polyps on flexible proctosigmoidoscopy reveals synchronous neoplasms proximal to the sigmoid colon in about 40% to 50% of patients.[75, 84, 103] From 6% to 10% of the proximal lesions discovered in this way are highly significant, including cancers, large adenomas, and adenomas with severe dysplasia.[75, 102, 104–106] Epithelial dysplasia, whether in flat mucosa or other lesions, is a precancerous condition.[19] Patients with multiple polyps are of particular concern; approximately 25% of patients who have five or more adenomatous polyps have a synchronous colon cancer at the initial colonoscopy.[107]

One study with a different slant on the issue assessed the long-term risk of cancer of the colorectum after rigid sigmoidoscopy and polypectomy in 1618 patients who did not subsequently undergo colonoscopy.[108] The risk of cancer of the proximal colon was related to the size and extent of villous change in the distal adenoma. Adenomas that were tubular and small (<1 cm) were low risk, and adenomas that were large (≥1 cm) or had a villous component were high risk. The number of adenomas in the rectum or sigmoid did not influence risk.[108] The authors suggested that the need for colonoscopy can be determined by estimating the risk of synchronous lesions in this way.[108]

The issue of barium enema versus colonoscopy to search for synchronous lesions was discussed earlier. Prospective trials comparing the two methods give the edge to colonoscopy because it is more sensitive and more specific, and these characteristics outweigh the greater cost and larger risk of colonoscopy in the view of most analysts.[27, 75, 82–85, 99] Unfortunately, subjectivity colors arguments on both sides of this controversy.

The importance of detecting and removing small polyps is debated, but some small polyps (up to 60% of those ≤1 cm in diameter) are neoplastic, and presumably all neoplastic polyps have some potential for harm if left alone.[106] In the National Polyp Study carried out in the United States, adenoma size and the extent of the villous component were found to be the major independent polyp risk factors associated with high-grade dysplasia.[18] So-called flat adenomas, which are small, flat, or depressed tubular adenomas that tend to occur in the ascending colon, may become malignant when still only a few millimeters in diameter.[109] In one series of flat adenomas, the overall malignancy rate was 13.3%, much higher than the 2.8% rate of cancer in ordinary small polypoid adenomas.[110] Barium enema cannot detect flat adenomas as reliably as colonoscopy can. Some flat adenomas can be removed by snare or strip biopsy during colonoscopy (see further on).[110]

Previous Colorectal Neoplasm

Colonoscopy is useful in screening another high-risk group—that is, patients who have had a colorectal adenoma or carcinoma in the past. The endoscopist misses at least 20% to 30% of polyps 2 to 5 mm in diameter, and therefore a second endoscopy is advised 1 year after polypectomy.[75]

Colonoscopy detects metachronous polyps and cancers.[111, 112] Patients with a previous colorectal adenoma are at a threefold greater risk for the development of colorectal cancer than is the general population.[113] The detection rate for new adenomas ranges from 13% to 50% after resection of polyps or cancer.[112, 114–116] Polyp multiplicity is a predictor of metachronous polyps.[117, 118] Other variables that have been reported to increase the prevalence of neoplasms detected at follow-up include increasing age, male sex, black race, and the size of the index adenoma.[118] New adenomas are significantly more common in patients who had carcinoma in situ or a villous component in the index polyp.[5, 114] A subgroup of subjects whose worst index lesion was a single small (≤1 cm) tubular adenoma and who had no first-degree relatives with colorectal cancer had only a 3% prevalence of advanced colonic neoplasms (tubular adenoma $\geq$1 cm, villous component, severe dysplasia, or invasive cancer) on follow-up colonoscopy—a prevalence no greater than that in the general population.[118]

Policies for follow-up of patients after excision of a colorectal adenoma have not been strictly determined.[5] The first postpolypectomy colonoscopy is at 1 year in most programs. Thereafter, colonoscopy at longer intervals usually suffices, perhaps every 2 to 3 years.[75, 114] The National Polyp Study suggests that intervals may be prolonged to 3 to 4 years in most patients, without an increase of important new neoplasia, and colonoscopy every 5 years may be enough in some patients, especially if the index lesion was a single small tubular adenoma.[93, 118, 119] Those with multiple or large adenomas, or both, with or without dysplasia may require more frequent examination, perhaps every 2 to 4 years.[93] The occurrence of new significant polyps detected by colonoscopy continues indefinitely (Table 22–2).[120] A common pattern of follow-up after curative resection of colorectal carcinoma is total colonoscopy 6 months to 1 year after operation; if this examination is normal, colonoscopy is repeated at 2 year intervals.[121, 122] Recommended follow-up care for patients who have had colorectal cancer also includes tests for metastatic disease (*e.g.,* CEA).[123]

The cost-effectiveness of colonoscopic surveillance is very sensitive to estimates of the cumulative remaining risk of death from cancer after polypectomy, as well as to surveillance efficacy. In one study, it was calculated that colonoscopy every 3 years for 30 years in a 50-year-old man after colonoscopic polypectomy would incur a cumulative 1.4% risk of perforation, an 0.11% risk of death from perforation, and a cost of $2071 in fees for the colonoscopic procedures.[8] If a 50-year-old man's cumulative remaining risk of death from cancer is 2.5% after the removal of a single small adenoma, and if effectiveness of colonoscopic surveillance

every 3 years is 100%, one death from cancer could be prevented by doing 283 colonoscopies, incurring 0.6 perforations, 0.04 perforation-related deaths, and direct physician costs of $82,000. If surveillance were 50% effective and the cumulative remaining risk for death from cancer were 1.25% (a plausible scenario), 1131 colonoscopies would be required to prevent one death from cancer, incurring 2.3 perforations, 0.17 perforation-related deaths, and physician costs of $331,000.[8] The authors concluded that recommendations for colonoscopic surveillance at fixed and regular intervals may be excessively costly for patients whose remaining risk for death from cancer is low.[8]

Metachronous cancer develops in 2% to 3% of patients after curative resection.[5] A recent unconfirmed report found an astonishingly high cumulative risk of metachronous colorectal cancer of 30% after 40 years of follow-up.[124] The risk appeared to be higher in this study if adenomas also were present at the initial operation.

Anastomotic recurrence rates range from 5% to 15%.[115, 125] Endoscopic evidence of anastomotic recurrence is seen in 30% to 90% of these patients.[115, 122, 125] The prognosis for anastomotic recurrence is poor because it often indicates unresectable disease, and therefore the benefits of making the diagnosis may be questioned.[93, 111, 119, 125] Potentially curative resections are possible in as few as 0% and as many as 50% of patients with anastomotic recurrence.[120, 125, 126] Survival is prolonged in up to 80% of patients in whom resection of localized recurrence is carried out.[120, 125, 126] Because so few patients are in this category, however, some authors have concluded that colonoscopic follow-up of patients to examine the anastomosis is not worth the cost.[93, 119]

A recent study evaluated the benefits of regular follow-up with physical examination, CEA determination, flexible sigmoidoscopy, and colonoscopy after curative resection for colorectal cancer.[127] The cancer-related 5-year survival rate

Table 22–2. COLON FINDINGS DURING STUDY

	Time After Curative Resection (mo)							
	0–6	6–12	12–18	18–24	24–36	36–48	48–60	60–72
No. of patients entering interval	174	174	166	145	116	96	40	37
Anastomotic recurrences	—	1	2	4	2	—	—	—
Metachronous cancer	—	—	—	3	—	1	—	—
Polyps	6	21	30	23	34	30	12	4
Significant polyps	3	6	7	5	7	6	2	1
Interval occurrence rate of significant polyps (%)	1.7	3.4	4.2	3.4	6.0	6.2	5	2.7

From Juhl G, Larson GM, Mullins R, et al. Six-year results of annual colonoscopy after resection of colon cancer. World J Surg 14:255–261, 1990.

was 72% in 368 patients who were followed closely and 62% in 139 patients who were outside the follow-up program. This difference was not significant.[127] Follow-up did have consequences, however. Recurrence was detected in 32% of the follow-up group and 21% of the others ($p < .02$), and curative reoperations were performed in 21% of the follow-up group with recurrent cancer compared with 7% of those with recurrent cancer in the other group.[127] Thus, in this study, regular follow-up detected more recurrent cancers and enabled radical reoperations to be performed significantly more often.[127]

Conclusion

The weight of opinion favors colonoscopic follow-up after excision of a polyp or cancer, but objective data suggest that not all patients need be treated alike in this regard. A single small tubular adenoma is a weak indication for colonoscopic follow-up, and colonoscopy certainly need not be performed often in these patients. Multiple polyps, a villous component in a previous polyp, and family history (see further on) are factors predictive of a favorable risk–benefit ratio for colonoscopy. Follow-up of cancer is mainly directed toward detection of metachronous lesions. Despite reports of successful reoperation for anastomotic recurrence detected by colonoscopy, most such tumors are unresectable for cure. Moreover, it is likely that these recurrences can be detected at just as favorable a stage by rising levels of CEA, symptoms, or radiologic tests. Metachronous cancers and polyps are worthwhile targets of follow-up. Colonoscopy need not be performed more often than every 2 to 3 years after an initial postoperative check.

Inherited Colorectal Cancer

Familial Adenomatous Polyposis

Familial adenomatous polyposis (FAP) is an autosomal dominant inherited disorder that results in more than a hundred and up to several thousand adenomatous polyps in the colon and rectum with a high likelihood of cancer if colectomy is not performed.[128] FAP is rare; at most, 0.5% of all colorectal carcinomas are associated with this condition.[129] The gene for FAP has been localized to the long arm of chromosome 5, and it has been sequenced recently.[130] Gene mapping of FAP and Gardner's syndrome sup-

ports the view that the two syndromes are identical.[131]

If a patient with FAP is discovered, first-degree relatives should be screened.[128, 131] There is little question that screening for FAP is beneficial because it leads to early diagnosis and treatment by colectomy before cancer can develop.[128] Screening of relatives of patients with FAP among 82 families in a central registry in the Netherlands revealed colorectal carcinoma at the time of diagnosis in 5 of 126 patients (4%) compared with 49 of 104 patients with FAP (47%) who were referred because they were symptomatic.[128] A study from Finland reported that 66% of symptomatic patients had colorectal carcinoma compared with only 6.6% of patients with FAP detected during screening of family members.[129]

Screening should start at 10 to 12 years of age and continue up to age 50 years.[128] By the age of 40 years, 90% of asymptomatic relatives with FAP will have been diagnosed. In rare cases of families with a late onset of FAP, screening should continue up to age 60 years.[128]

Endoscopic screening for FAP usually takes the form of annual flexible proctosigmoidoscopy.[131] Colonoscopy is seldom necessary to make the diagnosis because polyps almost invariably can be seen in the rectum or sigmoid colon. Very rare patients may have polyps in the ascending colon without distal evidence of FAP. Colonoscopic polypectomy is unimportant in management except to provide biopsy material. Endoscopic screening of the upper gastrointestinal tract in FAP has been recommended, but there is no evidence of benefit.[132] Endoscopic surveillance of the small intestine in individuals with FAP has been suggested, but this procedure too has no established role.[132] Newer screening methods include ophthalmoscopic examination for congenital hypertrophy of the retinal pigment epithelium, which is present in about 65% of families, and gene probes.[130, 131, 133]

Hereditary Nonpolyposis Colon Cancer

Research into inherited colorectal cancer has intensified in the past decade. Estimates of the proportion of patients with colorectal cancer having an inherited basis range enormously from 1% to 30%.[97, 134–136] FAP is the best known syndrome, but it is much less common than hereditary nonpolyposis colon cancer (HNPCC).[13, 137]

At least two varieties of HNPCC have been identified: (1) hereditary site-specific nonpolyposis colorectal cancer (Lynch syndrome I) and (2) colorectal cancer in association with other types of cancer, especially endometrial carcinoma (cancer family syndrome, Lynch syndrome II).[13, 137] The development of cancer at a young age, multiple synchronous or metachronous cancers, and proximal dominance of colonic cancer are characteristics of both syndromes.[13] Adenomas do not occur in large numbers in HNPCC, but they develop at a young age, attain a large size, often show a villous configuration, and are more prone to malignant conversion than are sporadic adenomas.[138] Hereditary flat adenoma syndrome has been described recently.[139] It is separable from FAP and is either a variant of HNPCC or a distinct entity.

Periodic screening examination of family members at risk has the potential benefit of detecting life-threatening tumors at an early stage; disadvantages include costs, inconvenience, and risks.[13, 140] To evaluate the effectiveness of a screening program, one study involved colonoscopy or a combination of flexible sigmoidoscopy and double-contrast barium enema in 22 families.[13] Two groups were studied: group A consisted of patients with symptomatic colorectal cancer, and group B was made up of family members who were found to have a colorectal lesion by screening. Overall, cancers were proximal to the splenic flexure in 60% of these individuals, and multiple synchronous primary colorectal carcinomas were found in 26% of those with malignancy.[13] In group A, the cancer was Dukes' stage A in 7%, Dukes' stage B in 43%, Dukes' stage C in 24% and Dukes' stage D in 12%; the staging was unknown in the remainder.[13] By contrast, in group B patients, an adenoma was found in 70% and carcinoma in 30% of individuals, and of this small group, one third were Dukes' stage A and two thirds were Dukes' stage B.[13] The authors concluded that screening should be initiated at the age of 20 years and continued for life.[13]

In another study, 44 asymptomatic putative Lynch syndrome patients participated in a colonoscopy screening program.[141] Thirty percent of these individuals were found to have at least one adenoma, and 20% had multiple adenomas. In 18% of the patients, adenomas were discovered proximal to the splenic flexure. In a group of age- and sex-matched controls, 11% had adenomas, 4% had multiple adenomas, and 1% had adenomas in the ascending colon. Thus, the prevalence of adenomas in the Lynch syndromes was greater than in controls, and the adenomas were more proximally located, corresponding to the site distribution of cancer in HNPCC.[141] A high rate of synchronous and metachronous lesions was found also.[141]

HNPCC calls for a FOBT annually and colonoscopy every 2 years beginning at age 25 years or at an age 5 years younger than the age at which the earliest colon cancer was diagnosed in a family member.[1]

First-degree Relatives

First-degree relatives of patients with colorectal cancer have a threefold increased risk of acquiring the disease compared with the general population—that is, around 10% instead of 4%.[86, 104, 142] Some of these patients have unrecognized HNPCC. The American Cancer Society recommends that a person with a family history of colorectal cancer in one or more first-degree relatives should undergo annual digital rectal examination and a FOBT beginning at age 40 years, with either total colonoscopy or barium enema and sigmoidoscopy every 3 to 5 years.[5] Numerous appraisals of this policy have been reported.

In one study, flexible sigmoidoscopy was performed in first-degree relatives after full bowel preparation, followed immediately by either therapeutic colonoscopy if polyps were seen or barium enema if sigmoidoscopy examination was normal.[104] Adenomas were found in 19% of 88 first-degree relatives compared with the expected finding of adenomas in 8% of those screened. The authors concluded that this protocol was workable, but they encountered many problems with compliance of referring physicians and patients.

Colonoscopy alone identifies neoplastic polyps in 10% to 63% of individuals with affected first-degree relatives.[105, 142–150] The definition of a polyp and other methodologic differences may explain some of the wide variations in these reports. Control patients of the same age but without a family history of colorectal cancer generally have a 10% or lower prevalence of neoplastic colonic polyps.[104, 150] More than 20% of polyps in first-degree relatives are proximal to the splenic flexure.[104, 105, 142, 148] The prevalence of adenomas increases significantly with the age of the subjects.[143] Male sex is an independent risk factor as well.[150] The prevalence of adenomas on colonoscopic screening increases with the number of affected first-degree relatives (Table 22–3).[144, 147, 150] Cancer is detected by screening colonoscopy in 1.3% to 2% of subjects.[105, 144, 147, 149]

At present, data are conflicting on the role of colonoscopy in screening persons who have one first-degree relative with colorectal cancer. The majority of authors favor colonoscopy for this indication,[6, 86, 105, 144, 150] but others do not.[143, 145, 146]

Table 22–3. PREVALENCE OF ASYMPTOMATIC ADENOMAS AS A FUNCTION OF FAMILIAL RISK

Afflicted FDR	Subjects with Adenomas/Total No. of Subjects (%)
0	7/83 (8.4%)
1	21/160 (13.1%)
≥2*	5/21 (25.0%)

From Guillem JG, Forde KA, Treat MR, et al. Colonoscopic screening for neoplasms in asymptomatic first-degree relatives of colon cancer patients. A controlled, prospective study. Dis Colon Rectum 35:523–529, 1992. © by American Society of Colon and Rectal Surgeons.

FDR = first-degree relative with histologically proven colorectal cancer.

*Of 21 subjects with ≥2 FDRs affected with colorectal cancer, 20 had 2 and 1 had 3 affected FDRs.

There is near unanimity of opinion, however, that persons who have two or more afflicted first-degree relatives should have screening colonoscopy.[93, 151] Cost considerations are influential in making these judgments. One group calculated that screening of asymptomatic adults by colonoscopy is markedly (fourfold) more cost-effective if they have two or more first-degree relatives with colon cancer.[151] One recommended program is colonoscopic examination every 2 years beginning at 30 to 40 years of age, depending on the age at which cancer developed in the relatives.[144]

Cancer of Other Organs

Patients who have had endometrial, ovarian, or breast cancer have a two to three times greater than average risk of acquiring large bowel cancer.[5, 13, 152] Authorities agree, however, that these patients should not be screened by colonoscopy because the yield of colorectal neoplasms is too low to justify the costs and risks.[5, 13, 93, 152] Guidelines for persons at average risk of disease are sufficient for these patients.

Inflammatory Bowel Disease

Cancer in Inflammatory Bowel Disease

UC predisposes to malignancy of the colon or rectum.[153] Crohn's colitis also can lead to cancer, but the tendency is less pronounced (see further on). The cumulative probability of the development of colorectal carcinoma in extensive UC using the life table method overestimates the risk when the proportion of patients undergoing surgery is high or the population contains many older patients who die from other causes.[154] The best data suggest that long-standing UC is associated with a cancer risk in the range of 0.5% to 1%/year after the first 10 years of disease.[154–158] This cumulative risk is considerably higher, by a factor of up to 20, than the risk in the general population, and the possibility of dying of colorectal cancer is increased four to five times.[154, 157]

The single strongest risk factor for cancer in UC is the duration of disease, and the risk is relatively independent of the age at onset of colitis.[157] Extent of disease also is a risk factor, although patients with disease limited to the distal bowel can develop cancer too.[155, 157] Colitis-associated cancers are more often multiple, broadly infiltrating, anaplastic, and uniformly distributed throughout the colon than are other colorectal cancers. Also, cancers in UC typically arise from flat mucosa instead of following the usual adenoma-cancer sequence, and they occur in much younger patients. Stage for stage, the prognosis is the same.

The risk of a patient with UC dying of colorectal carcinoma can be reduced in one of three ways: (1) the performance of colectomy before the precancerous phase develops, (2) the detection of the precancerous phase, advising surgery at that time, or (3) the detection of cancer at an early and surgically curable stage.[154] The first strategy is impractical because patients usually resist prophylactic colectomy if their symptoms are not disabling. Current surveillance programs pursue the second strategy, preferably, or the third strategy. There is enough hope for improved survival to make some kind of surveillance technique worthwhile.[157]

Epithelial Dysplasia in Ulcerative Colitis

Epithelial dysplasia is a nonpolypoid adenomatous change that predicts malignant degeneration in colorectal mucosa.[156] Pathologists have reached agreement on the classification of dysplasia in UC, and the terminology listed in Table 22–4 is now standard.[159, 160] Although the presence of inflammation makes these changes more difficult to interpret, active disease does not negate the significance of this finding.[161]

There is a strong association between high-grade dysplasia and cancer. From 75% to 90% of patients with carcinoma arising in UC have high-grade dysplasia within the resected specimen, and up to 40% of patients with high-grade dysplasia have a focus of carcinoma in the resected colon.[156] Low-grade dysplasia is a precursor of high-grade dysplasia and cancer.[156, 161]

Table 22–4. CLASSIFICATION OF DYSPLASIA IN INFLAMMATORY BOWEL DISEASE

1. Mucosa negative for dysplasia	Regular follow-up
2. Mucosa indefinite for dysplasia	Increased surveillance

3. Mucosa positive for dysplasia
   a. Low grade
   b. High grade
	Consider colectomy after histologic confirmation of the diagnosis

From Bramwell NH, Riddell RH. Cancer and dysplasia. In: Gitnick G, ed. Inflammatory bowel disease. Diagnosis and treatment. New York: Igaku-Shoin, 1991:503–516.

The lead time between low-grade dysplasia and the development of high-grade dysplasia or cancer is about 3 years.[156] When accompanied by a *dysplasia-associated lesion or mass* (DALM), low-grade dysplasia is closely associated with malignancy.[162]

It is possible that dysplasia can disappear spontaneously, although there is no conclusive evidence that it does so.[163] It is inevitable that dysplasia is demonstrated inconsistently from one colonoscopy to the next because of the limitations of visual inspection and biopsy.[163]

Surveillance for Cancer in Ulcerative Colitis

Surveillance for colorectal dysplasia and cancer usually takes the form of periodic colonoscopy with biopsy of suspicious lesions and random biopsy of other areas of mucosa. The initial prevalence or screening colonoscopy is performed about 10 years after the onset of UC if it was not necessary before. Colonoscopy is always preferable to double-contrast enema in patients with colitis because dysplasia often develops in flat mucosa and cannot be detected radiographically.[75]

Rigid or flexible proctosigmoidoscopy also can be used for surveillance. In some studies, more lesions are discovered by sigmoidoscopy than by colonoscopy, partly because sigmoidoscopy is performed more often.[154, 161] Colonoscopy is more time-consuming and potentially more dangerous than sigmoidoscopy and, of course, colonoscopy requires bowel preparation and usually sedation.[154] Proctosigmoidoscopy cannot replace colonoscopy, however, because up to 60% of dysplasia specimens are obtained from the ascending colon. Perhaps sigmoidoscopy and biopsy during the interim between colonoscopies should be part of the routine management of UC.[161, 164]

Endoscopy may discover frank carcinoma or suspicious elevated or polypoid velvety lesions.[165] Detection of such abnormalities is more difficult in the midst of colitis than in the normal colon because the mucosa is hyperemic, inflammatory polyps may be present, and mucus or blood may obscure detail.[154] Biopsy specimens should be taken from representative areas of flat mucosa in each portion of the colon and rectum and from suspicious lesions.[166] Supplementation of biopsies by cytologic examination of brushings has no advantage.[167]

Strictures in UC can make it difficult to examine the entire colon. Of course, strictures themselves may be malignant. The distal aspect of a malignant stricture may appear normal grossly and histologically, so if a stricture cannot be negotiated, no conclusions can be drawn about the diagnosis.[75] Small diameter endoscopes may be helpful in assessing tight strictures.[75] Even if the colonoscope passes through the stricture, however, its maneuverability may be restricted so that adequate biopsies cannot be obtained.[75] Also, the mucosa may appear benign, although cancer is infiltrating in the submucosa.

Management of patients with epithelial dysplasia depends on the grade and persistence of the abnormality (see Table 22–4). Before taking action, it is recommended that the finding of dysplasia be confirmed by more than one pathologist.[154] In general, if the patient has low-grade dysplasia, colonoscopy and biopsies should be repeated in 6 to 12 months. Confirmed high-grade dysplasia requires colectomy.

Results of long-term surveillance programs vary, in part because of differences in patient eligibility, protocols employed, interpretation of tests, and action required for a positive test result.[156] Periodic colonoscopic surveillance of ulcerative pancolitis of more than 7 to 10 years' duration detects dysplasia or neoplasia in 10% to 22% of patients cumulatively after a mean of 15 to 20 years.[161, 164, 168, 169] Dysplasia and neoplasia are less prevalent in left-sided colitis.[164] When dysplasia is present, it is low grade in 60% to 80% of patients and high grade in the remainder.[161, 169] Adenomas are discovered in 2% of screened colitis patients.[161]

Carcinoma occurs in as few as 0% and as many as 17% of patients in surveillance programs.[161, 164, 168–173] Dysplasia precedes carcinoma in 15% to 20% of patients with either dysplasia or neoplasia, and carcinoma develops without prior dysplasia in 2.5%.[161] When colectomy is performed for high-grade dysplasia detected in a surveillance program, 17% of specimens contain carcinoma.[169] Some carcinomas have metastasized to lymph nodes or distant sites at the time of colectomy.[154, 174, 175] Overall, however, there seems to be a reduction in the proportion of advanced carcinomas in surveillance studies.[154, 175] An increase in the proportion of patients with early carcinoma should translate to reduced mortality in patients with colitis, just as it should in the general population.[154]

A normal examination is no cause for relaxation of vigilance.[161] If initial colonoscopy reveals no gross or histologic dysplasia or neoplasia, colonoscopy is repeated. The second examination detects dysplasia or neoplasia in 7% of those who had normal initial colonoscopic examinations, and 4% of patients will show dysplasia or neoplasia after multiple normal examinations.[161] The optimum interval between colonoscopies is unknown, but colonoscopy every 2 years is recommended commonly.[154, 160, 175] Annual or more frequent examinations are required if low-grade dysplasia is found.[154] According to one view, as the hazard rate increases with duration of disease, the screening interval should shorten accordingly.[156]

The majority of authorities have concluded that a colonoscopic surveillance program is a safe and effective alternative to prophylactic colectomy in long-standing UC.[85, 154, 161, 162, 164, 169-173, 175, 176] From 0.5% to 2% of patients die of cancer despite the surveillance program.[168, 175] In one study of more than 200 patients, all 4 patients who died of cancer had high-grade dysplasia at the initial colonoscopy.[175] A surveillance program of annual colonoscopy in 91 patients with pancolitis for at least 8 years compared differences in survival, cancer detection, and colectomy rates in the screened group with those in 95 control patients with UC.[177] In the surveillance group, there were eight fewer deaths ($p < .05$ by survival curve analysis) but two more cancer deaths (not significant). Colectomy was less common ($p < .05$) and was performed 4 years later in the surveillance group. The authors concluded that screening for cancer in UC was associated with improved survival and delayed colectomy, but the improvement was not attributable to better cancer-related survival.[177]

Surveillance for cancer by colonoscopy in patients with UC has limitations of several kinds.[11, 93, 160] Clinical limitations include the skill of the colonoscopist and the technical constraints of colonoscopy.[160] For whatever reason, the colonoscope may not reach all of the colon. Cancer or dysplasia, or both, may be overlooked or may not be visible. The impact of colonoscopist observer variation on the detection of dysplasia has never been examined, but it is likely that the appearance of dysplasia and

DALM is unfamiliar to many colonoscopists.[165] Observer variation impedes cancer surveillance for several reasons: (1) mistaking a DALM for an inflammatory mass may lead to fewer or no biopsies, (2) failing to appreciate an altered (velvety) flat mucosa could result in a missed opportunity for dysplasia detection, and (3) misinterpreting an inflammatory polyp for a DALM might lead to inappropriate surgery.[165] Dysplasia may be irregular or patchy, and sampling errors may occur.[93, 160] The optimum number of biopsy specimens to minimize sampling errors is unknown.[160] The current practice is one or two specimens every 10 cm throughout the colon. This method samples only 5 to 10 mm^2 from each 100 cm^2 of colon, so perhaps the number of specimens from each segment should be increased.[93]

Pathologic limitations derive from the relationship of dysplasia to carcinoma.[160] Cancer can and does occur without dysplasia in patients with UC. One group of investigators extensively and systematically sampled specimens of colon that were resected for established colitis-associated cancer and found that 26% of these colons harbored no dysplasia in any sample from any region.[178] The sensitivity and specificity of random colonic biopsies to detect concomitant carcinoma were 0.74 and 0.74, respectively, in this study, and the authors concluded that reliance on random biopsies during colonoscopic surveillance may be misplaced.[178] Also, there still is some degree of observer variation in pathologists who interpret the slides.[160] Patient compliance is another kind of limitation. Compliance with surveillance is diminished when patients are asymptomatic.[161] They may drop out or relocate, and some patients are unwilling to accept advice based on surveillance findings.[160]

In addition to the limitations listed, the value of colonoscopic surveillance has been challenged on other grounds.[11, 178, 179] The design of some studies and the conclusions drawn from the data are invalid according to critics.[11, 179] Patients seen at referral centers, the source of most published reports, are a highly selected group that may introduce bias into the results of surveillance.[11] Some patients who are seen for the first time at a specialist center may have symptoms of cancer already, and detection of the cancer is inappropriately credited to surveillance.[11] Individuals operated on because of disease activity who are found to have cancer incidentally do not represent successful surveillance.[11] Patients with extensive cancer must be regarded as failures of a surveillance program.[179] Patients who are found to have cancer as a result of investigations other than the surveillance technique should be excluded too.[11, 179] Finally, critics note that it takes many colonoscopies to find a cancer, and colonoscopy is expensive and carries risks.[11, 179]

Surveillance strategies that employ a more sensitive marker than biopsy detection of dysplasia or cancer are greatly needed.[177] One promising tool is flow cytometric DNA analysis of mucosal biopsy specimens.[169, 180] Aneuploidy in patients with colitis correlates with histologic grade and identifies a subset of patients without dysplasia who are more likely to acquire it.[180] If biopsy specimens from the initial colonoscopy in a patient with long-standing UC are diploid and negative for dysplasia, colonoscopy every 2 to 3 years is sufficient because these patients are unlikely to acquire cancer during the interval.[180] Aneuploidy without dysplasia suggests a need for more frequent follow-up because of a greater risk of future dysplasia. Flow cytometry may be useful to guide a program that reduces cost and detects more curable lesions.[180]

For now, surveillance by colonoscopy and biopsies to detect dysplasia is standard practice. Cancers can be missed despite appropriate screening studies, however, and surgeons at referral centers sense that the pendulum is swinging back toward prophylactic colectomy in more patients.[179] Colectomy obviates the need for future colonoscopies and eliminates the risk of missing a curable carcinoma, and the functional results of ileoanal pouch procedures are excellent.[181]

Screening for Cancer in Crohn's Disease

The risk of colorectal cancer in patients with Crohn's disease is 4 to 20 times greater than in the general population.[182] Most patients have had the disease for a long time, averaging 20 years, but in about 20% of the reported cases, the diagnoses of carcinoma and Crohn's disease were made simultaneously.[182] Approximately 50% of carcinomas associated with Crohn's disease are of the colloid type compared with 9% colloid cancers in the general population.[182] A gross intraluminal lesion usually is present, approximately 10% are multifocal, and about 20% of colorectal cancers in Crohn's disease occur in an excluded rectum. The prognosis for Crohn's disease–associated colonic carcinoma is the same, stage for stage, as for colonic cancer in the general population.[182]

Recently, dysplasia has been identified as a regular associate of carcinoma complicating Crohn's disease, suggesting a dysplasia-carcinoma sequence similar to that for UC.[182] Dysplasia distant from the colonic carcinoma is less extensive than in UC.[182] Whether dysplasia or carcinoma relates to the duration or the extent of Crohn's disease, as it does in UC, has not been determined.[182]

There is no consensus in favor of cancer surveillance in Crohn's colitis at this time.[182, 183] Since dysplasia probably precedes the development of invasive carcinoma, and the association of carcinoma and dysplasia in Crohn's disease is as strong as it is in UC, theoretically surveillance would be of some benefit.[182, 183] Conversely, the true incidence of carcinoma in Crohn's disease is unknown but is probably quite low; only about 100 Crohn's disease–associated colorectal carcinomas have been reported to date.[182] Dysplasia is less extensive in Crohn's disease and may be a less useful marker than in UC.[182] It is unlikely that an endoscopic cancer surveillance program will justify the cost and effort.[182]

Patients with recrudescence of colitis-like symptoms and a background of long-standing (15 to 20 years) Crohn's disease should have colonoscopy.[182] A change in a fistula should be investigated and strictures must be examined.[184] Yearly surveillance of a diverted rectum seems appropriate, although retained rectal stumps often have strictures and are difficult to examine.[182] The presence of high-grade dysplasia should be managed like dysplasia in UC.[182]

Ureterosigmoidostomy

Ureterosigmoidostomy predisposes to cancer of the colon.[75] The risk is hundreds of times greater than could be expected as a chance event.[75] It is greatest 10 years or more after surgery. Local bacterial production of nitrosamines from urinary nitrates and nitrites is believed to be part of the mechanism of carcinogenesis. Surveillance every 2 to 3 years by flexible sigmoidoscopy or colonoscopy is sufficient. The finding of adenomas should trigger plans to resect the colon and establish another type of urinary conduit.

Conclusions Regarding Colonoscopy in Screening

There is little support for colonoscopy as the initial screening test in asymptomatic persons at average risk of acquiring colorectal cancer. The FOBT detects early lesions, but a benefit in terms of lower mortality has yet to be proved.

Flexible proctosigmoidoscopy is reported to confer a survival benefit, but this finding needs to be confirmed by controlled studies. Barium enema has few proponents as a screening test in patients at average risk.

Colonoscopy is central in screening persons at high risk. Patients with a polyp or cancer should have colonoscopy to search for synchronous lesions. Colonoscopic follow-up is recommended after excision of a cancer and after removal of multiple polyps or polyps that were large or had a villous component. A single small tubular adenoma is a weak indication for colonoscopic follow-up. First-degree relatives of patients with FAP are screened by flexible proctosigmoidoscopy. Individuals from families with HNPCC should have an FOBT annually and colonoscopy every 2 years beginning at age 25 years or at an age that is 5 years younger than the age at which the earliest colon cancer was diagnosed in a family member. Screening colonoscopy is warranted in persons with two or more first-degree relatives with colorectal cancer.

Although many questions remain, colonoscopy for surveillance of chronic UC is recommended by most authorities. Initial colonoscopic screening is performed about 10 years after disease onset, and if the examination is normal, colonoscopy is repeated every 2 years. Surveillance colonoscopy in Crohn's colitis is not required at this time. Patients who have a ureterosigmoidostomy are evaluated by periodic flexible proctosigmoidoscopy.

COLONOSCOPY IN THE MANAGEMENT OF CANCER

Diagnosis

Most cancers of the colon and rectum present with symptoms (mainly rectal bleeding, stool changes, and abdominal pain) or anemia.[50] Symptoms or signs suggestive of colorectal cancer require complete examination of the large bowel by total colonoscopy or by a combination of flexible sigmoidoscopy and barium enema.[5] The relative merits of these approaches as screening tools in asymptomatic individuals were compared earlier. In patients with symptoms, particularly bleeding, colonoscopy probably is the best choice because it achieves both goals of preoperative colonic evaluation—that is, histologic diagnosis and discovery of synchronous tumors.[24, 52, 72, 99, 100, 185] Some authors advocate flexible sigmoidoscopy plus barium enema.[64–67] In a prospective study of nonemergent rectal bleeding, colonoscopy was more cost-effective for detection of neoplasms in patients older than age 55 years, and flexible sigmoidoscopy plus air contrast barium enema was a more cost-effective strategy in patients younger than 55 years.[186]

Colonoscopy is performed preoperatively if possible, but a patient with distal obstruction must undergo intraoperative colonoscopy, or total colonoscopy must wait until the follow-up period.[187] One study documented that an aggressive policy of performing colonoscopy in response to symptoms improved the staging of cancers; early cancers increased from 12% of malignant lesions prior to initiation of this policy to 41% after the new philosophy was introduced.[188] Disseminated cancers dropped from 19% to 3% after the change.[188]

The colonoscopic diagnosis of adenocarcinoma of the colon or rectum is seldom difficult.[75] Cancer is a reddish, friable mass that projects into the lumen. Larger lesions have central ulceration with rolled edges. A malignant tumor is firm as judged by probing with the biopsy forceps. Tiny cancers and those infiltrating the submucosa can be more problematic. Early depressed cancer of the large intestine, typically in the proximal colon, is a reddish depression that looks like the sucker of an octopus.[25] Extramural cancers invading from adjacent organs may deform the lumen and leave the colonic mucosa intact.

Biopsy specimens of a cancer usually are abnormal if obtained at the rolled edge. The central ulceration may be so necrotic that no viable tumor remains. Several biopsy specimens should be obtained. Occasionally a large piece can be excised with a polypectomy snare. One must be careful to avoid bleeding or perforation.

It is important to pinpoint the location of the cancer within the colon to guide the surgeon to the appropriate segment. Usually it is sufficient to note the relationship of the tumor to endoscopic landmarks. If doubt remains, a barium enema may be helpful to avoid the improper placement of an incision or even resection of the wrong part of the colon. Intraoperative colonoscopy is an excellent solution to uncertain location of the tumor, but it is necessary to provide for this eventuality when positioning the patient. Submucosal injection of India ink during the initial colonoscopy has been recommended to mark small lesions for subsequent resection.[189, 190] India ink diluted with an equal volume of water and sterilized in an autoclave can be injected via a standard sclerotherapy injector passed through the biopsy channel of the colonoscope.[190] Approximately 0.2 to 0.5 mL is injected in each of four sites around the circumference, raising a wheal in each location. One group reported the use of this technique in 40 patients, and in every instance the ink stain was helpful.[190] Ink remains in the site for at least 12 years.

Endoscopic ultrasound is a new procedure that may prove worthwhile in diagnosing or staging colorectal cancers in the future (see Chap. 9).[191]

Treatment

Malignant Polyps

Excision of malignant polyps is an important part of colonoscopic management of colorectal cancer. This topic is covered in Chapter 21.

Strip Biopsy

Strip biopsy through the colonoscope has been described as a means of removing flat adenomas and early invasive carcinomas.[192] The technique is illustrated in Figure 22–2. Saline solution (2 to 3 mL) is injected into the submucosa near the lesion using a needle passed through the biopsy channel. This elevates the mucosa containing the lesion so that a snare can

Table 22–5. OUTCOME OF LASER TREATMENT IN 38 PATIENTS

	No. of Small Tumors (N = 6)	No. of Large Tumors (N = 32)
Complete resolution	3	0
Residual disease, symptoms controlled	1	8
No improvement, symptomatic treatment	0	6
No improvement, surgery	0	11
Unassessable	2	6
Unsuitable for laser treatment	0	1

From Bright N, Hale P, Mason R. Poor palliation of colorectal malignancy with the neodymium yttrium-aluminum-garnet laser. Br J Surg 79:308–309, 1992. By permission of the publishers, Butterworth-Heinemann Ltd.

be placed around it for excision.[192] A larger specimen is recovered when compared with one obtained with biopsy forceps. Lesions suitable for this technique are uncommon in the experience of endoscopists in Western countries.

Laser Photocoagulation

Endoscopic neodymium:yttrium-aluminum garnet (Nd:YAG) laser photocoagulation of small distal rectal cancers may be curative.[193, 194] Trans-

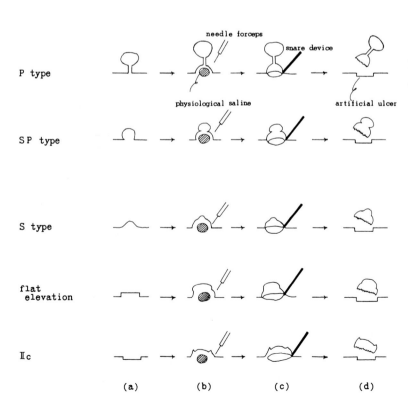

Figure 22–2. Technique of endoscopic strip biopsy resection. **(Column a)** The same procedure is used for strip biopsy of lesions identified as pedunculated (P), semipedunculated (SP), or sessile (S) polyps and for elevated, flat and IIC carcinoma. **(Column b)** Needle forceps puncture the mucosa near the lesion, and 2 to 3 mL of physiologic saline are injected into the submucosa. The lesion and the surrounding mucosa are elevated like a submucosal tumor. **(Column c)** A snare device is placed around the elevated tissues. **(Column d)** The elevated tissues are excised using electrocoagulation. (From Karita M, Tada M, Okita K, et al. Endoscopic therapy for early colon cancer: The strip biopsy resection technique. Gastrointest Endosc 1991; 37:128–132. © by the American Society for Gastrointestinal Endoscopy.)

anal excision usually is possible for the same kind of lesions, however, and excision has the advantage of providing the entire tumor for histologic examination. Subsequent or adjuvant therapy depends in large measure on the histopathologic details. Laser photocoagulation of rectal cancer with curative intent should be reserved for patients whose lesions for some reason are unsuitable for management by local excision.

Laser photocoagulation is used for palliation of obstructing rectal cancers that cannot be treated definitively by other means.[194, 195] Unfortunately, many large circumferential tumors and those close to or involving the anal sphincters show poor results with laser treatment (Table 22–5).[193] Laser photocoagulation cannot destroy all of an advanced rectal cancer, and therefore tenesmus often is not relieved even if the lumen is kept patent. Tenesmus is such a distressing symptom that patients will do almost anything to be free of it, some even accepting a palliative abdominoperineal resection that they formerly rejected. Lasers are also used by a few experts to palliate obstructing colonic cancer.[194, 196] This procedure is potentially hazardous.

Interestingly, the success of laser photoablation for gastrointestinal cancer was rated lower by referring physicians than by the endoscopists who treated the patients in one study.[194] The authors believe that referring physicians had unrealistic expectations; also, symptoms that continued to trouble patients after laser treatment may have been due to progression of disease rather than laser therapy itself.[194]

Dilation of Obstruction

Complete colonic obstruction secondary to colorectal cancer is usually managed by a staged operative approach. The colon containing the lesion is resected emergently, a colostomy is established to avoid the risks of anastomotic leak in unprepared bowel, and intestinal continuity is reestablished later. Transendoscopic balloon dilation of complete malignant colonic obstruction has been reported.[196–198] A guidewire is inserted through the obstructing lesion, balloon dilation is carried out, and a tube is placed through the bowel proximal to the tumor. If successful, balloon dilation makes it possible to prepare the bowel and then perform elective one-stage resection.[196] This procedure has not been applied widely because of the perceived risks of perforation during insertion of the guidewire and perforation of the bowel as the lesion is stretched.[198]

References

1. Hardcastle J, Winawer S, Burt R, et al. Screening for colorectal neoplasia. In: Working Party Reports. Melbourne: Blackwell Scientific Publications, 1990:27–35.
2. Silverberg E, Lubera J. Cancer statistics, 1989. CA 39:3–20, 1989.
3. Pollock A, Quirke P. Adenoma screening and colorectal cancer. The need for screening and polypectomy is unproved. Br Med J 303:3–4, 1991.
4. Schrock T. Conceptual developments through colonoscopy. Surg Endosc 2:240–244, 1988.
5. Decosse J. Early cancer detection: colorectal cancer. Cancer 62:1787–1790, 1988.
6. Levin B. Screening sigmoidoscopy for colorectal cancer (editorial). N Engl J Med 326:700–702, 1992.
7. Winawer S, Schottenfeld D, Flehinger B. Colorectal cancer screening. J Natl Cancer Inst 83:243–253, 1991.
8. Ransohoff DF, Lang CA, Kuo HS. Colonoscopic surveillance after polypectomy: considerations of cost effectiveness. Ann Intern Med 114:177–182, 1991.
9. McGill D, Ahlquist D. Screening for colorectal disease. In: Phillips S, Pemberton J, Shorter R, eds. The Large Intestine: Physiology, Pathophysiology, and Disease. New York: Raven Press, 1991:335–355.
10. Winawer S, Kerner J. Sigmoidoscopy: case finding versus screening (editorial). Gastroenterology 95:527–530, 1988.
11. Axon A. Surveillance in ulcerative colitis does not work and cannot work. In: Riddell R, ed. Dysplasia and Cancer in Colitis. New York: Elsevier, 1991:43–48.
12. Wilson J, Junger G. Principles and practise of screening for disease. Geneva, Switzerland: World Health Organization, 1968.
13. Vasen H, den Hartog Jager F, Menko F, et al. Screening for hereditary nonpolyposis colorectal cancer: a study of 22 kindreds in the Netherlands. Am J Med 86:278–281, 1989.
14. Roulston J. Limitations of tumour markers in screening. Br J Surg 77:961–962, 1990.
15. Neugut A, Pita S. Role of sigmoidoscopy in screening for colorectal cancer: a critical review. Gastroenterology 95:492–499, 1988.
16. Tierney R, Ballantyne G, Modlin I. The adenoma to carcinoma sequence. Surg Gynecol Obstet 171:81–94, 1990.
17. Stryker S, Wolff B, Culp C, et al. Natural history of untreated colonic polyps. Gastroenterology 93:1009–1013, 1987.
18. O'Brien M, Winawer S, Zauber A, et al. The National Polyp Study. Patient and polyp characteristics associated with high-grade dysplasia in colorectal adenomas. Gartroenterology 98:371–379, 1990.
19. Jass J. Do all colorectal carcinomas arise in preexisting adenomas? World J Surg 13:45–51, 1989.
20. Hermanek P. Dysplasia-carcinoma sequence, types of adenomas and early colo-rectal carcinoma. Eur J Surg Oncol 13:141–143, 1987.
21. Simons B, Morrison A, Lev R, et al. Relationship of polyps to cancer of the large intestine. J Natl Cancer Inst 84:962–966, 1992.
22. Colorectal cancer: new evidence for the adenoma/carcinoma sequence (editorial). Lancet 340:210–211, 1992.
23. Bedenne L, Faivre J, Boutron M, et al. Adenoma-carcinoma sequence or "de novo" carcinogenesis? A study of adenomatous remnants in a population-based series of large bowel cancers. Cancer 69:883–888, 1992.

24. Williams C, Bedenne L. Management of colorectal polyps: is all the effort worthwhile? J Gastroenterol Hepatol 1(Suppl):144–165, 1990.
25. Iishi H, Tatsuta M, Tsutsui S, et al. Early depressed adenocarcinomas of the large intestine. Cancer 69:2406–2410, 1992.
26. Shimoda T, Ikegami M, Fujisaki J, et al. Early colorectal carcinoma with special reference to its development de novo. Cancer 64:1138–1146, 1989.
27. Fleischer D, Goldberg S, Browning T, et al. Detection and surveillance of colorectal cancer. JAMA 261:580–585, 1989.
28. Smart C. Screening and early diagnosis. Cancer 70:1246–1251, 1992.
29. Hardcastle J, Chamberlain J, Sheffield J, et al. Randomised, controlled trial of faecal occult blood screening for colorectal cancer. Results for first 107,349 subjects. Lancet 1:1160–1164, 1989.
30. Simon J. Occult blood screening for colorectal carcinoma: A critical review. Gastroenterology 88:820–837, 1985.
31. Petrelli N, Palmer M, Michalek A, et al. Massive screening for colorectal cancer. A single institution's public commitment. Arch Surg 125:104–105, 1990.
32. Bertario L, Spinelli P, Gennari L, et al. Sensitivity of Hemoccult test for large bowel cancer in high-risk subjects. Dig Dis Sci 33:609–613, 1988.
33. Reilly J, Ballantyne G, Fleming F, et al. Evaluation of the occult blood test in screening for colorectal neoplasms. A prospective study using flexible endoscopy. Am Surg 56:119–123, 1990.
34. Rozen P, Ran E, Fireman Z, et al. The relative value of fecal occult blood tests and flexible sigmoidoscopy in screening for large bowel neoplasia. Cancer 60:2553–2558, 1987.
35. Hardcastle J, Pye G. Screening for colorectal cancer: a critical review. World J Surg 13:38–44, 1989.
36. Mandel J, Bond J, Bardley M, et al. Sensitivity, specificity, and positive predictivity of the Hemoccult test in screening for colorectal cancers. The University of Minnesota's Colon Cancer Control Study. Gastroenterology 97:597–600, 1989.
37. Ahlquist D. Occult blood screening. Obstacles to effectiveness. Cancer 70:1259–1265, 1992.
38. Ahlquist D, McGill D, Fleming J, et al. Patterns of occult bleeding in asymptomatic colorectal cancer. Cancer 63:1826–1830, 1989.
39. Foutch P, Manne R, Sanowski R, et al. Risk factors for blood loss from adenomatous polyps of the large bowel: a colonoscopic evaluation with histopathological correlation. J Clin Gastroenterol 10:50–56, 1988.
40. Herzog P, Holtermuller K, Preiss J, et al. Fecal blood loss in patients with colonic polyps: a comparison of measurements with ^{51} chromium-labelled erythromycin and with the Haemoccult test. Gastroenterology 83:957–962, 1990.
41. Ransohoff D, Lang C. Small adenomas detected during fecal occult blood test screening for colorectal cancer. The impact of serendipity. JAMA 264:76–78, 1990.
42. Schrock T. Colon and rectum: diagnostic techniques. In: Condon R, ed. Shackelford's Surgery of the Alimentary Tract. Vol 4: Colon and anorectum. 3rd ed. Philadelphia: WB Saunders, 1991:22–37.
43. Thomas W, Pye G, Hardcastle J, et al. Screening for colorectal carcinoma: an analysis of the sensitivity of Haemoccult. Br J Surg 9:833–835, 1992.
44. Kewenter J, Engaras B, Haglind E, et al. Value of retesting subjects with a positive Hemoccult in screening for colorectal cancer. Br J Surg 77:1349–1351, 1990.
45. Goldschmeidt M, Ahlquist D, Wieand H, et al. Measurement of degraded fecal hemoglobin-heme to estimate gastrointestinal site of occult bleeding: appraisal of its clinical utility. Dig Dis Sci 33:605–608, 1988.
46. Miyoshi H, Ohshiba S, Asada S, et al. Immunological determination of fecal hemoglobin and transferrin levels: a comparison with other fecal occult blood tests. Am J Gastroenterol 87:67–73, 1992.
47. Miller M, Stanley T. Results of a mass screening program for colorectal cancer. Arch Surg 123:63–65, 1988.
48. McGarrity R, Long P, Peiffer L. Results of a repeat television-advertised mass screening program for colorectal cancer using fecal occult blood tests. Am J Gastroenterol 85:266–270, 1990.
49. Simon J. Colonic polyps, occult blood, and chance (editorial). JAMA 264:84–85, 1990.
50. Ahlquist D, Klee G, McGill D. Colorectal cancer detection in the practice setting. Impact of fecal blood testing. Arch Intern Med 150:1041–1045, 1990.
51. Nord H, Zuckerman G. The workup of a patient with a positive fecal occult blood test: one procedure? Two procedures? Am J Gastroenterol 86:542–545, 1991.
52. Schrock T. Colonoscopic diagnosis and treatment of lower gastrointestinal bleeding. Surg Clin North Am 69:1309–1325, 1989.
53. Barry M, Mulley A, Richter J. Effect of workup strategy on the cost-effectiveness of fecal occult blood screening for colorectal cancer. Gastroenterology 93:301–310, 1987.
54. Gilbertsen V, Nelms J. The prevention of invasive cancer of the rectum. Cancer 41:1137–1139, 1978.
55. Dunaway M, Webb W, Rodning C. Intraluminal measurement of distance in the colorectal region employing rigid and flexible endoscopes. Surg Endosc 2:81–83, 1988.
56. Wilking N, Petrelli N, Herrera-Ornelas L, et al. A comparison of the 25-cm rigid proctosigmoidoscope with the 65-cm flexible endoscope in the screening of patients for colorectal carcinoma. Cancer 57:669–671, 1986.
57. Kee F, Wilson R, Gilliland R, et al. Changing site distribution of colorectal cancer. Br Med J 305:158, 1992.
58. Ghahremani G, Dowlatshahi K. Colorectal carcinomas: diagnostic implications of their changing frequency and anatomic distribution. World J Surg 13:321–325, 1989.
59. Crerand S, Feeley T, Waldron R, et al. Colorectal carcinoma over 30 years at one hospital: no evidence for a shift to the right. Int J Colorectal Dis 6:184–187, 1991.
60. Selby J, Friedman G. Sigmoidoscopy in the periodic health examination of asymptomatic adults. JAMA 261:594–601, 1989.
61. Gupta TP, Jaszewski R, Luk GD. Efficacy of screening flexible sigmoidoscopy for colorectal neoplasia in asymptomatic subjects. Am J Med 86:547–550, 1989.
62. Selby J, Friedman G, Quesenberry CJ, et al. A case-control study of screening sigmoidoscopy and mortality from colorectal cancer. N Engl J Med 326:653–657, 1992.
63. Newcomb P, Norfleet R, Storer B, et al. Screening sigmoidoscopy and colorectal cancer mortality. J Natl Cancer Inst 84:1572–1575, 1992.
64. Simpkins K. What use is barium? Clin Radiol 39:469–473, 1988.

65. Margulis A, Thoeni R. The present status of the radiologic examination of the colon. Radiology 167:1–5, 1988.
66. Isabel-Martinez L, Chapman A, Hall R. The value of a barium enema in the investigation of patients with rectal carcinoma. Clin Radiol 39:531–533, 1988.
67. Spencer N, Richards D, Bartlett P, et al. Colorectal polyps: a correlation of radiological and pathological findings. Clin Radiol 39:407–411, 1988.
68. Clayman C. Mass screening for colorectal cancer: are we ready? (editorial). JAMA 261:609, 1989.
69. Gelfand D, Ott D. The economic implications of radiologic screening for colonic cancer. Am J Roentgenol 156:939–943, 1991.
70. Jensen J, Kewenter J, Asztely M, et al. Double contrast barium enema and flexible rectosigmoidoscopy: a reliable diagnostic combination for detection of colorectal neoplasm. Br J Surg 77:270–272, 1990.
71. Keeffe D, Schrock T. Complications of gastrointestinal endoscopy. In: Sleisenger M, Fordtran J, eds. Gastrointestinal disease. Pathophysiology. Diagnosis. Management. 5th ed. Philadelphia: WB Saunders, 1993:301–308.
72. Church JM. Analysis of the colonoscopic findings in patients with rectal bleeding according to the pattern of their presenting symptoms. Dis Colon Rectum 34:391–395, 1991.
73. Hixson LJ, Fennerty MB, Sampliner RE, et al. Prospective blinded trial of the colonoscopic miss-rate of large colorectal polyps. Gastrointest Endosc 37:125–127, 1991.
74. Warneke J, Petrelli N, Herrera L, et al. Accuracy of colonoscopy for the detection of colorectal polyps. Dis Colon Rectum 35:981–985, 1992.
75. Williams C, Price A. Colon polyps and carcinoma. In: Sivak MJ, ed. Gastroenterologic endoscopy. Philadelphia: WB Saunders, 1987:921–945.
76. Foutch P, Mai H, Pardy K, et al. Flexible sigmoidoscopy may be ineffective for secondary prevention of colorectal cancer in asymptomatic, average-risk men. Dig Dis Sci 36:924–928, 1991.
77. Schuman B, McKay M, Griffin JJ. The use of the 130-cm colonoscope for screening flexible sigmoidoscopy. Gastrointest Endosc 34:459–460, 1988.
78. Agrez M, Evans D, Duggan J. Faecal occult blood testing for colorectal cancer: luxury or necessity? Aust NZ J Surg 60:451–454, 1990.
79. Forde K, Webb W. Acute lower gastrointestinal bleeding. Perspect Colon Rectal Surg 1:105–112, 1988.
80. Van Ness N, Chobanian S, Winters CJ, et al. A study of patient acceptance of double-contrast barium enema and colonoscopy. Arch Intern Med 147:2175–2176, 1987.
81. Glick S, Teplick S, Balfe D, et al. Large colonic neoplasms missed by endoscopy. Am J Radiol 152:513–517, 1989.
82. Schrock T. Lower gastrointestinal bleeding. In: Sivak MJ, ed. Gastroenterologic endoscopy. 2nd ed. Philadelphia: WB Saunders, in press.
83. Irvine E, O'Connor J, Frost R, et al. Prospective comparison of double contrast barium enema plus flexible sigmoidoscopy v colonoscopy in rectal bleeding; barium enema v colonoscopy in rectal bleeding. Gut 29:1188–1193, 1988.
84. Norfleet RG, Ryan ME, Wyman JB, et al. Barium enema versus colonoscopy for patients with polyps found during flexible sigmoidoscopy. Gastrointest Endosc 37:531–534, 1991.
85. Lashner B, Silverstein M. Evaluation and therapy of the patient with fecal occult blood loss: a decision analysis. Am J Gastroenterol 85:1088–1095, 1990.
86. Dunlop M. Screening for large bowel neoplasms in individuals with a family history of colorectal cancer. Br J Surg 79:488–494, 1992.
87. Gane EJ, Lane MR. Colonoscopy in unexplained lower gastrointestinal bleeding. NZ Med J 105:31–33, 1992.
88. Guillem J, Forde K, Treat M, et al. The impact of colonoscopy on the early detection of colonic neoplasms in patients with rectal bleeding. Ann Surg 206:606–611, 1987.
89. DiSario J, Foutch P, Mai H, et al. Prevalence and malignant potential of colorectal polyps in asymptomatic, average-risk men. Am J Gastroenterol 86:941–945, 1991.
90. Eddy D. David Eddy ranks the tests. Harvard Health Letter 10–11, 1992.
91. Lieberman DA, Smith FW. Screening for colon malignancy with colonoscopy. Am J Gastroenterol 86:946–951, 1991.
92. Lieberman D. Cost-effectiveness of colon cancer screening. Am J Gastroenterol 86:1789–1794, 1991.
93. Hunt R. Screening by colonoscopy—has the time arrived? Can J Gastroenterol 4:527–532, 1990.
94. Rex D, Lehman G, Hawes R, et al. Screening colonoscopy in asymptomatic average-risk persons with negative fecal occult blood tests. Gastroenterology 100:64–67, 1991.
95. Zuckerman G, Benitez J. A prospective study of bidirectional endoscopy (colonoscopy and upper endoscopy) in the evaluation of patients with occult gastrointestinal bleeding. Am J Gastroenterol 87:62–66, 1992.
96. Shapiro S. Goals of screening. Cancer 70:1252–1258, 1992.
97. Eddy D, Nugent F, Eddy F, et al. Screening for colorectal cancer in a high-risk population: results of a mathematical model. Gastroenterology 92:682–692, 1987.
98. Kronborg O, Hage E, Deichgraeber E. The clean colon. Scand J Gastroenterol 16:879–884, 1981.
99. Barillari P, Ramacciato G, De AR, et al. Effect of preoperative colonoscopy on the incidence of synchronous and metachronous neoplasms. Acta Chir Scand 156:163–166, 1990.
100. Slater G, Aufses AJ, Szporn A. Synchronous carcinoma of the colon and rectum. Surg Gynecol Obstet 171:283–287, 1990.
101. King's Fund Centre. Cancer of the colon and rectum; the seventh King's Fund consensus statement. Br J Surg 77:1063–1065, 1990.
102. Ryan ME, Norfleet RG, Kirchner JP, et al. The significance of diminutive colonic polyps found at flexible sigmoidoscopy. Gastrointest Endosc 35:85–89, 1989.
103. Opelka FG, Timmcke AE, Gathright JJ, et al. Diminutive colonic polyps: an indication for colonoscopy. Dis Colon Rectum 35:178–181, 1992.
104. Stevenson G, Hernandez C. Single-visit screening and treatment of first-degree relatives. Colon cancer pilot study. Dis Colon Rectum 34:1120–1124, 1991.
105. Baker J, Gathright JJ, Timmcke A, et al. Colonoscopic screening of asymptomatic patients with a family history of colon cancer. Dis Colon Rectum 33:926–930, 1990.
106. Cosgrove J, Wolff W, Tenenbaum N, et al. An appraisal of small and diminutive colonic polyps. Surg Endosc 5:143–145, 1991.

107. Schuman B, Simsek H, Lyons R. The association of multiple colonic adenomatous polyps with cancer of the colon. Am J Gastroenterol 85:846–849, 1990.
108. Atkin W, Morson B, Cuzick J. Long-term risk of colorectal cancer after excision of rectosigmoid adenomas. N Engl J Med 326:658–662, 1992.
109. Muto T, Kamiya J, Sawada T. Small "flat adenoma" of the large bowel with special reference to its clinicopathologic features. Dis Colon Rectum 28:847–851, 1985.
110. Adachi M, Muto T, Okinaga K, et al. Clinicopathologic features of the flat adenoma. Dis Colon Rectum 34:981–986, 1991.
111. Kelly C, Daly J. Colorectal cancer: principles of postoperative follow-up. Cancer 70:1397–1408, 1992.
112. Olsen H, Lawrence W, Snook C, et al. Review of recurrent polyps and cancer in 500 patients with initial colonoscopy for polyps. Dis Colon Rectum 31:222–227, 1988.
113. Lofti A, Spencer R, Ilstrup D, et al. Colorectal polyps and the risk of subsequent carcinoma. Mayo Clin Proc 61:337–343, 1986.
114. Yashiro K, Nagasako K, Sato S, et al. Follow-up after polypectomy of colorectal adenomas. The importance of total colonoscopy. Surg Endosc 3:87–91, 1989.
115. Barkin J, Cohen M, Flaxman M, et al. Value of a routine followup endoscopy program for the detection of recurrent colorectal carcinoma. Am J Gastroenterol 12:1355–1359, 1988.
116. McFarland RJ, Becciolini C, Lallemand RC. The value of colonoscopic surveillance following a diagnosis of colorectal cancer or adenomatous polyp. Eur J Surg Oncol 17:514–518, 1991.
117. Woolfson IK, Eckholdt GJ, Wetzel CR, et al. Usefulness of performing colonoscopy one year after endoscopic polypectomy. Dis Colon Rectum 33:389–393, 1990.
118. Grossman S, Milos M, Tekawa I, et al. Colonoscopic screening of persons with suspected risk factors for colon cancer. II. Past history of colorectal neoplasms. Gastroenterology 96:299–306, 1989.
119. Jahn H, Joergensen O, Kronborg O, et al. Can Hemoccult-IITM replace colonoscopy in surveillance after radical surgery for colorectal cancer and after polypectomy? Dis Colon Rectum 35:253–256, 1992.
120. Juhl G, Larson G, Mullins R, et al. Six-year results of annual colonoscopy after resection of colorectal cancer. World J Surg 14:255–261, 1990.
121. Weber C, Deveney K, Pelegrini C, et al. Routine colonoscopy in the management of colorectal carcinoma. Am J Surg 152:87–92, 1986.
122. Granqvist S, Karlsson T. Postoperative follow-up of patients with colorectal carcinoma by colonoscopy. Eur J Surg 158:307–312, 1992.
123. Fantini G, DeCosse J. Surveillance strategies after resection of carcinoma of the colon. Surg Gynecol Obstet 171:267–273, 1990.
124. Bulow S, Svendsen L, Mellemgaard A. Metachronous colorectal carcinoma. Br J Surg 77:502–505, 1990.
125. Himal H. Anastomotic recurrence of carcinoma of the colon and rectum. The value of endoscopy and serum CEA levels. Am Surg 57:334–337, 1991.
126. Stulc J, Petrelli N, Herrera L, et al. Anastomotic recurrence of adenocarcinoma of the colon. Arch Surg 121:1077–1080, 1986.
127. Ovaska J, Jarvinen H, Kujari H, et al. Follow-up of patients operated on for colorectal carcinoma. Am J Surg 159:593–596, 1990.
128. Vasen H, Griffioen G, Offerhaus G, et al. The value
of screening and central registration of families with familial adenomatous polyposis. A study of 82 families in the Netherlands. Dis Colon Rectum 33:227–230, 1990.
129. Jarvinen H. Epidemiology of familial adenomatous polyposis in Finland: impact of family screening on the colorectal cancer rate and survival. Gut 33:357–360, 1992.
130. Burn J, Chapman P, Delhanty J, et al. Genetic registers for familial adenomatous polyposis: use of age of onset, CHRPE's and DNA markers in risk calculation. J Med Genet 28:289–296, 1991.
131. Rhodes M, Bradburn D. Overview of screening and management of familial adenomatous polyposis. Gut 33:125–131, 1992.
132. Norfleet R. Screening for upper gastrointestinal neoplasms in patients with familial adenomatous polyposis and Gardner's syndrome (editorial). J Clin Gastroenterol 14:95–96, 1992.
133. Heyen F, Jagelman D, Romania A, et al. Predictive value of congenital hypertrophy of the retinal pigment epithelium as a clinical marker for familial adenomatous polyposis. Dis Colon Rectum 33:1003–1008, 1990.
134. Kee F, Collins B. Families at risk of colorectal cancer: who are they? Gut 33:787–790, 1992.
135. Lynch P, Lynch H. Hereditary nonpolyposis colon cancer epidemiological and clinical-genetic features. In: Lynch P, Lynch H, eds. Colon cancer genetics. New York: VN Reinholt, 1985:99–110.
136. Stephenson B, Finan P, Gascoyne J, et al. Frequency of familial colorectal cancer. Br J Surg 78:1162–1166, 1991.
137. Lynch H. The surgeon and colorectal cancer genetics. Arch Surg 125:698–701, 1990.
138. Jass J, Stewart S. Evolution of hereditary non-polyposis colorectal cancer. Gut 33:783–786, 1992.
139. Lynch H, Smyrk T, Watson P, et al. Hereditary flat adenoma syndrome: a variant of familial adenomatous polyposis? Dis Colon Rectum 35:411–421, 1992.
140. Itoh H, Houlston R, Slack J. Risk of cancer death in first-degree relatives of patients with hereditary non-polyposis cancer syndrome (Lynch type II): a study of 130 kindreds in the United Kingdom. Br J Surg 77:1367–1370, 1990.
141. Lanspa SJ, Lynch HT, Smyrk TC, et al. Colorectal adenomas in the Lynch syndromes. Results of a colonoscopy screening program. Gastroenterology 98:1117–1122, 1990.
142. Love R, Morrissey J. Colonoscopy in asymptomatic individuals with a family history of colorectal cancer. Arch Intern Med 144:2209–2211, 1984.
143. Grossman S, Milos M. Colonoscopic screening of persons with suspected risk factors for colon cancer. I. Family history. Gastroenterology 94:395–400, 1988.
144. Meagher A, Stuart M. Colonoscopy in patients with a family history of colorectal cancer. Dis Colon Rectum 35:315–321, 1992.
145. Luchtefeld M, Syverson D, Solfelt M, et al. Is colonoscopic screening appropriate in asymptomatic patients with family history of colon cancer? Dis Colon Rectum 34:763–768, 1991.
146. McConnell J, Nizin J, Slade M. Colonoscopy in patients with a primary family history of colon cancer. Dis Colon Rectum 33:105–107, 1990.
147. Brzezinski W, Orrom W, Wiens E. Prospective and retrospective analysis of colonoscopy findings in patients with a history of colorectal carcinoma in first-degree relatives. Can J Surg 33:314–316, 1990.
148. Gryska P, Cohen A. Screening asymptomatic patients

at high risk for colon cancer with full colonoscopy. Dis Colon Rectum 30:18–20, 1987.

149. Houlston R, Murday V, Harocopos C, et al. Screening and genetic counselling for relatives of patients with colorectal cancer in a family cancer clinic. Br Med J 301:366–368, 1990.

150. Guillem JG, Forde KA, Treat MR, et al. Colonoscopic screening for neoplasms in asymptomatic first-degree relatives of colon cancer patients. A controlled, prospective study. Dis Colon Rectum 35:523–529, 1992.

151. Rozen P, Ron E. A cost analysis of screening methodology for family members of colorectal cancer patients. Am J Gastroenterol 84:1548–1551, 1989.

152. Rozen P, Fireman Z, Figer A, et al. Colorectal rumor screening in women with a past history of breast, uterine, or ovarian malignancies. Cancer 57:1235–1239, 1986.

153. Ekbom A, Helmick C, Zack M, et al. Ulcerative colitis and colorectal cancer. A population-based study. N Engl J Med 323:1228–1233, 1990.

154. Lennard-Jones J. Cancer surveillance in ulcerative colitis appears to work and can be made to work better. In: Riddell R, ed. Dysplasia and cancer in colitis. New York: Elsevier, 1991:11–18.

155. Lashner BA, Silverstein MD, Hanauer SB. Hazard rates for dysplasia and cancer in ulcerative colitis. Results from a surveillance program. Dig Dis Sci 34:1536–1541, 1989.

156. Lashner B. Recommendations for colorectal cancer screening in ulcerative colitis: a review of research from a single university-based surveillance program. Am J Gastroenterol 87:168–175.

157. Sachar D. Cancer risk in inflammatory bowel disease: myths and metaphors. In: Riddell R, ed. Dysplasia and cancer in colitis. New York: Elsevier, 1991:5–9.

158. Gilat T, Fireman Z, Grossman A, et al. Colorectal cancer in patients with ulcerative colitis: a population study in central Israel. Gastroenterology 94:870–877, 1988.

159. Riddell R, Goldman H, Ransohoff D, et al. Dysplasia in inflammatory bowel disease: standardized classification with provisional clinical implications. Hum Pathol 14:931–968, 1983.

160. Bramwell N, Riddell R. Cancer and dysplasia. In: Gitnick G, ed. Inflammatory bowel disease. Diagnosis and treatment. New York: Igaku-Shoin, 1991:503–516.

161. Woolrich AJ, DaSilva MD, Korelitz BI. Surveillance in the routine management of ulcerative colitis: the predictive value of low-grade dysplasia. Gastroenterology 103:431–438, 1992.

162. Blackstone M, Riddell R, Rogers B, et al. Dysplasia-associated lesion of mass (DALM) detected by colonoscopy in longstanding ulcerative colitis: an indication for colectomy. Gastroenterology 80:366–374, 1981.

163. Yardley J. How can dysplasia "disappear" at colectomy? In: Riddell R, ed. Dysplasia and cancer in colitis. New York: Elsevier, 1991:49–53.

164. Leidenius M, Kellokumpu I, Husa A, et al. Dysplasia and carcinoma in longstanding ulcerative colitis: an endoscopic and histological surveillance programme. Gut 32:1521–1525, 1991.

165. Blackstone M. Endoscopy in chronic colitis: is quality assurance achievable? In: Riddell R, ed. Dysplasia and cancer in colitis. New York: Elsevier, 1991:55–59.

166. Melville D, Richman P, Shepherd N, et al. Brush cytology of the colon and rectum in ulcerative colitis: an aid to cancer diagnosis. J Clin Pathol 41:1180–1186, 1988.

167. Isbister WH, Gupta RK. Colonoscopy, mucosal biopsy and brush cytology in the assessment of patients with colorectal inflammatory bowel disease. Surg Endosc 3:159–163, 1989.

168. Lennard-Jones J, Melville D, Morson B, et al. Precancer and cancer in extensive ulcerative colitis: findings among 401 patients over 22 years. Gut 31:800–806, 1990.

169. Löfberg R, Broström O, Karlën P, et al. Colonoscopic surveillance in long-standing total ulcerative colitis—a 15-year follow-up study. Gastroenterology 99:1021–1031, 1990.

170. Bröstrom O, Löfberg R, Ost A, et al. Cancer surveillance of patients with longstanding ulcerative colitis: a clinical, endoscopical, and histological study. Gut 27:1408–1413, 1986.

171. Jones H, Grogono J, Hoare A. Surveillance in ulcerative colitis: burdens and benefit. Gut 29:325–331, 1988.

172. Manning A, Bulgim O, Dixon M, et al. Screening by colonoscopy for colonic epithelial dysplasia in inflammatory bowel disease. Gut 29:1489–1494, 1987.

173. Rutegard L, Ahsgren R, Stenling R, et al. Ulcerative colitis: cancer surveillance in an unselected population. Scand J Gastroenterol 23:139–145, 1988.

174. Collins R, Feldman M, Fordtran J. Colon cancer, dysplasia and surveillance in patients with ulcerative colitis: a critical review. N Engl J Med 316:1654–1658, 1987.

175. Nugent F, Haggitt R, Gilpin P. Cancer surveillance in ulcerative colitis. Gastroenterology 100:1241–1248, 1991.

176. Rosenstock E, Farmer R, Petras R, et al. Surveillance for colonic carcinoma in ulcerative colitis. Gastroenterology 89:1342–1346, 1985.

177. Lashner BA, Kane SV, Hanauer SB. Colon cancer surveillance in chronic ulcerative colitis: historical cohort study. Am J Gastroenterol 85:1083–1087, 1990.

178. Taylor B, Pemberton J, Carpenter H, et al. Dysplasia in chronic ulcerative colitis: implications for colonoscopic surveillance. Dis Colon Rectum 35:950–956, 1992.

179. Gyde S. Screening for colorectal cancer in ulcerative colitis: dubious benefits and high costs. Gut 31:1089–1092, 1990.

180. Rubin C, Haggitt R, Burmer G, et al. DNA aneuploidy in colonic biopsies predicts future development of dysplasia in ulcerative colitis. Gastroenterology 103:1611–1620, 1992.

181. Morrissey J, Reichelderfer M. Gastgrointestinal endoscopy (second of two parts). N Engl J Med 325:1214–1222, 1991.

182. Petras R. Dysplasia and cancer in Crohn's disease. In: Bayless T, ed. Current management of inflammatory bowel disease. Philadelphia: BC Decker, 1989:360–363.

183. Stahl T, Schoetz DJ, Roberts P, et al. Crohn's disease and carcinoma: increasing justification for surveillance? Dis Colon Rectum 35:850–856, 1992.

183. Yamazaki Y, Ribeiro M, Sachar D etal. Malignant colorectal strictures in Crohn's disease. Am J Gastroenterol 86:882–885, 1991.

185. Brenna E, Skreden K, Waldum HL, et al. The benefit of colonoscopy. Scand J Gastroenterol 25:81–88, 1990.

186. Rex DK, Weddle RA, Lehman GA, et al. Flexible sigmoidoscopy plus air contrast barium enema versus colonoscopy for suspected lower gastrointestinal bleeding. Gastroenterology 98:855–861, 1990.

187. Whelan RL, Buls JG, Goldberg SM, et al. Intra-operative endoscopy. University of Minnesota experience. Am Surg 55:281–286, 1989.
188. Longo W, Ballantyne G, Modlin I. Colonoscopic detection of early colorectal cancers. Impact of a surgical endoscopy service. Ann Surg 207:174–178, 1988.
189. Hilliard G, Ramming K, Thompson JJ, et al. The elusive colonic malignancy. A need for definitive preoperative localization. Am Surg 56:742–744, 1990.
190. Hyman N, Waye JD. Endoscopic four quadrant tattoo for the identification of colonic lesions at surgery. Gastrointest Endosc 37:56–58, 1991.
191. Rösch T, Lorenz R, Classen M. Endoscopic ultrasonography in the evaluation of colon and rectal disease. Gastrointest Endosc 36:382–386, 1990.
192. Karita M, Tada M, Okita K, et al. Endoscopic therapy for early colon cancer: the strip biopsy resection technique. Gastrointest Endosc 37:128–132, 1991.
193. Bright N, Hale P, Mason R. Poor palliation of colorectal malignancy with the neodymium yttrium-aluminium-garnet laser. Br J Surg 79:308–309, 1992.
194. Mathus-Vliegen E, Tytgat G. Palliation by laser photoablation: a multidisciplinary quality assessment. Gastrointest Endosc 38:365–368, 1992.
195. Brunetaud J, Maunoury V, Ducrotte P, et al. Palliative treatment of rectosigmoid carcinoma by laser endoscopic photoablation. Gastroenterology 92:663–668, 1987.
196. Stone JM, Bloom RJ. Transendoscopic balloon dilatation of complete colonic obstruction. An adjunct in the treatment of colorectal cancer: report of three cases. Dis Colon Rectum 32:429–431, 1989.
197. Lelcuk S, Ratan J, Klausner J, et al. Endoscopic decompression of acute colonic obstruction: avoiding staged surgery. Ann Surg 203:292–294, 1986.
198. Rattan J, Klausner JM, Rozen P, et al. Acute left colonic obstruction: a new nonsurgical treatment. J Clin Gastroenterol 11:331–334, 1989.

23

Anoscopy and Flexible Fiberoptic Sigmoidoscopy
Evaluation of the Distal 50 Cm of Colorectum

Gerald Marks and John Marks

The prevalence of cancers arising in the distal 50 cm of colorectum and the frequency of troublesome and sometimes serious non-malignant anorectal disorders underscore the importance of accurate assessment of the terminal portion of the gastrointestinal tract.

Most critical to this assessment is endoscopy, but it is only one component in the comprehensive approach to the evaluation and treatment of the colorectal surgery patient. A detailed patient history, carefully conducted physical examination, and related laboratory evaluations are other factors essential to an accurate diagnosis. Endoscopic examination, in the hands of a well-trained physician, can be conducted safely, quickly, and effectively. Because in many instances the quality of care offered to the surgical patient is determined by the expertise of the endoscopist, the goal of the surgeon is to achieve such expertise. This chapter is designed to enhance the surgeon's proficiency in addressing the endoscopic evaluation of the terminal 50 cm of the colorectum and anal canal exclusive of colonoscopy.

ANATOMY AND PHYSIOLOGY

The anal canal and rectum comprise a hollow, muscular viscus that represents the termination of the gastrointestinal tract. Their close anatomic relationship to certain osseous and soft tissues of the pelvis and perineum affects many aspects of anorectal disorders. The transition from sigmoid to rectum is not always visually identifiable, although a physiologic sphincter can occasionally be identified either endoscopically or radiographically. The rectum is 12 to 15 cm long and descends from the pelvis through the musculotendinous pelvic diaphragm. It is fixed by various fascial and muscular attachments, which aid in maintaining the sacral curve of the rectum and contribute to both continence and the ability to defecate. The rectum descends to the anorectal junction, which is located at the upper border of the puborectal muscle in the anal canal (Fig. 23–1).

The anal canal is divided into roughly two equal parts by the dentate or pectinate line. The distal portion of the canal is approximately 2 cm long and is normally lined with pink, stratified, non-keratinized squamous epithelium. The mucosa above the dentate line appears deep purple or plum colored. The rectal columns of Morgagni contained in the mucosal lining proximal to the dentate line are united at their lower ends by the anal valves and form the anal crypts. Anal glands with ducts that are important to the pathogenesis of anorectal infection, abscesses, and fistulas reside deep in these crypts.

The internal sphincter is the downward continuation of the circular muscular coat of the rectum. It begins 6 to 8 cm above the anal orifice and ends 1 to 2 cm below the level of the anal valves with a well-defined edge that

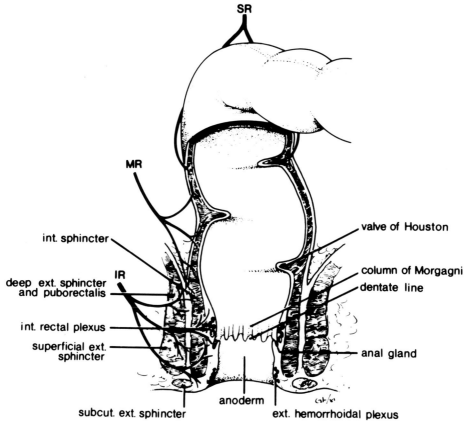

Figure 23–1. Anatomy of anal canal and rectum. SR = superior rectal artery; MR = middle rectal artery; IR = inferior rectal artery.

can be palpated at the upper margin of the intersphincteric groove. The external sphincter, which is the principal element in fecal continence, is skeletal muscle and is composed of three parts—superficial, subcutaneous, and deep. The levator ani is another three-part muscle and forms the pelvic floor. It also provides divergent forces that fix the rectum, and it plays a role in the act of defecation and in maintaining continence.

Anorectal spaces exist that are of importance in the potential development of abscesses. These spaces are marginal perianal, ischiorectal, intersphincteric, submucosal, superficial and deep postanal, and retrorectal. The superior, middle, and inferior rectal arteries; the middle sacral artery; and corresponding veins supply the anorectum. The lymphatic vessels of the anorectum follow the visceral or somatic vascular pathways (see Fig. 23–1).

Although changes in intraluminal pressure are felt, the rectum and rectal mucosa are relatively insensitive to pain. Sensory innervation is limited primarily to the skin of the anal canal and perianal region, but sensory fibers may extend as high as 2 cm above the pectinate line in some individuals, which explains why in exceptional instances submucosal sclerosing injection or rubber band ligation produces pain.[1] Reflex sphincter spasm following trauma is produced by the rich sensory innervation of the anus and the sensitivity of the tissue to increased interstitial pressure.

The reservoir capacity of the rectum and the competence of the external sphincter and puborectal muscles are the two elements of fecal continence. The afferent proprioceptive sensor is now believed to originate in the puborectal muscle, and although its role is not fully understood, the internal sphincter is believed to contribute to the ability to distinguish among gaseous, liquid, and solid materials. The integrity of both muscle and neural pathways is necessary for competent muscular action.

SYMPTOMATOLOGY

The thesis that a complete understanding of the nature and cause of symptoms leads to a more accurate diagnosis demands that a proper history be elicited. The quality of sensations perceived, temporal relationships, and the nature of signs are most meaningful.[2]

Pain is a frequent and distressing symptom. As an aid in diagnosis, the quality of the pain must be carefully analyzed. Cutting, tearing, burning pain may result from anal fissures (Fig. 23–2); abrasions; lacerations at the base of a prolapsed, hypertrophied anal papilla; and excoriations in the anal or perianal skin. A constant superficial ache indicates increased interstitial tension in the anal and perianal subcutaneous tissue. External thrombotic hemorrhoids or small abscesses may cause this type of sensation. Throbbing associated with a constant ache signifies an abscess. A deep aching pain without a throbbing quality, whether wavelike or not, suggests muscle spasm and is often perceived as such by the patient. Severe spasm of the levator ani muscle produces proctalgia fugax, which is described as a shooting pain in the rectum. Less severe levator ani spasm is often described by the patient as a deep perineal ache and is likened to the sensation of sitting on a ball. This sensation is also present with occult rectal prolapse. The discomfort produced by anorectal trauma; anal fissure; prolapsed, strangulated internal hemorrhoids; and anorectal surgery as the result of sphincter spasm is intermittent and can be triggered merely by a change in body position. A herpes simplex, type 2 viral infection is accompanied by inordinately severe pain. Pelvic and presacral metastatic disease that involves sacral nerves is often associated with ill-defined but deep and severe presacral and perineal pain. Ill-defined burning pain in the perineum and rectum may be the result of disease of the lumbosacral spine.

When bleeding occurs, the color and quantity of blood issued via the anus should be evaluated for clues to its origin. It is important to determine whether the blood is marbleized in the feces or is merely on the surface, whether it is present solely on the toilet tissue or drips into the toilet bowl, and whether it occurs spontaneously or with defecation.

Blood streaked on the stool surface originates from the distal rectum, hemorrhoidal zone, or anal canal, and blood marbleized in the stool is presumed to issue from a site proximal to the distal rectum. Bleeding from the hemorrhoidal zone has been known to fill the entire colon before stimulating evacuation, a fact that may produce dire consequences by delaying or distorting the diagnosis. Bleeding that drips into the toilet bowl or soils undergarments is from a point distal to the grasp of the sphincters, and a prolapsing internal hemorrhoid, polyp, or perirectal laceration may be the cause.

Hemolyzed blood can originate in any segment of the gastrointestinal tract, whereas clotted blood usually originates in the distal portion of the colorectum. Bright red blood indicates an arterial bleeding point, but hemorrhoidal blood can also be bright red because of arteriovenous communication. Blood from the proximal gastrointestinal tract, although ordinarily tarry, may be bright red if bleeding is massive and transit is brisk. Systemic signs of exsanguinating blood loss must be recognized immediately. Life-threatening hemorrhage can originate in the anorectum, and because this site may be overlooked, careful anoscopic inspection of this area must precede sigmoidoscopy and colonoscopy.

The sensation of needing to evacuate but passing only mucoid material or blood is, by common usage, the definition of tenesmus. An intraluminal or intramural obstruction, such as a fecal impaction or neoplasm, may produce this symptom. An inflammatory process in any portion of the rectal wall, such as proctitis or pelvic abscess, can also produce tenesmus.

A number of cutaneous lesions may produce perianal irritation. This symptom complex includes mild burning, chafing, or actual pain, depending on the degree of integumental disturbance or destruction. Perianal irritation may be produced by an infection; herpes simplex, type 2; fecal debris with proteolytic enzymes; accumulation of moisture; contact dermatitis;

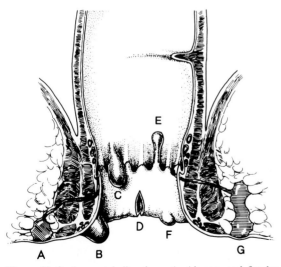

Figure 23–2. Anorectal disorders. *A,* Abscess and fistula; *B,* external thrombotic hemorrhoids; *C,* internal hemorrhoids; *D,* fissure; *E,* hypertrophied anal papilla; *F,* skin tag; and *G,* abscess and fistula.

or trauma caused by sexual contact or overzealous cleansing. The sensation of itching is mediated through pain fibers and results from a low-intensity pain stimulus. Mild trauma of any kind will initiate pruritus. Proteolytic enzymes that remain on the skin, the result of faulty cleansing, may well be the most common cause of pruritus ani.

Patients often do not distinguish among frank suppuration, a moist discharge, and fecal staining. A funnel-shaped perineum and obesity are major causes of accumulated perineal moisture. Fecal seepage occurs in individuals with postoperative anal defects or incompetent sphincter mechanisms but also may result merely from watery fecal contents. Suppuration results from any infected lesion in the anal or perianal region. These lesions include pilonidal cysts and abscesses, fistula-in-ano with abscess, hidradenitis suppurativa, and infected inclusion cysts. Excellent lighting is required to exclude the presence of a secondary opening of a fistula.

EXAMINATION

A complete patient history is crucial to making an accurate diagnosis and should be obtained prior to carrying out the anorectal examination.

Preparation of Patient

To accomplish a complete and adequate inspection, the rectal vault and distal sigmoid must be free of fecal material and excessive quantities of liquid.[3] One or two Fleet enemas (sodium biphosphate and sodium phosphate) usually suffice when administered 0.5 hour apart and as close to examination as is practical. It is not necessary for the patient to abstain from food nor is sedation ordinarily required unless the patient has a painful condition. It is important to remember that even significant disease in the anorectal zone and distal rectum is commonly overlooked when flexible sigmoidoscopy alone is used, highlighting the importance of anoscopy and careful digital examination. Cathartics should be avoided in the 24 hours prior to examination to preclude the accumulation of a large amount of liquid fecal material, which can obscure disease and is annoying to the endoscopist.

Position of the Patient

A perfectly adequate examination can be carried out with the patient in the Sims position, with the buttocks drawn over the edge of an ordinary examining table, or with the patient in the knee-chest position. The Sims position is considerably more comfortable for the patient and may be preferred by the examiner. The knee-chest position, which produces a negative intraperitoneal pressure that distracts the walls and widens the lumen of the rectum, is advantageous in certain situations, such as for biopsy purposes.

Instruments and Materials

Materials needed to perform an anorectal and rectal examination include disposable gloves, water-soluble lubricant, an anoscope, a rigid sigmoidoscope, a stricturescope, and a bright light source. It is also desirable to have a suction apparatus, cotton swabs, a topical anesthetic of either 10% cocaine solution or lidocaine jelly, flexible fiberoptic sigmoidoscope, 20% silver nitrate solution, and silver nitrate sticks. Other instruments such as biopsy forceps, malleable probes, and an electrocautery unit offer the endoscopist additional latitude in treating the patient.

Visual Inspection

The initial step is inspection of the skin in the postsacral, perineal, perianal, and buttock areas. The skin at the anal verge must be distracted to adequately assess the anal canal for the presence of a fissure or exudate. Distortion of anal symmetry, indicating sphincter disruption and muscle contracture as part of the anal reflex, is also noted. Excellent illumination is needed to detect small but important changes.

Palpation and Internal Digital Examination

Perianal sensory perception is determined by palpation and point of tenderness or induration noted. Internal digital examination is initiated by gently pressing anteriorly at the opening of the anal canal to overcome the resistance of the anal sphincter with a well-lubricated, gloved index finger. The patient can help to initiate sphincter relaxation by bearing down as light digital pressure is exerted. The quality of the anal mucosa, the adequacy of the lumen, and the tone of the sphincter are noted on digital examination. The rectal vault is palpated by a circumferential sweeping motion of the examining digit. Because visualization of the posterior wall of the rectum is made difficult by the posterior sacral curve, this area must be palpated with care to exclude significant disease. Straining effort by the patient produces an intussusception effect that may bring lesions located beyond 7 to 8 cm to within reach of the examining finger. Submucosal, intramural, and extramural masses often go undetected on endoscopic examination but can be appreciated with careful palpation. An experienced examiner can palpate the subtleties of mucosal edema, intramural fibrosis, extramural lymph nodes, and indurated lymphatics. Pain elicited in the anal canal or perianal area may indicate the presence of a fissure, thrombosis, or an abscess. Pelvic peritonitis, retroperitoneal suppuration, or a lesion of the lumbosacral plexus produces tenderness high in the rectum. All material retrieved on the examining finger should be inspected for the presence of blood and purulent discharge.

ANOSCOPY

Anoscopy is essential to the complete evaluation of the anorectum and the treatment of specific conditions. The patient's tolerance for the anoscope can be estimated during the visual and digital examination. The diameter of the anoscope should not exceed the patient's tolerance level; the author's scope of choice is the Martin-Davis type. Severe pain or stricture may make it necessary to use a stricturescope or anesthesia. Our rule is, "Never cause the patient discomfort in the office or at the bedside." With the patient in the Sims position and the upper buttock elevated, a lubricated anoscope with its obturator in place is inserted in the same manner as the examining digit. The obturator is removed and examined for the presence and quality of stool, pus, or blood. Careful inspection of the mucosa in the hemorrhoidal zone is then carried out. Slow withdrawal of the anoscope allows the lumen to be observed for the presence of mucosal friability, neoplasms, internal hemorrhoids, exudate, erythema, hypertrophied anal papillae, fissures, or excoriation. Prolapsing redundant mucosa and internal hemorrhoids can be demonstrated if the patient can be encouraged to bear down as the scope is being removed.

RIGID SIGMOIDOSCOPY

The indications for rigid sigmoidoscopy have become less clear since the advent of flexible fiberoptic sigmoidoscopy (see further on). Rigid sigmoidoscopy may be used as an adjunctive procedure prior to flexible fiberoptic sigmoidoscopy under certain circumstances. It may permit fine delineation, site localization, and critical measurements in planning surgery.[3] It is appropriate when the point of interest is within its reach.

Rigid sigmoidoscopes are available in plastic disposable and standard metal models. The outside diameter of rigid scopes varies from 15 to 20 mm, and the outside diameter of disposable scopes is usually 20 mm. The outside diameter of the stricturescope is only 10 mm. Rigid scopes are also available in various lengths, but the standard scope is 25 cm long. Both fiberoptic and incandescent light sources are available either in a proximal or distal position. Although distal lighting provides illumination that is superior to proximal lighting, the presence of debris or blood in the lumen may diminish that advantage.

Disposable scopes are useful for examining patients who have, or are suspected of having, a communicable process. When there is no blood, fecal debris, or contagious disorder, the thinner metal scope is used to provide greater patient comfort. For therapeutic use, the instrument of choice is that of the shortest length and greatest diameter.

Digital examination always precedes instrumentation. The instrument is lubricated and inserted into a lubricated anal canal in a direct line from the anal verge to the umbilicus. Sphincter resistance is overcome in the same manner as described for digital and anoscopic examinations. Once the resistance of the sphincter is overcome and the distal rectum entered, the tip of the scope with the obturator in place is pointed posteriorly into the sacral hollow. To prevent any fluid that is present in the rectum from flowing out, the sigmoidoscope handle is elevated prior to removing the obturator. The rigid scope is advanced only if the lumen can be clearly visualized. When the patient is in the Sims position, visualization can be achieved only by insufflation. If the lumen becomes obscured, the endoscope can be withdrawn as much as 3 to 5 cm to achieve orientation of the tip. As long as the lumen can be visualized and the patient is comfortable, the entire length of the endoscope can be passed. Once the limit of introduction has been reached, withdrawal is begun. Slowly rotating the tip permits the examiner to visualize the entire circumference of the lumen. Special care is then taken to visualize the superior surface of each valve of Houston. In a healthy bowel, the architecture of the submucosal vasculature is clearly delineated. The presence of mucosal friability, ulceration, edema, purulence, neoplasia, and lumenal blood and mucus should be sought.

Painful conditions may prevent the patient from tolerating anything more than the stricturescope without the use of anesthesia. An anal block may enable the patient to tolerate a complete anorectal examination, otherwise regional or general anesthesia may be used.

Several caveats governing the use of rigid endoscopy should be obeyed: never advance a rigid scope without clear visualization of the lumen; gentle pressure can be applied against an area of spasm only if the lumen can be seen; pain is a signal to stop the examination immediately; and actual or suspected peritonitis and pelvic cellulitis are contraindications for all but the most minimal endoscopic inspection of the distal rectum.

FLEXIBLE FIBEROPTIC SIGMOIDOSCOPY

The rigid sigmoidoscope, the traditional mainstay in the armamentarium of the surgeon treating colorectal disease, served so well for so long that the introduction of the flexible sigmoidoscope, an instrument that served a similar purpose but was many times more expensive, initially met with little acceptance. Physicians were reluctant to endorse, without proved benefit, an instrument that not only was far more expensive than the old reliable rigid scope but also permitted the physician to examine less of the colon than the already available colonoscope. Other reasons given for the reluctance to accept the flexible fiberoptic sigmoidoscope were the low cost-effectiveness, bothersome patient preparation, increased time required for both the procedure and sterilization of the instrument, potential hazards, difficulty in use, lack of instrument durability, and questionable patient acceptance. It was also suggested that since total colonoscopy could be so expeditiously and safely performed, it would be unreasonable to provide the patient with less than a complete examination.[3]

The development of flexible fiberoptic technology and the introduction of the colonoscope in 1969 and the flexible fiberoptic sigmoidoscope in its commercial mode around 1976 to 1977 brought us to a new level of assessment and treatment of colorectal disorders. The flexible fiberoptic sigmoidoscope has become the standard of distal colorectal evaluation and treatment. The transition, however, from routine evaluation with rigid sigmoidoscopes to that with the flexible models required extensive application, evaluation, and review before many clinicians were comfortable accepting the flexible sigmoidoscope as the standard.

Many of the early studies reported circa 1976 to 1977 not only failed to convincingly present the advantages of the flexible scope but also drew negative conclusions as to its feasibility.[4–6] A cooperative study on the use of the early production model of the flexible fiberoptic sigmoidoscope not only showed convincingly that the presumed disadvantages of the instrument were invalid but also that striking advantages were often derived from its use.[7] The examination could be conducted simply and cleanly in the office, with minimal preparation of the patient, no sedation, and the expectation of an extremely high yield of information. Strong reasons support flexible fiberoptic sigmoidoscopy as the standard for examination of the distal colorectum.

Controversy exists about the value of screening colorectal cancers with the flexible fiberoptic sigmoidoscope. Although there is a general lack of evidence on this topic, a case control study by Selby and colleagues[8] indicated that benefit is derived from sigmoidoscopic screening. Their review of nearly 300 patients in whom the efficacy of sigmoidoscopic screening was tested showed that sigmoidoscopic evaluation of asymptomatic patients could reduce mortality from cancer of the rectum and distal colon. The study suggested that a randomized trial might further clarify the issue.

A critical evaluation of the comparative effectiveness of the rigid sigmoidoscope and the flexible fiberoptic sigmoidoscope was undertaken to identify patient subsets and the relative yield of information. A prospective, comparative computerized study was begun in October 1977 with the cooperation of six colorectal surgeons who examined and collected data on 3000 patients in their offices.[9] Patients seen in a surgeon's office are preselected, and a high incidence of clinically significant colorectal abnormality, particularly neoplasia, might be expected. When the initial arm of the study reported data on the first 1012 patients in June 1978, the advantages were so impressive that the value of flexible fiberoptic sigmoidoscopy was never again in doubt. Information from this and other clinical studies and programs proves that the flexible scope is an instrument of extraordinary capability in detecting colorectal neoplasms, with yields two to three times greater than those achieved with the rigid sigmoidoscope in symptom resolution and in the surveillance of patients with polyps and cancer.[7] In addition, the practical advantages of the narrow diameter, flexibility, and length of the fiberoptic sigmoidoscope were readily appreciated by surgeons as they determined that patients could be examined satisfactorily despite rectal or sigmoid strictures, marked angulations, or contracted lumens in which a rigid scope would be unsuitable.

On the basis of the data, guidelines were developed for the application of the flexible fiberoptic sigmoidoscope.[7] Appreciation of the role of the rigid sigmoidoscope and the proper relationship between the rigid and flexible instruments was identified as well. It was realized that precise indication categories exist for sigmoidoscopy, and within each of these categories, the yield can justify the identified use of flexible fiberoptic sigmoidoscopy. Recognition that colorectal cancer was becoming less common in the rectum and more common in the sigmoid colon, and the discovery of an even distribution of benign premalignant neoplasms through the distal 50 cm of colorectum, emphasized the need to examine as much of the colorectum as possible in the initial sigmoidoscopic examination.[10]

There has never been any disagreement about the potential danger of flexible fiberoptic sigmoidoscopy when performed by untrained individuals. The anxieties regarding possible jeopardy to patients and the overuse of this more expensive study have been met by the establishment of training and practice standards and guidelines for use.[10] It is fair to presume that through training and clinical experience, the surgeon is well prepared to achieve proficiency in flexible fiberoptic sigmoidoscopy, but a commitment of time and effort to achieve the level of skill necessary to safely perform the procedure is still required. The rewards that accrue to both surgeon and patient amply justify the use of flexible fiberoptic sigmoidoscopy in the treatment of all patients with, or in danger of having, colorectal disorders.

Indications for Flexible Fiberoptic Colonoscopy

The indications for flexible fiberoptic sigmoidoscopy are best understood when the roles of both the rigid sigmoidoscope and the flexible fiberoptic colonoscope are clearly delineated. The application of the rigid sigmoidoscope has been addressed.

Briefly, there are three major categories of indications for flexible fiberoptic colonoscopy: diagnosis, surveillance, and therapy.

Diagnosis

The indications for diagnostic flexible fiberoptic colonoscopy include symptoms that are inconsistent with negative results from sigmoidoscopic and barium enema studies, unexplained blood in the colonic lumen, unexplained chronic gastrointestinal blood loss, indeterminate radiographic findings, acute undiagnosed colonic hemorrhage, the need for confirmation of radiographic findings, colorectal neoplasia at any site, preoperative colectomy clearance, mapping the extent of inflammatory bowel disease, and familial polyposis progeny.

Surveillance

Indications for surveillance include postpolypectomy patients, following resection for a polyp or cancer, a history of breast or uterine cancer, a family history of colonic cancer, prior radiation therapy, chronic ulcerative colitis, Crohn's disease, a family history of polyposis, cancer family syndrome, and uveal tract melanoma (See Chap. 7).

Therapy

Therapeutic indications include polypectomy, electrocoagulation of bleeding sites, anastomotic dilation, reduction of volvulus, ileus decompression, and foreign body removal, among others.

Flexible fiberoptic sigmoidoscopy has an important role when used interactively with colonoscopy in surveillance. The need for total colonoscopy should never be preempted by flexible fiberoptic sigmoidoscopy.[3]

Indications for Flexible Fiberoptic Sigmoidoscopy

An outgrowth of the original comparative study was the identification of specific indications for flexible fiberoptic sigmoidoscopy, which include routine screening, high-risk status screening, symptom resolution, polyp surveillance, cancer surveillance, confirmation of radiographic findings, resolution of questionable radiographic findings, preoperative clearance of the colon, anastomotic inspection or dilation, inflammatory bowel disease monitoring, and rigid sigmoidoscopy failure.

Routine Screening

Sigmoidoscopy should be performed in all adults undergoing a complete physical examination. The advantages of discovering premalignant polyps and early malignant neoplasms in the asymptomatic patient have been thoroughly established. Cancers almost always arise from polyps, and early detection of these premalignant lesions, even in young adults, should be the goal. With the site distribution of colorectal cancer moving upward, discovery and visualization rates achieved with the rigid sigmoidoscope have decreased. In the Thomas Jefferson University Hospital study, 69% of colorectal cancers could be detected with the 25-cm rigid sigmoidoscope prior to 1955, whereas only 45% could be seen in the subsequent study period of 1959 to 1977.[11] Despite fewer cancers being accessible to the rigid scope, 67% of colorectal neoplasms are found distal to the sigmoidocolic junction, a point that is within reach of the flexible scope. In 13% of the asymptomatic patients examined in the cooperative comparative study, one or more polyps were discovered with the flexible scope, whereas polyps were detected in only 5% of these patients with the rigid scope.[9] It is recommended that routine screening begin at age 35 years and be repeated at 3 to 5-year intervals until age 45 years and at 3-year intervals to age 50 years. Annual examinations should begin after age 50 years. This is at variance with the recommendations of the American Cancer Society.

Symptom Resolution

Flexible fiberoptic sigmoidoscopy can be expected to provide a rich harvest of benign, premalignant, and malignant lesions in the symptomatic patient. A 4.6:1 yield advantage was achieved over the rigid scope in the aforementioned cooperative study. Significant disease was discovered with the flexible scope in 46% of patients in this group, whereas significant disease was discovered with the rigid scope in only 9%.

Polyp Surveillance and Cancer Surveillance

At high risk for recurrence or new neoplasms are patients who have or have had polyps or cancer, and inspection at regular intervals is imperative. Sigmoidoscopy is only one element in the surveillance scheme, which includes colonoscopy and selective barium enema studies. Data indicate that these patients are two to three times more likely to have polyps discovered with the flexible sigmoidoscope than with the rigid sigmoidoscope.[4]

Radiographic Confirmation and Resolution

The sigmoid colon, frequently a site of confusion to the radiologist, is the area of greatest radiographic inaccuracy. Resolution of a questionable finding in the sigmoid colon can be achieved rapidly with the flexible scope without subjecting the patient to the expense and inconvenience of formal colonoscopy. With the flexible scope, a 10-fold advantage has been achieved over the rigid scope in this category.[9]

High-risk Status Screening

A personal history of polyps; colonic, breast, and uterine cancer; ulcerative colitis; Crohn's disease; radiation therapy; a first-degree relative with a history of colonic cancer or polyps; a family history of adenomatous familial polyposis coli; cancer family syndrome; or uveal tract melanoma places a patient at high risk for colorectal cancer. Sigmoidoscopy in conjunction with flexible fiberoptic colonoscopy and selective barium enema examination should be used at appropriate intervals in managing such patients.

Anastomotic Inspection or Dilation

Colonic anastomoses beyond the reach of the rigid scope that require inspection, strictures or luminal restrictions that limit the use of the rigid sigmoidoscope, or the need for magnification of details are indications for flexible fiberoptic instrumentation. Flexible sigmoidoscopy may, in itself, be helpful in the dilation of a stricture, or it may be used in conjunction with a balloon catheter or esophageal dilator.

Monitoring Inflammatory Bowel Disease

At intervals between total colonoscopy examinations, inflammatory bowel disease can be observed satisfactorily with the flexible scope.

Rigid Sigmoidoscopy Failure

Even when a problem is within reach of the 25-cm rigid sigmoidoscope, the presence of strictures, angulations, discomfort, or a contracted lumen may prohibit the use of the rigid scope.

In this setting, the flexible scope is of great value.

The geographic distribution of 827 colorectal neoplasms detected in the study of 3000 patients clearly proves the advantages provided by the flexible scope. The distribution density of the 827 benign and malignant neoplasms is expressed as the number of neoplasms/10-cm length of distal colorectum/100 diagnostic intubations. The density of neoplasms was 3.57 in the rectum and varied from 4.68 to 5.57 through the 15- to 55-cm range, which indicates an essentially homogeneous distribution of neoplasms. Thirty-three percent of these 827 neoplasms would have gone undetected with a 35-cm scope and 44% would have gone undetected with a 30-cm scope. These data are vital to the issue of what constitutes the ideal length of a sigmoidoscope. The distribution density of benign and malignant colorectal neoplasms that can be discovered with a conventional 65-cm flexible fiberoptic sigmoidoscope in this study proves the exceptional advantage of using a longer sigmoidoscope.

The Examination

Flexible fiberoptic sigmoidoscopy should be performed as part of a traditional comprehensive proctosigmoidoscopic examination. It is important to remember that significant disease occurring in the anorectal zone and distal rectum can easily be overlooked by even experienced examiners. A careful digital rectal examination and anoscopy are necessary preliminaries to flexible fiberoptic sigmoidoscopy. A complete history is important for diagnostic accuracy, and it is assumed that such will be elicited prior to the examination, with careful notation of the familial incidence of colorectal neoplasia.

Instruments and Materials

Disposable gloves, a water-soluble lubricant, a rigid sigmoidoscope (metal and disposable), an adequate light source, basic instruments and materials for an anorectal examination, an anoscope, a suction apparatus with adequate suction tips, and cotton swabs are required in addition to the basic equipment necessary for performing flexible fiberoptic sigmoidoscopy. Silver nitrate sticks and 10% or 20% silver nitrate solution should also be conveniently at hand. Biopsy forceps, lacrimal duct probes, rubber band ligators, sclerosing solution, and an electrosurgical

unit allow the examiner greater latitude in both the examination and treatment.

The conventional flexible fiberoptic sigmoidoscope has all the qualities of a colonoscope, is 60 or 65 cm in length, and has an effective working length of 55 cm. Instrument lengths of 30 and 35 cm have been promoted by some groups, but we do not endorse using instruments of these lengths. Four major flexible endoscope manufacturers produce flexible fiberoptic sigmoidoscopes, and all are satisfactory. Available light sources range from a simple, inexpensive, low-capacity model to the computerized high-intensity type that is suitable for various methods of photography. All scopes are adaptable to photographic equipment, video cameras, and teaching attachments. A full spectrum of ancillary endoscopic equipment is available. Digitized electronic video endoscopes offer sigmoidoscope models that provide technologic advantages. The cost of this equipment is difficult to justify in the customary office setting.[12]

Preparation of the Patient

For complete and adequate inspection, the rectal vault and distal sigmoid colon should be free of fecal debris and fluid. Adequate preparation is accomplished with two disposable enemas, administered 0.5 hour apart and as close to the examination time as is practical. It is not necessary to withhold meals or sedate the patient. Patients should be advised to avoid a cathartic the night before the examination because this too often leads to the accumulation of a large quantity of liquid fecal material, which presents an annoying obstacle.

Position

The anorectal examination preceding flexible fiberoptic sigmoidoscopy can be conducted in either the Sims or the knee-chest position, depending on personal preference. It is not essential to have a mechanized or breaking procto-sigmoidoscopic table, since an adequate sigmoidoscopic examination can be conducted with the patient in the Sims position, with buttocks drawn over the edge of either an ordinary examining table or litter. The Sims position has been found to be considerably more comfortable for the patient and for the examiner. The knee-chest position, which produces negative intraperitoneal pressure that distracts the walls and widens the lumen of the rectum may be advantageous in certain situations; this issue was addressed earlier.

Inspection

The skin of the perianal, perineal, and post-sacral regions is inspected as the initial step. Digital examination requires the insertion of a well-lubricated, gloved index finger into the rectum by pressing anteriorly on the anal canal to overcome the resistance of the anal sphincter while the patient strains to initiate sphincter relaxation. The details of digital anoscopic and rigid sigmoidoscopic examination have been fully described.

Flexible Fiberoptic Sigmoidoscopic Procedure

The electric power and light source for the flexible fiberoptic sigmoidoscope are turned on and the instrument is carefully checked before it is inserted to make certain that it is fully operational. Suction and air insufflation are checked and the buttons are properly positioned. The two modes of holding the instrument are the customary left-handed holding method and the chest brace-harness right-handed control method.[13] Although both a single-examiner mode and a dual-examiner mode are present, the only justification for the two-person approach is for teaching, and even that seems unnecessary. With the index finger in the anal canal, the tip of the instrument, well lubricated with a water-soluble jelly, is inserted over the finger into the rectum. Fluid is used to clean the lens and then air is insufflated to distract the rectal walls. If the walls do not separate, the usual cause is faulty air insufflation caused by an imperfect connection. The scope is brought back to the hemorrhoidal zone and inspection of the rectum is begun as the instrument is introduced. Insufflation and tip manipulation allow adequate visualization, particularly of the superior surface of the rectal valves. If debris remains in the rectal vault, a choice must be made whether to circumnavigate the debris, aspirate and clog the channel, or remove the instrument and administer an enema. The rectosigmoid is reached at approximately the 15-cm level, and traversing this area is the most difficult feature of the examination. The rectosigmoid junction appears as either a concentric sphincter-type configuration or a slit-like channel. The sphincter-type configuration can be addressed by moderate insufflation of air and gentle pressure to advance the instrument tip under direct visualization with a slight axial rotation. For the slit-like channel, it is advantageous to introduce large volumes of air and to rotate the instrument axially in alternate directions while manipulating the dual control knobs to visualize the lumen. If the lumen is still not apparent, the tip may be placed at a right angle and, with a hook-like action, withdrawn slightly. When all of these measures are non-productive, forward pressure can be exerted within the tolerance level of the tissues and the patient's comfort while axial rotation in alternating directions is performed. As long as the mucosa slides by, the tip of the instrument can be advanced cautiously.

Difficulty in advancing the instrument beyond the rectosigmoid is found most frequently in individuals who have had either pelvic surgery or diverticulitis. It should be remembered that there are individuals in whom passage of the scope beyond the rectosigmoid cannot be safely accomplished. Advancing the instrument through the sigmoid colon is sometimes facilitated by slightly withdrawing and inserting the instrument in a push-pull manner as the lumen is sought and pursued. "Jiggling" the instrument for the purpose of advancing the tip, although advocated by some, is not recommended as a routine maneuver.[3] Air insufflation and axial rotation in either a counterclockwise or clockwise direction, withdrawing and sliding the scope, and manipulation of the dual knobs are all part of the insertion technique. Concentric circles with highlights occur at right angles to the longitudinal axis of the bowel and are helpful in finding the lumen. Glucagon, although used freely in the endoscopic suite, might be used in exceptional situations in the office. Diverticular disease, manifested by segmentation and spasm, and fixation require additional patience on the part of the examiner. In the presence of diverticular disease, the hazard of perforation exists without introducing the instrument forcefully; even minimal air insufflation or the gentlest introduction has the potential of disrupting a sealed, silent perforation or causing a weakened diverticulum to perforate.

Pelvic peritonitis and, in particular, diverticulitis and peridiverticulitis are relative contraindications to flexible sigmoidoscopy, which, as a diagnostic study, must be applied consistent with mature surgical judgment. Brief inspection of the mucosa of the rectum may be permissible in this situation. Free blood in the lumen must be pursued to its source. The full spectrum of inflammatory changes from punctate hemorrhages to severely ulcerative processes must be recognized sigmoidoscopically with the same accuracy as with the colonoscope. Reinspection of the lumen is conducted as the instrument is withdrawn, and an attempt is made to visualize the full circumference of bowel wall. Polyps often hide behind mucosal curtains, and fecal debris may cling to and obscure polypoid lesions. Retroflexion of the instrument for the purpose of examining the hemorrhoidal zone is an improper method of viewing this area. Air is aspirated on withdrawal. A thoughtful concluding touch is to provide a bathroom facility so that the patient can eliminate the air that has accumulated during the procedure.

The examiner should not expect to be able to fully introduce the instrument in every individual. Pain is the most important signal of possible injury. Furthermore, to promote compliance in patients who require further examinations, it is mandatory that the procedure be comfortable. The use of sedation, anodynes, or glucagon should be reserved for exceptional instances.

Mucosal biopsy, brush cytology, and the removal of small foreign bodies are procedures that are suitable for flexible sigmoidoscopy in an office setting. If procedures are to be carried out in the office, however, strict attention to infection control must be observed. The removal of polyps with the flexible sigmoidoscope is not advisable inasmuch as total colonoscopy must be performed and there is also a lack of complete bowel preparation.

The key word for the appropriate use of a flexible fiberoptic sigmoidoscope is practicality. The procedure, whether performed in a hospital or in an office setting, must not be burdensome to the patient, the physician, or support personnel. To facilitate its use in the office, the flexible scope must be kept in readiness. Hanging the scope on the wall next to the examining table or on a mobile trolley with the light source and suction apparatus connected at all times has proved convenient. With a single motion, the instrument can be made ready for insertion. The need to deliberate about performing the procedure and hurried, harried setting up are to be avoided. The arrangement should permit quick and easy cleaning of the instrument between uses. Mechanical cleansing and thorough irrigation should be performed in conjunction with disinfection. What constitutes adequate disinfection is controversial. Consensus holds that limited contact with 2% activated glutaraldehyde or a solution of hydrogen peroxide is appropriate. The issue is the length of time the scope must be in contact with the disinfectant.

Environmental considerations are not to be overlooked, for which ever-changing guidelines should be observed. The flexible fiberoptic endoscopist is urged to remain alert to the recommendations of the two major endoscopic societies—the American Society of Gastrointestinal Endoscopy and the Society of American Gastrointestinal Endoscopic Surgeons.

References

1. Duthie HL, Gairns FW. Sensory nerve endings and sensation in the anal region of man. Br J Surg 47:585, 1960.
2. Marks G. Acute anorectal disorders. In: Nord HJ, Brandy PG, eds. Critical Care Gastroenterology. New York: Churchill Livingstone, 1982.
3. Marks G, Eisenstat T, Borenstein B. Flexible fiberoptic sigmoidoscopy. In: Dent TL, Strodel WE, Turcotte JG. Surgical Endoscopy. Chicago: Year Book Medical Publishers, 1985.
4. Bohlman TW, Daton RM, Lipshutz GR, et al: Fiberoptic pansigmoidoscopy: An evaluation and comparison with rigid sigmoidoscopy. Gastroenterology 72:644, 1977.
5. Hilsabeck JR. Experience with routine office sigmoidoscopy using the 60 cm flexible colonoscope in private practice. Dis Colon Rectum 26:314, 1983.
6. Marino AW Jr. Looking ahead: Types of flexible sigmoidoscopes and preparation of the patient (symposium). Dis Colon Rectum 20:91, 1977.
7. Marks G, Boggs HW, Castro AF, et al. Sigmoidoscopic examination with rigid and flexible fiberoptic sigmoidoscopes in the surgeons's office: A comparative prospective study of effectiveness in 1012 cases. Dis Colon Rectum 22:162, 1979.
8. Selby JV, Friedman GD, Quesenberry CP, Weiss NS. A case-control study of screening sigmoidoscopy and mortality from colorectal cancer. N Engl J Med 326(10):653, 1992.
9. Marks G, Boggs HW, Castro AF, et al. Distribution density of 827 colorectal neoplasms detected by flexible fiberoptic sigmoidoscopy. Presented to the annual meeting of the Society of American Gastrointestinal Endoscopic Surgeons, Philadelphia, April 8, 1984.
10. Marks G, Gathright JB, Boggs HW, et al. Guidelines for use of the flexible fiberoptic sigmoidoscope in the management of the surgical patient. Dis Colon Rectum 25:187, 1982.
11. Rosato FE, Marks G. Changing site distribution patterns of colorectal cancer at Thomas Jefferson University Hospital. Dis Colon Rectum 24:93, 1981.
12. Satava RM, Poe W, Joyce G. Current generation video endoscope. A critical evaluation. Am Surg 54(2):73, 1988.
13. Marks G. A new technique of hand reversal using a harness-type endoscope holder for twin-knob colonoscopy and flexible fiberoptic sigmoidoscopy. Dis Colon Rectum 24:567, 1981.

24

Diagnostic Laparoscopy for Benign and Malignant Disease

Thomas A. Stellato

ORIGINS OF LAPAROSCOPY

Laparoscopy was conceived and first performed by Kelling, who reported the examination of the abdominal cavity of a live canine using a Nitze cystoscope in 1901 (Fig. 24–1).[1, 2] Kelling created a pneumoperitoneum via a puncture needle and introduced the laparoscope (cystoscope) through a larger trocar. Thus the essential elements and technique for diagnostic laparoscopy were born at the beginning of the 20th century. The appellation laparoscopy is one of several designations for the procedure; Kelling termed the operation koelioskopie (coelioscopy). Kelling subsequently reported his laparoscopy experience in humans, but the first major clinical series is attributed to Jacobaeus,[3, 4] who coined the term "laparothorakoskopie," since he devised methods to examine both the abdominal and thoracic cavities. He reported on 115 laparothorascopic examinations in 72 patients and was able to identify syphilis, tuberculosis, cirrhosis, and malignancy.

One of the earliest experiences in the United States with this new procedure was reported by Bernheim from the Johns Hopkins University,[5] who called the procedure organoscopy and reported his experience with two patients, one of whom was under the care of Halsted. This patient had a cancer of the pancreas with jaundice. Bernheim used laparoscopy to confirm the lack of metastasis. The accuracy of this laparoscopy (organoscopy) was subsequently verified by laparotomy. In the second case, Bernheim was able to identify chronic appendicitis and rule out gastric ulcer disease.

From this early beginning, numerous reports followed, many consisting of a few case reports such as Bernheim's.[5] One notable publication is by Short, a surgeon from the Bristol Royal Infirmary. Short reported his experience with coelioscopy in 1925 and listed as one of its advantages over exploratory laparotomy the fact that "it can be done at the patient's own house."[6] More importantly for the modern day diagnostic laparoscopist, Short made the important observation that coelioscopy is "principally valuable for what is definitely seen and not for what is apparently absent."[6]

Several major advances in diagnostic laparoscopy were introduced by the German hepatologist Kalk.[7, 8] They included the development of a 135°-angle laparoscope and the dual trocar technique. The latter not only allowed for a more thorough abdominal examination but also provided the foundation for later efforts in therapeutic laparoscopy. In 1951, Kalk reported that his personal series of 2000 laparoscopies were without mortality.

A landmark article from the United States was published in 1937 in the journal *Surgery, Gynecology, and Obstetrics*, authored by the internist Ruddock.[9] Entitled simply Peritoneoscopy, Ruddock detailed his experience with 500 laparoscopies over a 4-year period. In this series, 39 biopsies were performed. This is one of the earliest reports of laparoscopic biopsy and thus represents a milestone in the history of diagnostic laparoscopy.

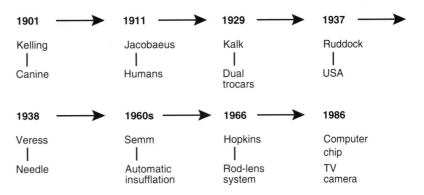

Figure 24-1. Some of the major personalities and technologic milestones that have shaped laparoscopy from its origins in 1901 to modern videolaparoscopy. (From Stellato TA. History of laparoscopic surgery. Surg Clin North Am 72:997–1002, 1992.)

An ingenious application of laparoscopy and endoscopy was proposed by Anderson from Corpus Christi, Texas, in 1937.[10] Anderson described the use of endoscopy of the urinary bladder, stomach, and rectosigmoid combined with laparoscopy to allow transillumination of the walls of these structures so that they could be more thoroughly evaluated laparoscopically. This technique has application today in both diagnostic and therapeutic laparoscopy.

Safety in the performance of laparoscopy was provided by the development of a spring-loaded needle by Veress in 1938[11] and controlled automatic insufflation by Semm in the 1960s.[12]

The modern era of laparoscopy necessitated improvement in optics, which was accomplished with the Hopkins rod-lens system and the subsequent development of the computer chip television camera. It is somewhat paradoxical that these advances and the development of laparoscopic cholecystectomy (therapeutic laparoscopy) in the late 1980s provided the impetus for rediscovering diagnostic laparoscopy. The explosion in the application of laparoscopy for therapy has provided a natural opportunity for the use of laparoscopy as an important diagnostic tool.

PREOPERATIVE PREPARATION

Although laparoscopy can be performed under local, regional, or general anesthesia, a thorough preoperative evaluation is still essential because the major risk to the patient is secondary to the cardiopulmonary effects of the pneumoperitoneum, which is independent of the type of anesthetic used. Because carbon dioxide (CO_2) is well tolerated biologically and does not support combustion, it is the gas most commonly used for creation of pneumoperitoneum. However, CO_2 is highly diffusible, and its absorption across the peritoneal membrane can result in an elevated arterial CO_2.[13]

Hemodynamic and pulmonary alterations in healthy (American Society of Anesthesiologists categories I and II) individuals undergoing laparoscopy and laparoscopic cholecystectomy have been shown to produce a significant decrease in cardiac index and arterial pH and an increase in mean arterial pressure, systemic vascular resistance, and end tidal CO_2 and arterial CO_2.[14, 15] Although these changes may go unnoticed in the healthy individual, especially if the laparoscopic procedure is of short duration, their impact on persons with preexisting cardiopulmonary disease may be significant and lead to acute cardiopulmonary decompensation (see Chap. 34).

With the broader application of laparoscopy, especially therapeutically, increased laparoscopic operating times are not uncommon. Hypothermia has been identified with laparoscopy and is felt to represent the differential between the insufflation temperature of CO_2 at 21.1°C and the core abdominal temperature of the patient. A decrease of 0.3°C in the core temperature was observed for each 50 L of CO_2 delivered.[16] The volume of CO_2 delivered is directly proportional to the length of the operative procedure. This phenomenon will have little impact in the healthy individual undergoing a procedure of short duration. However, it is obvious that these and other effects yet to be appreciated may have serious sequelae, especially if underlying systemic disease exists or if an excessively lengthy procedure is undertaken in a patient who is otherwise in a compensated state. Therefore, all individuals undergoing laparoscopic surgery must have a complete history taken and a physical examination with attention to cardiopulmonary and hematologic systems.

TECHNIQUE OF LAPAROSCOPY

Whether laparoscopy is performed in the endoscopy suite, intensive care unit, emergency room, or operating room, adequate monitoring of the patient is essential, as already indicated, and sterility of the instruments and field must be maintained throughout the procedure. The operating room most readily meets these requirements, but laparoscopy has been performed successfully outside the operating room by experienced laparoscopists.

A table with tilting capability will allow a more complete diagnostic evaluation. The patient should be strapped to the table; positioning in the Trendelenburg position to evaluate pelvic structures or the reverse Trendelenburg position to visualize the upper abdomen (*e.g.*, spleen) will be necessary.

Diagnostic laparoscopy may be performed with local anesthesia combined with intravenous sedation, regional anesthesia, or general anesthesia. The sine qua non is a cooperative patient. Peritoneal biopsies will be felt by the unanesthetized patient, and straining or sudden movements by the patient may cause serious intraabdominal injury from trocars or other instruments.

Since pneumoperitoneum impairs venous return, which may be further compromised by positions such as the reverse Trendelenburg, consideration should be given to some form of antithrombotic prophylaxis such as sequential compression boots. The need for a nasogastric or orogastric tube to decompress the stomach and a Foley catheter to decompress the urinary bladder may be individualized depending on the method used for creating the pneumoperitoneum. If the pneumoperitoneum is created using a Veress-type needle (Fig. 24–2), the stomach and bladder should be decompressed because both the Veress needle and the initial trocar are placed into the abdominal cavity "blindly." If

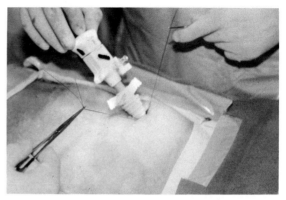

Figure 24–3. Trocar for open laparoscopy. Fascial traction sutures are secured around the "wings" of the tapered core, which prevents pneumoperitoneum leakage.

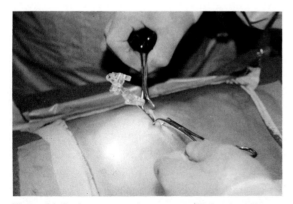

Figure 24–2. A pneumoperitoneum needle has been introduced into the abdominal cavity. Towel clips provide counteraction. The needle introduced at the umbilicus is toward the pelvis, away from the aortic bifurcation.

the Hasson open technique[17] is used (Fig. 24–3), a Foley catheter may be avoided if the patient has voided immediately prior to the procedure and the procedure will not be lengthy. The nasogastric tube in this situation can be used selectively.

Regardless of the indications for the procedure, the type of anesthesia used, or the location where the laparoscopy is performed, the entire abdomen is cleansed with a suitable agent using sterile technique as for an open abdominal operation. Once the area is cleansed and draped, the pneumoperitoneum can be created. The choice between the closed Veress needle technique versus the open Hasson technique is based on multiple variables. All laparoscopists should be familiar with the open technique. The open technique should be considered in patients who have had prior abdominal procedures, especially multiple prior procedures, and in patients who have had prior peritonitis. The Veress closed technique has the advantages of speed and simplicity. The needle is most commonly introduced at the umbilicus, although this area should be avoided if there have been prior incisions in the vicinity or if portal hypertension exists. The umbilicus is the thinnest area of the abdominal wall. If the umbilicus is unacceptable, the lower quadrants may be used if no masses are present.[18] Verification of the intraperitoneal position of the Veress needle is made by a number of maneuvers: the water drop test, aspiration of the needle, injection with saline, and measuring pressure through the needle (Fig. 24–4). None of these measures is infallible, however, and any concern about the placement of the needle should prompt its reinsertion or the abandonment of the closed technique and conversion to the open technique.

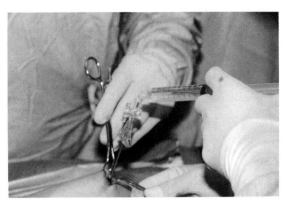

Figure 24–4. Water drop test. If the needle is placed intraperitoneally, a drop of water (or saline) introduced into the needle should "fall" into the peritoneal cavity when the towel clips are lifted upward.

If the laparoscopist is comfortable with the placement of the Veress needle, a pneumoperitoneum can be created with CO_2. The initial insufflation flow should be no greater than 1.5 L/minute. Intraabdominal pressure is usually kept at less than 15 mm Hg. Once an adequate pneumoperitoneum is created (judged by the intraperitoneal pressure and the tympany and tenseness of the abdomen), the incision at the umbilicus can be enlarged to accommodate the trocar. The trocar (and Veress needle) must be introduced toward the pelvis and away from the bifurcation of the aorta. Despite the safety sheath that is present on disposable trocars, serious life-threatening injury can occur if uncontrolled introduction of the trocar (or needle) is performed.

In open laparoscopy (Hasson technique), a blunt trocar is introduced through a minilaparotomy (see Fig. 24–3).[17] Its advantages include the almost complete elimination of possible visceral or vascular injury. It is slightly more time-consuming than the closed technique and requires some means to prevent insufflation gas leakage, which is accomplished by using the Hasson trocar or one of its commercial variants.

Once the initial trocar is placed, all additional trocars are introduced under direct vision, which should eliminate the possibility of injury. Inspection of the abdominal cavity should be performed in an orderly fashion. One simple method is to mimic the hands of the clock. Since the trocar is directed toward the pelvis, examination begins at the 6 o'clock position, proceeds toward the right to view the ascending colon, followed by the liver, diaphragm, and stomach at the 12 o'clock position, and then proceeds to the examination of the descending and sigmoid colon. After the initial inspection, probes may be introduced through accessory trocars to manipulate bowel or organs to complete the examination. The patient with ascites poses special problems. Efforts should be made not to insufflate into the ascitic pool because this will cause bubbling, which will interfere with the examination. By removing some of the ascites prior to insufflation and tilting the patient to direct ascites away from the area to be viewed, a thorough examination can be performed.

At the completion of the examination, accessory trocars should be removed under direct vision. Fascial incisions larger than 1 cm should be closed.

INDICATIONS FOR LAPAROSCOPY

Prior to the development of video laparoscopy and laparoscopic cholecystectomy, the majority of laparoscopic procedures in the United States were performed by gynecologists, with laparoscopy performed by general surgeons and gastroenterologists being more the exception than the rule. In the brief period since the development of video laparoscopy, a renewed interest in the application of laparoscopy to general surgery, urologic surgery, and pediatric surgery has occurred. Any list of indications for diagnostic laparoscopy will be incomplete. However, an attempt will be made to address the use of laparoscopy for diagnosis for the following problems.

Liver Disease and Ascites

Evaluation of liver disease and determination of the cause of ascites that may or may not be related to a hepatic pathologic condition represent the most frequent indications for performing diagnostic laparoscopy. In the past, laparoscopy has been an important modality in the evaluation of the jaundiced patient. Laparoscopy may occasionally still assist in the diagnosis of cholestasis.[19] However, the introduction and refinement of ultrasonography has relegated laparoscopy to a secondary role.[20] Laparoscopy remains superior in providing a detailed view of the liver surface and thus is irreplaceable in the diagnosis of cirrhosis (Fig. 24–5).[21] Blind percutaneous liver biopsy will yield an accurate diagnosis in diffuse diseases such as fatty metamorphosis and acute hepatitis, but sampling errors are to be expected in less diffuse, patchy diseases such as chronic hepatitis and cirrhosis.[22] In the patient with cirrhosis, blind percutaneous

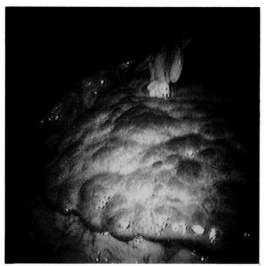

Figure 24-5. Macronodular cirrhosis is seen laparoscopically.

biopsies may sample a regenerating nodule (which can be completely normal) or may slide off hard fibrous tissue and sample the softer parenchyma. Laparoscopic biopsy has the advantage of visualizing the liver surface and provides a much more adequately sized biopsy specimen to confirm the diagnosis of cirrhosis.

Laparoscopy may not only confirm cirrhosis but may also provide prognostic information. Of eight laparoscopic parameters, the following three were most important in predicting a deleterious outcome: degree of development of regenerating nodules, formation of small lymphatic vesicles, and splenomegaly.[23]

The diagnosis of primary and metastatic liver tumors is most commonly evaluated by ultrasound, computed tomography (CT), and laparoscopy. It has been suggested that ultrasound may serve as a screening and staging modality for hepatocellular carcinoma.[24] Ultrasound not only can detect cancers below the surface but also can provide information regarding portal vein patency. However, ultrasound usually fails to identify cirrhosis or peritoneal involvement by hepatoma.[25, 26] Ultrasound and laparoscopy are more appropriately viewed as complementary procedures in the evaluation of hepatocellular carcinoma. Ultrasound may be used for screening, and if unresectability can be documented, laparoscopy is not needed. However, laparoscopy is indicated if the ultrasound examination is normal when hepatocellular carcinoma is suspected clinically or when a curative resection is contemplated. Laparoscopy can evaluate not only the extent of the cancer but also the presence and degree of cirrhosis.

Laparoscopy is also highly accurate in the diagnosis of metastatic tumors to the liver. Of 65 malignant metastatic neoplasms, laparoscopy was able to identify and provide tissue for histologic examination in 60 of them (92% sensitivity and 100% specificity).[27] One third of these tumors originated from breast and colon primary lesions.

Laparoscopy may also be used to evaluate benign hepatic tumors when scanning is nondiagnostic.[28] Liver abscess can be confirmed by laparoscopy, and laparoscopically guided puncture can provide material to determine the cause of the abscess.[29] When medical therapy fails to heal amebic abscesses, or when they are in imminent danger of rupturing out of the liver, laparoscopy can be used to aspirate and drain these collections.[30, 31]

The initial evaluation of ascites is nonoperative. If paracentesis and scanning fail to identify the cause of the ascites, laparoscopic exploration is indicated.[32] Not uncommonly, the reason that scanning fails to identify the cause is the peritoneal involvement by diffuse, minute malignant implants (e.g., pancreas, ovary, breast, colon, mesothelioma,[33–35] and others) or minute benign implants (tuberculosis,[36–39] Listeria,[40] Opisthorchis viverrini—liver fluke,[41] and others). In each of these cases, minute rice- or millet-like implants cover the peritoneal, diaphragmatic, and serosal surfaces (Fig. 24–6), which are below the limits of resolution of ultrasound or CT (Fig. 24–7). Laparoscopy allows complete abdominal evaluation, characterization of the miliary nodules (the uniform size of tuberculosis versus the varying sizes of malignant implants[37]), collection of large volumes of ascites for cytologic and microbiologic examination and biopsy of multiple nodules.

Tumor Staging

Use of laparoscopy in the evaluation of hepatocellular carcinoma has already been addressed. A number of other tumors have been evaluated by laparoscopy.[42–44]

Esophagus

The frequent association between esophageal cancer and alcohol abuse, as well as the common occurrence of metastasis with this tumor, makes laparoscopy valuable in decisions regarding resection. In a series of 369 patients with cancer of the esophagus, laparoscopy identified cirrhosis in 14.3% and severe portal hypertension in 6.7%. In addition, laparoscopy identified me-

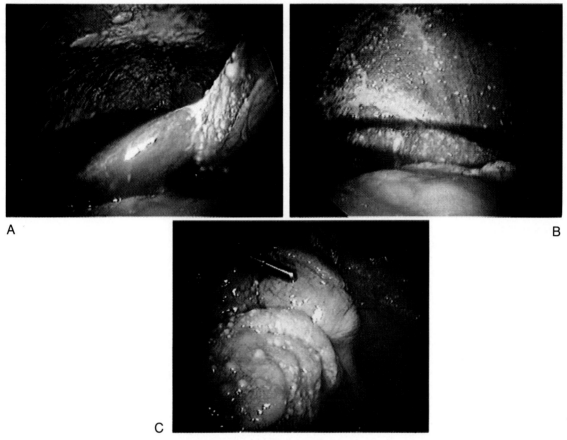

Figure 24–6. A 38-year-old man with vague abdominal pain. The diagnosis of mesothelioma was made by laparoscopy. **(A)** Diffuse large and small implants along the diaphragm and falciform ligament. **(B)** Implants on the diaphragm and liver, with the liver submerged in ascites. **(C)** Mesothelioma implants on the cecum *(probe)*, mesentery, and peritoneum.

tastasis to the liver, peritoneum, omentum, stomach, and lymph nodes in 14%.[45] In a prospective trial, laparoscopy significantly improved the sensitivity and specificity of CT scanning.[46] Laparoscopy may allow the exclusion of patients with intraabdominal spread and thus improve resectability rates.[47]

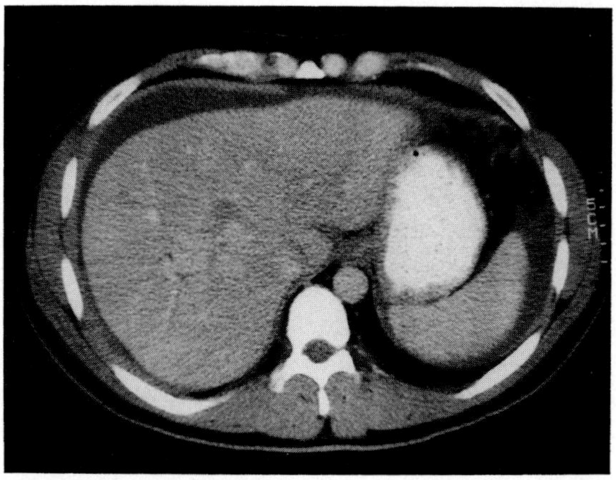

Stomach

Laparoscopy appears to be an excellent tool for evaluating tumor fixation and liver and peritoneal metastasis.[48] It has been proposed that laparoscopy can prevent futile laparotomy in 40% to 50% of patients with gastric cancer.[49, 50]

Gallbladder

Carcinoma of the gallbladder is commonly advanced at the time of presentation. Therefore laparoscopy can be helpful in confirming the diagnosis and identifying the extent of the disease. Local or distant metastasis can be identified in more than 85% of patients with this malignancy using the laparoscope.[51, 52] Laparotomy may be avoided in more than 80% of patients by the laparoscopic identification of

Figure 24–7. CT scan of the patient in Figure 24–6 with mesothelioma shows nonspecific ascites around the liver and spleen. Laparoscopy was diagnostic.

advanced disease.[53] A recent case report describes the definitive management of a carcinoid tumor of the gallbladder by laparoscopic resection.[54]

Pancreas

Despite its retroperitoneal location, access to the pancreas can be accomplished laparoscopically. Meyer-Burg presented the first description of the laparoscopic examination of the pancreas in 1972.[55] Cuschieri and associates approached the pancreas through an infragastric exploration of the lesser sac. This was successful in 6 of 10 patients.[56] Ishida used a supragastric approach and was able to observe carcinoma in the head of the pancreas in 32% of 71 patients and carcinoma in the body of the pancreas in 85%. He also demonstrated that liver metastasis and peritoneal spread were present in 11% and 24% of patients, respectively, from cancers in the head of the pancreas and in 50% and 61% of patients, respectively, from cancers in the body and tail.[57] Warshaw and associates have shown the limitations of ultrasound and CT in staging pancreatic cancer. In patients in whom ultrasound and CT showed no metastasis, laparoscopy identified metastasis in 17 of 40 cases (43%).[58, 59]

Hodgkin's and Non-Hodgkin's Lymphoma

Shortly after the first report in 1969 suggesting a value of diagnostic laparotomy in Hodgkin's disease,[60] attempts were made to substitute laparoscopy for laparotomy to obviate the risk associated with laparotomy and splenectomy. DeVita and associates performed peritoneoscopy in 38 patients with advanced Hodgkin's disease in 1971.[61] Liver involvement was identified in 6 of 38 patients (16%). All patients with liver involvement had subdiaphragmatic lymph node involvement. Clinically, liver enlargement correlated poorly with true involvement. Of 14 patients with Hodgkin's disease who were thought to have involvement of the liver prior to laparoscopy, only 2 (14%) had evidence of disease at biopsy. Of 24 patients who were thought not to have liver involvement based on normal liver size or liver function tests, 4 (16%) proved to have tumor in the liver at biopsy.

Beretta and colleagues from the National Cancer Institute in Milan evaluated liver and spleen biopsy specimens in 121 patients with Hodgkin's disease.[62] All patients with normal liver or spleen biopsy results at laparoscopy were subjected to laparotomy to evaluate for false-negative laparoscopy results. All 121 patients underwent laparoscopic liver biopsy, and seven specimens were abnormal (6%). At laparotomy, only 2 patients were found to have abnormal liver biopsy specimens (2%). One hundred eight of the 121 patients underwent one to three spleen biopsies at laparoscopy and 14 specimens (13%) were abnormal. However, an additional 37 patients (20%) were found to have splenic involvement at laparotomy. Thus, laparoscopy is useful for staging the liver but cannot be recommended for evaluating the spleen. The high diagnostic accuracy of laparoscopy for hepatic disease has been confirmed by others.[63]

Prior to the availability of CT, the combination of lymphangiography, bone marrow biopsy, and laparoscopy was shown to be effective in identifying disseminated disease in the majority of patients with non-Hodgkin's lymphoma.[64] More recently, laparoscopy has been used to biopsy retroperitoneal processes, including involvement by carcinoma and non-Hodgkin's lymphoma.[65] Patients with palpable retroperitoneal processes or those who undergo noninvasive studies such as CT or barium contrast enema that identify displacement of viscera are most likely to have successful laparoscopic biopsies.[65]

In summary, laparoscopy is useful in patients with Hodgkin's disease to evaluate liver involvement. This may permit the avoidance of laparotomy and splenectomy. However, a normal laparoscopic examination does not prove the lack of stage III or stage IV disease. Laparoscopy will be needed less frequently for non-Hodgkin's lymphoma but may be valuable if other staging modalities are normal.

Ovary

Laparoscopy has had the greatest impact on the management of ovarian cancer. Prior to the incorporation of laparoscopy in the management of ovarian cancer, surgery consisted of infraumbilical exploration that did not allow evaluation of the diaphragm and the majority of the peritoneal surface. A preliminary report in 1973 by Bagley and colleagues from the National Cancer Institute demonstrated that ovarian cancer metastatic to the diaphragm could be identified by laparoscopy.[66] When laparoscopy was performed less than 1 month after definitive ovarian surgery through the infraumbilical incision, 11 of 14 patients were found to have abnormal diaphragm implants. All 11 patients were upstaged because of laparoscopy, and 7 of these

11 individuals had diaphragm involvement as the only site of metastasis outside the pelvis.[67] Laparoscopy has been valuable not only in staging but also in restaging of ovarian cancer. Despite prior laparotomy, laparoscopic examination can usually be performed adequately.[68] As in all other tumors, an abnormal laparoscopic examination is valuable in documenting the extent or recurrence of disease, but a normal laparoscopic examination, especially in the patient with prior abdominal surgery, can never completely rule out recurrent disease. The experience with laparoscopy in ovarian cancer and other gynecologic malignancies is extensive and has been nicely summarized by Gelman.[44]

Evaluation of Appendicitis

Appendicitis has long been considered a clinical diagnosis, and varying percentages for misdiagnosis have been accepted. A higher percentage of misdiagnosis has been accepted for women because tubal infertility rises with rupture of the appendix but not with uncomplicated appendicitis.[69] A variety of nonsurgical and surgical pelvic abnormalities can mimic appendicitis in the female patient. Thus, laparoscopy can play an important role, especially in the female patient. In nearly all reports in which laparoscopy was incorporated into the workup for right lower quadrant pain, the laparotomy rate was decreased or the diagnosis was altered. In one early and widely quoted study, Leape and Ramenofsky reported that 37.5% of their patients avoided a laparotomy, and the rate of appendectomies that should not have been performed decreased from 10% to 1% with the use of laparoscopy for questionable appendicitis.[70] Similarly, Deutsch and colleagues reported a decrease in laparotomy by one-third in women with the diagnosis of appendicitis who were evaluated by laparoscopy.[71] Others have concurred with the benefits of laparoscopy in identifying gynecologic pathologic conditions but have failed to demonstrate a decrease in the rate of improperly performed appendectomies.[72] Laparoscopy is most helpful in patients with atypical presentations rather than in those with classic appendicitis.[73] It may also be invaluable in assessing the patient who is immunocompromised.[74]

Chronic Abdominal Pain

Chronic abdominal pain poses a difficult problem for both the surgeon and the internist. This is especially true when it occurs in the patient who has had prior abdominal surgery. If the usual evaluation, consisting of a careful history taking and physical examination supplemented by a focused radiologic evaluation, is unrewarding, laparoscopy may provide insight into the cause of the pain. Easter and colleagues demonstrated that laparoscopy yielded abnormal findings in 47% of cases of chronic abdominal pain.[75] Most patients with significant adhesions at laparoscopy were in the group of subjects with chronic pain. Laparoscopy was used therapeutically to perform adhesiolysis, but follow-up was inadequate to judge the results. Postappendectomy pain has been attributed to adhesions and laparoscopic diagnosis; lysis of adhesions may ablate the symptoms.[76] Although the benefit of laparoscopy for chronic pain may not be as demonstrable as its use in acute processes, it will nonetheless resolve a substantial percentage of difficult diagnostic problems.

Miscellaneous

Numerous other nonemergency indications for diagnostic laparoscopy exist. Laparoscopy has been used to evaluate malfunctioning peritoneal dialysis catheters,[77] as well as a variety of urologic disorders such as undescended testes and the depth of mural involvement of bladder cancer.[78] Applications of diagnostic laparoscopy will continue to grow, as will the number of proponents of this very powerful diagnostic tool. Without a doubt, the laparoscope will be a major diagnostic instrument for the 21st century.

References

1. Stellato TA. History of laparoscopic surgery. Surg Clin North Am, 72:997–1002, 1992.
2. Kelling G. Ueber oesophagoskopie, gastrokopie und koelioskopie. Munch Med Wochenschr 49:21–24, 1901.
3. Jacobaeus HC. Ueber die moglichkeit die zystokopie bei untersuchung seroser hohlungen anzuwenden. Munch Med Wochenschr 57:2090–2092, 1910.
4. Jacobaeus HC. Kurze uebersicht uber meine erfahrungen mit der laparothorakoskopie. Munch Med Wochenschr 58:2017–2019, 1911.
5. Bernheim BM. Organoscopy. Cystoscopy of the abdominal cavity. Ann Surg 53:764–767, 1911.
6. Short AR. The uses of coelioscopy. Br Med J 2:254–255, 1925.
7. Kalk H. Erfahrungen mit der laparoskopie. Z Klin Med 111:303–348, 1929.
8. Kalk H, Bruhl W, Brugmann W. Leitfaden der laparoskopie und gastroskopie. Stuttgart, Thieme; New York, Grune & Stratton, 1951.
9. Ruddock JC. Peritoneoscopy. Surg Gynecol Obstet 65:623–639, 1937.

10. Anderson ET. Peritonoscopy. Am J Surg 35:136–139, 1937.

11. Veress J. Neues instrument zur ausfuhrung von brust-oder banchpunktionen und pneumothoraxbehandlung. Dtsch Med Wochenschr 41:1480–1481, 1938.

12. Semm K (translated by Friederich ER). Operative manual for endoscopic abdominal surgery. Chicago, Year Book Medical Publishers, 1987.

13. Baratz RA, Karis JH. Blood gas studies during laparoscopy under general anesthesia. Anesthesiology 30:463–464, 1969.

14. Torrielli R, Cesarini M, Winnock S, et al. Modifications hemodynamiques durant la coelioscopie: etude menee par bioimpedance electrique thoracique. Can J Anaesth 37:46–49, 1990.

15. Lin SY, Leighton T, Davis I, et al. Prospective analysis of cardiopulmonary responses to laparoscopic cholecystectomy. J Laparoendoscopic Surg 1:241–246, 1991.

16. Ott DE. Laparoscopic hypothermia. J Laparoendoscopic Surg 1:127–131, 1991.

17. Hasson HM. Open laparoscopy: a report of 150 cases. J Reprod Med 12:234–238, 1974.

18. Sackier JM, Berci G, Paz-Partlow M. Elective diagnostic laparoscopy. Am J Surg 161:326–331, 1991.

19. Schier F, Waldschmidt J. Experience with laparoscopy for the evaluation of cholestasis in newborns. Surg Endosc 4:13–14, 1990.

20. Gandolfi L, Rossi A, Leo P, et al. Indications for laparoscopy before and after the introduction of ultrasonography. Gastrointest Endosc 31:1–3, 1985.

21. Fornari F, Rapaccini GL, Cavanna L, et al. Diagnosis of hepatic lesions: ultrasonically guided five needle biopsy or laparoscopy? Gastrointest Endosc 34:231–234, 1988.

22. Nord HJ. Biopsy diagnosis of cirrhosis: blind percutaneous versus guided direct vision techniques—a review. Gastrointest Endosc 28:102–104, 1982.

23. Tanneda Y, Yoshizawa N, Takase K, et al. Prognostic value of peritoneoscopic findings in cirrhosis of the liver. Gastrointest Endosc 36:34–38, 1990.

24. Brady PG. Laparoscopy and ultrasonography in the diagnosis of hepatocellular carcinoma. Gastrointest Endosc 35:577–578, 1989.

25. Brady PG, Goldschmid S, Chappel G, et al. A comparison of biopsy techniques in suspected focal liver disease. Gastrointest Endosc 33:289–292, 1987.

26. Jeffers C, Spieglman G, Reddy R, et al. Laparoscopically directed fine needle aspiration for the diagnosis of hepatocellular carcinoma: a safe and accurate technique. Gastrointest Endosc 34:235–237, 1988.

27. Lightdale CJ, Winawer SJ, Kurtz RS, et al. Laparoscopic diagnosis of suspected liver neoplasms. Value of prior liver scan. Dig Dis Sci 24:588–593, 1979.

28. Bhargava DH, Verma K, Malaviya AN. Solitary tuberculoma of liver: laparoscopic, histologic and cytologic diagnosis. Gastrointest Endosc 29:329–330, 1983.

29. Hitanant S, Trong DT, Damrongsak C, et al. Peritonoscopy in the diagnosis of liver abscess. Experience with 108 cases during a 10 year period. Gastrointest Endosc 30:234–236, 1984.

30. Staples DC, Dale JA. Peritoneoscopically guided needle aspiration of anuresic liver abscess. Gastrointest Endosc 26:21–22, 1980.

31. Salky B, Finkel S. Laparoscopic drainage of amebic liver abscess. Gastrointest Endosc 31:30–32, 1985.

32. Brady PG, Peebles M, Goldschmid S. Role of laparoscopy in the evaluation of patients with suspected hepatic or peritoneal malignancy. Gastrointest Endosc 37:27–30, 1991.

33. Eslami B, Cutcher CL. Antemortem diagnosis in two cases of malignant peritoneal mesothelioma. Am J Med Sci 267:117–121, 1974.

34. McCallum RW, Maceri DR, Jensen D, et al. Laparoscopic diagnosis of peritoneal mesothelioma. Dig Dis Sci 24:170–174, 1979.

35. Salky B. Laparoscopic diagnosis of peritoneal mesothelioma. Gastrointest Endosc 29:65–70, 1983.

36. Wolfe JHN, Behn AR, Jackson BT. Tuberculous peritonitis and the role of diagnostic laparoscopy. Lancet 1:852–853, 1979.

37. Geake TMS, Spitaels JM, Moshal MG, et al. Peritoneoscopy in the diagnosis of tuberculous peritonitis. Gastrointest Endosc 27:66–68, 1981.

38. Alberti-Flor JJ, Vaughan S, Dunn GD. Laparoscopy and tuberculous peritonitis. Gastrointest Endosc 31:106–107, 1985.

39. Willis SM, Brewer TG. More on tuberculous peritonitis and laparoscopy. Gastrointest Endosc 34:151, 1988.

40. Larson CC, Baine WB, Ware AJ, et al. Listeria peritonitis diagnosed by laparoscopy. Gastrointest Endosc 34:352–354,1988.

41. Hitanant S, Trong DT, Damrongsak L, et al. Peritoneoscopic findings in 203 patients with *Opisthorchis viverrini* infection. Gastrointest Endosc 33:18–20, 1987.

42. Sugarbaker PH, Wilson RE. Using celioscopy to determine stages of intra-abdominal malignant neoplasms. Arch Surg 111:41–44, 1976.

43. Lightdale CJ. Clinical applications in patients with malignant neoplasms. Gastrointest Endosc 28:99–101, 1982.

44. Gelman EP. The role of laparoscopy in cancer management. Updates. Cancer Principles Pract 2:1–11, 1988.

45. Dagnini G, Caldironi MW, Marin G. Laparoscopy in abdominal staging of esophageal carcinoma. Report of 369 cases. Gastrointest Endosc 32:400–402, 1986.

46. Lightdale CJ, Kelsen DP, Kurtz RC, et al. Staging of the liver in patients with carcinoma of the esophagus with CT and laparoscopy. Gastrointest Endosc 30:147, 1984.

47. Shandall A, Johnson C. Laparoscopy or scanning in oesophagesal and gastric carcinoma? Br J Surg 72:449–451, 1985.

48. Possik RA, Franco EL, Pires DR, et al. Sensitivity, specificity and predictive value of laparoscopy for the staging of gastric cancer and the detection of liver metastases. Cancer 58:1–6, 1986.

49. Kriplani AK, Kapur ML. Laparoscopy for preoperative staging and assessment of operability in gastric carcinoma. Gastrointest Endosc 37:441–443, 1991.

50. Gross E, Bancewicz J, Ingram O. Assessment of gastric cancer by laparoscopy. Br Med J 288:1577, 1984.

51. Dagnini G, Marin G, Patella M, et al. Laparoscopy in the diagnosis of primary carcinoma of the gallbladder. A study of 98 cases. Gastrointest Endosc 30:289–291, 1984.

52. Kriplani AK, Jayant S, Kapur BML. Laparoscopy in primary carcinoma of the gallbladder. Gastrointest Endosc 38:326–329, 1992.

53. Bhargava DK, Sarin S, Verma K, et al. Laparoscopy in carcinoma of the gallbladder. Gastrointest Endosc 29:21–22, 1983.

54. Porter JM, Kalloo AN, Abernathy EC. Carcinoid tumor of the gallbladder: laparoscopic resection and review of the literature. Surgery 112:100–105, 1992.

55. Meyer-Burg J. The inspection, palpation and biopsy of the pancreas by peritoneoscopy. Endoscopy 4:99–101, 1972.

56. Cuschieri A, Hall AW, Clark J. Value of laparoscopy in the diagnosis and management of pancreatic cancer. Gut 19:672–677, 1978.

57. Ishida H. Peritoneoscopy and pancreas biopsy in the diagnosis of pancreatic disease. Gastrointest Endosc 29:211–218, 1983.
58. Warshaw AL, Tepper JE, Shipley WA. Laparoscopy in the staging and planning of therapy for pancreatic cancer. Am J Surg 151:76–80, 1986.
59. Warshaw AL, Gu Z, Wittenberg J, et al. Preoperative staging and assessment of resectability of pancreatic cancer. Arch Surg 125:230–233, 1990.
60. Glatstein E, Guernsey JM, Rosenberg SA, et al. The value of laparotomy and splenectomy in the staging of Hodgkin's disease. Cancer 24:709–718, 1969.
61. DeVita VT, Bagley CM, Goodell B, et al. Peritoneoscopy in the staging of Hodgkin's disease. Cancer Res 31:1746–1750, 1971.
62. Beretta G, Spinelli P, Rilke F, et al. Sequential laparoscopy and laparotomy combined with bone marrow biopsy in staging Hodgkin's disease. Cancer Treat Rep 60:1231–1237, 1976.
63. Coleman M, Lightdale LJ, Vinciguerra VP. Peritoneoscopy in Hodgkin's disease confirmation of results by laparotomy. JAMA 236:2634–2636, 1976.
64. Chabner BA, Johnson RE, Young RL, et al. Sequential nonsurgical and surgical staging of non-Hodgkin's lymphoma. Ann Intern Med 85:149–154, 1976.
65. Salky BA, Bauer JJ, Gelernt IM, et al. The use of laparoscopy in retroperitoneal pathology. Gastrointest Endosc 34:227–230, 1988.
66. Bagley CM, Young RC, Schein PS, et al. Ovarian cancer metastatic to the diaphragm—frequently undiagnosed at laparotomy. Am J Obstet Gynecol 116:397–400, 1973.
67. Rosenoff SH, Young RC, Anderson T, et al. Peritoneoscopy: a valuable staging tool in ovarian cancer. Ann Intern Med 83:37–41, 1975.
68. Dagnini G, Marin G, Caldironi MW, et al. Laparoscopy in staging, follow-up, and restaging of ovarian cancer. Gastrointest Endosc 33:80–83, 1987.
69. Mueller BA, Daling JR, Moore DE, et al. Appendectomy and the risk of tubal infertility. N Engl J Med 315:1506–1508, 1986.
70. Leape LL, Ramenofsky ML. Laparoscopy for questionable appendicitis. Can it reduce the negative appendectomy rate? Ann Surg 191:410–413, 1979.
71. Deutsch AA, Zelikovsky A, Reiss R. Laparoscopy in the prevention of unnecessary appendicectomies: a prospective study. Br J Surg 69:336–337, 1982.
72. Whitworth CM, Whitworth PW, Sanfillipo J, et al. Value of diagnostic laparoscopy in young women with possible appendicitis. Surg Gynecol Obstet 167:187–190, 1988.
73. Anteby SO, Schenker JG, Polishuk WZ. The value of laparoscopy in acute pelvic pain. Ann Surg 181:484–486, 1975.
74. Shenk R, Stellato TA. Surgical abdominal emergency in patients undergoing treatment with malignant lymphoma. Surg Oncol Clin North Am 2:267–282, 1993.
75. Easter DW, Cuschieri A, Nathanson LK, et al. The utility of diagnostic laparoscopy for abdominal disorders. Audit of 120 patients. Arch Surg 127:379–383, 1992.
76. Kleinhaus S. Laparoscopic lysis of adhesions for postappendectomy pain. Gastrointest Endosc 30:304–305, 1984.
77. Smith DW, Rankin RA. Value of peritoneoscopy for nonfunctioning continuous ambulatory peritoneal dialysis catheters. Gastrointest Endosc 35:90–92, 1989.
78. Winfield HN. Suddenly, urology takes up the laparoscope. Contemp Urol 70–80, 1991.

25

Emergent Laparoscopy

Jonathan M. Sackier

As has been detailed in Chapter 1, endoscopic surgery has a colorful history; laparoscopy, specifically, was born at the turn of the 20th century. However, despite the enthusiasm of many authors and multiple publications detailing the benefits of diagnostic laparoscopy, it was not until the arrival of laparoscopic cholecystectomy[1-3] that interest in this modality for diagnostic purposes was revived. The works of Carnevale,[4] Gazzaniga,[5] Berci[6] and their associates all proclaimed that laparoscopy was useful in the evaluation of the traumatized patient. Although many surgeons now use the laparoscopic approach to the biliary tree, this does not automatically imply that the laparoscope should become the first tool of investigation in the emergency setting. Just as the assessment and treatment of patients with trauma or an acute abdomen demands a special degree of interest and skill, so does laparoscopy in this setting.

It is vital that a surgeon be more than conversant in laparoscopic techniques and have all the support systems in place before commencing a career as an emergent laparoscopist.

The indications for emergent laparoscopy are discussed and appropriate techniques detailed in this chapter, and although this author is enthusiastic about this form of appraisal, one should constantly bear in mind that the laparoscope is not a panacea—it merely has a role to play that is sometimes better defined than at other times. These deficiencies will be alluded to.

LOGISTICS

For the laparoscope to be of value in ensuring the rapid triage of injured or emergency patients, it should be as readily available to the surgeon as other modalities, such as computed tomography (CT). This requires dedication on the part of the hospital and the paramedical staff. First, sufficient and appropriate equipment must be purchased, correctly stored, maintained, and sterilized. Second, there must be an appreciation of techniques on the part of those who will assist the surgeon in making an endoscopic diagnosis under stressful circumstances—for example, in the middle of the night when the staff on duty may be unfamiliar with one another.

As has been mentioned, only surgeons who are well trained in laparoscopy and dedicated to its routine use should carry out the examination in these tense circumstances, and they should be able to decide on the suitable technique and location for the examination.

Under many circumstances, diagnostic laparoscopy may take place in the emergency room, and this will determine whether a patient should be transferred to the operating room, undergo further tests, be examined by another specialist, or be discharged home. Laparoscopy may also take place in the intensive care unit if it has been necessary to transfer a patient to such a setting for observation, ventilation, or stabilization. Of course, in many circumstances the patient's condition may militate against the luxury of using the emergency room; the patient may in fact need to go to the operating room. This will commonly be the case in patients who have sustained multiple system trauma and require, for instance, thoracotomy or craniotomy.

The endoscopic examination should be performed as soon after the patient's admission as possible, finding an early place in the management of the acutely ill patient, perhaps being substituted for diagnostic peritoneal lavage (DPL) or CT.

EQUIPMENT

Although most hospitals have one operating room in which laparoscopic cholecystectomies are performed and in which equipment is installed, this may not be the room used when a patient requires emergency laparoscopy. Should the injured patient need a major vascular, orthopedic, or neurosurgical procedure, the specialists performing these procedures will wish to use their own room, which may be distant from the general surgical suite. For this reason, and to enable laparoscopy in the emergency room or the intensive care unit, the equipment should be placed on a mobile cart. The location of this cart should be well known to all staff; it is useful to post a sign at the nursing station in the emergency room as to the location of the cart. Locks should be used to secure it to the wall and ensure that its contents remain as they should be. The cart should be of sturdy construction with large wheels and a handle that allows easy movement. This cart should contain a television monitor bolted to its uppermost surface, a light source, camera control unit, insufflator, cylinders of carbon dioxide, video recorder, or still printer, or both, and trays of instruments (Fig. 25–1).

Each of these components will now be considered in turn. The light source should ideally be a 300-W xenon cold light source, for although the smaller and lighter 150-W sources are appropriate for the elective situation, they may not be suitable for the patient with hemoperitoneum in whom maximal illumination is required. Together with the light source, at least two cables—preferably fluid-filled (which provide up to 30% more illumination)—should be available in case of breakage, and they should be individually sterilized and wrapped. The television monitor need be no larger than 20 inches and must be securely attached to the cart so that it is not dislodged when the cart is moved from one location to another. Some carts have a platform with an articulated arm that allows the monitor to be moved closer to the operator, which is obviously advantageous. The insufflator need not be the high-flow variety used in laparoscopic cholecystectomy, as one will rarely need more than two ports. Carbon dioxide is still the insufflating gas of choice, and at least two cylinders should be on the cart: one joined in series with the insufflator and the second sealed full cylinder kept as a spare. A wrench should be attached to the cylinder by a metal cable, along with spare gaskets, and the surgeon should be familiar with the techniques of chang-

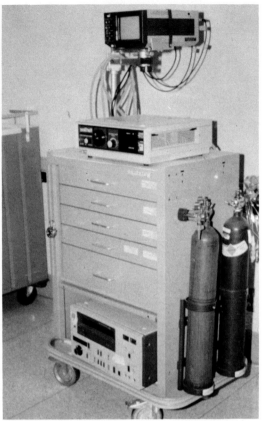

Figure 25–1. The mobile emergency diagnostic laparoscopic cart with a fixed television monitor, an insufflator, a light source, and drawers to contain ancillary equipment.

ing from an empty to a full cylinder (Fig. 25–2).

Documentation of emergency procedures is invaluable for teaching residents, medical students, and one's attending colleagues, and it is an impressive way of sharing information about the patient's condition with referring physicians. Videotapes are obviously bulky, and decisions should be made about storage, although legal implications must be taken into account, as such tapes become a part of the patient's record. The use of still printers is gaining popularity; they have the facility to generate a number of copies of a given photograph so that one may be placed in the patient's chart, one may be shown to the referring physician, and one may be kept in the surgeon's office.

At least two trays of equipment should be available in the cart so that, immediately upon the completion of one laparoscopy, the cart remains available if another case should follow quickly. In the interim, the first tray and contents should be sterilized, rewrapped, and returned to the cart. The tray should contain two

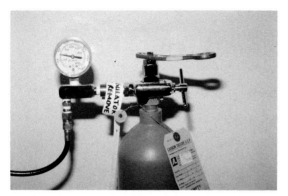

Figure 25–2. The top of a carbon dioxide cylinder, showing the attached wrench and spare gaskets.

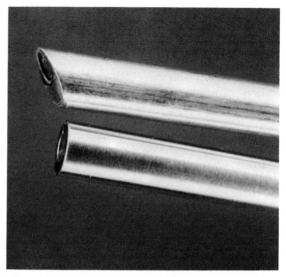

Figure 25–3. The tips of the 0° and 30° 10-mm laparoscopes.

Veress needles unless one elects to use a disposable product. If reusable needles are used, they must be well maintained, cleaned, and periodically sharpened. One 10-mm and three 5-mm trocars should be included. This will allow the surgeon to choose the larger or smaller laparoscope and still allow for up to three accessory portals. Appropriate reducers should obviously be present, and either disposable or reusable trocars may be chosen—this is purely a matter of the surgeon's preference.

The choice of telescope is the next important consideration, for the smaller 4-mm scope allows one to place a 5-mm trocar, which is obviously easier. However, the 10-mm scope allows much more light and therefore provides a better image, although it does require that the larger trocar be inserted. One must then decide on the viewing angle. The 0° scope is easier to use, for one need not concentrate on the orientation of the telescope. Although the 30° scope requires the surgeon to maintain the correct positioning, it allows several perspectives of the structures and enables the surgeon to look up at the abdominal wall and "around corners" (Fig. 25–3).

The set should also include a blunt palpation probe, which is valuable in lifting loops of bowel, liver, and other organs, and atraumatic bowel graspers, which allow one to "run the bowel" when looking for less obvious pathologic conditions (Fig. 25–4).

The workhorse of emergency laparoscopy is the suction, coagulation, and irrigation probe; this may be of the reusable or disposable variety. At the time of the procedure, this probe should be connected to the wall suction, a standard monopolar electric cautery generator to which the patient should be grounded, and a form of irrigation (Fig. 25–5). The simplest irrigation is

a liter of saline placed inside the pressure bag that is available in every emergency room.

The optic of the telescope is liable to fog from condensation, which will obscure vision. This is especially likely during an emergency procedure when the abdomen may contain blood or intestinal fluid; therefore, it is useful to have a system to clean and defog the telescope. A number of alternatives exist, such as commercial antifog solutions or water heated to greater than body temperature. This latter solution is preferable, as the scope is washed and antifogged at the same time. It may be difficult to ensure a constant supply of hot water; therefore, a thermos flask, specifically designed for the laparoscope, is a useful adjunct (Fig. 25–6).

It is valuable to have a system to routinely check the cart for function and completeness of instrumentation, such as pressure within the gas

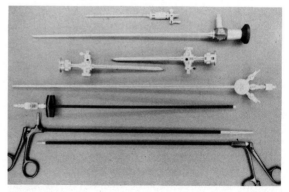

Figure 25–4. The tray of instruments used in diagnostic laparoscopy in emergencies.

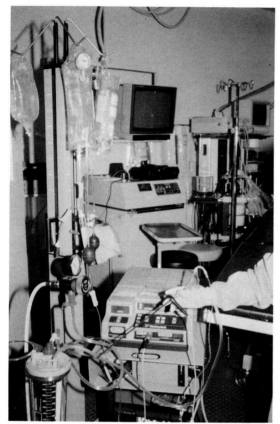

Figure 25-5. The electrocautery generator, suction, and pressure bag used to deliver irrigation. These three pieces of equipment are attached to the "workhorse" of diagnostic laparoscopy.

and passage of an oral or nasogastric tube to deflate the stomach. If the patient requires endotracheal intubation and general anesthesia for other reasons—such as major chest or neurosurgical injury—this obviously facilitates laparoscopy. If there are no concerns about damage to the lower extremities, deep venous thrombosis prophylaxis with sequential compression stockings is to be encouraged.

In many cases it is possible to perform the procedure in the emergency room with local anesthesia and intravenous sedation with diazepam and meperidine. The ideal situation is for the patient to be somnolent but responsive. One should be certain to have drugs available to reverse the before-mentioned agents, specifically naloxone and flumazenil. The patient should receive oxygen through nasal specula, and the clinical status should be monitored with blood pressure, pulse, and respiratory rate determinations and pulse oximetry. These measurements should be obtained by a nurse trained in critical care, a member of the house staff or, ideally, an anesthesiologist if one is available.

cylinders and presence of disposable supplies. One such approach is to have a card attached to the cart, much like those used on fire extinguishers for routine checks, and to have one member of the emergency room nursing staff responsible for this function.

TECHNIQUES

Preoperative investigations will be dictated by the patient's clinical presentation. It is an essential part of performing a laparoscopy to obtain the patient's informed consent; the detail into which one goes depends on the circumstances and the patient's mental state, although if relatives or friends are available they should be consulted. The patient and family should also be made aware of the occasional necessity to convert the procedure to open surgery. As a matter of routine, the patient should undergo bladder decompression with a Foley catheter

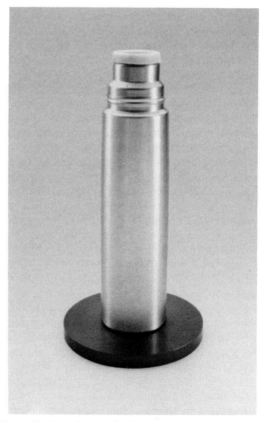

Figure 25-6. A thermos flask laparoscope warmer simultaneously washes and defogs the lens.

The abdomen should be shaved, prepared with povidone-iodine, and draped in the usual fashion. The ideal site for trocar insertion is at the inferior crease of the umbilicus, although previous surgery may suggest the left iliac fossa or hypochondrium as more appropriate. The site should be anesthetized with 1% lidocaine with adrenaline, and the Veress needle should be inserted through a small incision. It is essential to perform all the tests to confirm needle position; by lifting the abdominal wall with the tap open, a "hiss" may be heard, initially. A syringe with saline should then be attached and aspirated (hopefully with no return) and injected twice with no resistance. If saline is retrieved, this implies the needle is in the preperitoneal space; if blood has been aspirated, this means that either there is a hemoperitoneum or the needle has penetrated a vessel. If intestinal contents are aspirated, it means that this material is free within the peritoneal cavity or that the needle is within part of the gastrointestinal tract. The water drop test is also valuable. When the surgeon is convinced that the needle is in the peritoneal cavity, insufflation takes place, usually to no more than 8 to 10 mm Hg. It is important not to insufflate the abdomen too rapidly, as this may cause vagal stimulation, pain, or diaphragmatic rupture.[7]

In the case of previous surgery, failure to pass the Veress needle, or surgeon preference, the Hasson technique of trocar placement may be used.[8]

Once pneumoperitoneum has been established, the chosen trocar is inserted at the primary puncture site and the warmed telescope with attached camera is introduced. After surveying the abdominal wall, the accessory trocar position is chosen; this is usually in the right midclavicular line just superior to the anterior superior iliac spine. Obviously, it is important to anesthetize this area first if the procedure is not taking place under general anesthesia. It is vital to introduce the trocar under vision to prevent inadvertent bowel injury. At the completion of the procedure, the accessory trocar is removed and the telescope withdrawn. The pneumoperitoneum should be fully evacuated either into a suction bottle or by placing damp gauze over the valve mechanism of the trocar. The surgeon should not breathe the gas, as it may contain blood and viral particles. The puncture site should be closed with a secure suture to the fascia of the umbilical incision, subcuticular sutures to the skin, and adhesive strips to cover these sutures. Antibiotics should be administered as indicated but are not used as a matter of routine.

INDICATIONS

Broadly speaking, indications for this procedure may be divided into traumatic and nontraumatic ones, and each will be considered in turn. In certain circumstances, the diagnostic laparoscopy will provide the vehicle for further therapy and, when this is feasible, due mention will be made.

Traumatic Indications

Blunt Abdominal Trauma

Patients who have sustained nonpenetrating trauma may have injuries to other parts of the body, and the trauma surgeon is obliged to determine treatment priorities. Sometimes injuries are obvious, such as extruding brain with skull fractures, flail chest from a crushing injury, or the bruised and rapidly expanding abdomen seen with massive hepatic disruptions. This is not always the case, however, and one may have a patient who has a pressing need for treatment of injuries in different systems. When there is doubt as to the presence of an intraabdominal lesion, the laparoscope is an effective instrument. In 1965, Root and associates[9] introduced DPL. This blind technique allows one to detect the presence of blood in retrieved infused saline. In the United States, it is customary to interpret a level of 100,000 red cells/mL as an abnormal result. However, the presence of red cells in the fluid does not mean that there is active bleeding, and normal laparotomy may ensue in 11% to 25% of patients.[10–12] The 4-mm diagnostic laparoscope and trocar is little larger that the DPL equipment and provides so much more valid information (Fig. 25–7).

In many centers, such patients are assessed

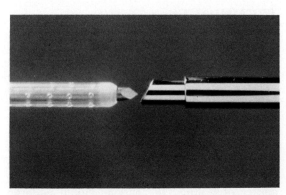

Figure 25–7. The comparative sizes of the diagnostic peritoneal lavage needle and diagnostic laparoscope. The latter is similar but provides much more information.

with a CT scan, but this, too, has its problems. The patient must be moved from the emergency room to the radiology suite, which can be especially worrisome if the patient is unstable. One has to rely on another practitioner for the investigation and interpretation of the study. Indeed, there are problems once the study is completed because the result is highly observer-dependent and, again, even if fluid is seen, this does not imply active bleeding or organ perforation; as a result, roughly one in five laparotomies will produce normal results.[13] Such laparotomies have numerous negative connotations, such as the morbidity of the procedure and possible mortality for the patient, unnecessary investment of time for the surgeon and paramedical staff, and financial implications for the patient, surgeon, and hospital. Therefore, the laparoscope may be used to select which patients do or do not need laparotomy; in order to do this more effectively a classification system has been developed, discussion of which follows.[14]

If, on introducing the laparoscope, small flecks of blood are seen on intestinal loops, they should be washed clear and a careful search made for a bleeding source. If after 10 minutes of observation no source is seen and no blood reaccumulates, this may be deemed a minimal hemoperitoneum and the procedure terminated. The patient should be admitted and observed for at least 24 hours. If one sees a pool of blood in the paracolic gutters, it should be aspirated, the area irrigated, and a search made. (The patient may have moderate hemoperitoneum.) It is in such circumstances that one may well find a small liver laceration, which may be coagulated with the electrosurgical tool, probably thereby avoiding a laparotomy (Fig. 25–8). When the Veress needle is introduced and fresh blood is retrieved, or a large pool of blood is seen on entering the abdomen, the patient should have immediate laparotomy, as a major injury is probably present (severe hemoperitoneum).

Injuries to the spleen may manifest themselves with major hemoperitoneum, or one may see the omentum raised over this organ, perhaps with a blue tinge of underlying blood clots. It is important to note that the spleen is not usually visible in laparoscopy. Frequent sites of laceration to the liver are the dome of the right lobe and the area of attachment to the falciform ligament, especially in deceleration injuries. In patients with possible pelvic fractures, there may be some intraperitoneal blood and a bulging peritoneum, implying injuries to the major vessels with retroperitoneal hematoma. Laparos-

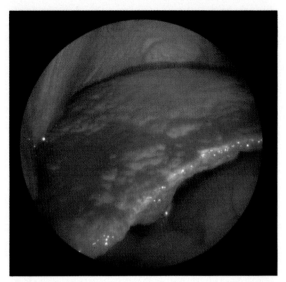

Figure 25–8. Laparoscopic view of a liver laceration showing sufficient blood to have caused a positive peritoneal lavage. However, it was possible to secure hemostasis with laparoscopic electrocautery.

copy should be supplemented with angiography and embolization, as appropriate.

Penetrating Trauma

Penetrating trauma is most applicable to knife wounds of the abdomen. Initially one should close the site of penetration then perform laparoscopy. Using the 30° telescope and moving the patient will allow the peritoneum underlying the stab wound to be seen when it is indented with the surgeon's finger. If no penetration of the parietal peritoneum is seen, one may complete the laparoscopy and discharge the patient. If the peritoneum has been breached, the underlying organs should be carefully inspected for damage. Obviously, the presence of blood or intestinal fluid in the abdomen or pelvis is a good indication that there has, in fact, been damage.

The next step will depend largely on the skill of the surgeon, the tools available, and the nature of the injury. It is possible to repair a number of injuries inflicted by a knife—for example, suturing perforations of the anterior wall of the stomach. One area of concern is a knife wound entering between the nipples and the costal margin, as injury to the diaphragm may be missed unless a very careful search is made for telltale flecks of blood—the 30° telescope is invaluable here. If the surgeon does not feel adept or able to position additional trocars and suture injuries, the laparoscopic diagnosis will at least guide the surgeon in placing an incision, or one of course may perform a laparoscopically guided repair by bringing the bowel out through a trocar site to repair an enterotomy.

In most circumstances, gunshot wounds to the abdomen demand immediate surgery, but laparoscopy may have a role to play in a small, carefully selected group of patients. When a bullet takes a seemingly tangential course across the abdomen of an obese patient, and a plain x-ray film does not reveal either any free gas or bullet fragments seeming to lie within the peritoneum, one should consider that this bullet has passed merely through the pannus. In this circumstance, laparoscopy may save an unnecessary and frustrating operation.[15]

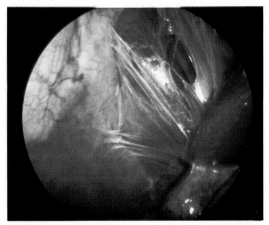

Figure 25–9. Laparoscopic view of adhesions between the liver and parietal peritoneum in a case of Fitz-Hugh–Curtis syndrome.

Nontraumatic Indications

Abdominal Pain

The young woman of childbearing age who presents to the emergency room with right iliac fossa pain often has a complex differential diagnosis, which includes appendicitis, ectopic pregnancy, pelvic inflammatory disease, torsion of an ovarian cyst, and numerous other conditions such as Crohn's disease or inflammation of a Meckel's diverticulum.

Occasionally, the patient may have a chronic history of abdominal pain of unknown origin, which has been extensively investigated. If the pain is situated in the right upper quadrant and ultrasound examination has been normal, it is worth remembering the diagnosis of Fitz-Hugh–Curtis syndrome, which may be detected and treated laparoscopically (Fig. 25–9).

On many occasions, an erroneous diagnosis is reached based on clinical criteria, which may lead to unnecessary laparotomy and appendectomy, with a consequence of adhesion formation and the impediment of future fertility. Indeed, the number of appendixes that are removed and subsequently found to be normal is as high as 30%.[16, 17]

It is in this clinical arena that emergent diagnostic laparoscopy is extremely valuable. Such patients may undergo endoscopy, resulting in the correct diagnosis. Of course, if an inflamed appendix is seen, it may be removed under laparoscopic control[18] (see Chap. 28). Certainly, if the laparoscopy reveals no obvious abnormality, laparoscopic appendectomy is a reasonable next step, as this would follow naturally if open exploration had been performed. It has

been shown repeatedly that such patients often have improvement of clinical symptoms even if the appendix is histologically normal.[19] The value of laparoscopy as a diagnostic aid in this setting has been demonstrated.[20, 21]

In a patient with an obscure diagnosis because of age, senility, obfuscation from alcohol or narcotics, or the severity of the clinical picture, such as with sepsis, laparoscopy may be a saving grace. In these difficult diagnostic dilemmas, the surgeon may avoid the morbidity of a laparotomy incision, which often results in normal findings. Perhaps not as bad, but certainly irritating or embarrassing for the surgeon, is to make an inappropriately placed incision, which may be better directed by laparoscopic surveillance preoperatively. Such a scenario may include a patient with a perforated duodenal ulcer who, because of a stoic nature, may not present until fluid in the right paracolic gutter causes localized peritoneal signs (Fig. 25–10). This may lead the surgeon to fashion a gridiron incision only to discover that it is, in fact, an upper midline approach that is required. In elderly patients who present with a likely diagnosis of diverticulitis, laparoscopy may allow for less invasive treatment by confirming the diagnosis, allowing for the placement of percutaneous drainage or even a defunctioning colostomy.[22, 23]

Occasionally, the patient in the intensive care unit may present with rising levels of liver enzymes and a clinical picture that implies acalculous cholecystitis. However, in such patients this diagnosis is fraught with difficulty and the use of [99m]technetium dimethyl iminodiacetic acid (HIDA) is not totally reliable. Laparoscopic evaluation, which may even be performed in the intensive care unit, allows for this diagnosis

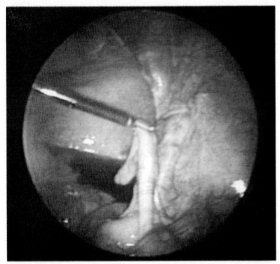

Figure 25–10. The laparoscopic view of a normal appendix with brown fluid in the right paracolic gutter, implying duodenal perforation, prevented an unnecessary laparotomy.

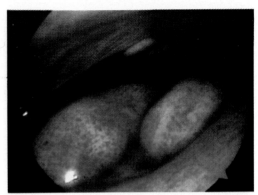

Figure 25–11. Laparoscopic view demonstrates small bowel ischemia, which required early operation.

to be confirmed or refuted and, if necessary, for percutaneous cholecystostomy to be instituted.[24]

Unexplained Shock

Occasionally, a young patient may present with seemingly profound hemodynamic shock that has no discernible reason. The clinical scenarios to remember are spontaneous splenic rupture from viral infection (infectious mononucleosis, cytomegalovirus) or delayed rupture of the spleen after trauma with subcapsular hematoma formation. The laparoscope is one way to assess this situation and decide whether conservative or operative therapy is required. Of course, laparoscopic splenectomy is now an area under exploration; for the time being, however, it should not be attempted in the emergent situation.

Mesenteric Ischemia

Mesenteric ischemia usually presents in elderly patients, who often have coexistent disease of the cardiorespiratory system. Laparotomy has a high morbidity and mortality rate in these individuals. If the clinical picture leads one to suspect this diagnosis, the laparoscope effectively opens a window of opportunity during which effective surgical therapy, such as embolectomy, may be instituted with good outcome (Fig. 25–11). When the ischemia affects the colon, this is a different disease entity that will very often resolve with resuscitation and con-

servative measures. Laparoscopy will allow one to view the colon at first hand (Fig. 25–12).

Fever of Unknown Origin

Patients with fever of unknown origin have often undergone an extensive workup with cultures, labeled white cell scans, CT scans, and ultrasound studies, from which no answer may be found. In the critical situation, laparoscopy may provide the answer, the likely diagnoses being tuberculosis (Fig. 25–13), brucellosis, unsuspected abscess (especially in the immunocompromised patient), and lymphoma.

Gastrointestinal Bleeding

The diagnosis in the vast majority of individuals with gastrointestinal bleeding will be reached by a combination of upper and lower gastrointestinal endoscopy, labeled red cell scans, and angiography. However, in the young patient who has never had a laparotomy, it is

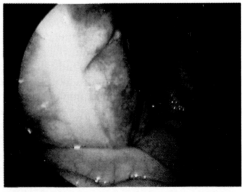

Figure 25–12. Laparoscopic view of ischemic colitis that was managed conservatively.

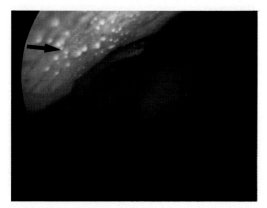

Figure 25–13. Laparoscopic view of miliary tuberculous deposits of the parietal peritoneum.

extremely likely that a Meckel's diverticulum or small bowel tumor will be responsible, and these conditions may be located and treated laparoscopically. Of course, an elective laparoscopic Meckel's diverticulum or small bowel resection may be planned in combination with angiography.

EMERGENCY CONCERNS

In order to ensure that laparoscopy is not misused, the patient should be carefully selected and prepared for this procedure. However, there are a number of issues that remain unanswered at this time.

In the assessment of the patient with multiple system trauma, the effect of carbon dioxide pneumoperitoneum on intracranial pressure has not been characterized. Using experimental animals in our laboratory, we have ascertained that pneumoperitoneum greater than 12 mm Hg does raise the intracranial pressure, although if the animal remains in the reverse Trendelenburg position, the effect is negated.[25] Further work is needed to clarify this. Additionally, if a knife wound below the nipple but above the costal margin necessitates laparoscopy because of questionable abdominal findings, it should be preceded by a chest x-ray study to exclude pneumothorax; otherwise the potential exists that a tension pneumothorax might be induced, and chest drainage might need to be instituted.

The safety of laparoscopy in the pregnant patient has been detailed in the gynecologic literature, but general surgeons have been loathe to undertake laparoscopic cholecystectomy in this group of patients, as the operative time is longer. Some experimental work has been done that demonstrates that pneumoperi-

toneum may have an effect on the fetal blood flow unless gas exchange in the mother is appropriately modified, which may mitigate against diagnostic emergency laparoscopy under local anesthesia.[26] However, it should be borne in mind that laparoscopy is an extremely safe modality when used correctly by well-trained surgeons and should certainly become a part of the surgeon's armamentarium.[27]

CONCLUSION

Emergency diagnostic laparoscopy requires dedicated equipment, well-trained surgical and allied health care professionals, and a critical appraisal of the individual clinical situation. It is extremely valuable in the assessment of patients with blunt and penetrating abdominal trauma, as it can help to reduce the number of unnecessary laparotomies by up to 20%. In patients with abdominal pain, unnecessary appendectomies may be avoided, thereby minimizing subsequent pelvic adhesions. For the evaluation of patients with obscure pain, fever, mesenteric ischemia, or hypotension, it is also of benefit and is a valued adjunct to CT scanning and other diagnostic tests.

Acknowledgments

I am most grateful to my colleagues for allowing me to discuss their cases and for their assistance in evaluating laparoscopy and laparoscopic instruments—most specifically George Berci, M.D., David Easter, M.D., and Steven Shoop, M.D.

References

1. Reddick E, Olsen DO. Laparoscopic laser cholecystectomy. A comparison with minilap cholecystectomy. Surg Endosc 3:131–133, 1989.
2. Dubois F, Icard P, Berthelot G, Levard H. Coelioscopic cholecystectomy: preliminary report of 36 cases. Ann Surg 211:60–62, 1990.
3. Berci G, Sackier JM. The Los Angeles experience with laparoscopic cholecystectomy. Am J Surg 161:382–384, 1991.
4. Carnevale N, Baron N, Delany HM. Peritoneoscopy, as an aid in the diagnosis of abdominal trauma: a preliminary report. J Trauma 17:634–641, 1977.
5. Gazzaniga AB, Slanton WW, Bartlett RH. Laparoscopy in the diagnosis of blunt and penetrating injuries to the abdomen. Am J Surg 131:315–318, 1976.
6. Berci G, Dunkelman D, Michel SL, et al. Emergency minilaparoscopy in abdominal trauma. An update. Am J Surg 146:261–265, 1983.
7. Doctor HN, Hussain Z. Bilateral pneumothorax associated with laparoscopy: a case report of a rare hazard and review of the literature. Anesthesiology 28:75–81, 1973.

8. Hasson HM. Open laparoscopy versus closed laparoscopy. A comparison of complication rates. Adv Planned Parenthood 13:41–44, 1978.
9. Root HO, Hauser CW, McKinley CR, et al. Diagnostic peritoneal lavage. Surgery 57:633–637, 1965.
10. Cox EF. Blunt abdominal trauma: a five year analysis of 870 patients. Ann Surg 199(4):467–474, 1984.
11. DuPriest RW, Rodriguez A, Khaneja SC, et al. Open diagnostic peritoneal lavage in blunt abdominal trauma victims. Surg Gynecol Obstet 148:890–894, 1979.
12. Peterson SR, Sheldon GF. Morbidity of a negative finding at laparotomy in abdominal trauma. Surg Gynecol Obstet 148(1):23–26, 1979.
13. Federle MP, Crass A, Brooke J, Trunkey DO. Computed tomography in blunt abdominal trauma. Arch Surg 117:645–650, 1982.
14. Berci G, Sackier JM, Paz-Partlow M. Emergency laparoscopy. Am J Surg 161:332–335, 1991.
15. Sosa JL, Sims D, Martin L, Zeppa R. Laparoscopic evaluation of tangential abdominal gunshot wounds. Arch Surg 127:109–110, 1992.
16. Paterson-Brown S, Eckersley JRT, Sim AJW, et al. Laparoscopy as an adjunct to decision making in the acute abdomen. Br J Surg 73:1022–1024, 1986.
17. Clark PJ, Hands LJ, Gough MH, et al. The use of laparoscopy in the management of right iliac fossa pain. Ann R Coll Surg Engl 68:68–69, 1986.
18. Semm K. Endoscopic appendectomy. Endoscopy 15:59–64, 1983.
19. Götz F, Pier A, Bacher C. Modified laparoscopic appendectomy in surgery: a report of 388 operations. Surg Endosc 4:6–9, 1990.
20. Paterson-Brown S, Vipond MN, Simms K, et al. Clinical decision making and laparoscopy versus computer prediction in the management of the acute abdomen. Br J Surg 76:1011–1013, 1986.
21. Nagy A, James D. Diagnostic laparoscopy. Am J Surg 157:490–493, 1989.
22. Sackier JM. Perforated diverticulitis. In: Dudley H, Carter D, Todd IP, Fielding LP, eds. Operative Surgery. London: Butterworth, in press.
23. Sackier JM. Laparoscopy: applications to colorectal surgery. Semin Colon Rectal Surg 3(1):2–8, 1992.
24. Berci G, Cuschieri A. Laparoscopic cholecystostomy. In: Berci G, Cuschieri A, eds. Practical laparoscopy. London: Bailliere Tindall, 1986:103–107.
25. Sackier JM. Laparoscopy for trauma. Presented at the Postgraduate Course of the Ninth Annual Meeting of the Society of American Gastrointestinal Endoscopic Surgeons. April 1992, Washington DC.
26. Hunter JH. Laparoscopy in the pregnant patient. Presented at the Postgraduate Course of the Eighth Annual Congress of the Society of American Gastrointestinal Endoscopic Surgeons. April 1991, Monterey, CA. Surg Endosc 6(1):52–53, 1992.
27. Chamberlain GVP, Carron Brown JA. Report of the working party of the confidential inquiry into gynaecological laparoscopy. R Coll Obstet Gynaecol, 1978.

26

Laparoscopic Cholecystectomy

Jacques Périssat, Michael Edye, and Denis Collet

HISTORICAL NOTE

In his thesis for the diploma of Doctor of Medicine from the University of Paris, which was first presented at 1 P.M. on December 12, 1890, François Calot described the anatomic boundaries of a hepatobiliary triangle, which is now named after him.[1, 2] While an anatomy assistant, he performed cholecystectomy, cholecystostomy, and cannulation of the cystic and common bile ducts, as well as experiments to determine the effects of free bile in the peritoneal cavity, in laboratory animals. What Calot has not been credited with since is the uncanny foresight that he displayed of the present-day problems of laparoscopic cholecystectomy. He noted that the gallbladder was always scarred and surrounded by dense adhesions, making dissection difficult and very time-consuming, clearly an indication of the complicated nature of the gallstone disease that came to surgical treatment at that time. The attachments of the gallbladder to the liver were frequently so dense that a scalpel was required to divide them. He advised against the use of thermocautery, as the insulating sleeve made the instrument difficult to sterilize, which is very relevant when comparing the merits of disposable and nondisposable laparoscopic equipment. Moreover, he described the problems and dangers of inadequate visualization of his triangle (which he refrained from naming after himself!) from differing angles, which is reminiscent of the imaging problems experienced during laparoscopic cholecystectomy with 0° or 30° scopes.

François Dubois first performed a laparoscopic cholecystectomy (LC) in Paris in 1988.[3] He had heard of the procedure from an operating room nurse who had worked with Mouret in Lyon, who as yet had not published his work. Périssat in Bordeaux furthered the truly minimally invasive concept of the operation by pioneering in situ lithotripsy so that little or no dilation of a 10-mm puncture was necessary to remove a gallbladder already emptied of its calculi. LC developed more or less concurrently on both sides of the Atlantic. McKernan[4] performed the first LC in the United States, and the procedure was then developed and popularized by Olsen and Reddick.[5] What is interesting in this evolution is that Dubois[3] and Olsen and Reddick[5] had already started cholecystectomy by minilaparotomy and had written about this intermediate procedure either alone or in comparison with LC. Not surprisingly, the enthusiasm with which surgeons embraced the laparoscopic procedure has largely overshadowed the merits of minilaparotomy, for which a well-defined role (to be discussed briefly later in this chapter) still exists.

The best current data indicate that as a method for removing a patient's gallbladder (in 75% of women and 25% of men), LC is associated with a slightly greater risk of common bile duct injury than is open cholecystectomy, but when it is performed without complication, it is vastly more acceptable. Common bile duct injury rates between 0.2% and 0.5%[6, 7] have been reported, although these are cumulative series from multiple operators or institutions. Detailed information on duct injuries is frequently unreliable or unavailable, so an increase in bile duct reconstructions, the figures for which can be obtained from insurance databases, may be an indirect guide to numbers, although there will be a lag period.

EQUIPMENT

The tools needed to operate are used by the surgeon to irrigate, suck, cut, grasp, clip, ligate, and coagulate. Operating cannulas are not included in this category. A vast array of tools has become available in a short time. Many are identical instruments stamped with different brands. Other are newly conceived and original and represent a positive step in the evolution of the instrumentation. The ergonomics and practical requirements of instruments intended for laparoscopic use are such that traditional approaches to dimensions, blades, joints, hinges, ratchets, catches, and jaws are frequently inappropriate. Unfortunately, many surgeons or hospitals have purchased universally expensive equipment that can only be described as interim technology.

Some of the general qualities of an ideal tool may be as follows:

- It should have a 5-mm diameter to fit through the smallest cannula.
- It should possess intuitive and consistent action properly suited to the ergonomics of hand-arm positioning, which is different from that in open surgery.
- It should have undamageable insulation.
- It should be easily distinguishable from other instruments of similar shape but different function (*e.g.,* scissors from grasper).
- It should be completely cleanable without time-consuming disassembly.
- It should be autoclavable.
- It should be modular so that worn jaws, ratchet assembly, or blades can be easily replaced without expensive repairs or complete replacement.

Without attempting to belabor the obvious, tools should be selected that perform the function for which they were designed; therefore, scissors should cut right to the tip and graspers should hold in as atraumatic a fashion as possible without slipping off. The functionality of all available tools increases with operator experience. Once the skill of operating in the foreign videoscopic environment has been mastered, the ability to make instruments work as they should improves. Nonetheless, many instruments are still not ideal for reasons such as

- Their mechanisms snag and puncture rubber gloves.
- Their ratchet assemblies are overly complex and difficult to operate, and they spring apart.
- Being derived from an earlier instrument, they impose an unnatural hand position on the operator when used laparoscopically.

INDICATIONS

It is now clear that in experienced hands, LC is the operation of choice for symptomatic cholelithiasis. Except in unusual circumstances, asymptomatic gallstones are still best treated expectantly. Even in the presence of acute cholecystitis or a known duct stone, with sufficient experience the biliary surgeon should at least begin with a laparoscopy, as many of the more complicated presentations of gallstones can be managed laparoscopically.

CONTRAINDICATIONS

Specific contraindications to LC are unusual. Suppurative cholangitis due to a stone occluding the lower end of the common bile duct should be dealt with urgently by endoscopic sphincterotomy and the gallbladder removed, if still indicated, when the acute inflammation has settled.

Carcinoma of the gallbladder can occur in 1% to 2% of cases, of which 60% to 90% present with acute cholecystitis. Ultrasonography is not diagnostic, and preoperative diagnosis is rare (10% of cases).[8] Since an operative diagnosis is made in less than half of those patients operated on, the carcinoma will commonly be identified first by the histopathologist. Hence, it is illusory to consider such a lesion a strict contraindication to LC unless a strong preoperative suspicion of carcinoma exists. A recent report of seeding of a gallbladder carcinoma at the umbilical and left abdominal cannula sites suggested that surgical resection or postoperative irradiation of the cannula sites should be included in supplementary treatment.[8] To this could be added the operative precaution of enclosing all acutely inflamed gallbladders in an extraction bag prior to removal at laparoscopy in view of the frequent presentation of carcinoma as acute cholecystitis.

The presence of a biliary-enteric fistula will challenge even the most experienced operators, so although successful laparoscopic management of a cholecystoduodenal fistula has been reported,[9] it is likely that most operators will manage this type of lesion in the traditional manner.

Of a more general nature, cardiac or respiratory disease that may decompensate with positive pressure pneumoperitoneum may be a contraindication, depending on the attitude of the anesthesia team. Use of an abdominal wall lifting device enables a laparoscopic approach in these patients, although postoperative abdominal wall pain may be more marked. Undoubtedly, so-called contraindications may become mere precautions with wider experience.

ANTICOAGULANT THERAPY

By avoiding a major abdominal incision, and thus the possibility of a substantial wound hematoma, patients undergoing LC may benefit from a reduced risk of wound complications if they have had anticoagulant therapy. LC has been performed in patients who have undergone anticoagulation treatment for a wide variety of conditions, including the presence of aortic and mitral valve prostheses, chronic atrial fibrillation, and thromboembolic disease.[10] Administration of oral anticoagulants should be ceased prior to surgery, which is scheduled when the prothrombin ratio is around a factor of 1.2 or less. Whether heparin anticoagulation is added and in what regimen depends on the patient's risk for thrombosis. To date, in our series of more than 800 cases, all patients who did not undergo anticoagulant therapy received prophylactic low molecular weight heparin, and those taking oral anticoagulant medication discontinued it until the second postoperative day and received subcutaneous heparin (Calciparine) dependent on body mass and the clinical indication. There were no thromboembolic complications in the prophylactic group, nor were there any complications related to the therapeutic anticoagulation group (heparin window). Meticulous hemostasis is a prerequisite for good laparoscopic surgical technique but two points need emphasis: (1) transillumination of the abdominal wall will help to prevent trocar injury of parietal vessels and (2) the path of trocar insertion should avoid traversing the body of either rectus muscle to be certain to miss the epigastric vessels coursing within its substance.

OBESITY

Far from obesity being a contraindication to LC, obese patients stand to benefit doubly from a laparoscopic procedure. We have found that the procedure takes about the same time in these patients and that discharge and return to normal activities occur at about the same time as in nonobese patients.[11] Although there are insufficient data at present to substantiate it scientifically, it would be reasonable to postulate that the complications of surgery and anesthesia related to obesity are thereby reduced. Certainly the surgery can be more tedious, as special techniques are necessary to deal with a thickened abdominal wall. The cannula for the laparoscope should be sited well above the umbilicus, which is frequently low in relation to the operative field. Some nondisposable cannulas necessitate traversing abdominal wall obliquely so that the axis of the cannula is directed toward the operative field. Otherwise, the force required to pass the instrument through the cannula to come to this position can distort the seal in the cannula, causing an elusive and annoying gas leak. Other authors feel that a perpendicular puncture of the abdominal wall is necessary so that relatively short cannulas do not tend to slip back into the preperitoneal plane,[12] although this can be prevented by using longer (150 mm) ports. Undoubtedly, the most awkward part of the procedure is the removal of calculi and the gallbladder because of resistance in the lengthy track to the skin surface.

PREGNANCY

Acute cholecystitis or recurrent biliary colic is second only to appendicitis as a surgical condition complicating pregnancy and may be unresponsive to medical therapy, tempting the surgeon to intervene before term. Although we have no experience with this situation, two recent reports[13, 14] suggest that with appropriate fetal monitoring, tocolytic therapy if warranted, and careful cannula placement designed to avoid the gravid uterus (which is level with the umbilicus at around 20 weeks' gestation), LC can be safely performed in the second trimester. Whether this can be extrapolated to surgical intervention in the first trimester is unknown. Antibiotic therapy carries the theoretic risk of fetal abnormality, whereas the effects of prolonged carbon dioxide pneumoperitoneum and anesthesia are less clear. Any surgery during pregnancy for a biliary pathologic condition that is sufficiently severe to warrant intervention is likely to be more technically challenging and thus more lengthy. For this reason, only the most experienced operators should embark upon this type of procedure, with background obstetric support. Clearly, trocars must be placed with extreme care to avoid damage to the uterus.[13]

LAPAROSCOPIC CHOLECYSTECTOMY IN CHILDREN

We have had very limited experience with LC in the pediatric age group, but a recent report[15] indicates that the procedure can be performed safely for the hemolytic or glycogen storage disorders that form the usual indications in these patients. LC was performed in 12 children, with operative cholangiography performed in 6 of them using adult instrumentation. None of these children had obstructive jaundice preoperatively. The authors caution that umbilical hernia is not uncommon, and open laparoscopy may be the wisest way to start the procedure. The liver is frequently enlarged, necessitating adjustment of gallbladder retraction. Small ductal calculi seen at operative cholangiography can usually be flushed into the duodenum. Separate repair of an umbilical hernia, if present, is performed at closure.

PREPARATION

The Patient

The clinical history will provide vital clues as to the nature of the underlying gallbladder pathologic condition. A few episodes of biliary colic without fever or systemic toxicity that resolve rapidly after administration of an antispasmodic agent or a dose of parenteral analgesia and are punctuated by periods of being completely well are more likely to be associated with a thin-walled gallbladder. It is unusual for there to be tenderness in the right subcostal region in this situation. Repeated attacks over months or years associated with fever and necessitating antibiotic therapy and time away from work or normal activity or hospitalization will inevitably have led to scarring and contraction of the gallbladder. If local tenderness is present, it is a sign of acute inflammation superimposed on chronic inflammation, and the going is likely to be tougher. Conversely, a tense, distended, exquisitely tender gallbladder may prove relatively easy to remove, especially if located on a mesentery. The lack of worrisome symptoms and clinical signs is nonetheless quite consistent with a contracted, fibrosed gallbladder buried deep within the liver substance.

In spite of ever-increasing experience, a number of patients (5% to 10%) will undergo conversion to open cholecystectomy. It is therefore mandatory that this be explained during the initial consultation, mentioned specifically on any informed consent document, and repeated prior to anesthetic premedication. This is also the time to begin encouraging the patient to believe that a prolonged hospitalization is unusual and that discharge is planned on whatever postoperative day is the norm for a given unit. From the time of admission, in the recovery room, and continuing until the patient returns to the ward, the staff must maintain a positive attitude, using supportive terminology so that the attitude of confidence that was hopefully established in the patient is not compromised.

When interpreted in the light of the clinical history, the most significant examination is the ultrasound. Certain features such as a scarred, contracted (scleroatrophic) gallbladder or acute cholecystitis are associated with a rate of conversion of 20% or more and should alert the surgeon to give a less optimistic evaluation of laparoscopic operability. Preoperative identification of ductal stones is the ideal situation. The ultrasound report not only should make mention of the calculi in the gallbladder but also list their number and diameter, gallbladder wall quality (edema) and thickness, the presence or paucity of contained bile, and the measured diameter of the bile duct if it is identifiable. If this information is not available from the report or is not obvious from the films, they should be reviewed. It is not overuse of diagnostic services to have the ultrasound repeated if technical difficulties prevented the correct visualization of essential features on the first attempt.

Levels of γ-glutamyltransferase and alkaline phosphatase must be interpreted along with other clinical data, but an elevation of one or both occurs in the presence of the majority of ductal stones, although 10% to 15% will be silent.

Careful preoperative outpatient evaluation of other gastrointestinal symptoms and performance of appropriate examinations such as upper or lower gastrointestinal endoscopy, or computed tomography if clinically indicated, will give confidence to patient and surgeon, both of whom are to be deprived of the benefit of direct palpation of the abdominal viscera, which is possible only at laparotomy. Naturally any intercurrent medical problems need to be documented and allowance made. Of note, preexisting cardiovacular disease may indicate poor tolerance of pneumoperitoneum, especially if it is induced too quickly. Oral anticoagulant therapy is no more a contraindication to a laparoscopic procedure than it is to open surgery and can be replaced by a heparin window, as discussed previously. Antiplatelet drugs, such as aspirin and the nonsteroidal anti-inflammatory agents, should be ceased 10 days prior to surgery.

It is not strictly necessary to shave even hirsuit individuals.[16] With many of the unpleasant postoperative sequelae reduced or lacking, the regrowth of abdominal wound hair may seem more arduous. In older patients there is frequently a concretion of sebaceous material in the umbilicus, which should be removed well before the planned procedure.

In view of the small risk of colonic injury during LC, orthograde colonic cleansing with 3 L of a polyethylene glycol preparation is a wise precaution and should begin on the evening prior to surgery. With adequate explanation, this can be taken at home. Individual practices and hospital routines will vary, but although many young and fit patients can prepare themselves and arrive well rested for an early morning procedure, older and more frail patients will need to be admitted the day before surgery. It seems that some centers are determined to break the 24-hour barrier and have patients out of the hospital before their wounds are dry. The mere presence of a patient in a general hospital setting can generate accessory expenditure by medical attendants on behalf of their patients ("routine" postoperative tests), which is usually unjustified by the clinical condition. If a policy of preoperative outpatient workup is applied, with results that are available and sufficiently recent, no inpatient investigations will be necessary. All patients thus need to be reminded to bring all radiographs in their possession with them to the hospital.

LC is a major and sometimes prolonged operative procedure performed under general anesthesia with muscle relaxation. Prophylactic anticoagulants should be used, although there is as yet little direct evidence of benefit. Low-molecular-weight heparin is administered subcutaneously with the premedication and will usually continue in the recommended dose and frequency until discharge. The patient is requested to void just before premedication, and the volume is recorded.

The Operating Room

A quick check by the surgeon or assistant should be performed before scrubbing. The following should be ascertained:

- The insufflator should be connected, have a viable gas supply, and blow gas.
- The correct static pressure limit should be selected and the alarm should sound when this is exceeded.
- The video camera, monitor, and light source should produce a satisfactory image, which will avoid annoying delays once the operation is under way.

The patient is positioned supine on an operating table with cholangiography capability and is sufficiently immobilized to allow 20° of reverse Trendelenburg and lateral tilt. Depending on the operative technique used, the lower limbs are parallel or spread. If lithotomy positioning is used, the hips should be flexed as little as possible to minimize venous outflow impairment and avoid blocking access to the cannulas for long instruments. Compression stockings or intermittent calf compression or stimulation devices can be used, depending on personal preference. Following induction of anesthesia, a gastric tube is inserted to keep the stomach flat and is removed immediately after the procedure. Whether or not a urinary catheter is inserted can also be left to the surgeon's preference. If a purely biliary procedure is planned and is unlikely to last more than 2 hours, there is little to justify the added potential complication of a urinary catheter. Trocars need not be directed toward the urinary bladder during placement, so if the patient has recently voided, there is no risk of a bladder perforation.

Disposable drapes are light and easy to use but are expensive, and towel clips tend to tear through them. A single, very large nondisposable drape can easily be modified in the hospital sewing room with a fenestration 40 cm × 20 cm, the long side of which is oriented across the abdomen. An adhesive plastic drape fixes the other drapes in place and prevents a radiopaque towel clip from spoiling the cholangiogram.

THE OPERATION

Insufflation

Having draped the patient, induction of a pneumoperitoneum can proceed slowly while tubes, cables, and instruments are arranged. A long quiver fashioned from a sterile cotton drape and suspended close to the dominant hand of the operator is ideal to stock a small range of the most commonly used instruments. Care should be taken to avoid damage to plastic insulation sleeves and delicate tips when replacing or removing instruments. Rigid plastic or metal quivers need to be long enough so that the tip of an instrument dropped in does not hit bottom on a hard surface.

Unless the nondisposable Veress needle is sharpened frequently, a new disposable needle is advisable for each case, especially in the early learning stages. Although umbilical puncture is advocated by many, the most reliable site, especially in obese patients, is in the left hypochondrium, 3 to 5 cm below the costal margin over the lateral border of the rectus muscle. Here the muscles of the anterior abdominal wall are relatively fixed, and three distinct "pops" are felt as the needle passes progressively through anterior sheath, posterior sheath, and peritoneum. It is unusual for this area to be the site of adhesions unless there has been previous upper abdominal surgery, in which case an open laparoscopy and insertion of a Hasson-type cannula is the wisest option. Some authors advocate routine open laparoscopy,[17] arguing that once mastered it is rapidly performed and allows immediate insufflation at high flow rates. A gas seal is ensured by the firm insertion of the conical sleeve of the cannula into the small wound, and the muscular aponeurosis is easily repaired at closure by tying the stay sutures or fascial pursestring sutures placed at the beginning. Apart from extremely obese patients and those in whom rapid insufflation is poorly tolerated, the technique is relatively easy and extremely safe. If a needle has been inserted and the tests for tip position carried out (aspiration and gravity injection), the static pressure gauge of the insufflator and position of the needle should be carefully watched by at least one of the team during the entire insufflation. If the static pressure control has been set to 10 mm Hg, for example, the expected readings are as follows: 0 mm Hg prior to connection and 8 to 10 mm Hg on starting insufflation at 1 L/minute, which should drop after a few seconds to about 2 to 4 mm Hg and then rise slowly as the volume insufflated accumulates. If the pressure remains around 7 to 10 mm Hg, it is likely that the needle tip is enmeshed with omentum or bowel and should be withdrawn 1 or 2 cm or the abdominal wall tented up by firmly grasping it around the needle. Conversely, the needle is in an extraperitoneal position and needs to be reinserted and the test procedure repeated before attempting insufflation again.

Once insufflation is proceeding normally, the abdomen will swell symmetrically and liver dullness will disappear after administration of about 200 mL of gas. At this point, the needle should be withdrawn about 10 to 15 mm to clear its tip, which impales the omentum with surprising frequency and inflates the lesser sac. If the pressure alarm of the insufflator sounds at any time during the procedure, the following routine will quickly identify the problem: One should first check that the stopcock of the cannula has not been inadvertently closed or that the tubing is not kinked close to the cannula (the usual site); next it must be determined that the cannula itself has not slipped out so that the tip is in the preperitoneal space; lastly, contraction of the abdominal wall muscles, which indicates that the patient is not sufficiently anesthetized, may be the first sign the surgeon notices.

Siting of Cannulas

Three or more liters of insufflated gas is ample before insertion of the first cannula (Fig. 26–1). Usually this will be of 10-mm diameter and is inserted through a circumumbilical or midline umbilical incision (cannula No. 1). A midline incision allows for easy extension in the linea alba and if sited actually within the umbilicus will retract with healing and be effectively invisible. Incisions should be just long enough to ensure a very snug fit around the cannula to discourage it from slipping out but not so short that excessive force is required for insertion. Except for a midline incision, the incisions should be made parallel to the lines of skin cleavage. Two schools of thought apply to trocar placement. The trocar can be directed well to the right, taking an oblique course through the abdominal wall so that when the cannula is removed the anterior and posterior aponeurotic defects do not overlap, reducing the possibility of incisional hernia. It may prove more difficult to extract a gallbladder full of stones through the oblique track thus created. Alternatively, the trocar takes a more direct path through the abdominal wall, ensuring that the structures of the posterior abdominal wall, such as bowel and great vessels, are avoided with the point. In most instances a compromise must be reached, which will depend on the thickness of the abdominal wall and the length of the available cannulas. As stated previously, if the cannula is poorly positioned relative to the operative field in an obese patient, the gas seal of some nondisposable cannulas tends to distort and leak from the firm leverage required to correctly orient an instrument passing through it. In all cases the outer sleeve of the cannula must extend beyond the peritoneum.

If the abdomen is scarred, the first trocar is ideally placed as far away from the scar as

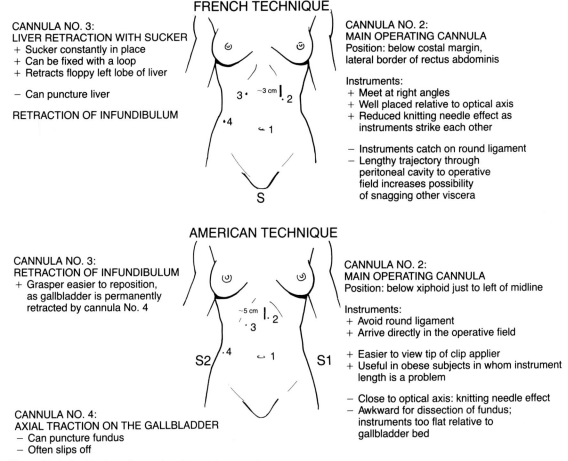

Figure 26–1. Positioning of cannulas. 2 = main operating cannula; 3 = midclavicular cannula; 4 = midaxillary cannula; S = position of surgeon; S1 and S2 = optional positions for surgeon.

possible. If the site chosen is on the right side, a 5- or 8-mm cannula inserted at a resonant point[18, 19] and a narrow, rigid endoscope are used to check for adhesions to the anterior abdominal wall. On the left side, assuming the French technique (see further on), the usual 10-mm cannula (cannula No. 2) is used. If adhesions are identified, but the contralateral side is clear, they are taken down by siting a 5-mm cannula in a free zone for the scissors. It is often the case in this adhesiolysis that the operator is not positioned in front of the adhesions and instrument responses are back to front. A handy technique is to rotate the laparoscope through 180°, which, although putting the abdominal wall at the bottom of the screen, makes instruments appear to respond in the normal way.

Having cleared the posterior aspect of the umbilicus, a 10-mm cannula can then be sited there (cannula No. 1).

There is no doubt that laparoscopy wounds cause soreness in the postoperative period. If a

long-acting local anesthesic such as bupivacaine, 0.5%, is to be used, the logical technique is to pass the needle directly through the proposed puncture site, raise a generous bleb of peritoneum, and then infiltrate the skin before removing the needle. Pain fibers are then blocked from the outset. A 5-mm cannula (cannula No. 3) is sited directly over the fundus of the gallbladder (usually in the midclavicular line) about 3 cm below the costal margin, although if this cannula is to be used for liver retraction using the sucker it will need to be closer to the costal margin. The position of the second 5-mm cannula (cannula No. 4) depends on the space between the costal margin and the iliac crest, but in general it will be in the anterior axillary line roughly level with the umbilicus.

A general laparoscopy is then performed to visualize all available abdominal viscera. How complete this needs to be depends on clinical parameters, including the age of the patient, how exhaustive the preoperative workup has been, and the presence of other unexplained symptoms. It is wise not to embark upon a laparoscopic cholecystectomy unless all reasonable cost-effective investigations have been completed. It is possible to palpate the liver by stroking it with the shaft of a 5-mm palpator. Once three cannulas are sited, using gentle graspers, the small bowel and colon can be inspected from the ligament of Treitz to the rectosigmoid junction, although this is time-consuming and requires the full range of table positions to see adequately. The pelvic viscera are well seen in the Trendelenburg position. The table is then positioned with 15° to 20° of reverse Trendelenburg and tilted to the patient's left.

Before blood staining can occur, an attempt should be made to locate the course of the common bile duct in the hepatoduodenal ligament. In thin subjects, it can often be seen as a darkening just deep to the peritoneum. A gentle pull on the gallbladder in its long axis may help to highlight it. Adhesions between the gallbladder and infrahepatic structures, if present, are then divided. If they are filmy, traction on the omentum, pericolic fat, or duodenum with a 5-mm grasper through the anterior axillary cannula (cannula No. 4) may be sufficient. Otherwise, scissor dissection just superficial to the plane of the visceral peritoneum of the gallbladder or electrocautery if the adhesions are vascular can be employed. It is often necessary to provide countertraction of the liver and gallbladder through cannula No. 3 during this maneuver.

Grasping the Gallbladder

Apart from the position of the operator, the chief differences between the so-called American and French techniques relate to the position of the operating cannula (cannula No. 2) and the method of displaying the triangle of Calot (see Fig. 26–1). Even after their early laparoscopic apprenticeship, a surprising number of surgeons continue to use a one-handed dissection technique, preferring to hold the camera in their nondominant hand. A skilled assistant, usually a second surgeon, is necessary to provide countertraction during dissection, which could otherwise be provided by the operator's other hand, which is occupied with the camera. This practice should be discarded as soon as possible. If not, dexterity remains dependent on skills over which the operator has no direct control. Operating one handed in classic surgery has

little to recommend it, and the same applies laparoscopically.

The American Technique

In the American technique, cannula No. 2 is sited about 5 cm below the xiphoid process just to the left of the midline and directed obliquely through the abdominal wall toward the hilum of the liver. It should exit in or just below the angle between the falciform ligament and the parietal peritoneum. Instruments passed through it arrive immediately in the operative field without having to skirt under the free edge of a pendulous round ligament. The gallbladder fundus is grasped firmly with an atraumatic grasper having as broad a tip as will fit through a 5-mm cannula (cannula No. 4) and is pushed up and laterally under the diaphragm, just far enough to cause the infundibulum of the gallbladder to lift gently. The gallbladder bed will have rotated anteriorly toward the abdominal wall. Traction on the infundibulum is provided by a grasper inserted through cannula No. 3. Operative cholangiograms performed with this degree of fundic retraction in normal tissues show that there is no tenting of the common bile duct (Edye et al., unpublished data) despite such an appearance clearly depicted in a recent publication,[34] which also appears in a popular manual of laparoscopic surgery. It has been suggested that this misrepresentation may have contributed to the higher incidence of bile duct injury in the United States compared with European reports, although it has not been reliably established that a difference does in fact exist.

The French Technique

In the French technique, the main operating instruments, such as dissector, diathermy hook, and scissors, pass through cannula No. 2 in the left hypochondrium. If the cannula tip is long enough, it will protrude beyond the edge of the round ligament. As any instrument is removed, the assistant holds the cannula in position to prevent it from slipping back and to fix its axis. This helps to avoid snagging the ligament or other structures with the next instrument introduced, which should arrive directly in the operative field. If the ligament is pendulous, and assuming an adequate pneumoperitoneum, the instrument should first be introduced in the direction of the right iliac fossa and then swept clockwise in an arc keeping close and parallel to the abdominal wall. Once practiced, this maneuver becomes automatic. If instruments still snag, a heavy thread on a long curved needle can be passed through the skin, under the ligament, back out through the skin, and tightened, which helps to retract both ligament and the left lobe of the liver (staying close to the midline will avoid injury to the epigastric vessels).

The sucker inserted through cannula No. 3 and positioned with its tip near the hilum or along the round ligament retracts the liver cephalad to provide countertraction for an infundibular grasper inserted through cannula No. 4. Care must be taken not to damage the liver parenchyma with the sucker, which approaches at a better angle if the cannula is close to the costal margin.

Pros and Cons of the American and French Techniques

It is instructive to analyze the reasons behind the evolution of each technique. As Reddick has explained regarding the American technique, the positions of the cannulas in the right subcostal region, apart from access factors, were largely determined by the need to join up the incisions should the case require conversion to laparotomy. In designing the French technique, it was planned that by siting the main operating cannula in the left hypochondrium, instruments would meet roughly at right angles and at an optimal angle relative to the optical axis, thereby making operating easier.

Figure 26–1 indicates the chief differences between cannula placement, function, and instrument access. Without repeating what is highlighted in the diagrams, it is interesting that when comparing the two approaches, the operative field *looks different* because of the different methods of exposure of the triangle of Calot. Familiarity with the normal appearance in both will help to prevent incorrect identification of vital structures. It will be a matter of personal preference and training as to which is used, but there is much to be said for a mixture of both.

Certainly it is quite feasible for the surgeon to sit between the patient's legs but use American cannula sites. Surgeons who prefer to stand on the patient's left side tend to bump elbows with the assistant, who is also standing on the left to avoid neck strain if there is only one monitor. This problem can be solved by the assistant standing between the patient's legs.

At times it is not possible to abduct a patient's legs because of ankylosis or hip replacement, so

the surgeon used to the French approach is obliged to stand at the patient's side, which can be disorienting.

Dissection of the Triangle of Calot

Whichever technique is preferred, once countertraction is in place, infundibular traction must be roughly at right angles to the new position of the gallbladder bed—that is, laterally, down, and forward. This is the key to a safe dissection. Beginners tend to neglect the left hand, which manipulates the infundibulum. Deprived of a three-dimensional view, this helps to replace the unconscious movements of the surgeon's head, which are used to see on all sides of the gallbladder in an open procedure.

The Easy Case

The cystic lymph node is identified if possible. Dissection starts at the junction of gallbladder and cystic duct staying just to the (anatomic) right of the node. With upward and outward traction of the infundibulum, the inferior peritoneal leaf is incised with scissors or hook diathermy from close to the gallbladder to the site of the peritoneal reflection on the liver. This is carried as far laterally as possible, freeing both peritoneal and areolar attachments. With downward and outward traction, the superior peritoneal leaf is similarly incised (Fig. 26–2) and the plane of separation further developed. At

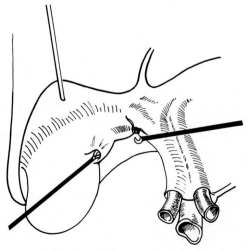

Figure 26–2. The superior peritoneal leaf is incised as far up as possible onto the liver (French exposure).

each cut, the infundibulum lifts out further, displaying the triangle and its contents. If conditions are ideal, a window is created between the infundibulum–presumed cystic duct and the liver. The scissors or hook in cannula No. 2 is replaced with a curved dissector, and the cleft between the cystic duct and the artery is developed by spreading the jaws first at right angles to, then along the axis of, the duct. If done gently, the small branches of the artery to the duct can be demonstrated and coagulated before they snap. If this happens, bleeding will stop with local pressure. The space between the artery and liver is then precisely dissected and the artery is gently skeletonized. Its course directly to the gallbladder must be confirmed before any further damage to it is contemplated. If the dissection has started right on the infundibulum, the cystic artery proper—that is, a vessel 1 mm or more in diameter—is not commonly seen, but smaller branches traverse this space. Those that are the diameter of the hook itself are best coagulated, as the application of clips to small vessels is merely a prelude to them falling off later. The hook gently skeletonizes each branch by being stroked behind the vessel, preferably with the tip in view. The vessel is then loosely tented away from the surrounding structures and coagulated over several millimeters. This should not be done under excessive tension or with too high a diathermy setting, as the vessel is likely to be divided and will rapidly retract. In the event of an arterial bleeding episode, direct pressure on the bleeding site with the flat of the hook or scissor (closed!) is the best immediate action. This is maintained for a few minutes while the sucker is positioned in cannula No. 3, if it is not already there. The spot can be irrigated and, if safe, precisely coagulated with the elbow or very tip of the hook.

The sheath of peritoneal, lymphatic, and fatty tissue around the cystic duct is stripped sharply or bluntly toward its junction with the common hepatic duct to a point at which the cystic duct just begins to flare. This represents the junction itself, or the site at which the cystic duct will run behind or parallel to the common duct, and dissection need proceed no further. If the surgeon must expose the junction, a good deal more dissection will be required if the cystic duct is long. There is no good reason to do this routinely. Dissection near the common bile duct may cause bleeding, the control of which increases the risk of injury to the duct wall either by electrocautery burn, devascularization, or mechanical effect. About 10 to 15 mm of exposed cystic duct makes for comfortable cholangiography, although it is possible with less. A site for opening the duct is selected on its upper anterior aspect and is spot coagulated with diathermy. Bleeding from the small vessel that runs in the wall is often hard to distinguish from bile and can obscure the opening, making cannulation more difficult.

A cystic artery of greater than 1 mm in diameter should now be divided between two firmly applied titanium clips (see Fig. 26–2). Double clipping the proximal side of the artery is unnecessary if the clips are secured well, as application of a second clip may dislodge the first. Ideally, the tip of each clip should be visible and observed to close before its body is finally squeezed. Disposable appliers containing up to 20 clips shorten this procedure but are a luxury, especially if fired only three to five times in the procedure. With division of the artery, the triangle of Calot loses a boundary, but the window necessary for safe cholecystectomy is now wide open and the infundibulum will hang freely on a pedicle containing only the cystic duct.

Division of the artery prior to cholangiography facilitates cannulation of the cystic duct, which can be stretched and positioned more effectively than with the artery intact but is only reasonable provided anatomic identification is satisfactory. It carries the further advantage that if a clip is poorly applied and impinges on the biliary tree, it will be visible on the films. Conversely, when there is genuine doubt as to the identity of a tubular structure thought to be the artery, it is better to perform the cholangiogram first, assuming adequate identification of the cystic duct. Prior to disposing of the applicator, a clip is also placed across the origin of the cystic duct at the infundibulum.

Operative Cholangiography

Operative cholangiography is described in detail elsewhere in this volume, and it is not proposed to discuss the indications or technique in detail here. Suffice it to say, it has been our practice to attempt operative cystic duct cholangiography routinely except in patients who have undergone successful preoperative endoscopic sphincterotomy. This is for two reasons. First, this most resembles our routine in open cholecystectomy. Second, it is an essential technique to master if we are to develop laparoscopic exploration of the common bile duct.[20]

In brief, a transverse opening in the cystic duct (Fig. 26–3) generous enough to allow introduction of the cholangiography catheter is

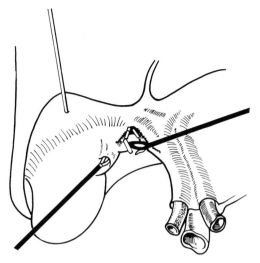

Figure 26–3. A short incision is made in the cystic duct, which is then milked from the common duct toward the ductotomy to expel any calculi.

made through cannula No. 2 with scissors, which are then replaced with a narrow-tipped grasper. The cystic duct is milked from the bile duct toward the opening. If a calculus is present in the accessible portion of the duct, bile will not drip from the opening until the calculus is expelled. Difficulty with cannulation may be due to an impacted stone but is more likely due to mucosal valves.

The narrow grasper in cannula No. 2 (in the surgeon's right hand) retracts the infundibulum to the right to keep the duct on stretch, and a duct cannulation forceps (Olsen forceps, Karl Storz, Tutlingen, Germany) loaded with a saline-purged ureteric catheter (No. 4 or No. 5 French) is advanced through cannula No. 3. The axes of the forceps and the duct are then aligned. Cannulation of the duct is more easily performed by the dominant hand of a surgeon standing between the legs, although with practice, a right-handed surgeon can learn to manipulate the forceps with his or her left hand, and orient the duct with the right hand. Left-handed surgeons are at a rare advantage, although both will remain at the mercy of the mucosal valves. Contrast injections proceed in the normal way and, assuming the cholangiogram is satisfactory, the catheter and forceps are removed and the graspers are replaced in their usual positions. It should be noted that incorrect interpretation of abnormal cholangiograms was a common associated feature of ductal injuries. Lack of filling of the upper ducts must be interpreted as an abnormality and action taken to determine the cause.

This does not mean that the procedure must be converted to open surgery, although some operators will only feel comfortable with this option. Laparoscopic removal of incorrectly placed hemostatic clips may correct the radiographic abnormality and allow assessment of duct wall damage (this is a point in favor of clipping the cystic artery before cholangiography in an uncomplicated case).

Cholangiography can be associated with a ductal injury. In one of our recent cases, what was thought to be the cystic duct wall was incised for a cholangiogram before it became apparent that it was the common duct. Mindful of the reported experience of others,[21] it was possible to repair this laparoscopically around a narrow latex T tube with no subsequent complication.

Management of a ductal calculus identified at cholangiography is discussed elsewhere in this volume. Beware that a liberal policy of endoscopic retrograde cholangiopancreatography (ERCP) and endoscopic sphincterotomy will ensure that the surgeon will not garner the experience in laparoscopic choledochotomy and transcystic bile duct exploration that is necessary to offer these confidently as options.

Completion of the Dissection

If the operative cholangiogram is satisfactory, the cystic duct is clipped doubly on the remaining side and divided (Fig. 26–4). Removal of the gallbladder from its bed is then accomplished exactly as in open surgery, using a combination of sharp, blunt, and electrocautery

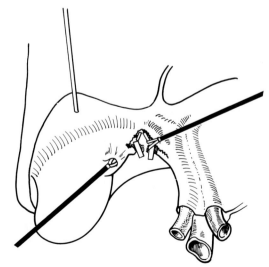

Figure 26–4. The cystic duct is divided between clips, two of which are applied on the proximal side.

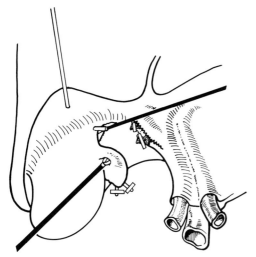

Figure 26–5. Electrocautery scissor dissection considerably speeds removal of the gallbladder from its bed (French exposure).

dissection. With confidence, this process can be sped up using electrocautery scissors (Fig. 26–5), with the usual proviso of staying close to the gallbladder wall and leaving a fringe of peritoneal coat on the liver to facilitate hemostasis.

The More Difficult Case

Dissection is relatively straightforward if the tissues are supple and uninflamed. In the presence of induration or inflammation, conditions rapidly deteriorate if hemostasis, frequently difficult under these circumstances, is not maintained. As tissues become blood-stained, a near-perfect video image progressively degrades as the camera's CCD chip struggles with an overload of reflected light wavelengths in the red band. In addition, the infundibular grasper will frequently slip off and inevitably punch a hole in the gallbladder wall. As in open surgery, the more recent the inflammation, the less difficult is the dissection.[22]

If the gallbladder is tense and distended, it should be decompressed by direct needle puncture of the fundus through the abdominal wall. Aspirated white bile or pus should be cultured. If the puncture is reasonably watertight, the gallbladder is washed out with several exchanges of saline and the needle is removed having gathered a good piece of fundus around the puncture with a grasper. Thickening of the gallbladder will now determine whether the 5-mm instruments are too pointed to avoid tearing a hole in its wall. If so, depending on the

retraction method used, now is the time to substitute one of the 5-mm cannulas for a 10-mm cannula. This will allow a heavier instrument that can distribute the load through its jaws over a wider area and hopefully avoid perforation.

Dissection in the Presence of Acute and Chronic Inflammation

Adequate retraction of the infundibulum is the key to safe dissection of the triangle of Calot. This can only be obtained with a grasper that will not slip off and is suited to the thickness of the gallbladder wall. The same rules as in open surgery apply. No structure is divided until its identity is confirmed anatomically. Dissection should proceed parallel to the presumed structures in the pedicle of the gallbladder until a firm identification is made. Diathermy creates smoke, which coats the end of the laparoscope, necessitating frequent removal and cleaning. Constant suction to clear smoke or blood eliminates the pneumoperitoneum and thus visibility unless the insufflator provides a very high gas flow. Blunt dissection by spreading dissector jaws or scissors must be performed gently and patiently.

Finding the plane of cleavage between gallbladder and liver is the next important step. Diathermy coagulation alters tissue color and texture so that the initial sight of the correct plane may be obscured. Moreover, effective diathermy dissection requires the use of the high-current density that is provided by a narrow-pointed instrument, which tends to puncture the gallbladder wall if it strays. For this reason, the best instrument is a pair of large, curved, round-tipped endoscopic scissors, which require a 10/11-mm cannula.[23] The scissors can be used to spread tissues and cut. In addition, if electrically insulated, precise electrocoagulation is possible using the tip with the blades closed to prolong instrument life.

If patience and reasonable persistence fail to define the anatomy, or if it is impossible to confidently identify a structure without damaging it, an orthograde, "fundus first," approach as in open surgery is possible. Some surgeons use this routinely to free the fundus from its liver attachments at the end of an uncomplicated cholecystectomy (Salky, personal communication). If performed for anatomic difficulty, the dissection may be more bloody, as the cystic artery should not have been divided. The sucker or a grasper passed through cannula No. 3

elevates the liver at the fundus and a grasper through cannula No. 4 provides downward traction on the fundus, enabling dissection of the plane between each side of the gallbladder and the liver. This dissection is carried toward the infundibulum, staying close to the gallbladder wall, until a pedicle containing only the cystic duct can be defined.

When to Convert to Laparotomy

Assuming a degree of expertise in laparoscopic surgery, except when there are anesthetic contraindications to positive pressure pneumoperitoneum, it is logical to commence even potentially difficult cases with a diagnostic laparoscopy to assess the feasibility of completing the cholecystectomy laparoscopically. The surgeon will be guided only by experience gained in previous difficult cases. Clearly, if the complexity of the problems encountered is well in excess of anything the surgeon has experienced in the past, prompt conversion is the wisest option. The following comments are not intended as hard and fast rules but simply as a guide for those who have not amassed a lot of experience. Therefore, consider conversion if

1. At first sight the gallbladder is surrounded by very dense inflammatory adhesions that are difficult to take down and hemorrhage may result.

2. The gallbladder is contracted, buried deeply in the liver substance.

3. No progress has been made in exposing the cystic duct or artery over 20 to 30 minutes.

4. A gallbladder carcinoma is suspected.

5. There is no filling of the upper ducts on the operative cholangiogram. (Beware when patients have had a preoperative endoscopic sphincterotomy; filling of the upper biliary tree in these patients needs to be encouraged by pressure occlusion of the common duct during contrast injection).

6. The patient will not tolerate positive pressure pneumoperitoneum even when reduced, and other anesthetic manipulations are unsuccessful.

7. Venous cavernoma of the portal vein is present. It is a rare but very hazardous abnormality that may be encountered during any cholecystectomy and occurred once during our series, prompting immediate conversion. Massive transfusion and abdominal packing were ultimately necessary for control. Positive pressure pneumoperitoneum may reduce the apparent size of these vessels so that severe or persistent bleeding from tissues that do not ordinarily bleed may be the only clue. In this case, unless irrevocably committed (cystic artery ligation, gallbladder perforation), deferral of the operation until this abnormality has been fully worked up or excluded is advised.

Vigorous bleeding from the main trunk or a branch of the cystic artery, although dramatic, should not prompt immediate conversion. Local pressure, irrigation, and patience will usually allow the bleeding vessel to be identified and controlled with precision. Clearly, if despite adequate exposure, irrigation, and suction, the hematoma is expanding, conversion is warranted.

The Role of Minilaparotomy

Exposure of the essential structures for a safe cholecystectomy is surprisingly good through the short, high, transverse incision of a minilaparotomy. Depending on the reason for conversion, this option, which needs to be in the armamentarium of any surgeon who performs minimally invasive biliary surgery, should be considered.

Once the peritoneal cavity is opened, dissection starts at the fundus and proceeds toward the pedicle, freeing the gallbladder from its bed. If the conversion is for hemorrhage, a pack can be placed at the appropriate site to compress the bleeding vessel prior to beginning the dissection. Hemostasis is usually then a simple matter when the gallbladder is on a pedicle.

Avoidance of Bile Duct Injury

If indeed there is a major increase in ductal injuries, why is this not well reflected in the published series? Ironically the radiographic appearance of a dilated duct above a cluster of surgical clips on the ERCP in a patient with a biliary fistula following LC illustrates a good use for such radiopaque markers. Useful analysis of a series of duct injuries referred to a single center was enhanced by the videotape available in 9 of the 12 cases documented.[24] Visualization of the bile duct by ERCP and video replay of the injury permitted precise identification of its mechanism, which in two thirds of cases consisted of mistaking the common duct for the cystic duct, resection of part of the common and hepatic ducts, and a right hepatic artery injury. Thermal injury is a potent cause of duct wall injury, although the precise mechanism is not always clear. In five of six cases, laser was the energy source used in a series of duct injuries referred for management, suggesting that laser use may be associated with a higher incidence of such injury.[25] Weeks or months may elapse before a stricture manifests itself.[26] Even intraperitoneal bile collections can present late, although inordinate diffuse postoperative abdominal pain is usually present. The most worrisome conclusion, consistent with all other series, is that the injury will probably not be recognized intraoperatively, especially if cholangiography is omitted. Conversely, the performance of an operative cholangiogram provides no guarantee that a ductal injury will be avoided, the most common mistake being to assume that nonfilling of the upper biliary tree is due to something other than iatrogenic occlusion. Hence, the single most important principle in avoiding ductal injury is a *confident anatomic identification of the cystic duct–gallbladder junction prior to ligation or division of any structure.* This will depend on the correctness of the technique of exposure and dissection employed. Moreover, visualization but *not* dissection of the cystic duct–common duct junction and a dissection that is carried away from the gallbladder and toward the common duct are important additional safety measures.[24]

The first 13 cases that a surgeon performs seem to be at highest risk, with an incidence of ductal injury of 2%, dropping to 0.1% thereafter for an overall rate of 0.5%.[27] A rate of 0.1% is consistent with the best reported series in open surgery and could be considered a reasonable if not perfect target when all presenting pathologic conditions are taken into account.

These and other findings suggest that to reduce the risks of ductal injury and other hazards in hospitals in which LC is performed, the following principles could be used to develop local credentialing requirements. Beginners should

- Learn to find their way around in a videoscopic environment and, following a period of bench training, should assist an experienced laparoscopist
- Learn camera operating techniques
- Be assisted in the first 12 to 15 cases by an experienced colleague, especially during dissection of the cystic duct
- Select uncomplicated gallstone cases until good operative proficiency and confidence is acquired—for example, after the first 25 cases
- Learn and practice the technique of laparoscopic cholangiography, be proficient in inter-

pretation of the images obtained, and be prepared to convert to open surgery if an unexpected abnormality is unexplained
- Keep a videotaped record of each case early in the learning period; review the tape after each case with an experienced colleague and ask for advice

Specific practices and techniques that may help to reduce ductal injury have been elaborated elegantly by Hunter.[28] Although we have found no particular advantage to using a 30° laparoscope as he advocates, we would agree that correct traction on the gallbladder fundus and infundibulum to present the cystic duct safely so that dissection commences at its junction with the infundibulum, as well as routine fluoroscopic cholangiography, are ways of avoiding mishaps.

Management of the Cystic Duct Stump

Under normal circumstances the duct is doubly clipped just proximal to the ductotomy and is divided. This is safe if the tips of each clip extend just beyond the edge of the compressed duct and the ductal tissue is uninflamed and resilient. If the duct is thickened and inflamed, it is ligated proximally using an intra- or extracorporeal knotting technique prior to division. This is preferred if a voluminous stomach, duodenum, or omentum are likely to obscure the duct should traction be released. Alternatively, the duct is temporarily clipped, divided, and then secured proximal to the clip with a loop of absorbable material. Indeed a case could be made for routine thread ligation of the cystic duct in view of the frequency of leakage from the cystic duct stump following LC.[29, 30]

Extraction of Stones and Gallbladder

Once the cholecystectomy is completed, extraction of the gallbladder can be a frustratingly lengthy business if the stones are large or numerous or if the gallbladder wall is thickened. A wise precaution in difficult cases is to introduce an extraction bag early on in the procedure to collect stones that spill from a rent in the gallbladder wall. A number are available commercially, but the most useful are self-opening, which facilitates the "arcade game style" exercise that placing stones or a bulky gallbladder becomes.

Our initial routine for large calculi was to perform lithotripsy with the gallbladder in situ,[31-33] thoroughly washing the lumen of the organ so that any subsequent spillage was of minimal consequence. It soon became apparent that this was a time-consuming procedure that could be achieved just as well once the gallbladder was available at an extraction orifice. A narrow-tipped, toothed clamp such as a Kocher forceps is easily introduced into the gallbladder through the infundibulum available at the skin surface, secured at the skin, and incised to open the orifice enough to allow fragments of stone to be extracted. The teeth help to grab calculi that tend to slip out of the jaws, and the instrument itself is solid enough to allow forceful crushing of hard stones.

Initial experience with a high-speed mechanical lithotripter (Laparolith, Endomedics, Los Angeles, CA) analogous to a shielded domestic whisk has been encouraging. The gallbladder is filled with saline through the hollow shaft of the instrument inserted through the gallbladder neck. We have found that the inertia of very large, smooth stones (>2 cm diameter) seems to prevent them from being lured into the fluid vortex created by the propellor, and these stones need to be broken into smaller, irregular fragments for the device to work. This should be used without an extraction bag technique only if the wall of the gallbladder is sound and undamaged by disease or dissection. At the first sign of difficulty during the cholecystectomy, and especially if the gallbladder wall is damaged during the dissection, we opt to use an extraction bag.

Drainage, Removal of Cannulas, and Closure

The subhepatic and infradiaphragmatic spaces are carefully irrigated with saline and any stone fragments are removed. If any liver parenchyma has been exposed during the dissection, if there is ooze from the gallbladder bed, if the gallbladder was inflamed, or if the procedure was difficult and prolonged, a No. 8 or No. 10 French suction drain is fed into the subhepatic space through one of the 5-mm cannulas on the right side. The end with side holes should be trimmed to length first;[34] a clamp on the extremity of the drain will prevent a sudden gas leak.

The head-up position of the patient is reversed and any blood or irrigant is aspirated from above the liver. The cannula puncture sites are inspected from inside for bleeding. If all is well, insufflation is terminated and the pneumoperitoneum deflated from as many of the 10-mm cannulas as there are hands to go around. Many surgeons insist on meticulous evacuation of all gas, citing it as a contributor to postoperative pain, although it is hard to understand the mechanism of this given the free solubility of carbon dioxide. Assuming normal coagulation, persistent bleeding from a puncture merits attention, either by a direct approach from the skin or with traction hemostasis using a small Foley balloon catheter, which is removed in the recovery room 2 to 3 hours later.

An attempt should be made to close the main musculofascial layer of the 10-mm incisions with a strong (1-0 or 2-0) absorbable stitch. Small right-angle retractors and thread loaded onto a stout, narrow-diameter (15 mm or less), half-circle–eyed needle will facilitate this process.

The wound itself should be irrigated if particulate matter or bile has contaminated it prior to closure with subcuticular absorbable sutures and adhesive strips.

Management of Complications

Intraoperative

Visceral injury by a direct mechanical effect such as a Verres needle stab at insufflation or inadvertent puncture or laceration from a pointed instrument can be managed with simple laparoscopic inversion or repair, assuming adequate suturing skills. The advantage of preoperative mechanical bowel preparation is obvious should the injury be in the colon.

Diathermy burns often are not obvious and may only become manifested later. Every effort must be made to avoid unintended current application by ensuring that the instrument is never activated out of the observed field. Electrical insulation of instruments becomes defective with sterilization, abrasion in metal cannulas, and contact with other instruments. If arcing occurs away from the active tip, the instrument must be changed immediately and repaired. Particular attention should be paid during dissection close to the bile duct when monopolar current is used. We prefer to perform most cystic duct dissection without diathermy, which is reserved for accurate coagulation of fine, individually displayed vessels, which are observed to poach and divide with short bursts at high current density.

Postoperative

On rare occasions, it is necessary to return a patient to the operating room, either to deal with suspected hemorrhage or a hollow visceral leak, usually biliary. The latter may be suggested by marked abdominal (nonwound) tenderness with peritonism, fever, leukocytosis, and elevated levels of serum alkaline phosphatase and bilirubin on the first or second postoperative day. It is quite feasible to manage this laparoscopically and, at least initially, for diagnostic purposes. A 10-mm incision is reopened, the little finger is inserted into the peritoneal cavity and swept in an arc to free any adherent structures, a securing stitch is placed to reduce gas leaks, a 10-mm cannula is inserted, and insufflation is commenced directly as in open laparoscopy.

We have observed a small number of patients with severe abdominal pain (when compared with the norm after laparoscopy) on the first postoperative day, as well as tenderness, tachycardia, and sweating, without elevation of the bilirubin or alkaline phosphatase level, who responded to symptomatic treatment with no complicating sequelae. Initially we investigated this syndrome with diagnostic laparoscopy and found no bile leak, so we later treated similar presentations expectantly with antiinflammatory suppositories (indomethacin). However, we would not advise expectant management as a routine; a clear diagnostic laparoscopy has minimal morbidity and is very reassuring for surgeon and patient alike.

Intraabdominal abscesses can be opened, irrigated, and drained laparoscopically. The frequent finding of calculous debris in the fluid obtained suggests that lost stones are less innocuous than sometimes thought. Ultrasound-guided drainage of intraabdominal collections is another option that we have used on three occasions.

The most common complication of LC is wound inflammation or infection. This is clearly not as serious as infection of the long incision of an open cholecystectomy and in our series has been exclusively managed by suture or tape removal, probing, and drainage without further surgery. It is not uncommon for gallstone fragments to be found during this toilet.

On one occasion we have had to repair an incisional hernia at the lateral border of the rectus, the position of cannula No. 2 (10 mm), about a year after the initial operation, hence, our insistence on careful closure of the larger punctures.

Role of Assistant

Laparoscopic surgery is changing our notions of operative technique. Whereas in open surgery it is good practice for the surgeon to maintain a constant view of the operative field and exchange instruments blindly in an outstretched hand, in videoscopic surgery the extra- and intraocular muscles and head position of the surgeon are replaced by the hand controlling the camera and laparoscope. The quality of the screen image and thus what the operator can see is the direct responsibility of the camera operator. Apart from actually requesting a specific camera adjustment, the control over the displayed image depends on the understanding between surgeon and camera operator. Alternatively, if sufficiently mobile, the operative target can be physically moved into the center of the picture. Hence, the necessity for the surgeon to maintain a constant view of the operative field is reduced, allowing greater reliance on a self-service approach to instrument choice. It is conceivable that the total number of personnel (P) scrubbed for a laparoscopic procedure need not depend on its complexity but on the number (N) of mobile (*i.e.,* nonfixed) cannulas used: $P \approx N \div 2$.

CONCLUSION

Once mastered, laparoscopic cholecystectomy is an elegant and logical technique for the management of gallstones. It is clear that what initially were thought to be contraindications to the procedure (cholecystitis, anticoagulant therapy, pregnancy, and so on) are now being managed confidently and safely by laparoscopy. It becomes apparent with this evolution that even more is possible, but progress will be hampered by complications. It has been shown that the rate of bile duct injury diminishes significantly after the early surgical apprenticeship. As surgeons take on more difficult cases, it is not unreasonable to expect an increase in the number of complications. Ideally, the nature of these complications should be related to the pathologic condition encountered rather than the surgical technique employed. Intelligent preparation of the patient both medically and mentally, meticulous attention to detail during the operative steps of the procedure, clear anatomic and radiologic identification of vital structures, and prompt conversion to laparotomy if difficulties well beyond the experience of the operator are encountered will guarantee the safety margin demanded in what is surgery for benign disease.

References

1. Calot F. De la cholécystectomie (ablation de la vésicule biliaire). Doctoral thesis presented at the University of Paris, December 12, 1890.

2. Rocko JM, Di Gioia JM. Calot's triangle revisited. Surg Gynecol Obstet 153:410–414, 1981.

3. Dubois F, Icard P, Berthelot G, et al. Coelioscopic cholecystectomy: preliminary report of 36 cases. Ann Surg 191:271–275, 1990.

4. McKernan JB. Laparoscopic cholecystectomy. Am Surg 57(5):309–312, 1991.

5. Reddick EJ, Olsen DO. Laparoscopic laser cholecystectomy. A comparison with mini-lap cholecystectomy. Surg Endosc 3:131–133, 1989.

6. Collet D, Crozat T, Alhi S. Incidents et complications de la cholecystectomie coelioscopique. L'enquête de la SFCERO. Lyon Chir 87(6):463–466, 1991.

7. Cuschieri A, Dubois F, Mouiel J, et al. The European experience with laparoscopic cholecystectomy. Am J Surg 161:385–387, 1991.

8. Pezet D, Fondinier N, Rotman N, et al. Partial seeding of carcinoma of the gallbladder after laparoscopic cholecystectomy. Br J Surg 79(3):230, 1992.

9. McKernan JB, Laws H. Laparoscopic cholecystectomy in the presence of cholecystoduodenal fistula. Submitted for presentation at the Third World Congress of Endoscopic Surgery, Bordeaux, June 1992.

10. Fitzgerald S, Bailey P, Liebscher G, Andrus C. Laparoscopic cholecystectomy in anticoagulated patients. Surg Endosc 5:166–169, 1991.

11. Collet D, Edye M, Magne E, et al. Laparoscopic cholecystectomy in the obese patient. Surg Endosc 6:186–188, 1992.

12. Unger SW, Scott JS, Unger HM, Edelman DS. Laparoscopic approach to gallstones in the morbidly obese patient. Surg Endosc 5:116–117, 1991.

13. Arvidsson D, Gerdin E. Laparoscopic cholecystectomy during pregnancy. Surg Laparosc Endosc 1:193–194, 1991.

14. Soper NJ, Hunter JG, Petrie RH. Laparoscopic cholecystectomy during pregnancy. Surg Endosc 6:115–117, 1992.

15. Davidoff AM, Branum GD, Murray EA, et al. The technique of laparoscopic cholecystectomy in children. Ann Surg 215(2):186–191, 1992.

16. Cruse P, Foord R. The epidemiology of wound infection: a 10 year prospective study of 62,939 wounds. Surg Clin North Am 60:27–47, 1980.

17. Fitzgibbons RJ, Schmid S, Santoscoy R, et al. Open laparoscopy for laparoscopic cholecystectomy. Surg Laparosc Endosc 4:216–222, 1991.

18. Grace PA, Leahy A, McEntee G, Bouchier-Hayes D. Laparoscopic cholecystectomy in the scarred abdomen. Surg Endosc 5:118–120, 1991.

19. Reddick EJ, Olsen D, Spaw A, et al. Safe performance of difficult laparoscopic cholecystectomies. Am J Surg 161:377–381, 1991.

20. Berci G. Biliary ductal anatomy and anomalies: the role of intraoperative cholangiography during laparoscopic cholecystectomy. Surg Clin North Am 72(5):1069–1075, 1992.

21. Lepsien G, Lüdtke FE, Neufang T, et al. Treatment of iatrogenic common bile duct injury during laparoscopic cholecystectomy through laparoscopic insertion of a T-tube stent. Surg Endosc 5:119–122, 1991.

22. Fletcher DR, Jones RM, O'Riordan B, Hardy K. Laparoscopic cholecystectomy for complicated gallstone disease. Surg Endosc 6:179–182, 1992.

23. Hugh TB, Li B. Scissor dissection technique for laparoscopic cholecystectomy: an alternative to laser and electrocautery. Aust NZ J Surg 62:738–740, 1992.

24. Davidoff AM, Pappas TN, Murray EA, et al. Mechanisms of major bile duct injury during laparoscopic cholecystectomy. Ann Surg 215(3):196–202, 1992.

25. Moosa AR, Easter DW, van Sonnenberg E, et al. Laparoscopic injuries to the bile duct. Ann Surg 215(3):203–208, 1992.

26. Cheslyn-Curtis S, Emberton M, Ahmed H, et al. Bile duct injury following laparoscopic cholecystectomy. Br J Surg 79(3):231–232, 1992.

27. Southern Surgeons Club. A prospective analysis of 1518 laparoscopic cholecsytectomies. N Engl J Med 324(16): 1073–1078, 1991.

28. Hunter JG. Avoidance of bile duct injury during laparoscopic cholecystectomy. Am J Surg 162(7):71–76, 1991.

29. Collet D, Edye M, Périssat J. Complications and conversions of laparoscopic cholecystectomy: a report of the French Association of Endoscopic Surgeons and Interventional Radiologists SFCERO. Surg Endosc 7:334–338, 1993

30. Ralph-Edwards T, Himal T. Bile leak after laparoscopic cholecystectomy. Surg Endosc 6:33–35, 1992.

31. Périssat J, Belliard R, Collet D. Lithiase vésiculaire. Lithotritie interne sous laparoscopie. Technique personnelle. Chirurgie 115:140–141, 1989.

32. Périssat J, Collet D, Belliard R. Gallstones: laparoscopic treatment—cholecystectomy, cholecystostomy, and lithotripsy. Our own technique. Surg Endosc 1:1–5, 1990.

33. Périssat J, Collet DR, Belliard R. Gallstones: laparoscopic treatment, intracorporeal lithotripsy followed by cholecystostomy or cholecystectomy—a personal technique. Endoscopy 21:373–374, 1989.

34. Zucker KA, Bailey RW, Flowers J. Laparoscopic management of acute and chronic cholecystitis. Surg Clin North Am 72(5):1045–1067, 1992.

27

Laparoscopic Approaches to the Common Bile Duct

Edward H. Phillips

BACKGROUND

The application of video endoscopic techniques to gallbladder and biliary surgery is a recent development, and the field is still evolving rapidly. Continued development and improvements in instrumentation enable the endoscopist–surgeon to deal more creatively and successfully with many different intraabdominal conditions.

Initial efforts in biliary laparoscopic surgery focused mainly on gallbladder removal and safety issues.[1-3] With the performance of more procedures and refinement of laparoscopic skills, a broadened range of clinical applications has emerged. Now patients with acute cholecystitis,[4] those who have had prior abdominal surgery, and individuals with common bile duct (CBD) stones are managed with laparoscopic techniques. Since CBD stones occur in at least 10% of patients undergoing laparoscopic cholecystectomy (LC), any approach to biliary stone disease must take these patients into account.[5, 6]

From a historical point of view, new modalities for treating cholelithiasis and choledocholithiasis have appeared in rapid succession, including endoscopic retrograde cholangiopancreatography (ERCP) and endoscopic sphincterotomy (ES), intracorporeal and extracorporeal lithotripsy, and dissolution of stones with medications and chemical solvents. The role of these newly developed therapies in relation to surgical common bile duct exploration (CBDE), and their relation to each other, is still evolving.[9-12] With the widespread adoption of laparoscopic techniques for cholecystectomy, various strategies have been attempted or proposed to combine these different modalities in the safest and most efficient manner. Yet there is little randomized prospective data or experience on which to base such clinical decisions. For instance, some have recommended preoperative ERCP with ES if CBD stones are suspected. In other situations, postoperative ES has been advised.[6, 13]

To deal with the problem of CBD stones, our institution has also considered various strategies to integrate ERCP and ES with LC. Unfortunately, preoperative prediction of CBD stones is less accurate than hoped.[11, 14] Routine preoperative ERCP and ES would result in a 40% to 70% rate of normal studies, and thus unnecessary preoperative endoscopic procedures with resultant morbidity and expense. Our attempts to perform intraoperative ES were discouraging because of the markedly increased technical complexity and the logistic difficulty in coordinating the proper personnel and equipment. In addition, adverse clinical outcomes convinced us to seek a better approach.

Postoperative ERCP-ES in those patients found to have CBD stones at LC has become a commonly chosen option and, if successful, avoids the abdominal incision. However, it adds another procedure and has the potential for added morbidity, as well as for failure. Failure of ES in this setting, of course, could lead to open CBDE, and thus a third major procedure for such patients. This would hardly be an improvement on traditional methods.

Techniques and equipment currently used in urologic surgery—specifically serial ureteral dilators and the flexible ureteroscope—as well as our experience in flexible choledochoscopy in open surgery, encouraged us to apply flexible choledochoscopic techniques to the problem of CBD stones encountered during LC.[15] By performing flexible endoscopy of the CBD during open CBDE, surgeons wishing to develop their laparoscopic skills can make a smooth transition from open surgical technique to the laparoscopic approach.[16–18]

Our group has performed more than 950 LCs. During LC, as in open cholecystectomy, we perform routine intraoperative cholangiography (IOC). In the laparoscopic approach, routine IOC helps prevent injury to the CBD and better defines the biliary anatomy.[5, 7] To avoid excisional CBD injuries, we recommend that a cholangiogram be obtained routinely before any tubular structures are divided. In addition to the beneficial anatomic information this study yields for the LC itself, the presence of CBD stones can also be assessed. Performing IOC can be technically difficult at first, which has delayed its initial acceptance. As more surgeons gain experience and confidence with LC, however, use of routine cholangiography is likely to increase. Since we perform routine IOC, we have had to develop several approaches to the management of CBD stones encountered during LC.

We saw an 11% incidence of CBD stones in our patients undergoing LC.[8] This is consistent with an ample body of data from previous surgical experience. Additionally, routine use of cholangiography has disclosed the presence of CBD stones in 4% of our patients who had no clinical or laboratory findings that suggested CBD stones.

Our approach and current techniques for laparoscopic exploration of the CBD, primarily via the transcystic duct (TCD), are explained further on. In the subsequent discussion, various potential management schemes for overall efficiency and safety, based on estimates of total morbidity and mortality, are compared.

TRANSCYSTIC DUCT CHOLEDOCHOSCOPY

The TCD technique offers a "one procedure cures all" approach to CBD stones while avoiding a choledochotomy and the difficulty of suturing laparoscopically. In our technique, a small, flexible endoscope (3.2 mm or smaller) is passed into the CBD through the cystic duct. Stones 8 mm or smaller can be retrieved using wire baskets under direct vision. Larger stones can be fragmented with a pulse-dye laser or electrohydraulic lithotripsy (EHL) and either retrieved with a wire basket or flushed through the ampulla. Because of limitations imposed by the size of the cystic duct, it is sometimes better to proceed to choledochotomy to treat these larger stones. Another limitation of TCD CBDE is the inability to manipulate the choledochoscope into the proximal CBD in approximately 90% of cases (depending on the angle of insertion of the cystic duct on the CBD), limiting the usefulness of this technique to those cases in which stones are in the distal CBD.

Nevertheless, the advantage of this technique is that a T tube is not required, and the cystic duct opening can be closed with the ease of an Endoloop (Ethicon-Endosurgery, Cincinnati, OH). This can also be a disadvantage in cases of cholangitis, postoperative edema of the ampulla, pancreatitis, or multiple stones when decompression of the CBD is indicated. In addition, in cases of retained stones, there is no ready access to the CBD. However, in these complex cases, a latex catheter can be left in the CBD via the cystic duct stump, but it must be secured well with one or two Endoloops. This catheter can also be used for postoperative cholangiography and even percutaneous intervention for retained stones via the established tract.

The TCD approach requires additional instrumentation. A separate mobile cart with all the necessary supplies and equipment facilitates the logistics when a CBD stone is encountered. This cart can also be used as an "emergency" or backup laparoscopy cart. The cart should include a high-definition television monitor, a 300-W xenon light source, an additional camera and controller, a video cassette recorder, balloon dilating catheters, wire baskets, guidewires, and a flexible endoscope. The endoscope should have at least a 1-mm working channel and preferably a 1.2-mm channel. The outer diameter (OD) should be between 2.7 and 3.2 mm, and it should have bidirectional deflection.

Because any patient can have unsuspected CBD stones, trocar location is critical (Fig. 27–1). The most medial subcostal trocar should always be placed in as lateral a position as possible and as close to the costal margin as possible. This facilitates insertion of the scissors for incising the cystic duct and introduction of the cholangiogram catheter. It eventually also provides the best angle of approach for the flexible choledochoscope.

After dissecting the cystic duct and the cystic artery, a "sentinel" clip is placed on the proximal cystic artery, and a clip is placed on the

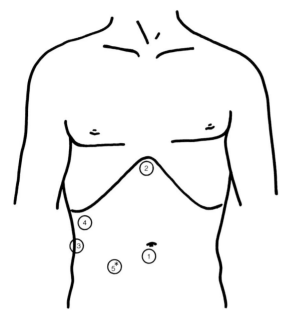

Figure 27–1. Trocar locations for laparoscopic cholecystectomy to facilitate transcystic duct common duct exploration.

junction of the gallbladder with the cystic duct, as high as possible on the gallbladder. A cholangiocatheter or a No. 4 "end hole" ureteral catheter is inserted into the cystic duct and secured in place with a clip or cholangiocatheter clamp, and cinefluoroscopic cholangiography is performed. Although the procedure can be performed solely with static films, we recommend the use of a mobile digital fluoroscopic unit. Considerable time is saved during the cholangiogram, and this equipment greatly facilitates insertion of the guidewires, catheters, and other instruments during CBDE.

If it is difficult to intubate the cystic duct and a better intubation angle is needed, an additional 5-mm trocar should be inserted. This can be used for direct insertion or for a grasper to gently guide the endoscope into the cystic duct. When a stone or stones are seen on intraoperative cholangiography, their number, size, and location should be noted, as well as their relationship to the entrance of the cystic duct into the CBD. The anatomic pattern is studied with particular attention to the entrance of the cystic duct into the CBD. After the cholangiogram is completed, the catheter is removed. If the case is amenable to the cystic duct approach, the cystic duct should be carefully and bluntly dissected down to its junction with the CBD. Occasionally, an additional incision in the cystic duct closer to the CBD will be required. This second incision provides a shorter segment of cystic duct to traverse, which can be dilated

more easily, but enough length must be left for later application of an Endoloop ligature during closure.

The cystic duct must be dilated enough to remove the stones, not just enough to insert the scope. This can be accomplished with sequential bougie-type dilators, but we prefer balloon dilators; they are safer, more effective, and less likely to avulse the cystic duct from the gallbladder. A 0.035-inch floppy-tipped Glidewire (Microvasive, Watertown, MA) is placed inside a balloon catheter capable of dilating to the size of the largest stone but no larger than the inner diameter of the common duct. The balloon catheter and guidewire are placed in a reducing tube that goes from 5 mm to 3 mm. This assembly is inserted through the subcostal trocar, and the guidewire is passed through the cystic duct into the CBD (Fig. 27–2A). The location of the wire must be confirmed by fluoroscopy or a portable x-ray study before passing the balloon catheter over the wire to avoid puncturing the cystic duct or CBD. The balloon is advanced so that a portion of it is still visible outside the incision in the cystic duct.

Using a LeVeen inflator syringe (Microvasive, Watertown, MA) and a pressure gauge, the balloon is inflated with saline to the maximum pressure (12 atm) while the balloon catheter in the cystic duct is observed laparoscopically (Fig. 27–2B). Insufflation is performed slowly and carefully under direct visual monitoring through the laparoscope. If it appears that the cystic duct is beginning to tear, the balloon is deflated and then inflated again more slowly. The cystic duct is dilated to the size of the largest stone to be removed, unless that stone is significantly larger than the 7-mm balloon diameter. In such a situation, we rely on fragmentation or choledochotomy. Once the balloon catheter is maximally inflated, it is left in place for a full 3 minutes. The balloon is then deflated and removed with the guidewire.

A high-resolution video camera is attached to the flexible choledochoscope, which is then inserted freehand into the cystic duct. Although the endoscope can be inserted over a guidewire, this can be more difficult because the working channel of some endoscopes may be eccentric in relation to the scope's cross section. If an additional trocar is inserted, an "atraumatic" grasper can be used to insert the choledochoscope, but care must be taken not to crush the end of the scope.

Once the scope is in the cystic duct, it is advanced into the CBD while irrigation is accomplished using warmed saline through the working channel. In about 10% of cases, the

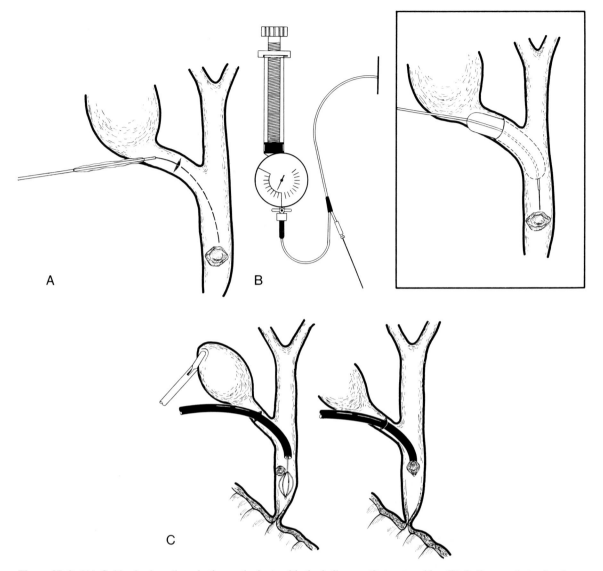

Figure 27–2. (A) Guidewire insertion via the cystic duct, with the balloon catheter as guide. **(B)** Balloon catheter in place in the cystic duct, inflated to 12 atm. One-third of the balloon is visible outside the incision in the cystic duct. **(C)** Endoloop closure of the cystic duct, and a rubber drainage tube in the cystic duct stump, held in place with two Endoloops.

choledochoscope can be passed into the proximal CBD, but usually the angle of approach allows inspection of only the distal portion of the CBD. Deflection of the scope tip can be controlled in either one or two planes; the scope is also steered by twisting its shaft in a torquing motion.

The CBD is explored under direct vision, and the stones are extracted. The stones are captured individually in a straight four-wire basket by advancing the basket beyond the stone, opening the basket, and withdrawing it until the stone is within the basket. The basket is closed around the stone and pulled up against the tip of the scope, which is then withdrawn together with the basket and the stone (Fig. 27–2C). The stones are gathered together for later removal. They can be set on the surface of the liver or stomach or inside an Endopouch (Ethicon-Endosurgery, Cincinnati, OH). This capturing maneuver is repeated until the last stone is removed. A completion cholangiogram is always performed.

Extraction of stones is clearly a skilled team effort requiring effective cooperation among three individuals to accomplish specific maneuvers. Once the operating room team is familiar with the technique, however, it can be a very rewarding procedure for all involved. Team member positions are occasionally changed so that the assistant surgeon stands on the patient's left side and holds the gallbladder–cystic duct junction on slight tension. The surgeon, now on the right side, inserts the preloaded dilating balloon catheter into a reducing tube that goes from 5 mm to 3 mm, and places the tip of the balloon catheter 1 mm from the incision in the cystic duct, so the wire can be seen. The surgeon then instructs the nurse or operating room technician to advance the guidewire. If it is difficult to pass, the nurse goes to the left side of the patient to hold the cystic duct under tension, and the assistant surgeon holds the balloon catheter near the cystic duct opening as the surgeon uses small in-and-out motions with the guidewire until it passes. The surgeon advances the balloon catheter over the wire and positions it in the cystic duct. The nurse or operating room technician inflates the balloon catheter slowly, monitoring the balloon pressure while the surgeon watches the effect of the dilation on the cystic duct. After the cystic duct is dilated, the surgeon inserts the endoscope, holding the shaft of the scope with the left hand to torque, advance, or withdraw it, while the right hand is used on the lever to deflect the tip.

During this part of the procedure, the assistant surgeon must be on the patient's left side controlling the cystic duct by holding it transversely under tension and holding the laparoscope in the left hand. Often it is necessary to intubate the opening at nearly right angles and then swing the duct toward and parallel to the scope so it can be inserted. Occasionally it takes two hands to torque the scope and advance it while the assistant surgeon operates the deflecting lever. Once the endoscope is positioned in the duct and a stone is encountered, the nurse or operating room technician can open and close the wire basket and entrap the stone with verbal guidance from the surgeon.

If the cystic duct cannot be dilated enough to allow insertion of an endoscope, or the cystic duct becomes transected, there are three other TCD techniques to employ. Intraoperative fluoroscopy is crucial for these maneuvers.

1. One milligram of glucagon is administered intravenously, 3 minutes are allowed to pass, and the CBD is forcibly lavaged to flush the stone through the ampulla into the duodenum. This may work with stones 2 mm or smaller and is usually tried before cystic duct dilation.

2. A spiral wire basket with a wire leader can be used fluoroscopically to entrap the stones. Again, the stones must be small enough to be retrieved via the cystic duct. Usually in this situation the surgeon can get an endoscope into the CBD and capture the stones under direct vision, but if an endoscope is lacking, this approach works occasionally (Fig. 27–3).

3. The third technique is controversial but allows clearance of the CBD stones in situations in which only a guidewire can be inserted via the cystic duct. Under fluoroscopic control, the dilating balloon catheter is passed over the guidewire until the radiopaque markers span the ampulla. The pressure is monitored closely while the balloon catheter is slowly dilated with 25% diatrizoate meglumine and diatrizoate sodium (Hypaque). The ampulla must not be dilated larger than the inside diameter of the distal CBD. The balloon catheter is left inflated for at least 3 minutes. The balloon is then deflated and pulled back into the cystic duct, and the CBD is forcibly lavaged. The cholangiogram is repeated (Fig. 27–4).

This last technique has been reported to be associated with a high incidence of pancreatitis when performed in a retrograde manner in association with ERCP. Our group has per-

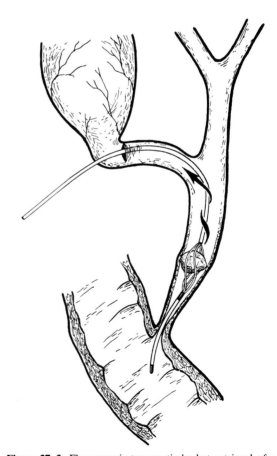

Figure 27–3. Fluoroscopic transcystic basket retrieval of a common bile duct stone.

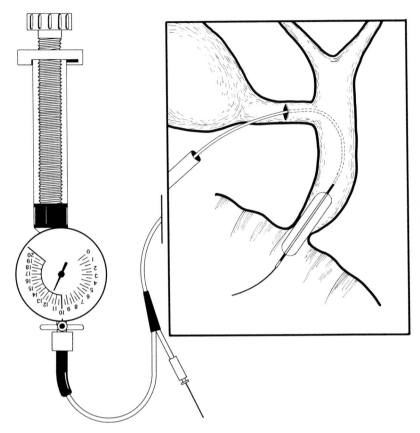

Figure 27–4. Technique of fluoroscopically guided transcystic duct ampullary balloon dilation.

formed it in only 20 cases.[19] Hyperamylasemia occurred 20% of the time, but mild clinical pancreatitis occurred three times (15%), and 1 of these patients had biliary pancreatitis preoperatively. We are closely monitoring the safety of this procedure in the laparoscopic setting. Until more data are available, this technique should be attempted as a last resort when ES is the alternative.

After TCD CBDE and a completion cholangiogram, but before ligating the cystic duct, one may consider placing a tube into the cystic duct to allow CBD decompression if the patient is septic, elderly, or immunocompromised. Such decompression also provides the means to perform a cholangiogram postoperatively. Usually there is no need for a tube, however, and the cystic duct is doubly ligated with polyglactin (Vicryl) or chromic Endoloops, as the cystic duct is usually too thinned from the instrumentation to hold clips (Fig. 27–5). At this point, both the cystic duct and the cystic artery are ligated and divided. The removal of the gallbladder is then completed laparoscopically, as described elsewhere.[1]

A Blake Edwards drain is almost always placed in the subhepatic space and is usually removed the next day. To place this drain, a toothed grasper is inserted through the most lateral of the 5-mm trocars and is then passed directly, in retrograde fashion, into the subxiphoid 10/11-mm trocar. The valve is opened, and the grasper is passed completely through this larger trocar, to grasp the drain. Because CO_2 is lost during this maneuver, the laparoscope should be pulled back into the trocar or removed to avoid burning the bowel. The drain is then pulled back into the abdomen, and the end is withdrawn, together with the 5-mm trocar, through its insertion site. The external end of the drain is clamped, and CO_2 is then insufflated to restore the pneumoperitoneum. The laparoscope is advanced once again. The drain can then be inspected through the laparoscope and positioned in the subhepatic space with a grasper. A skin suture is placed to secure the drain externally.

Postoperatively, the patient is observed for sepsis, bleeding, pancreatitis, or bile leak. These complications will usually occur within the first 24 hours. Postoperative laboratory tests should include a hematocrit determination, liver function tests, and amylase determination. If there is a question of a bile leak, ultrasound is the

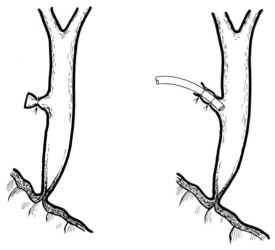

Figure 27–5. Technique of stone capture, opening the wire basket distal to the common bile duct stone, withdrawing the basket with the stone, and pulling the stone basket and choledochoscope out in unison.

best "first test" to look for a fluid collection; occasionally, cholescintigraphy using a derivative of ^{99m}technetium dimethyl iminodiacetic acid (HIDA) is helpful. ERCP is sometimes needed, not only to diagnose a leak but also to place a transampullary stent in association with percutaneous drainage. These steps usually control the leak. Reoperation is rarely necessary.

It is important to remember that in cases of cholangitis, the liver still harbors many bacteria, usually for weeks after the CBD has been cleared. That is why gallbladder and bile specimens should be cultured routinely. Elderly or immunocompromised patients should be administered antibiotics, sometimes for as long as 1 week and occasionally as long as 2 weeks, especially if the CBD is not decompressed. Antibiotics can be given orally on an outpatient basis if the patient is stable.

LAPAROSCOPIC CHOLEDOCHOTOMY

Other techniques for stone removal must be considered if the stone size cannot be reduced to allow withdrawal through the cystic duct, or if there are stones in the proximal ducts that are inaccessible with the choledochoscope using a TCD approach. In such cases, the patient can undergo exploration in the traditional open fashion, or postoperative ES can be planned. This decision should be made in advance, with the patient's participation if possible.

Another option is to proceed with laparoscopic choledochotomy, which provides access for an endoscope to remove stones, a laser fiber or an electrohydraulic probe to fragment them, or even a biopsy forceps to biopsy a tumor. Although this procedure has the advantage of minimally invasive surgery, its main drawback is that a T tube is required when the choledochotomy is closed, which requires considerable laparoscopic suturing and knot tying skills. However, placing a T tube has the advantage of decompressing the CBD while providing access to it postoperatively, should a retained stone be present.

In addition, a standard 8-mm OD flexible choledochoscope can be used via the subxiphoid trocar to explore the duct through a choledochotomy if the CBD is significantly dilated. This obviates the need for an additional endoscope (3.2 mm or less OD) and its smaller optics, working channels, and the more delicate wire baskets required for the TCD technique.

A laparoscopic choledochotomy is also preferred if the stones have to be fragmented with the dye pulse laser or EHL. We are hesitant to use EHL in a nondilated CBD because of potential thermal injury to the walls.[20] Also, when fragmentation is needed, a choledochotomy facilitates better lavage of the debris.

When performing a choledochotomy, the gallbladder should remain in situ so that a grasper, by way of the most lateral trocar, can be placed on it for upward retraction of the liver and the CBD by traction on the cystic duct. This grasper can be fixed to the abdominal wall with a towel clip. An additional 5-mm trocar is placed in the patient's right lower quadrant to accommodate an additional grasper, which will be used to hold a stay suture. The anterior wall of the CBD is exposed with blunt dissection. Two guy sutures of 4–0 chromic on a GU needle are placed on the lateral and medial sides of the CBD through the subxiphoid trocar, and held while the CBD is incised with a microscissors inserted through the anterior axillary line trocar (Fig. 27–6A). Electrocautery or laser should not be used. The length of the incision is kept as short as possible—that is, only large enough to remove the largest stone. This reduces the number of sutures needed later.

A 3- to 5-mm choledochoscope can be used by way of the anterior axillary line trocar, or a larger choledochoscope can be used through the 10-mm subxiphoid trocar to explore the CBD (Fig. 27–6B). The larger scope permits the use of a full-sized Segura wire basket, and stones as large as several centimeters have been removed

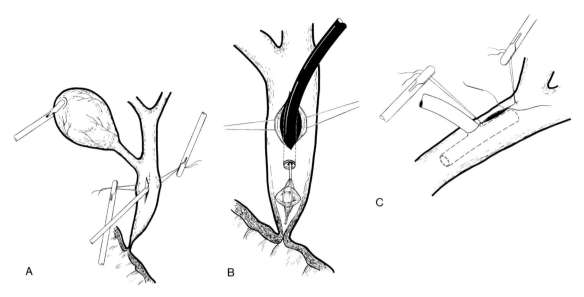

Figure 27–6. (A) Laparoscopic choledochotomy. Graspers are elevating the stay sutures. **(B)** Choledochoscope via choledochotomy, with wire basket stone retrieval. **(C)** Technique of closure of the choledochotomy with a T tube in situ.

in this way. The proximal portions of the biliary tree can also be inspected and cleared, and one can even pass another 1-mm endoscope through the larger scope's working channel to explore the smaller biliary radicles. Irrigation, Fogarty balloons, wire basket stone-capture techniques, or lithotripsy for impacted stones can be used.

After the biliary system is cleared, a T tube must be sewn in place. This is a rather demanding technical feat. The back wall of the T tube is trimmed and the T tube is inserted entirely into the abdominal cavity. The trimmed limb is inserted in the CBD (Fig. 27–6C). Chromic 4–0 or polyglactin laparoscopic sutures are then used to close the choledochotomy. The first suture is placed adjacent to the T tube at the distal end of the choledochotomy. The next suture is placed at the proximal end. Each is held up by a grasper as the others are placed. Intracorporeal knots are safer than extracorporeal knots on the delicate CBD. Suturing can be performed by way of the anterior axillary line or the subxiphoid trocar.

After the T tube is sewn in place, its side arm is brought out through the anterior axillary line trocar, and a completion cholangiogram is performed. If satisfactory, the cystic duct is divided, and the gallbladder is removed. The additional right lower quadrant trocar now serves as a retracting grasper on the gallbladder. Care must be taken not to dislodge the T tube. A subhepatic Blake Edwards drain is also used when a T tube is placed.

Although a more technically difficult procedure than the TCD approach, laparoscopic choledochotomy offers safe access and allows rapid removal of multiple CBD stones. Additionally, a T tube offers postoperative access in case of retained stones. Facility with laparoscopic suturing during CBDE gives the surgeon the future ability to perform laparoscopic choledochoduodenostomy and even Roux-en-Y jejunostomy should a biliary bypass be necessary.

Alternative methods of closing the choledochotomy are being developed, with the hope of eliminating either placement of the T tube or the difficult intracorporeal suturing. Research is under way using fibrin glue, or possibly some synthetic tube material, as a seal. It is premature at present to consider these options.

CLINICAL EXPERIENCE

We began performing LC at our institution in July 1989, and more than 950 cases had been performed as of November 1992. Laparoscopic cholangiography was attempted in all cases but was not accomplished in 11 of the first 100 cases. Since then, however, cholangiography was accomplished in all patients. Approximately 11% of these patients had CBD stones.

Early in our experience, we frequently opted for ERCP-ES or conversion of the laparoscopic procedure to an open CBDE when we found

CBD stones. In 1 patient, suspected CBD stones were successfully removed by preoperative ERCP, and LC was performed subsequently. The inability to accurately assess the presence of CBD stones with preoperative tests severely limited our confidence in the preoperative ERCP approach.

Two attempts at intraoperative ERCP were also disappointing. One attempt was unsuccessful; the other patient successfully underwent ES, but had a complicated postoperative course, with pancreatitis and a pseudocyst requiring percutaneous drainage. Intraoperative ERCP prolonged the surgery considerably. It was logistically very difficult, requiring a skilled endoscopist and the immediate availability of extra equipment. The supine position of the patient on the operating table was yet another complicating factor, since ERCP is normally performed with the patient prone.

We have used postoperative ES to manage some cases of CBD stones. However, we currently restrict this approach to older patients with a higher operative risk and those younger patients who refuse open CBDE after an unsuccessful TCD procedure.

We have followed 7 patients who did not undergo CBD stone removal, either because the stone was very small or because they changed their minds and later refused to go through with planned postoperative ES. These few patients have been asymptomatic to date.

We have used our TCD technique successfully to clear the ducts in 81 of 87 patients found on cholangiography to have CBD stones. The procedure in the other patients was converted to choledochotomy—three open and four laparoscopic procedures. In 2 patients in whom no attempt was made to remove the stones, a latex drain was inserted in the cystic duct for later extraction. All other cholangiograms at completion were clear of CBD stones, although we realize that both surgical and endoscopic experience has noted retained stones in some patients despite similar normal studies.[11]

In the group of 87 patients in whom we performed TCD CBDE, there was an 8% incidence of minor complications and a 6% incidence of major complications. Complications with the TCD technique can include perforation of the cystic or extrahepatic bile ducts, cystic duct stump leakage, pancreatitis, persistent cholangitis due to high intraductal pressures, delayed strictures due to mechanical injury or thermal injury from lithotripsy, and retained stones. All of these complications can be minimized by careful attention to detail and proper patient selection.

In our hands, surgical complications with the TCD approach were few and have been reported in detail.[15] Briefly, we have seen five very mild clinical cases of pancreatitis. Three of these patients had undergone ampullary dilation, and the others had not. There were 7 patients with new elevations of liver enzyme levels after exploration. One patient experienced an intraoperative pneumothorax, and another patient died of aspiration of tube feedings 32 days after surgery.

In a summary of cases collected from various centers consisting of 272 patients who underwent laparoscopic CBDE (Table 27–1),[36–41] the mortality rate was approximately 1%, usually resulting from comorbid illness—most commonly of the cardiac and pulmonary systems (Cuschieri, personal communication; Franklin, personal communication; Hunter, personal communication; Olsen, personal communication; Petelin, personal communication; Shapiro, personal communication). Myocardial infarction was the leading cause of postoperative mortality.[22] All deaths occurred in patients older than 65 years of age. Aspiration pneumonia occurred in 2% of our patients and was the cause of death in 1 patient. Retained stones occurred in approximately 4% of patients, and complications occurred in approximately 7%.

With respect to duration of hospitalization and return to work, the patients in our series who had a TCD CBDE can be separated into four groups: patients with suspected or unsuspected CBD stones and patients younger or older than 60 years of age. Patients who are sicker and have preoperatively suspected stones are discharged 3.6 days postoperatively on average. Patients with unsuspected stones are discharged 1.7 days postoperatively on average. Both groups tend to return to work or usual activities 10 days after surgery on average. Two cases of retained CBD stones were noted: one

Table 27–1. TRANSCYSTIC COMMON BILE DUCT EXPLORATION RESULTS

Surgeon	No. Patients	No. Complications	No. Deaths	No. Retained Stones
Cuschieri	8	0 (0%)	0 (0%)	1 (13%)
Franklin	2	1 (50%)	0 (0%)	0 (0%)
Hunter	25	5 (20%)	0 (0%)	0 (0%)
Olsen	39	0 (0%)	0 (0%)	6 (15%)
Petelin	80	5 (6%)	1 (1%)	2 (3%)
Phillips	81	5 (6%)	1 (1%)	2 (2%)
Shapiro	37	2 (5%)	0 (0%)	0 (0%)
TOTAL	272	18 (7%)	2 (1%)	11 (4%)

following TCD CBDE and one following laparoscopic choledochotomy. Both patients had more than 10 CBD stones and were thought likely to harbor more stones. A patient with a normal but suboptimal cholangiogram later had a clinical picture consistent with passage of a CBD stone but refused ERCP. No other patient is known yet to have recurrent symptoms. CBD stones were left intentionally in two patients, and a tube was left in the cystic duct for later access. One patient was pregnant and the other was a critically ill cardiac patient with gangrenous cholecystitis.

Four of our patients underwent laparoscopic choledochotomies. The procedures were successful, but the operative times were prolonged. Their length of stay in the hospital and time of disability from work were very close to those of our patients undergoing open CBDE. The 4 patients undergoing laparoscopic choledochotomy stayed an average of 8 days postoperatively and returned to work 25 days postoperatively on average, compared with 31 days postoperatively in 4 patients who underwent standard CBDE earlier in the series. In a cumulative world survey (Table 27–2), 102 patients underwent laparoscopic choledochotomy. Of these, 8% had complications and 2% had retained stones. One patient (1%) died of a myocardial infarction.

Understandably, operative time decreased as experience with these procedures accumulated. Currently, LC alone requires an average of 55 minutes in our hands, including cholangiography. When TCD CBDE was also performed laparoscopically, total operative time averaged about 140 minutes,[14] in substantial measure because of the need to bring in and set up additional equipment, as described previously. The three operations that included laparoscopic choledochotomy averaged 375 minutes, in part because of the technical demands relating to place-ment of the T tube, but Franklin and Cuschieri have each reported average operating times of 100 minutes (personal communication).

RISK ANALYSIS OF DIFFERING APPROACHES

There are several strategies one could advocate in dealing with CBD stones. Several of these will be compared against each other by calculating the relative risks to the patient (i.e., the rate of expected complications) for each approach. A similar decision analysis was published by Stalnikowicz and associates concerning the role of preoperative ES in patients with CBD stones.[23]

As described elsewhere,[24] the risk estimates derived in this analysis are based on assumptions of efficacy, accuracy, and the safety of individual procedures and do not include issues of cost nor the amount of physician or patient time involved in the procedures. In each of the proposed management strategies, we start with a group of 100 hypothetical patients definitely planning to undergo LC. No attempt is made here to apply these estimates to other clinical situations. The strategies compare various ways of identifying and handling the assumed 10% of patients that harbor CBD stones. The number and type of procedures needed in each scheme is estimated, based on the assumptions listed further on. The morbidity and mortality rates are totaled and weighted according to the number of each procedure required for the group of 100 patients. The summed risks for each strategy are then compared.

Because risk depends significantly on age for certain procedures, especially open CBDE, we have separated the younger and older patients. The assumptions used in the analysis come primarily from our data.[8]

Table 27–2. LAPAROSCOPIC CHOLEDOCHOTOMY RESULTS

Surgeon	No. Patients	No. Complications	No. Deaths	No. Retained Stones
Cuschieri	40	4 (10%)	0 (0%)	0 (0%)
Franklin	53	3 (5%)	1 (2%)	0 (0%)
Hunter	1	1 (100%)	0 (0%)	0 (0%)
Olsen	2	0 (0%)	0 (0%)	0 (0%)
Petelin	2	0 (0%)	0 (0%)	1 (50%)
Phillips	3	0 (0%)	0 (0%)	1 (33%)
Shapiro	1	0 (0%)	0 (0%)	0 (0%)
TOTAL	102	8 (8%)	1 (1%)	2 (1%)

Assumptions

1. Seventeen percent of patients undergoing LC have elevation in one or more liver function tests.

2. Six percent of patients undergoing LC have more than one abnormality in body chemistry.

3. Twenty-four percent of patients with any abnormal liver function test have CBD stones.

4. Thirty-six percent of patients with multiple abnormalities in body chemistry have CBD stones.

5. Ten percent (for ease of calculation) of

patients having LC are found to have CBD stones (4% unsuspected).

6. LC is successful in removing the gallbladder.

7. ES is 95% successful in clearing all CBD stones.

8. TCD CBDE fails to clear the CBD in 10% of cases (our current results are better than this).

9. Morbidity and mortality estimates for the various procedures are as listed in Tables 27–3 and 27–4.

Estimates of morbidity and mortality such as those shown in Tables 27–3 and 27–4 are not easy to agree upon. McSherry and Glenn noted a clear difference in mortality for cholecystectomy with CBDE before or after the age of 50 years, the rates being 0.9% and 4.4%, respectively.[25] These procedures took place from 1932 to 1978, so they likely overestimate today's mortality. A much more recent review of 1200 cholecystectomies on the teaching service at our own hospital just prior to the introduction of LC was performed by Morgenstern and colleagues.[26] The mortality rate for 220 patients undergoing CBDE was 0% in younger patients but was 4.1% in patients older than age 60 years. The overall mortality rate for the entire series was 1.8%. Most reviewers agree that CBDE roughly doubles the mortality rate compared with cholecystectomy alone and that age is a critical factor. Morbidity figures are somewhat less certain and depend on the definition of complications in various studies. Both morbidity and mortality rates seem higher when there is reoperation or secondary exploration than in primary operative procedures, and this likely holds true following ES as well as open surgery.[27]

Several studies and reviews place the risks of

Table 27–3. MORBIDITY AND MORTALITY ASSUMPTIONS USED IN RISK ANALYSIS IN PATIENTS LESS THAN AGE 60 YEARS

	% Morbidity	% Mortality
ERCP	3	0.1
ES	5	0.9
Conversion to open CC with CBDE	10	0.1
Salvage open CC with CBDE	20	1
LC	6	0.05
LC with TCD CBDE	7	0.1

ERCP = endoscopic retrograde cholangiopancreatography; ES = endoscopic sphincterotomy; CC = cholecystectomy; CBDE = common bile duct exploration; LC = laparoscopic cholecystectomy; TCD = transcystic duct.

Table 27–4. MORBIDITY AND MORTALITY ASSUMPTIONS USED IN RISK ANALYSIS IN PATIENTS AGED 60 YEARS AND OLDER

	% Morbidity	% Mortality
ERCP	5	0.2
ES	5	0.9
Conversion to open CC with CBDE	15	1.8
Salvage open CC with CBDE	20	4
LC	6	0.25
LC with TCD CBDE	10	1

ERCP = endoscopic retrograde cholangiopancreatography; ES = endoscopic sphincterotomy; CC = cholecystectomy; CBDE = common bile duct exploration; LC = laparoscopic cholecystectomy; TCD = transcystic duct.

ERCP with ES at roughly 8% to 10% major morbidity and 1% to 1.5% mortality.[12, 28] Cotton and associates' recent review of 7729 cases reports 8.2% major complications and 1.3% deaths.[28] There is not yet any indication of a clear difference with age.

Although LC is still quite new, estimates of its risks are already being derived. The Southern Surgeons Club reported 5.1% complications and 0.07% deaths in 1518 cases. In about 5% of cases, the procedures were converted to open surgery and included as complications if they resulted from an undesired event during LC. As experience with the procedure increases, one might expect the risk to decline somewhat. Our own series, dating from some of the earliest experience with LC, revealed major complications in 2% of patients and minor ones in 4%. One patient died of acquired immunodeficiency syndrome in the month after surgery, for a mortality rate of 0.2%.

Estimates of morbidity and mortality rates for TCD CBDE are certainly not clear at this point. Although cumulative data suggesting a 7% complication rate and a 1% mortality rate are promising, we do not yet know if the risk of this procedure is as close to that of LC as we have shown in this projection.

Strategies Being Compared

Strategy I

1. Before LC, screening ERCP is performed in patients with a recent elevation of any single liver function test (including amylase). In our group this would have been 17% of patients.

2. ES is also performed in patients found to have CBD stones on this ERCP—24% in our series.

3. The entire 100 patients have LC.

4. At LC, unsuspected stones are found in some patients who did not have preoperative screening. They receive postoperative ERCP and ES. (CBD stones are assumed to be present in 10% of the 100-patient group.)

5. ES fails to clear the CBD stones in 5% of the patients having the procedure postoperatively; these patients are referred for "salvage" open CBDE. (Failures of preoperative ES are not included in this analysis.)

Strategy II

1. Before LC, screening ERCP is performed in any patient with recent elevation of two or more liver function tests (including amylase). In our group this would have been 6% of patients.

2. ES is also performed in patients who are found to have CBD stones on this ERCP—36% in our series.

3. The entire 100 patients undergo LC.

4. At LC, unsuspected stones are found in some patients who did not have preoperative screening. They receive postoperative ERCP and ES.

5. In 5% of the patients having postoperative ES, the procedure fails to clear the CBD stones, and the patients are referred for salvage open CBDE. (Failures of preoperative ES are not included in this analysis.)

Strategy III

1. All 100 patients undergo LC without preoperative ERCP.

2. Patients who are found on intraoperative cholangiography to have CBD stones undergo postoperative ERCP and ES.

3. Open salvage CBDE is performed in the ES failures.

Strategy IV

1. LC is begun in 100 patients. It is completed in 90 patients, with no CBD stones found.

Table 27–5. RISK ANALYSIS OF STRATEGIES FOR COMMON BILE DUCT STONES ACCOMPANYING LAPAROSCOPIC CHOLECYSTECTOMY IN PATIENTS LESS THAN 60 YEARS

	Strategy	% Needed	No. of Patients	% Morbidity	% Mortality
I	Preoperative ERCP (any abnormal body chemistry)	17	17	0.51	0.017
	ES in those with stones	24	4.1	0.204	0.037
	LC	100	100	6	0.05
	Postoperative ERCP-ES (unsuspected stones)		5.9	0.474	0.059
	Salvage open CBDE (5% ES cases)	5	0.3	0.059	0.003
	TOTAL RISK			7.247	0.166
II	Preoperative ERCP (multiple abnormal body chemistries)	6	6.0	0.18	0.006
	ES in those with stones	36	2.2	0.108	0.019
	LC	100	100	6	0.05
	Postoperative ERCP-ES (unsuspected stones)		7.8	0.627	0.078
	Salvage open CBDE (5% ES cases)	5	0.4	0.078	0.004
	TOTAL RISK			6.993	0.157
III	LC	100	100	6	0.05
	Postoperative ERCP + ES for stones	10	10	0	0.1
	Salvage open CBDE (5% ES cases)	5	0.5	0.1	0.005
	TOTAL RISK			6.9	0.155
IV	LC if no CBDS at laparoscopic cholangiogram	90	90	5.4	0.045
	Convert to open CC-CBDE if stones	10	10	1	0.01
	TOTAL RISK			6.4	0.055
V	LC if no CBDS at cholangiogram	90	90	5.4	0.045
	TCD CBDE with LC	10	10	0.7	0.01
	Convert to open CC-CBDE if failed	10	1	0.1	0.001
	TOTAL RISK			6.2	0.056

ERCP = endoscopic retrograde cholangiopancreatography; ES = endoscopic sphincterotomy; LC = laparoscopic cholecystectomy; CBDE = common bile duct exploration; CBDS = common bile duct stones; CC = cholecystectomy; TCD = transcystic duct.

2. Immediate conversion to open cholecystectomy with CBDE is performed for the 10% of patients found on intraoperative cholangiography to have CBD stones.

Strategy V

1. LC is begun in 100 patients. It is completed in 90 patients, with no CBD stones found.
2. LC with TCD CBDE is performed in the 10% of patients found to have CBD stones.
3. In the 10% of these procedures that fail, open CBDE is performed. (Postoperative ES for certain failed procedures would be an alternative but is not calculated. This would affect only 1% of cases, so would have little effect on total risk.)

Tables 27–5 and 27–6 show the cumulative morbidity and mortality rates of the various management schemes considered, grouped by the patients' age. Although we have evolved our own strategy for management of CBD stones in a less mathematical fashion, these

estimates are thought-provoking and perhaps give added support to our approach. Of course, many of the preceding assumptions and estimates are far from certain, but with time, more data can help us refine these morbidity and mortality calculations. It should be remembered that this analysis presumes that the patient is going to have LC at a minimum, so the combined risk of any group cannot fall to less than that of LC alone. Seemingly close figures among some of the groups become much more disparate if the baseline risk of the 100 LC procedures is subtracted from the total risk of each group, yielding the incremental risk of the various options for management of CBD stones, as shown in Table 27–7.

The strategies that yield a lower risk are those that put the patients through the least number of procedures, particularly ones entailing higher risk. Clinically, other comorbid conditions such as heart disease, pulmonary disease, or obesity could also influence the choice of strategy for a particular patient. The relationship between age

Table 27–6. RISK ANALYSIS OF STRATEGIES FOR COMMON BILE DUCT STONES ACCOMPANYING LAPAROSCOPIC CHOLECYSTECTOMY IN PATIENTS AGED 60 YEARS AND OLDER

	Strategy	% Needed	No. of Patients	% Morbidity	% Mortality
I	Preoperative ERCP (any abnormal body chemistry)	17	17	0.850	0.034
	ES in those with stones	24	4.1	0.204	0.037
	LC	100	100	6	0.25
	Postoperative ERCP-ES (unsuspected stones)		5.9	0.592	0.065
	Salvage open CBDE (5% ES cases)	5	0.3	0.059	0.012
	TOTAL RISK			7.705	0.398
II	Preoperative ERCP (multiple abnormal body chemistries)	6	6	0.3	0.012
	ES in those with stones	36	2.2	0.108	0.019
	LC	100	100	6	0.25
	Postoperative ERCP-ES (unsuspected stones)		7.8	0.784	0.086
	Salvage open CBDE (5% ES cases)	5	0.4	0.078	0.016
	TOTAL RISK			7.27	0.383
III	LC	100	100	6	0.25
	Postoperative ERCP + ES for stones	10	10	1	0.11
	Salvage open CBDE (5% ES cases)	5	0.5	0.1	0.02
	TOTAL RISK			7.1	0.38
IV	LC if no CBDS at laparoscopic cholangiogram	90	90	5.4	0.225
	Convert to open CC-CBDE if stones	10	10	1.5	0.18
	TOTAL RISK			6.9	0.405
V	LC if no CBDS at cholangiogram	90	90	5.4	0.225
	TCD CBDE with LC	10	10	1	0.05
	Convert to open CC-CBDE if failed	10	1	0.15	0.018
	TOTAL RISK			6.55	0.293

ERCP = endoscopic retrograde cholangiopancreatography; ES = endoscopic sphincterotomy; LC = laparoscopic cholecystectomy; CBDE = common bile duct exploration; CBDS = common bile duct stones; CC = cholecystectomy; TCD = transcystic duct.

Table 27–7. EXCESS RISK GREATER THAN LAPAROSCOPIC CHOLECYSTECTOMY ALONE (%)

Strategy	Age Less Than 60 Years		Age 60 Years or More	
	% Morbidity	% Mortality	% Morbidity	% Mortality
I	1.247	0.116	1.705	0.148
II	0.994	0.108	1.27	0.133
III	0.9	0.105	1.1	0.13
IV	1	0.01	0.9	0.155
V	0.8	0.011	0.55	0.043

Conclusion: Strategy V appears to offer the lowest risk. When it is not available, strategy IV is preferred for younger patients and strategy III or IV for older patients.

and risk of laparoscopic surgery is still unresolved. Cost issues are not calculated here but would also likely favor an approach requiring the fewest major procedures/patient.

Our own preference, then, is to routinely perform intraoperative cholangiography during the LC procedure, without attempts at preoperative ES.[29] If stones are found, we currently proceed with TCD CBDE. In case this does not succeed, our attitude is that the risk of open CBDE is very low in young patients, probably less than that of ES; thus, we recommend immediate open CBDE for such patients, unless there is serious comorbidity. Some patients, of course, will still select postoperative ES, despite the higher risk of that strategy. For the older patient, especially one with frail health, we proceed with LC and recommend ES to follow if stones are present.

DISCUSSION

In a remarkably short time, the technique of LC has gained considerable acceptance among the surgical community and certainly among patients. There is now extraordinary interest in the application of less invasive endoscopic methods to numerous areas of surgical practice. Perhaps not since the introduction of anesthesia has surgical practice been so influenced by the patient's wish to reduce pain and disability from surgery. The accompanying cost savings often achieved by reduction of hospital use and recuperation time has further encouraged the development of these new methodologies. Many have said that we are witnessing a revolutionary phase in surgical practice, and there will likely be a rapid evolution of our ability to handle more surgical challenges via the emerging video endoscopic techniques.

As experience with LC grows, related biliary problems—particularly CBD stones—need to be addressed as well. Surgeons continue to analyze and refine approaches to CBD stones.

Alternative approaches must be compared with the standard of open CBDE, which has a proven low level of morbidity and mortality, at least in younger patients. Any other modality—endoscopic, laparoscopic, or otherwise—must have at least the same degree of safety.

Results of CBDE performed laparoscopically are comparable with those of conventional open CBDE. From 1982 to 1988, 216 open CBDEs were performed at Cedars-Sinai Medical Center, Los Angeles, with 0% mortality in patients younger than 60 years of age, and 1.3% mortality overall.

In contrast, ERCP-ES has 0.5% to 1% mortality in all age groups. Because the TCD technique of CBDE is effective and is relatively safe, especially in patients less than 65 years of age, we restrict preoperative ERCP and sphincterotomy to patients older than 65 years of age with significant cardiac and pulmonary disease who may not require cholecystectomy.

ES and extraction of CBD stones has been a valuable approach in patients at high surgical risk, particularly the elderly. In our fervor now to avoid open abdominal exploration and please the patient, many groups, including ours, have tried combining this endoscopic approach with LC. Neoptolemos and colleagues of Great Britain reported a prospective study of 120 patients in whom it was already known that CBD stones were present, comparing cholecystectomy combined with preoperative ES and surgery alone.[10] It must be emphasized that these patients had already undergone ERCP to be considered for the study, and the authors do not state how many other patients were similarly screened but found to be clear of CBD stones nor the complications present in those excluded patients. Despite this serious issue, their study still did not support the routine use of preoperative ES, even in patients already known to have CBD stones. An excess of deaths and complications in the combined modality group did not, however, reach statistical significance.

Neoptolemos and colleagues had previously

reported a review of 438 consecutive patients having CBDE or ES, or both, from 1981 to 1985.[30] The group of patients having preoperative ES had significantly more major complications than the group having surgery alone. ES alone, in other groups of patients with and without gallbladders, yielded a 17% to 19% major complication rate, although the patients with gallbladders left in situ were generally older and sicker.

Cotton has rightly pointed out the difficulty of comparing endoscopic management of ES with surgery.[9] He cites an 8% to 10% incidence of immediate major complications associated with ES—20% requiring surgery—and a mortality rate of about 1%. He also cites long-term problems in about 20% of patients following ES, including ductal stenosis or new stones, or both. Long-term complications of open surgical exploration were also noted.

A more recent report by Stain and coworkers[11] mirrored the findings of Neoptolemos and associates. ES before surgery was compared with surgery alone. CBD stones were found in 35% of patients at surgery following ES. Twelve of 26 patients in the group undergoing preoperative ES needed CBDE during surgery anyway for unsuccessful ES or additional CBD stones. Major complications were similar in the two groups, but were lower than in the earlier British studies. Cost was increased with preoperative ES, mostly because of the added screening of patients incorrectly suspected of harboring CBD stones. One major complication occurred in a patient not in the study during a normal screening ERCP examination. An additional point of interest is that CBDE was negative for stones in 7 of 26 patients in the surgery alone group, suggesting spontaneous passage following ERCP without ES. If these patients had undergone preoperative ES, they would have counted as successes for ES.

In a small series, Stiegmann and associates also found no clear advantage of the combined approach compared with surgery alone.[31] Three of their 8 patients who underwent preoperative attempts at endoscopic CBD stone extraction still needed open CBDE, one apparently for a cholangiocarcinoma. Morbidity and length of hospital stay, as well as cost, were not improved by this combined approach.

Monroe and colleagues came to different conclusions in a recent comparison of combined LC-ES with a retrospective series of CBDE cases.[32] Only 11 patients were in their study group; 5 patients underwent ES before LC, 6 patients underwent ES after LC. They found no complications in these 11 patients and noted a shorter length of stay and fewer days of work missed. However, their group undergoing CBDE had considerably longer hospital stays and convalescence periods than has been our own experience. They concluded that LC-ES was a preferred strategy.

In a series of 366 patients referred for cholecystectomy, Arregui and coworkers performed 38 ERCPs (29 preoperative and 9 postoperative) on 36 patients with suspected CBD stones.[33] Cannulation was successful in 95% of the procedures, and CBD stones were discovered in 17 patients. Of these patients, 10 underwent LC plus ES and extraction of the CBD stones. The gallbladder was left in situ in 1 high-risk elderly patient who underwent ES and endoscopic stone extraction. Two patients in whom cannulation failed and 2 patients who underwent successful cannulations but whose stones were too large for extraction underwent open cholecystectomy with CBDE. Two patients with impacted stones in the distal common duct underwent ES, but removal of the stones was incomplete and LC with flexible choledochoscopy and fragmentation of stones using EHL was performed. Complications related to ERCP occurred in 3 of the 38 cases (7.9%)—all three were preoperative ERCPs—one complication was pancreatitis, one was acute cholecystitis, and one was fever following ERCP, which was likely due to early ascending cholangitis. Each of these complications resolved without sequelae. The average length of stay for patients managed with ERCP-ES and LC was 4.5 days. Arregui and colleagues concluded that LC combined with ES is relatively safe, readily available, and effective management that is justified by patients' shorter hospitalization, reduced pain, and quicker recovery. Still, they predicted that LC with intraoperative cholangiography, choledochoscopy, and laparoscopic extraction of CBD stones will become the primary treatment for choledocholithiasis because it avoids the discomfort, morbidity, and cost of an extra procedure (preoperative ERCP).[33]

Our approach to CBD stones began with the routine use of laparoscopic cholangiography, which maximized our awareness of the prevalence and characteristics of this problem. We also attempted initially to merge the technologies of LC with ERCP and ES in an efficient manner.

If our ability to predict the presence of CBD stones could be nearly perfect, preoperative ERCP with ES might have seemed a more attractive approach. As noted also by others, there is no set of clinical parameters that can reliably predict CBD stones. Stiegmann and colleagues found no stones in 50% of 16 patients having preoperative ERCP, despite their inclusion in a group with clinically suspected CBD stones.[31] In our experience, any combination of chemical abnormalities used to predict CBD stones yielded a very high proportion of both false-negative and false-positive results. Selecting patients with jaundice, pancreatitis, dilated ducts on ultrasound, or multiple abnormal chemistry test results may increase one's yield in identifying CBD stones, but the majority of patients with CBD stones would still go undetected. Inevitably, many patients would have unnecessary preoperative ERCPs, with some risk; yet other patients would still be discovered at LC to harbor CBD stones and would require a separate management strategy at that point.

We have rejected the intraoperative use of ES. Still, postoperative ERCP is preferred by many groups in dealing with CBD stones after LC. It was disturbing to us, as well as to our patients, to be unable to fully resolve the patient's biliary pathologic condition with one procedure and one general anesthesia. Although seeming much less invasive to the patient, ES is a procedure that still adds substantial risk of morbidity and even mortality, apparently even at younger ages, and these risks may even exceed those of open CBDE in low-risk patients.

Our experience in using the TCD technique in 87 cases to date is encouraging. Extraction of these stones has been accomplished with a low level of morbidity and, except at the beginning of our series, an apparently high degree of success in clearing CBD stones. The shortened hospital stay and shortened period of disability in these patients, compared with open surgical cases, is dramatic.

Although cost would be reduced and convenience increased by this unified approach to cholecystectomy and CBD stones, clearly we must exercise caution before enthusiastically advocating widespread use of any newly developed methodology. For instance, careful antegrade dilation of the ampulla has appeared, so far, to be at least as safe as endoscopic dilation and sphincterotomy, but more data are needed. The incidence of CBD injury or pancreatitis following lithotripsy within the CBD is still not known, and at present we prefer to manually extract intact stones whenever possible, rather than fragment them.

Our 4 patients who underwent laparoscopic choledochotomy had rather long hospital stays and a delayed return to work, contrary to the experiences of Franklin and Cuschieri (personal communication), but the level of postoperative pain was diminished. Our current impression is that laparoscopic choledochotomy is possible, but very demanding technically, and seems to provide modest benefit over standard open CBDE. If the necessity for the T tube were to be eliminated, for example, patients could return to work considerably earlier even in these more complex cases. New developments in this area could prompt a reassessment.

As familiarity and experience increase among surgeons performing LC, we believe the TCD technique will be very efficient, relatively safe, and the primary approach to this difficult problem.

TRAINING

The rapid growth in demand for laparoscopic gallbladder surgery has tested the ability of the surgical community to adapt quickly to profound technologic change. Numerous courses have been offered to train surgeons in LC, representing the largest postgraduate training effort ever attempted. It is also well recognized that performance improves as experience increases.[5, 34] The laparoscopic techniques described in this chapter should be used only after achieving extensive experience and confidence in performing LC.

Laparoscopic cholangiography is being attempted with increasing frequency, which will eventually give practitioners confidence in some of the techniques used in the TCD approach. Other surgeons have already reported selected use of the TCD technique.[35] Routine IOC is recommended not only to avoid CBD injuries and identify CBD stones but also to gain the skill needed to perform TCD CBDE.

Flexible choledochoscopy is also very effective during open CBDE and not only enables relatively easy CBD examination and stone extraction but also provides valuable experience that can later facilitate the laparoscopic performance of TCD endoscopy and stone extraction procedures.

Techniques of TCD laparoscopic CBDE should be learned in the inanimate laboratory on simple models (Shapiro, personal communication) and then applied in "open" cases before attempting the procedure entirely laparoscopically. Endoscopic skills and stone-capturing skills appear to be more readily learned than laparoscopic suturing skills. Because suturing is so difficult and laparoscopic choledochotomy still requires a T tube, we encourage surgeons to learn the TCD technique first and rely on open CBDE for the 10% of cases of CBD stones that cannot be explored through the cystic duct (1% of all patients undergoing LC).

Ultimately, most surgeons will develop suturing skills and will perform laparoscopic choledochotomy in this subgroup of patients. Bench models have been developed for training surgeons in laparoscopic suturing manipulation, including intracorporeal and extracorporeal knot tying. Courses are available to teach such "advanced" skills and provide supervised laboratory practice, but weekly if not daily practice is needed.

CONCLUSION

LC has become the primary treatment for symptomatic cholelithiasis. CBD stones are present in many of these patients. Several approaches to their management are available, but the TCD technique for CBD exploration with choledochoscopy and stone extraction should become the primary technique. This procedure appears to be relatively safe and efficient and is perhaps the most cost-effective means of dealing with CBD stones. Availability of the TCD CBDE technique limits the role of ES for managing CBD stones in patients undergoing LC.

Acknowledgments

Special recognition belongs to Brendan J. Carroll, MD, FACS and Leon Daykhovsky, MD, who were involved with the development of our CBDE technique. Thanks to A. Randolph Pearlstein, M.D., Moses J. Fallas, M.D., Eric Partlow, Margaret Paz-Partlow, and Emma Matt.

Graphics and manuscript preparation were partly funded by a grant from Karl Storz and Ethicon.

References

1. Phillips E, Daykhovsky L, Carroll B, et al. Laparoscopic cholecystectomy: instrumentation and technique. J Laparoendosc Surg 1:3, 1990.
2. Reddick EJ, Olsen DO, Daniell J, et al. Laparoscopic laser cholecystectomy. Laser Med Surg News Adv p 38, 1989.
3. Peters JH, Ellison EC, Innes JT, et al. Safety and efficacy of laparoscopic cholecystectomy: a prospective analysis of 100 initial patients. Ann Surg 213:3, 1991.
4. Phillips EH, Carroll BJ, Bello JM, et al. Laparoscopic cholecystectomy in acute cholecystitis. Am Surg 58(5):273, 1992.
5. Berci G, Sackier JM. The Los Angeles experience with laparoscopic cholecystectomy. Am J Surg 161:382, 1991.
6. Reddick EJ, Olsen D, Spaw A, et al. Safe performance of difficult laparoscopic cholecystectomies. Am J Surg 161:377, 1991.
7. Phillips EH, Berci G, Carroll B, et al. The importance of intraoperative cholangiography during laparoscopic cholecystectomy. Am Surg 56:792, 1990.
8. Phillips EH, Carroll BJ. Experience in 400 laparoscopic cholecystectomies. Presented at meeting of southern California chapter of American College of Surgeons, January 1991.
9. Cotton PB. Endoscopic management of bile duct stones; (apples and oranges). Gut 25:587, 1984.
10. Neoptolemos JP, Carr-Locke DL, Fossard DP. Prospective randomized study of preoperative endoscopic sphincterotomy versus surgery alone for common bile duct stones. Br Med J 294:470, 1987.
11. Stain SC, Cohen H, Tsuishyosha M, Donovan AJ. Choledocholithiasis: endoscopic sphincterotomy or common bile duct exploration. Ann Surg 213:6, 1991.
12. Sivak MV. Endoscopic management of bile duct stones. Am J Surg 158:228, 1989.
13. Reddick EJ, Olsen D, Alexander W, et al. Laparoscopic laser cholecystectomy and choledocholithiasis. Surg Endosc 4:133, 1990.
14. Phillips EH, Carroll B, Fallas M. Laparoscopic cholecystectomy and common bile duct exploration: results from 453 consecutive patients. Am Surg 59, 1993, in press.
15. Phillips EH, Carroll BC. New techniques for the treatment of common bile duct calculi encountered during laparoscopic cholecystectomy. Probl Gen Surg 8(3):387, 1991.
16. Khanna TS, Falk SL. Exploration of the common bile duct through the cystic duct. Surg Gynecol Obstet 167:145, 1988.
17. Choi S, Choi TK, Wong J. Intraoperative flexible choledochoscopy for intrahepatic and extrahepatic biliary calculi. Surgery 101:571, 1987.
18. Nghiem DD. Choledochoscopy without choledochotomy. Surg Gynecol Obstet 164:377, 1987.
19. Carroll BJ, Phillips EH, Chandra M, Fallas M. Laparoscopic transcystic duct balloon dilatation of the sphincter of Oddi. Surg Endosc 7, 1993, in press.
20. Carroll B, Chandra M, Papaioannou T, et al. Biliary lithotripsy as an adjunct to laparoscopic common bile duct stone extraction. Surg Endosc 7, 1993, in press.
21. Carroll BJ, Phillips EH, Daykhovsky L, et al. Laparoscopic choledochoscopy: an effective approach to the common duct. J Laparoendosc Surg 2(1):15, 1992.
22. Phillips EH. The current spectrum of laparoscopic surgery (postgraduate course). Chicago, Annual Clinical Congress of the American College of Surgeons, October 1991.
23. Stalnikowicz R, Berger MY, Benbassat J. Management of common bile duct stones in patients with intact ladders: a decision analysis. Presented at Digestive Disease Week, New Orleans, May 1991.
24. Phillips EH, Carroll BJ, Pearlstein AR, et al. Laparoscopic choledochoscopy and extraction of common bile duct stones. World J Surg 17:22–28, 1993.
25. McSherry CK, Glenn F. The incidence and causes of death following surgery for nonmalignant biliary tract disease. Ann Surg 191:271, 1980.
26. Morgenstern L, Wong L, Berci G. Twelve hundred consecutive cholecystectomies before the laparoscopic era: morbidity, mortality, and general observations. Arch Surg 127(4):400–403, 1992.
27. Neoptolemos JP, Shaw DE, Carr-Locke DL. A multivariate analysis of preoperative risk factors in patients with common bile duct stones. Implications for treatment. Ann Surg 209:157, 1989.
28. Cotton PB, Lehman G, Vennes J, et al. Endoscopic sphincterotomy complications and their management: an attempt at consensus. Gastrointest Endosc 37:383, 1991.

29. Phillips EH. Routine versus selective intraoperative cholangiography. Am J Surg, 1993, in press.
30. Neoptolemos JP, Davidson BR, Shaw DE, et al. Study of common bile duct exploration and endoscopic sphincterotomy in a consecutive series of 438 patients. Br J Surg 74:916, 1987.
31. Stiegmann G, Goff J, Mansour A, et al. Pre-cholecystectomy endoscopic cholangiography and stone removal (ERCSR) is not superior to cholecystectomy cholangiography and common duct exploration (CC + CBDE): a prospective randomized trial. Presented at Digestive Disease Week, New Orleans, May 1991.
32. Monroe P, Kelley W, Sheridan V, et al. Comparison of laparoscopic cholecystectomy with endoscopic sphincterotomy (LC/ES) and cholecystectomy with common bile duct exploration (CDE). Presented at Digestive Disease Week, New Orleans, May 1991.
33. Arregui ME, Davis CJ, Arkush AM, Nagan RF. Laparoscopic cholecystectomy combined with endoscopic sphincterotomy and stone extraction or laparoscopic choledochoscopy and electrohydraulic lithotripsy for management of cholelithiasis with choledocholithiasis. Surg Endosc 6:10, 1992.
34. Southern Surgeons Club: A prospective analysis of 1518 laparoscopic cholecystectomies. N Engl J Med 324:1073, 1991.
35. Bagnato J. Laparoscopic common bile duct exploration. J Miss St Med Assoc 31:361, 1990.

28

Laparoscopic Appendectomy

J. Barry McKernan

Although the incidence of acute appendicitis has declined in recent years, as many as one in six individuals will have the appendix removed during his or her lifetime.[1] Thus, there is a wealth of surgical experience in the treatment of appendicitis, particularly considering that the open operative procedure most commonly used today, McBurney's muscle-splitting incisional approach, was originally described in 1894. Laparoscopic appendectomy was initially reported by Semm in 1983,[2] and O'Regan performed the first laparoscopic appendectomy for acute appendicitis in 1986,[1] years before the first reported laparoscopic cholecystectomy in 1988. Although the adoption of laparoscopic surgical techniques for appendectomy has not been as rapid as that for cholecystectomy, several groups throughout the world have reported on the safety of laparoscopic appendectomy.[3-6] This chapter briefly reviews the diagnostic and treatment roles for laparoscopy in the management of acute appendicitis and describes the procedure used at this institution for performing laparoscopic appendectomy.

DIAGNOSTIC LAPAROSCOPY FOR ACUTE APPENDICITIS

Despite its prevalence and the fact that it has been recognized and treated by surgeons for more than 100 years, the diagnosis of acute appendicitis remains elusive in many instances. The incidence of removing a normal appendix when acute appendicitis is suspected is embarrassingly high, particularly among women of childbearing age and young children. A review of the literature revealed that the rate of unnecessary appendectomy in these two groups was as high as 30% to 50%.[7] As Hoffmann and Rasmussen[7] succinctly point out, the dilemma surrounding the accurate diagnosis of appendicitis stems from the fact that the risk of perforation increases in tandem with the duration of the disease process. Thus, rather than hazard possible perforation and the significant mortality and morbidity associated with this complication, many surgeons act conservatively and operate, even if it means confronting a normal appendix. Unfortunately, however, removal of a histologically normal appendix is associated with a complication rate similar to that for removal of a diseased appendix. Immediate postoperative complications, including death,[8] have been reported in up to 15% of patients following unnecessary appendectomy,[9] and later complications, such as intestinal obstruction, sterility, and incisional hernias, are also seen.[7]

In the patient presenting with right lower-quadrant pain, diagnostic accuracy can be facilitated by supplementing a thorough history and physical examination with judicious use of laboratory tests. Although frequently used, a plain abdominal x-ray study is not a reliable indicator of appendicitis because currently accepted radiographic signs of appendicitis can also be present in patients with other causes of right lower quadrant pain and even in normal individuals.[10, 11] In contrast to plain abdominal x-ray film, ultrasound examination has been shown to be considerably more sensitive for detecting acute appendicitis.[12, 13] The primary disadvantage of ultrasound is that its accuracy is dependent on the expertise of the examiner. Barium enema has also been shown to be a sensitive indicator in about 90% of patients with acute appendicitis,[14, 15] although false-positive examinations have been reported, especially among patients with gynecologic disease.[7]

345

Because the diagnosis of acute appendicitis can be confirmed or refuted based on direct visualization of the region, laparoscopy is of considerable value in improving diagnostic accuracy. Paterson-Brown and colleagues[16] reported that of 40 patients with suspected appendicitis who underwent laparoscopy, only 3 had unnecessary appendectomies (7.5%). This was in contrast to the 22% rate of unnecessary appendectomies observed by this group among patients who underwent immediate laparotomy (11 of 50 patients). Similar low rates of removing a normal appendix following laparoscopy were reported by Graham and colleagues (2.2%)[17] and Nowzaradan and associates (5%).[18] Laparoscopy was also successful in preventing unnecessary appendectomy when another diagnostic test, fine-catheter peritoneal cytology, indicated appendicitis.[19] Of the 28 women who had positive results and underwent successful laparoscopy, 5 were found to have pelvic inflammatory disease and were spared laparotomy. Laparoscopy can be particularly valuable in preventing unnecessary appendectomy in women of reproductive age. Whitworth and colleagues[20] reported that operative intervention was avoided based on laparoscopic findings in 21 of the 51 young women in their series who presented with possible appendicitis. An initial study among patients with acquired immunodeficiency syndrome or human immunodeficiency virus–positive status,[21] in whom right lower quadrant abdominal pain presents a difficult diagnostic dilemma and for whom surgical intervention is associated with greatly increased mortality and morbidity, suggested that laparoscopy can result in earlier and more accurate diagnosis of appendicitis.

Removal of a normal appendix following laparoscopic evaluation typically occurs only in those cases in which the appendix cannot be directly visualized or when technical failure occurs. The rate of such procedural failures has generally been reported to be less than 10%. Given the substantially improved rate for correctly diagnosing acute appendicitis, particularly among patient groups in whom accurate diagnosis is difficult, most individuals deserving hospital admission for possible appendicitis should undergo laparoscopy. With laparoscopy, the diagnosis can be established and, if acute, the appendix can be removed at the same time. Moreover, diagnostic laparoscopy can facilitate the recognition and subsequent appropriate management of other disorders whose symptoms mimic those of appendicitis, such as salpingitis, a ruptured ovarian follicle, mesenteric adenitis, endometriosis, diverticulitis, Crohn's disease, and acute cholecystitis.

INDICATIONS FOR LAPAROSCOPIC APPENDECTOMY

As with the gallbladder, the appendix lends itself well to removal laparoscopically because it is an end organ. Several large series have recently been reported confirming the feasibility of laparoscopic appendectomy and demonstrating its safety,[3–5] even in a pediatric population[22] and among pregnant women.[23] Advantages of laparoscopic appendectomy include those associated with all laparoscopic surgical procedures described to date, namely, reduced morbidity and postoperative pain, a shortened hospital stay, a faster return to normal activities, and improved cosmetic appearance. Furthermore, laparoscopy provides good exposure of the appendix and permits complete examination of the abdominal region. Thus, complications of open appendectomy procedures, such as evisceration, herniation, and small bowel obstruction, are easier to avoid with the direct visualization afforded by the laparoscope. The incidence of wound infections may also be diminished with laparoscopic appendectomy because the size of the incision is less than that in open procedures and, importantly, the appendix is removed through a cannula or an Endopouch (Ethicon Endosurgery, Cincinnati, OH), minimizing tissue exposure. Additionally, suction of purulent material and irrigation of the pelvis are easier to accomplish with the improved visualization afforded by the laparoscope.

Among the published reports of laparoscopic appendectomy, either no postoperative complications were noted[18, 23–26] or complications were mild and consisted of nonspecific abdominal pain or slight fever in a few patients.[3, 27, 28] In his initial series of 70 women, Schreiber[6] reported the development of peritonitis with paralytic ileus in one patient in whom heat damage to the cecum occurred during endocoagulation, requiring further surgical intervention. Postoperative abscess formation requiring interval laparotomy has also been noted in a fraction of patients.[4, 29]

Three prospective studies have compared laparoscopic appendectomy to an open procedure.[27, 29, 30] Selection of the specific procedure performed was dictated by staff and equipment availability. Removal of the inflamed appendix by means of laparoscopic surgery was accomplished as easily as with the open procedure in these studies. The laparoscopic procedure was converted to an open one in 1 of 10 patients in Hill and associates' series[27] and in 2 of 27 patients in McAnena and colleagues' series[30] because of perforation in two cases and technical difficulties in one. In Gilchrist and colleagues' series[29] none of the 14 laparoscopic procedures was converted to an open appendectomy despite the occurrence of a ruptured appendix with abscess in 5 patients.

The length of hospitalization was shorter among patients undergoing laparoscopic appendectomy in all three studies. Gilchrist and colleagues[29] also noted that their pediatric patients returned to normal activities in a significantly shorter time (106 weeks in the group undergoing laparoscopy vs. 4 weeks in the group undergoing open appendectomy). Moreover, the same advantages for the laparoscopic procedure with respect to shorter hospital stay and quicker return to full activity were also noted for patients with complicated appendicitis (*i.e.,* gangrenous or perforated appendix).[29] Because of the limited number of patients in these three series, it is difficult to compare the incidence of postoperative complications in the laparoscopic and open surgery groups. Nevertheless, only 2 of the total 51 patients who underwent laparoscopic appendectomy in these studies had a significant postoperative complication; one pediatric patient in Gilchrist and colleagues'

series[29] experienced pneumonia, and another child in this series had a pelvic abscess that required operative drainage. In this pediatric series, pneumonia and pelvic abscess were also noted in 1 patient each among the group undergoing open surgery.

TECHNIQUE FOR LAPAROSCOPIC APPENDECTOMY

To perform our laparoscopic appendectomy procedure, male patients and female patients who have had a hysterectomy are placed in the supine position, whereas female patients who have not had a hysterectomy are positioned in low stirrups. A urinary catheter is inserted and patients are placed under general anesthesia. Preoperative antibiotic administration (intravenous cefoxitin sodium) is routine. The pelvis can usually be adequately inspected using a blunt probe through the suprapubic trocar (position #1 on Fig. 28–1); alternatively for some females who have not had a hysterectomy, it may be necessary to use a vaginal speculum, grasp the cervix with a single-toothed tenaculum, and introduce an intrauterine manipulator.

The surgeon stands at the patient's left, and the assistant, who stands at the patient's right, typically handles the camera, as well as the instruments in the right lower quadrant. The Hasson 11-mm trocar is introduced through a periumbilical incision. The peritoneal cavity is

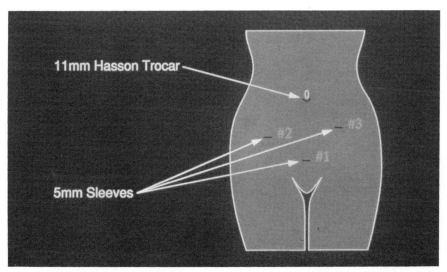

Figure 28–1. Trocar placement sites for laparoscopic appendectomy procedure.

then insufflated with carbon dioxide to an intraperitoneal pressure of 12 mm Hg. The laparoscope is inserted through the Hasson trocar along with the camera. To improve exposure, the table should be changed so that the patient is in the Trendelenburg position and rotated to the patient's left.

Under direct visualization, a 5-mm trocar is placed in the suprapubic area (position #1 on Fig. 28–1), and the pelvis and abdomen are visually explored using a blunt probe through this trocar. The uterus may have to be manipulated by the intrauterine manipulator in some females. After the need to remove the appendix is confirmed, attention should be directed to the small intestine. A 5-mm trocar is inserted above the cecum (in the area of the appendix), care being taken not to injure the inferior epigastric vessels (position #2 on Fig. 28–1). The small intestine is run with grasping forceps passed through position #1 (surgeon's left hand) and surgeon's right hand to make certain there is no other small bowel pathologic condition. The third 5-mm trocar (position #3 on Fig. 28–1) is placed halfway between the periumbilical Hasson trocar and the suprapubic trocar.

With the assistant elevating the appendix with a grasper by way of the second trocar, the surgeon holds the appendiceal mesentery with a grasper through the first trocar and makes windows in the avascular areas of the mesentery with the energy source passed through the third trocar. This can be effectively accomplished with endocautery and sharp dissection. As each vessel is exposed, it is grasped proximally through the first trocar, severed, and the grasper is transferred to the assistant. An Endoloop (Ethicon Endosurgery, Cincinnati, OH) ligature is passed through the second trocar. A grasper is inserted by way of the third trocar and the severed end of the vessels is grasped above or below the assistant's grasper. The Endoloop ligature is then tightened on the severed pedicle of the mesoappendix and the suture is cut with scissors passed through the first or third trocar. This process of clamping, severing, and ligating each vessel group is repeated sequentially until the appendix is completely freed down to its juncture with the cecum.

The appendiceal base is ligated with three Endoloop ligatures placed at 5-mm intervals, with the first ligature at the junction of the appendix and cecum. A grasper is inserted by means of the second trocar through the Endoloop ligature to hold the appendix as each Endoloop ligature is secured. The mesoappendix is carefully irrigated and inspected to be certain of hemostasis. The appendix is then severed between the two loops distally. The possibility of spillage from the appendix is controlled by the distal Endoloop.

A 5-mm laparoscope is passed through the suprapubic trocar. A 10-mm claw forceps is advanced through the Hasson trocar to take hold of the appendix just above the tie. The appendix is removed by bringing it out through the Hasson trocar, if feasible. If the appendix is too edematous and inflamed, it is placed in an endopouch, the Hasson trocar is removed, and the appendix in the Endopouch is carefully pulled through the periumbilical incision. It may be necessary to enlarge the fascial incision to do this. Upon completion of the operation, the Hasson trocar is reinserted into the abdominal cavity and the 5-mm laparoscope is removed. The mesoappendix and appendiceal stump are carefully inspected and the abdomen is irrigated with copious amounts of Ringer's solution. Lastly, the Hasson trocar is removed and the midline fascial puncture and all skin incisions are closed in the usual fashion.

ISSUES RELATED TO LAPAROSCOPIC APPENDECTOMY PROCEDURES

Laparoscopic appendectomy has clearly been shown by us and others to be a safe and effective alternative to traditional open appendectomy procedures. In addition to the benefits of diminished postoperative pain, shortened hospitalization, quicker return to normal activities, and minimization of cosmetic disfigurement, the laparoscope provides excellent visualization of the intraabdominal and pelvic regions, thereby facilitating accurate diagnosis. However, proficiency in the use of the laparoscope, as well as all accessory instruments, is essential to prevent the complications inherent in laparoscopy. Furthermore, dexterity in endoscopic bimanual surgery, proficiency in endosurgical suturing techniques (including intracorporeal and extracorporeal knot-tying), and the use of angle scopes are necessary skills for any surgeon performing operative laparoscopy.

From its inception, there have been arguments over the cost-effectiveness of laparoscopic surgery. Although surgeons should and must play a more prominent role in making certain that unnecessary costs are kept to a minimum, it is not clear that in the long run, open surgery has significant cost advantages over operative laparoscopy. Although the initial outlay for the equipment and training needed to perform laparoscopic surgery is considerable, the benefits of this type of surgery in terms of reduced hospitalization and lower morbidity may serve to diminish any cost differential between it and traditional open procedures. Moreover, costs associated with productivity loss during the recuperative period must be included in any comparison of expenses and, again, laparoscopic surgery has clear advantages over open procedures in terms of a significantly faster return to normal activities. In their analysis of hospital and operative costs associated with open and laparoscopic appendectomy procedures among a pediatric group, Gilchrist and colleagues[29] reported no difference in the average hospital costs and only about a $1000 difference in the average operative costs, with the laparoscopic procedure being more expensive. Interestingly, for patients with complicated appendicitis (*i.e.,* gangrenous or perforated appendix), average operative costs were approximately $1200 *less* for the laparoscopic group than for the traditional surgery group.

To share their responsibility with society in controlling medical care costs, surgeons must remain conscious of cost and should strive to develop or select procedures that balance the effectiveness of the surgical intervention with expense. In performing laparoscopic appendectomy, for example, the mesoappendix may be controlled by creation of mesenteric windows,

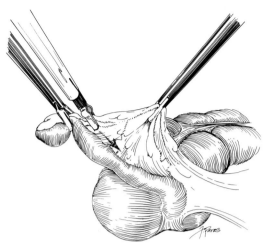

Figure 28–3. Bipolar electrocoagulation of the mesoappendix with Kleppinger forceps.

by suture ligation (Fig. 28–2), or by bipolar electrocautery (Fig. 28–3). Surgical options for creating mesenteric windows in the avascular area include the use of sharp dissection, laser, or electrocautery. After a mesenteric window is created, the surgeon may ligate the mesoappendix with metallic Endoclips (Ethicon Endosurgery, Cincinnati, OH) (Fig. 28–4), a vascular stapling device (Fig. 28–5), or by Endoloops using the two-grasper technique (Fig. 28–6 and 28–7). At this point, the base of the appendix is ready to be occluded, which can be accomplished with either Endoloop ligation (Fig. 28–8) or an automatic stapling device (Fig. 28–9). In deciding how to perform the specific procedure, each surgeon must weigh the speed of the operation against the expense of the equipment.

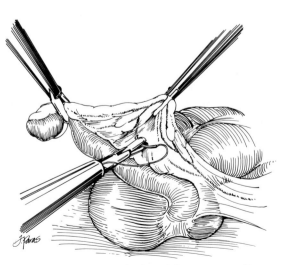

Figure 28–2. Suture ligation of the mesoappendix.

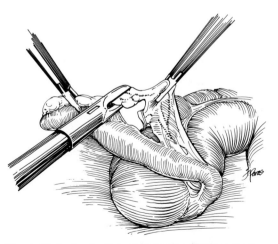

Figure 28–4. Application of Endoclips (Ethicon Endosurgery, Cincinnati, OH) for hemostasis of the mesoappendix.

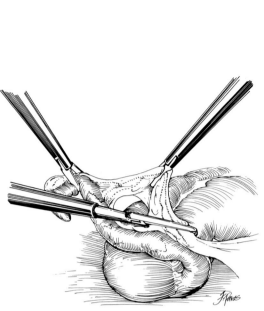

Figure 28–5. Stapling of the mesoappendix with a staple and linear cutter for control of hemostasis.

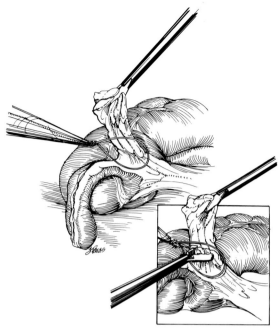

Figure 28–7. Two-grasper technique for using the Endoloop (Ethicon Endosurgery, Cincinnati, OH) on the mesoappendix.

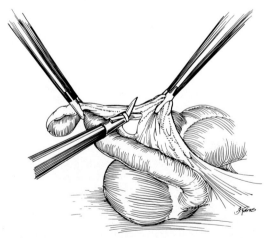

Figure 28–6. Cutting the mesoappendix while maintaining proximal control with tissue grasper.

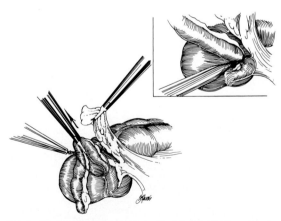

Figure 28–8. Application of an Endoloop (Ethicon Endosurgery, Cincinnati, OH) around the base of the appendix.

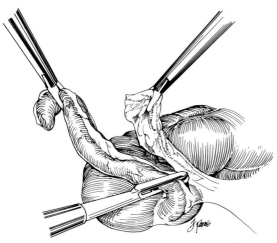

Figure 28–9. Stapling the base of the appendix.

CONCLUSION

Laparoscopic appendectomy has clearly been shown to be a safe and effective procedure that appears to offer significant potential benefits for patients in terms of lower morbidity, reduced hospitalization, a quicker return to normal activities, and improved cosmetic appearance. Diagnostic laparoscopy is clearly indicated for most patients with suspected appendicitis, whereas the choice between open and laparoscopic appendectomy is dictated by the complexity of the pathologic condition and the skill of the endoscopic surgeon.

References

1. Jess P. Acute appendicitis: epidemiology, diagnostic accuracy, and complications. Scand Gastroenterol 18:161–163, 1983.
2. Semm K. Endoscopic appendectomy. Endoscopy 15:59–64, 1983.
3. Nezhat C, Nezhat F. Incidental appendectomy during videolaseroscopy. Am J Obstet Gynecol 165:559–564, 1991.
4. Peir A, Gotz F, Bacher C. Laparoscopic appendectomy in 625 cases: from innovation to routine. Surg Laparosc Endosc 1:8–13, 1991.
5. Saye WB, Rives DA, Cochran EB. Laparoscopic appendectomy: three years' experience. Surg Laparosc Endosc 1:109–115, 1991.
6. Schreiber JH. Early experience with laparoscopic appendectomy in women. Surg Endosc 1:211–216, 1987.
7. Hoffmann J, Rasmussen OO. Aids in the diagnosis of acute appendicitis. Br J Surg 76:774–779, 1989.
8. Pieper R, Kager L, Nasman P. Acute appendicitis: a clinical study of 1018 cases of emergency appendectomy. Acta Chir Scand 148:51–62, 1982.
9. Lewis FR, Holcroft JW, Boey J, et al. Appendicitis: a critical review of diagnosis and treatment in 1000 cases. Arch Surg 110:677–684, 1975.
10. Campbell JPM, Gunn AA. Plain abdominal radiographs and acute abdominal pain. Br J Surg 75:554–556, 1988.
11. Graham AD, Johnson HF. The incidence of radiographic findings in acute appendicitis compared to 200 normal abdomens. Milit Med 131:272–276, 1966.
12. Adams DH, Fine C, Brooks DC. High-resolution real-time ultrasonography: a new tool in the diagnosis of acute appendicitis. Am J Surg 155:93–97, 1988.
13. Puylaert JBCM, Rutgers PH, Lalisang RI, et al. A prospective study of ultrasonography in the diagnosis of appendicitis. N Engl J Med 317:666–669, 1987.
14. Lewin GA, Mikity V, Wingert WA. Barium enema: an outpatient procedure in the early diagnosis of acute appendicitis. J Pediatr 92:451–453, 1978.
15. Rajogopalan AE, Mason JH, Kennedy M, Pawlikowski J. The value of the barium enema in the diagnosis of acute appendicitis. Arch Surg 112:531–533, 1977.
16. Paterson-Brown S, Thompson JN, Eckersley JRT, et al. Which patients with suspected appendicitis should undergo laparoscopy? Br Med J 296:1363–1364, 1988.
17. Graham A, Henley C, Mobley J. Laparoscopic evaluation of acute abdominal pain. J Laparoendosc Surg 1:165–168, 1991.
18. Nowzaradan Y, Westmoreland J, McCarver CT, Harris RJ. Laparoscopic appendectomy for acute appendicitis: indications and current use. J Laparoendosc Surg 1:247–257, 1991.
19. Baigrie RJ, Zaidan Z, Scott-Coombes D, et al. Role of fine catheter peritoneal cytology and laparoscopy in the management of acute abdominal pain. Br J Surg 78:167–170, 1991.
20. Whitworth CM, Whitworth PM, Sanfillipo J, Polk HC. Value of diagnostic laparoscopy in young women with possible appendicitis. Surg Obstet Gynecol 167:187–190, 1988.
21. Binderow SR, Shaked AA. Acute appendicitis in patients with AIDS/HIV infection. Am J Surg 162:9–12, 1991.
22. Valla JS, Limmone B, Valla V, et al. Laparoscopic appendectomy in children: report of 465 cases. Surg Laparosc Endosc 1:166–172, 1991.
23. Schreiber JH. Laparoscopic appendectomy in pregnancy. Surg Endosc 4:100–102, 1990.
24. Daniell JF, Gurley LD, Kurtz BR, Chambers JF. The use of an automatic stapling device for laparoscopic appendectomy. Obstet Gynecol 78:721–723, 1991.
25. McKernan JB, Saye WB. Laparoscopic techniques in appendectomy with argon laser. South Med J 83:1019–1020, 1990.
26. Wolenski M, Markus E, Pelosi MA. Laparoscopic appendectomy incidental to gynecologic procedures. Today's OR Nurse 13:12–18, 1991.
27. Hill ADK, Attwood SEA, Stephens RB. Laparoscopy appendicectomy is feasible and safe in acute appendicitis. Ir J Med Sci 160:268–270, 1991.
28. O'Regan PJ. Laparoscopic appendectomy. Can J Surg 34:256–258, 1991.
29. Gilchrist BF, Lobe TE, Schropp KP, et al. Is there a role for laparoscopic appendectomy in pediatric surgery? J Pediat Surg 27:209–214, 1992.
30. McAnena OJ, Austin O, Hederman WP, et al. Laparoscopic versus open appendicectomy. Lancet 338:693, 1991.

29

Laparoscopic Inguinal Hernia Repair

Riccardo G. Annibali, Robert J. Fitzgibbons, Jr.,
Charles J. Filipi, Bradley S. Litke, and Giovanni M. Salerno

If no other field were offered to the surgeon for his activity than herniotomy it would be worthwhile to become a surgeon and to devote an entire life to this service.[1]

M. RAVITCH

"Operations for the cure of hernia would seem to be established and well known beyond the possible need for further discussion and demonstration." This comment introduced the reader to a popular handbook of operative surgery on the repair of hernias in 1969.[1] In reality, more than 20 years later, the last word on the surgical treatment of groin hernias has yet to be written.

The excellent results obtained with laparoscopic cholecystectomy since its introduction in 1988 have influenced surgical opinion, resulting in a wide acceptance of other therapeutic laparoscopic methods for a variety of applications, including biliary tract surgery, appendectomy, gynecologic procedures, esophageal and antireflux surgery, bowel resections, and others.[2, 3] Laparoscopic herniorrhaphy is one of these new procedures. A number of surgeons, having become quite comfortable with the principles and practice of therapeutic laparoscopy, have begun to investigate laparoscopic herniorrhaphy, the goal being an operation that is associated with lower operative morbidity and a shorter time to return to normal activity, with a reduced recurrence rate when compared with conventional hernia repair.

At present, however, some important controversies remain, whereas the benefits of applying laparoscopic techniques to inguinal hernia repair may not be self-evident. The conventional operation is frequently performed under local anesthesia on an outpatient basis, whereas general anesthesia is generally recommended for the laparoscopic approach. Moreover, most conventional herniorrhaphies do not require entry into the peritoneal cavity, thus avoiding the possible risks and consequences that are inherent to laparoscopy.

For these reasons, laparoscopic inguinal herniorrhaphy is still under investigation, with intensive evaluation required to prove decreased morbidity and a reduced recurrence rate before its adoption can be recommended to the surgical community at large.

The purpose of this chapter is to examine the background of and justification for laparoscopic inguinal herniorrhaphy, as well as to discuss the pertinent anatomy, early types of repair, and specialized instrumentation required. The currently accepted techniques are highlighted and, finally, the possible role of laparoscopic herniorrhaphy in the future is discussed.

EPIDEMIOLOGY

The generally quoted average number of 500,000 to 550,000 inguinal herniorrhaphies performed yearly in the United States is probably an underestimate, as these figures refer only to patients discharged from short-stay, nonfederal hospitals.[4–8] A US Department of Health, Education, and Welfare study demonstrated in 1960 that hernia prevalence is approximately 15 cases/1000 population.[9] The prevalence is likely

352

to be higher, however, because this figure includes only hernias of which the respondents to an interview were aware. In a study conducted in Israel, the prevalence of inguinal hernia ranged from 5% among men aged 25 to 34 years to 45% among men aged 75 years and older; the ratio of right-sided hernia to left-sided hernias was 1.3:1.[10]

The incidence of the different types of abdominal hernias, compiled by Harkins, is shown in Table 29–1.[11] The condition afflicts far more men than women, with a ratio of 10.7:1.[12] Recurrent hernias account for 50,000 to 100,000 cases a year in the United States.[6, 13]

An apparent reduction in the total number of inguinal hernia repairs in the last decade (537,000 operations reported in 1980 compared with 243,000 in 1989, in nonfederal hospitals) probably reflects a change in the proportions managed by inpatient and outpatient surgeries (the average hospital stay in the United States for a unilateral groin hernia was 6.0 days in 1982 and 2.9 days in 1989).[8, 12, 14] In fact, this operation remains one of the most commonly performed surgical procedures worldwide.[5, 15–17] In 1987, it was the fourth most frequently performed operation in men, after cardiac catheterization, prostatectomy, and reduction of fractures, with a rate of 2.5 procedures/1000 population.[18] In addition, it is important to note that only one third of the "obvious" hernias in the Israeli study mentioned had been subsequently operated upon.[10] In the United States, approximately 800,000 subjects/annum who are found to have hernias choose not to have the condition repaired.[6]

ANATOMIC CONSIDERATIONS

No disease of the human body belonging to the province of the surgeon requires in its treatment a greater combination of accurate anatomic knowledge with surgical skill than hernia in all its varieties.[19]

SIR ASTLEY COOPER

The anatomy of the inguinal region is misunderstood by some surgeons at all levels of seniority.[20]

R. CONDON

A hernia is usually defined as the "protrusion of a viscus from the cavity in which it is normally contained" or more completely as "the protrusion of a loop or knuckle of an organ or tissue through an abnormal opening."[21]

Table 29–1. INCIDENCE OF DIFFERENT TYPES OF HERNIA

Type of Hernia	Incidence
Indirect inguinal	56
Direct inguinal	22
Femoral	6
Ventral and incisional	10
Umbilical	3
Esophageal hiatus	1
Others	2
TOTAL	100

From Gaster J. Hernia: One day repair. Darien, CT, Hafner Publishing, 1970.

Inguinal hernias have troubled humankind since time immemorial, and several hypotheses have been formed to explain the origins of this ailment. The one most credited today is the human phylogenetic theory, which ascribes the cause of development of inguinal hernias to the abandonment of the quadruped gait in order to gain the erect position.[6] The change from the horizontal position of the quadruped animal to the vertical position of *Homo erectus* resulted in the development of a weakness in the lower abdomen (Fig. 29–1). The groin area in quadrupeds is less affected by abdominal pressure because in the horizontal position, the maximum pressure is exerted toward the umbilicus. In addition, because in the quadruped the thigh is flexed against the trunk, firm support is provided to the inguinoabdominal region.[22] Moreover, in the bipedal erect position, the bony cavity of the pelvis resembles a right-side-up bowl, tilted forward. This results in an increase of abdominal pressure acting at the groin region.[23] It is not surprising that 90% of all hernias in the human body occur in the area of the inguinal canal and femoral canal.[24]

The study of anatomy of the groin and inguinal canal has always represented a stumbling block for medical students and residents alike. Most anatomic and groin hernia textbooks describe the critical layers in sequence as a dissection would proceed from the superficial layers to the deep ones, reserving little consideration for the internal view of the abdominal wall. Indeed, in 1945 Lytle wrote: "The operating surgeon knows little of the posterior wall of the inguinal canal, so well is it hidden from his view."[25] For laparoscopic herniorrhaphy, it would seem appropriate to reverse this approach and start from the inner layers, since laparoscopy provides an optimal panoramic view of the posterior surface of the abdominal wall.

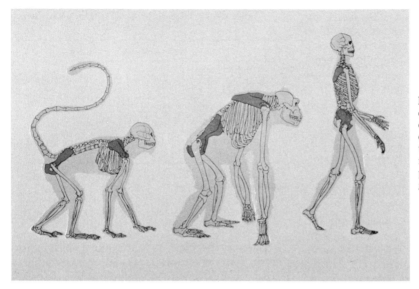

Figure 29–1. The groin area in quadrupeds is less affected by abdominal pressure. In the bipedal erect position, the bony cavity of the pelvis is tilted forward. This results in an increase of abdominal pressure acting at the inguinal region.

Peritoneum

The internal surface of the abdominal wall above the inguinal ligament is lined by peritoneum (Figs. 29–2 and 29–3). Below the umbilicus there are five peritoneal folds, uplifted by three convergent fibrous cords in the center and two vascular bundles peripherally. In the midline is the *median umbilical ligament,* which represents the obliterated remnant of the embryonic urachus and extends from the fundus of the bladder to the umbilicus. Two peritoneal folds, the medial and lateral umbilical ligaments, delineate three shallow fossae on either side of the midline. The *medial umbilical ligament* consists of a fold of peritoneum covering the obliterated distal portion of the umbilical artery. This is usually atrophic, cord-like, and obsolete in the adult. The umbilical artery is normally patent in its proximal tract and provides the *superior vesical arteries* to the urinary bladder (see Figs. 29–2 and 29–8*A*). Occasionally, the entire umbilical artery remains patent.[26] In some patients, this fold is particularly prominent and may hinder the laparoscopic surgeon in accomplishing a proper dissection.[27] The *lateral umbilical ligament* consists of a fold of peritoneum around the inferior epigastric vessels together with a variable amount of fatty tissue.

It should be noted that there is some confusion regarding the correct terminology of these folds, as some authors define the fold outlined by the umbilical artery as the *lateral umbilical ligament,* whereas the fold associated with the inferior epigastric vessels has been called the *plica epigastrica.*[21, 26, 28] For the purposes of this

chapter, the more consistent terminology described in the preceding paragraph, which conforms with that found in Nomina Anatomica, will be used (Table 29–2).[20, 23, 29–32]

As stated previously, the medial and lateral umbilical ligaments delineate three fossae on either side of the midline (see Fig. 29–3). The *lateral fossa* lies lateral to the inferior epigastric vessels and is the site of indirect hernias, because it contains the internal inguinal ring. The *medial* (or middle) *fossa* is defined as the space between the inferior epigastric vessels and the medial umbilical ligament and corresponds to the site of direct inguinal hernias. The location of the medial umbilical ligament, however, is variable; it sometimes is virtually superimposed over the lateral umbilical ligament and is not to be considered a consistent landmark. Finally, the *supravesical* (or internal) *inguinal fossa* lies between the medial and the median umbilical ligaments. The musculus rectus abdominis and

Table 29–2. DIFFERENT TERMINOLOGIES USED TO INDICATE THE PERITONEAL FOLDS OF THE DEEP SURFACE OF THE ANTERIOR ABDOMINAL WALL

Structure Determining the Fold	Nomina Anatomica Terminology	Alternative Terminology
Urachus	Median umbilical ligament	Median umbilical ligament
Obliterated umbilical artery	Medial umbilical ligament	Lateral umbilical ligament
Inferior epigastric vessels	Lateral umbilical ligament	Plica epigastrica

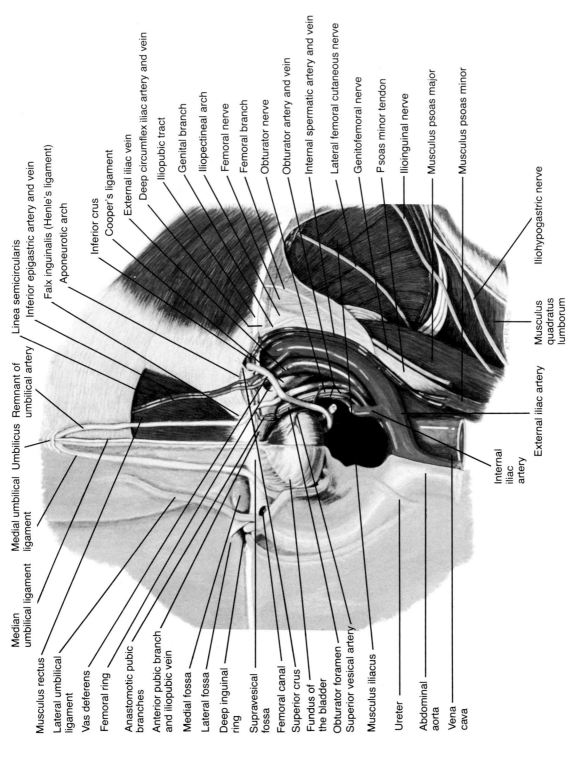

Figure 29–2. Anatomy of the inguinal region, lower deep abdominal wall, and lower trunk. Internal view.

Median
umbilical ligament

Medial umbilical
ligament

Umbilicus

Remnant of
umbilical artery

Musculus rectus

Lateral umbilical
ligament

Vas deferens

Femoral ring

Anastomotic pubic
branches

Anterior pubic branch
and iliopubic vein

Medial fossa

Lateral fossa

Deep inguinal
ring

Supravesical
fossa

Femoral canal

Superior crus

Fundus of
the bladder

Obturator foramen

Superior vesical artery

Musculus iliacus

Ureter

Abdominal
aorta

Vena
cava

Linea semicircularis

Inferior epigastric artery and vein

Falx inguinalis (Henle's ligament)

Aponeurotic arch

Inferior crus

Cooper's ligament

External iliac vein

Deep circumflex iliac artery and vein

Iliopubic tract

Genital branch

Iliopectineal arch

Femoral nerve

Femoral branch

Obturator nerve

Obturator artery and vein

Internal spermatic artery and vein

Lateral femoral cutaneous nerve

Genitofemoral nerve

Psoas minor tendon

Ilioinguinal nerve

Musculus psoas major

Musculus psoas minor

Iliohypogastric nerve

Musculus
quadratus
lumborum

External iliac artery

Internal
iliac
artery

355

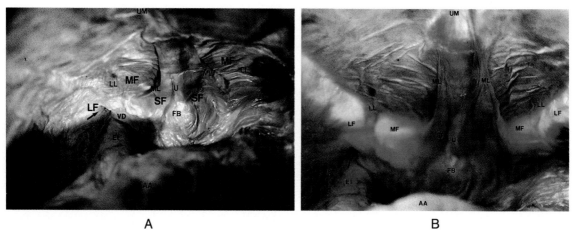

| A | B |

Figure 29–3. (A) Panoramic view of the deep surface of the anterior abdominal wall in a cadaver preparation. Peritoneal folds and fossae are demonstrated. The arrow indicates the deep inguinal ring. **(B)** The weak areas corresponding to the peritoneal fossae are better demonstrated with transillumination of the lower anterior abdominal wall.

UM = umbilicus; FB = fundus of the bladder; U = median umbilical ligament; ML = medial umbilical ligament; LL = lateral umbilical ligament (inferior epigastric vessels); SF = supravesical fossa; MF = medial fossa; LF = lateral fossa; IS = internal spermatic vessels; VD = vas deferens; EI = external iliac vessels; AA = abdominal aorta.

its sheath confer a greater strength to this area, making supravesical hernias rare.[23] Condon remarked in 1978 that "the umbilical fossae are rarely noted during intraabdominal operations and are of no surgical importance in regard to either the etiology or the repair of groin hernias."[20] The development of laparoscopic groin herniorrhaphy has changed this idea, as increased familiarity with the inside view of the abdomen has proved a consistent relationship between inguinal herniation and the umbilical fossae.

Preperitoneal Space

Beneath the peritoneum, a variable amount of connective tissue (which may be areolar, fatty, or semimembranous) is found in the preperitoneal space of Bogros (Fig. 29–4; see also Fig. 29–2).[21, 23, 29] The residua of the umbilical artery and the inferior epigastric vessels, which produce the two peritoneal folds on either side of the midline, are located here (Fig. 29–5; see also Figs. 29–8A and 29–13B). This space is important for the laparoscopic surgeon intending to perform a preperitoneal hernia repair. The *external iliac vessels* run along the musculus psoas major fascia, on the medial aspect of the musculus psoas major, pass under the iliopubic tract wrapped into the femoral sheath, and under the inguinal ligament, to become the *femoral vessels* (see Fig. 29–5; see also Figs. 29–8A and 29–13B). From the external iliac vessels originate the *inferior epigastric vessels* (see Fig.

29–5; see also Figs. 29–2 and 29–8); they run superiorly and medially toward the umbilicus from a point midway between the anterior superior iliac spine and the symphysis pubis, ascend obliquely along the medial margin of the internal inguinal ring between the fascia transversalis and the peritoneum, and finally pierce the fascia transversalis to enter the sheath of the musculus rectus abdominis. These vessels lie free in the preperitoneal space and have no

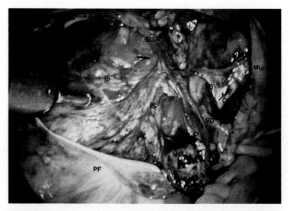

Figure 29–4. Preperitoneal space as seen laparoscopically during a transabdominal preperitoneal procedure (TAPP) hernia repair. The arrow points to the deep inguinal ring.

PF = peritoneal flap, reflected; IS = internal spermatic vessels; VD = vas deferens; CL = Cooper's ligament; ML = medial umbilical ligament; PB = anastomotic pubic branch; AP = iliopubic vein; IE = inferior epigastric vessels; SC = superior crus of the fascia transversalis sling; IP = iliopubic tract; AA = aponeurotic arch of the musculus transversus abdominis.

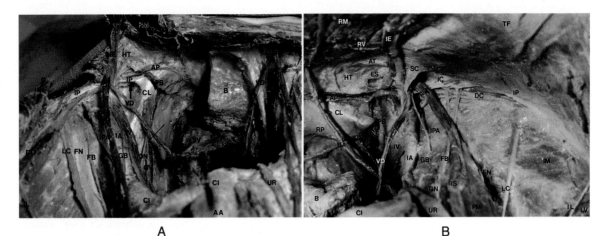

A   B

Figure 29–5. (A) Photograph of a cadaver dissection *(left side)* showing the inguinal (Hesselbach's) triangle, Cooper's ligament, the iliopubic tract, and the femoral region. The thick arrow indicates the femoral ring; the thin arrow points to the obturator foramen. **(B)** Photograph of a cadaver preparation *(right side)* showing the inguinal area at the level of the preperitoneal space after removal of the peritoneum and preperitoneal adipose tissue (the remnant of the urachus has been resected and the bladder retracted posteriorly). The arrow points to the femoral ring.

IR = deep inguinal ring; HT = inguinal (Hesselbach's) triangle; RM = musculus rectus abdominis muscle; RV = rectusial vein; IE = inferior epigastric vessels; IP = iliopubic tract; CL = Cooper's ligament; AT = aponeurotic arch of the musculus transversus abdominis; IS = internal spermatic vessels; ES = external spermatic vessels; VD = vas deferens; IA = external iliac artery; IV = external iliac vein; IPA = iliopectineal arch; ON = obturator nerve; OV = obturator vessels; GN = genitofemoral nerve; GB = genital branch of the genitofemoral nerve; FB = femoral branch of the genitofemoral nerve; FN = femoral nerve; LC = lateral femoral cutaneous nerve; IL = ilioinguinal nerve; DC = deep circumflex iliac vessels; SV = seminal vesicles; UA = umbilical artery; PB = anastomotic pubic branch; AP = anterior pubic branch and accompanying iliopubic vein; RP = retropubic vein; LV = iliolumbal vessels; B = bladder (the left half has been removed in **A**); CI = common iliac artery; AA = abdominal aorta; UR = ureter; IM = musculus iliacus; PM = musculus psoas major; TF = fascia transversalis.

intimate anatomic relationship with the fascia transversalis, a fact that is important to the laparoscopic surgeon.

The inferior epigastric arteries give rise to two collateral branches: the *external spermatic (or cremasteric) artery* and the *anastomotic pubic branch* (see Fig. 29–5; see also Figs. 29–2, 29–8A, and 29–13B). The former runs upward from its origin along the medial aspect of the internal inguinal ring, pierces the fascia transversalis, and crosses the preperitoneal space to join the spermatic cord. The latter runs to the obturator foramen, at which point it joins the obturator artery after giving rise to a small branch called the *anterior pubic branch,* where it crosses the superior ramus of the pubis. The anterior pubic branch runs along the superior ramus of the pubis toward the body of this bone. The anastomotic ring, formed by the pubic branch, normally paralleled by its corresponding venous system, is also known as the *corona mortis* (crown of death) because of the bleeding that occurs if it is injured while sutures or staples are applied to Cooper's ligament. An obturator artery originating from the inferior epigastric or external iliac vessel has been observed in approximately 30% of specimens studied.[33–35] This

origin is usually related to a considerable enlargement of the pubic branch from the inferior epigastric vessels (see Fig. 29–8A). Damage to this anomalous artery during surgical repair could lead to serious hemorrhage into the preperitoneal space. The anterior pubic branch is usually accompanied by a vein, called the *iliopubic vein* because it courses deep to the iliopubic tract (see Fig. 29–5A; see also Figs. 29–2, 29–4, 29–8A and B, and 29–13B). It either empties directly into the inferior epigastric vein or joins the venous anastomotic pubic branch to form a common trunk that drains into the inferior epigastric vein.[36] The *rectusial vein* is another affluent of the inferior epigastric vein and runs along, or embedded within, the lower lateral fibers of the musculus rectus abdominis (see Fig. 29–5B; see also Fig. 29–8A and B). According to Bendavid, who first gave a name to this vessel, it consistently forms a venous anastomotic ring by joining the iliopubic vein above the pubic crest.[36] During our cadaver dissections, in most cases we were able to demonstrate this connection. However, it should be noted that these venous anastomoses are better identified at the operating table, rather than in the anatomy laboratory, as the small veins are often collapsed and empty in the cadaver but are darkened and engorged in the patient undergoing surgical treatment. Finally, another small collateral branch of the anastomotic pubic vessel is commonly observed on the lower posterior aspect of the pubic ramus, beneath Cooper's ligament, and has been called the *retropubic vein* (see Fig. 29–5B; see also Figs. 29–8A and B and 29–13B). The importance of becoming familiar with the deep inguinal venous circulation for all surgeons interested in placing prosthetic materials inside the preperitoneal space for hernia repair is evident: damage to these structures is easy and usually leads to hematoma formation.

The external iliac vessels are also the origin of the *deep circumflex iliac artery and vein* (see Fig. 29–5; see also Figs. 29–2, 29–13B, and 29–14B and C), which cross laterally over the femoral sheath, run between the iliopubic tract and the iliopectineal arch, and pierce the fascia transversalis to finally end in the space between the musculus transversus abdominis and the musculus obliquus internus abdominis, at which point they anastomose with the *iliolumbar and superior gluteal vessels* (see Fig. 29–5; see also Figs. 29–2 and 29–14B).[20, 37] The laparoscopic surgeon needs to appreciate the relationship of these vessels because if they are inadvertently stapled during laparoscopic herniorrhaphy, a hematoma may result.

Fascia Transversalis

Proceeding outward, external to the preperitoneal space is the *endoabdominal fascia*. This fascia covers separate muscles or aponeuroses, or it becomes attached to the periosteum of interposed bony structures. It acquires different names corresponding to the external structure covered at that point (*i.e.*, transversalis, psoas, obturator, iliac, and so on) but belongs to a single fascial envelope that invests the entire abdomen.[21] The term fascia transversalis was coined by Sir Astley Cooper to designate the portion of the endoabdominal fascia that covers the internal surface of the musculus transversus abdominis.[24, 38]

Read has pointed out that the original description by Cooper suggested that the fascia transversalis was composed of an outer (or anterior) and an inner (or posterior) lamina.[38] This concept has been supported by Cleland and Mackay[39] but disputed by Condon[20] Anson and McVay.[40] Cooper felt that the anterior layer was closely related to the musculus transversus abdominis aponeurosis. It attached inferiorly to

Cooper's ligament and medially enveloped the musculus rectus abdominis (rectus fascia of McVay).[40] The posterior layer inserted superiorly to the linea semicircularis of Douglas, medially to the linea alba and inferiorly to the superior ramus of the pubis. Read pointed out that in this model, the inferior epigastric vessels do not actually lie within the preperitoneal space but instead are contained within the two layers of the fascia transversalis.[38] Other authors have identified what Read considers the posterior layer of the fascia transversalis as the *preperitoneal membrane* or *preperitoneal fascia*.[25, 41, 42]

The importance of the fascia transversalis is linked to the fact that it is a layer through which inguinal hernias must pass.[23] There is, however, significant confusion and uncertainty about the precise role the fascia transversalis plays in the origin and repair of inguinal hernias.[6, 19, 43] Some authors feel that the fascia transversalis is a thin and weak layer with no intrinsic strength.[6, 20, 24] Others argue that a resistant and strong fascia transversalis is essential to the avoidance of herniation.[23] Indeed, Griffith stated that "the fact that fascia transversalis may be destroyed by large direct hernias in obese elderly men has led to the concept that the fascia transversalis is unimportant. Nothing could be further from the truth."[44]

There is general agreement, however, that the combination of deep elements of the abdominal wall, including the musculus transversus abdominis with its aponeurosis and the fascia transversalis, is the firm, solid structure that supports the pressure from the intraabdominal organs and prevents herniation.[5, 16, 23, 45] The argument concerning the importance of the fascia transversalis is probably of academic interest, primarily because most surgeons include both the fascia and muscle when repairing a hernia.

The *internal inguinal ring* (or deep inguinal ring) is located in the lateral fossa about 1.25 cm above and slightly lateral to the middle of the inguinal ligament[5, 6, 15] (Fig. 29–6; see also Figs. 29–2, 29–3, 29–5, 29–8A and B, 29–12, and 29–13B). It is the internal opening of the inguinal canal and is a conduit for the vas deferens and the testicular vessels. It is usually reported as being 2 cm in circumference but appears nearly closed when viewed laparoscopically.

Fascia Transversalis Analogs

Various appendices, thickenings, and condensations of the fascia transversalis have specific

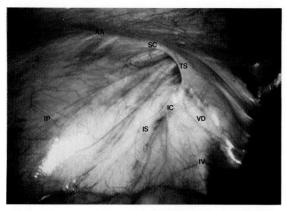

Figure 29–6. Laparoscopic view of the internal inguinal ring.
TS = fascia transversalis sling; SC = superior crus of the fascia transversalis sling; IC = inferior crus of the fascia transversalis sling; IS = internal spermatic vessels; VD = vas deferens; IV = external iliac vein; IP = iliopubic tract; IE = inferior epigastric vessels.

names and are important to the laparoscopic surgeon. These are the so-called *fascia transversalis analogs.*[5, 20]

One important analog is the *fascia transversalis sling* (see Fig. 29–6; see also Figs. 29–2, 29–4, 29–5B, 29–8A and B, and 29–13B). During fetal development, the testicle descends from its abdominal location to the scrotum, pulling with it a blunt, funnel-shaped, oblique cone of fascia transversalis.[6, 20, 44] This cone of fascia is not geometrically perfect in shape, as it is bent obliquely and orientated inferomedially. However, it is less oblique than the cord direction, thus being redundant on the medial side of the cord and forming a sling-shaped, thickened condensation in the fascia transversalis that reinforces the medial aspect of the deep ring (the "sling").[15, 37] The sling has superior and inferior extensions that are known as the *superior* and *inferior crura.*[20, 23]

The physiologic importance of this anatomic structure is significant, as it plays a key role in the *sphincteric* or *valvular mechanism* of the internal inguinal ring. When the muscular fibers of the musculus transversus abdominis contract, the fascia transversalis moves along with them, displacing the internal ring laterally and cephalad under the muscular edge of the musculus obliquus internus abdominis.[25, 46] This action also causes the crura to approximate each other, further reinforcing the internal ring closure and preventing indirect herniation.[5, 20, 29]

The *iliopubic tract* is a fascial condensation beginning laterally at the inner lip of the iliac crest, the anterior superior iliac spine, and the iliopectineal arch. It runs parallel to the inguinal ligament, crosses the femoral vessels anteriorly while bordering the deep inguinal ring inferiorly, curves around the medial surface of the femoral sheath, and finally fans out to attach to the medial portion of Cooper's ligament and the pubic tubercle (Figs. 29–7, 29–8A and B, and 29–9; see also 29–2, 29–4, 29–5A and B, 29–6, 29–12, and 29–14).[5, 6, 15, 24, 47] This structure has been given several other names such as bandelette de Thompson, bandelette ilio-pubienne, and deep femoral arch, but none of these terms is commonly used.[6] According to some authors, it is a tough elastic cord essential for hernia repair.[15, 48] Lichtenstein and colleagues, however, have found it to be of significant strength only in a small number (25%) of cases and do not regard it as a supportive structure.[13, 49] In a series of 151 dissections of embalmed inguinal regions and in serial sagittal sections of four body halves performed both in the United States and in China, Gilroy and coworkers could identify a substantial structure corresponding to the iliopubic tract in 42% of the specimens.[50]

Cooper's ligament is a structure easily identified at surgery but difficult to define anatomically, as the original description of Sir Astley Cooper has been often modified (see Figs. 29–2, 29–4, 29–5A and B, 29–7, 29–8A and B, and 29–13B).[19, 43] Some have described it as the fusion of the periosteum covering the superior ramus of the pubis lateral to the pubic tubercle with the fascia transversalis and the iliopubic tract.[5, 20, 24, 48, 51] Others feel it is simply a lateral extension of tendinous fibers from the lacunar ligament.[52] Still others have questioned whether it is appropriate to refer to it as a separate ligament.[24] Nevertheless, for surgical purposes, Cooper's ligament is the shiny fibrous structure covering the superior pubic ramus.[27]

The *iliopectineal arch* is a condensation of the fascia transversalis on the medial side of the iliac fascia and is connected laterally with the anterosuperior iliac spine and medially with the iliopectineal eminence after crossing the lateral aspect of the femoral sheath (see Figs. 29–2, 29–5B, 29–7, 29–13B, and 29–14B and C). It is the origin for parts of the fibers of the musculi obliquus externus abdominis, obliquus internus abdominis, and transversus abdominis and the iliopubic tract. It extends into the femoral triangle, where it is also an important landmark to separate the vascular compartment (lacuna vasorum medially) from the muscular partition (lacuna musculorum laterally) (see Fig. 29–13B). The former contains the femoral vessels and the femoral canal; the latter is mainly

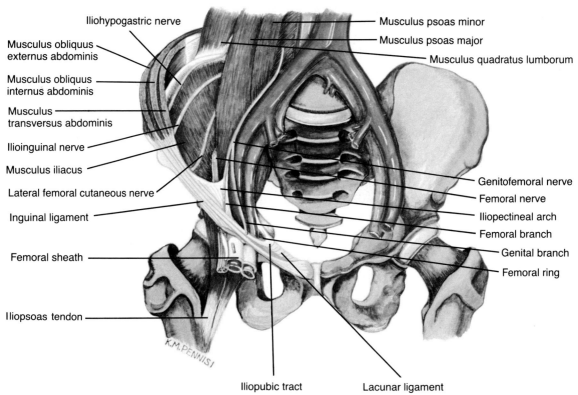

Figure 29–7. Anatomy of the inguinal and femoral region.

occupied by the musculus iliopsoas but also contains the femoral nerve and the lateral femoral cutaneous nerve (see further on).

Musculus Transversus Abdominis

The musculus transversus abdominis takes its origin from the lower six ribs, the lumbodorsal fascia, the iliac crest, the iliopubic tract, and the musculus iliopsoas fascia. These fibers pass transversely around the lateral abdomen to the midline. Lateral to the musculus rectus abdominis, the fibers of the musculus transversus abdominis transit into a tendinous aponeurosis. The lower fibers cross downward and medially to form an *aponeurotic arch,* which inserts at the pubic tubercle and the medial side of Cooper's ligament, thus forming the superior margin of the inguinal ring (see Fig. 29–9; see also Figs. 29–2, 29–4, 29–5*B*, 29–8, and 29–14*A* and *B*).[23] Occasionally, these fibers join with parallel lower fibers of the musculus obliquus internus abdominis as they insert on the pubic tubercle and the superior ramus of the pubis to form the so-called conjoined tendon.[20, 53] This combination, however, has been found in only 3% to

5% of cases.[5, 20, 52] In fact, McVay and others have contended that the conjoined tendon does not exist and is only an artifact of the dissection.[48, 53]

Direct and indirect herniation is prevented by a second important physiologic system known as the *shutter mechanism.* It is activated by the simultaneous contraction of the musculi obliquus internus abdominis and transversus abdominis to approximate the musculus transversus abdominis aponeurotic arch to the iliopubic tract and the inguinal ligament, thus reinforcing the posterior wall of the inguinal canal.[20, 29, 46] In approximately 25% of individuals, the arch cannot descend enough to reach the inguinal ligament. Sometimes, the arch is highly located or poorly developed.[29, 54] In these cases, part of the deep wall lacks the reinforcement of the aponeurotic arch and is supported only by the fascia transversalis in the area of Hesselbach's triangle.[45]

Cephalad to a line located approximately midway between the umbilicus and the symphysis pubis (called the *linea semicircularis of Douglas*),[23, 26, 30] the aponeurotic fibers of the musculus transversus abdominis pass posterior to the musculus rectus abdominis, thus contributing to the

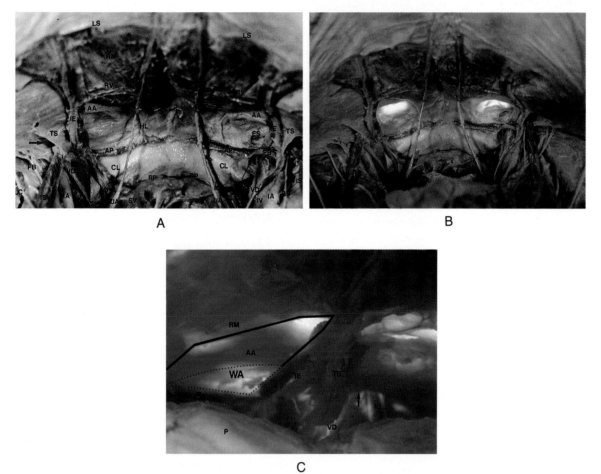

Figure 29–8. (A) The internal surface of the lower anterior abdominal wall prepared in a cadaver to demonstrate the areas corresponding to the inguinal (Hesselbach's) triangle (the remnant of the urachus and the bladder have been removed). The thick arrow points to the deep inguinal ring. The thin arrow indicates the femoral ring. **(B)** The weak areas inside the inguinal triangles through which direct herniations occur, which are located between the aponeurotic arch of the musculus transversus abdominis superiorly and the iliopubic tract inferiorly, are better demonstrated here by transillumination of the lower anterior abdominal wall. **(C)** Close-up of the area of the inguinal triangle transilluminated in a different cadaver dissection to demonstrate the weak area through which direct herniations occur. The thick arrow points to the deep inguinal ring.

RM = musculus rectus abdominis; LS = linea semicircularis (Douglas); IE = inferior epigastric vessels; ES = external spermatic vessels; RV = rectusial vein; CL = Cooper's ligament; IP = iliopubic tract; UA = umbilical arteries; SV = superior vesical arteries; HL = Henle's ligament (falx inguinalis); AA = aponeurotic arch of the musculus transversus abdominis; P = peritoneum; VD = vas deferens; IS = internal spermatic vessels; PB = anastomotic pubic branch; AP = anterior pubic branch and iliopubic vein; RP = retropubic vein; AO = anomalous obturator artery; GB = genital branch of the genitofemoral nerve; FB = femoral branch of the genitofemoral nerve; LC = lateral femoral cutaneous nerve; TS = fascia transversalis sling; WA = weak area.

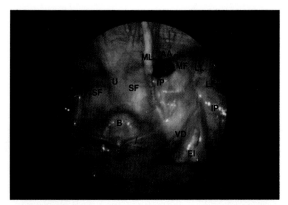

Figure 29–9. A bilateral direct hernia as seen at laparoscopy. The defects are visible bilaterally in the weak area between the aponeurotic arch of the musculus transversus abdominis and the iliopubic tract.

U = median umbilical ligament; ML = medial umbilical ligament; LL = lateral umbilical ligament; AA = aponeurotic arch of the musculus transversus abdominis; IP = iliopubic tract; SF = supravesical fossa; MF = medial fossa; LF = lateral fossa; VD = vas deferens; IS = internal spermatic vessels; EI = external iliac vessels; B = bladder with Foley catheter inserted.

posterior rectus sheath, whereas caudad to that level, they usually cross anteriorly as part of the anterior rectus sheath (see Figs. 29–2, 29–8A and B, and 29–14A and B). Consequently, only the fascia transversalis and the peritoneum make up the posterior portion of the musculus rectus abdominis sheath caudad to the linea semicircularis. In a minor number of cases, the aponeurotic lower portion of the musculus transversus abdominis does not end at the musculus rectus abdominis sheath but curves down to insert onto the superior ramus of the pubis.[20] This slip is defined by some as the *falx inguinalis.*[5, 15, 37] According to others, however, the term falx inguinalis should be reserved to indicate the *ligament of Henle,* which is a vertical extension of the tendon of rectus muscle (observed in 30% to 50% of patients) that attaches to the symphysis pubis and Cooper's ligament (see Figs. 29–2 and 29–8A and B).[24, 28]

Inguinal Triangle

The *inguinal triangle (Hesselbach's triangle)* is the "Achilles heel" of the groin (see Figs. 29–2, 29–5, and 29–8). According to the original description, its boundaries were described as the inferior epigastric vessels superolaterally, the musculus rectus abdominis sheath medially, and Cooper's ligament inferiorly.[15, 23, 24, 37] These limits were subsequently modified with the substitution of the inguinal ligament for Cooper's

ligament to allow easier identification of the area for the surgeon using an anterior approach for herniorraphy. For the laparoscopic procedure, however, it seems appropriate to return to the original Hesselbach's description, since the inguinal ligament is not visible from within the abdomen. Alternatively, the iliopubic tract can substitute the inguinal ligament as the inferior border. The triangle corresponds to the anatomic deep inguinal wall and includes in its lower portion the weak area of the medial umbilical fossa in which direct hernias develop.[20, 24] This weak area is in the lower half of the inguinal triangle, bordered by the aponeurotic arch superiorly and the iliopubic tract inferiorly (Fig. 29–9; see also Fig. 29–8).

Musculi Obliquus Internus Abdominis and Obliquus Externus Abdominis

The two most superficial abdominal wall muscles, namely, the *musculi obliquus internus abdominis* and *obliquus externus abdominis* constitute the anterior and lateral abdominal wall.[55, 56] They probably only play a role in modifying the direction of a hernial bulge and are not felt to be of great relevance in the etiology of inguinofemoral herniation.[24, 45] The lowermost part of the aponeurosis of the musculus obliquus externus abdominis forms the *inguinal (or Poupart's) ligament,* which extends from the anterior superior iliac spine laterally to the pubic tubercle medially. Medially, some of its fibers rotate to insert onto Cooper's ligament, forming the *lacunar ligament (of Gimbernat),* but the distinction appears to be clinically irrelevant (see Fig. 29–7).[20, 37]

Inguinal Canal and Spermatic Cord

The *inguinal canal* is an oblique passage approximately 4 cm long (Fig. 29–10). It begins at the deep inguinal ring and extends downward and medially through a gap in the musculi transversus abdominis and obliquus internus abdominis at a point approximately midway between the anterior superior iliac spine and the pubic tubercle to finally emerge at the *external (or superficial) inguinal ring.* This is a triangular opening formed by a defect in the fibers of the aponeurosis of the musculus obliquus externus abdominis above the inguinal ligament and lateral to its medial insertion on the pubic tubercle.

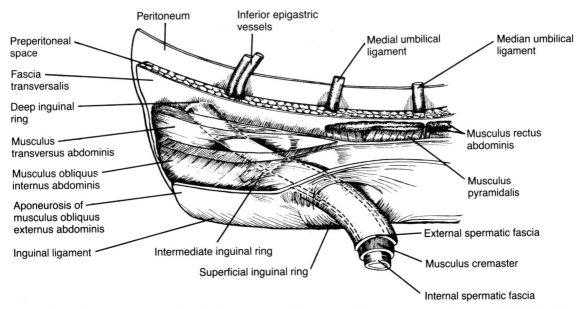

Figure 29–10. The inguinal canal. (Modified from Yaeger WL. Intermediate inguinal ring. Clin Anat 5:289–295, 1992. Copyright © 1992. Reprinted by permission of Wiley-Liss, a division of John Wiley and Sons, Inc.)

The inguinal canal is limited inferiorly by the inguinal ligament and the iliopubic tract, inferomedially by the lacunar ligament, anteriorly by the aponeurosis of the musculus obliquus externus abdominis, laterally and superiorly by the fibers of the musculus obliquus internus abdominis and the aponeurotic arch of the musculus transversus abdominis.[37] The posterior wall, between the aponeurotic arch superiorly and the iliopubic tract inferiorly, is formed only by fascia transversalis.

The inguinal canal is the passageway for the *spermatic cord,* which originates at the internal inguinal ring, at which point the vas deferens and the internal spermatic (or testicular) vessels join together with a matrix of connective tissue in continuity with the preperitoneal connective tissue. The *processus vaginalis*[5, 6, 23] is the portion of peritoneum that accompanies the testicle during its descent toward the scrotum in embryonic life. Its funicular portion is commonly obliterated in the adult, whereas the testicular portion constitutes the tunica vaginalis testis. However, 30% to 40% of children 3 to 4 months old have a patent processus vaginalis.[57] According to Russell, all indirect inguinal hernias have a congenital origin due to patency of all or part of the processus vaginalis.[58] The cord also includes the external spermatic vessels and the *artery of the ductus deferens,* as well as the genital branch of the genitofemoral nerve and the ilioinguinal nerve. The spermatic vein drains blood from the pampiniform plexus, a network

of smaller veins inside the cord, and empties into the renal vein on the left and into the inferior vena cava on the right.

The cord is covered by three layers acquired when crossing the abdominal wall (Fig. 29–10). The *internal spermatic fascia* is provided by the fascia transversalis at the deep inguinal ring and is the inner layer. The fibers of the *musculus cremaster* and its investing fascia are derived from the musculus obliquus internus abdominis and its fascia on the lateral aspect of the inguinal canal; this is the middle layer. Yeager introduced a new anatomic entity, the *intermediate inguinal ring,* to indicate the ovalis area in which the lower fibers of the musculus obliquus internus abdominis evaginate to form the musculus cremaster layer.[59] Finally, at the *external inguinal ring,* the musculus obliquus externus abdominis fascia reflects onto the cord, forming the *external spermatic fascia.*[5, 29, 37]

The Femoral Sheath and Femoral Canal

The *femoral sheath* is a tubular, funnel-shaped expansion of the endoabdominal fascia that encompasses the femoral artery, femoral vein, and femoral canal in the upper thigh (see Fig. 29–7). The lateral wall of the sheath is almost vertical, whereas the medial wall points obliquely downward and lateral.[6, 21] The anterior wall is formed by the fascia transversalis and is reinforced by the iliopubic tract. It is important to notice that the inguinal ligament is not in direct contact with the anterior surface of the femoral sheath, as the iliopubic tract is interposed between the two structures.[6, 23] Posteriorly, reinforcement is provided by a slip of the musculi pectineus and iliopsoas fascia.[23, 24, 48] The lateral wall is in contact with the ileopectineal arch and is pierced distally by the femoral branch of the genitofemoral nerve.[6, 21] The sheath is divided into three partitions by septae of connective tissue. The lateral compartment is occupied by the femoral artery and the femoral branch of the genitofemoral nerve. The femoral vein lies in the median compartment, whereas the medial area is called the *femoral canal* (see Fig. 29–7). The femoral canal is conical and approximately 1.25 to 2 cm long, with the apex at the fossa ovalis.[6, 29] Its base is a rigid ring known as the femoral ring (or crural ring) that is 1 to 1.5 cm in transverse diameter (see Figs. 29–2, 29–5, 29–8A and B, and 29–13B). According to different authors, the anterior border of the femoral ring is made up of the iliopubic tract, the inguinal ligament, or both.[6, 21, 23, 29] Posteriorly, it is delimited by the superior ramus of the pubis, the musculus pectineus and its fascia, and Cooper's ligament. The lateral boundary is the femoral vein. The medial border remains controversial. Traditionally, it has been considered to be the lacunar ligament.[21] Recently, however, some authors have stated that the reflected aponeurotic arch of the musculus transversus abdominis onto the pubic tubercle and superior ramus of pubis[23, 48] or the fan-shaped medial insertion of the iliopubic tract onto the Cooper's ligament is more accurate.[5, 20] The studies conducted in the anatomic laboratory lead us to agree with the latter statement. The femoral ring is usually closed by the *septum femorale,* composed by fatty tissue.[54] The femoral canal contains some connective tissue, small lymph nodes, and lymphatic vessels. A large lymph node is commonly present in the femoral triangle of the thigh, at the end of the femoral canal, and is known as the node of Cloquet. The femoral canal is clinically important because it is the outlet for femoral hernias.

Innervation

In the extraperitoneal space, five major nerves are responsible for the innervation of the lower abdominal wall, the inguinal and genital region, the thigh, and the leg: the ilioinguinal, iliohypogastric, genitofemoral, femoral, and lateral femoral cutaneous nerves (see Figs. 29–2, 29–5, 29–7, 29–13B, and 29–14B and C). All nerves originate from the lumbar plexus (T12, L1, L2, L3, L4).

The *iliohypogastric nerve* (see Figs. 29–2 and 29–7) appears at the lateral margin of the musculus psoas major and crosses obliquely on the musculus quadratus lumborum passing beneath the inferior pole of the kidney, pierces the musculus transversus abdominis, and then splits into two branches, the most important one being the hypogastric nerve. This branch lies between the musculi obliquus externus abdominis and obliquus internus abdominis at the level of the anterior superior iliac spine and reaches the suprapubic skin by piercing either the musculus obliquus externus abdominis aponeurosis above the external ring or the anterior musculus rectus abdominis sheath.[6, 20, 37] It innervates the skin of the anterior abdominal wall above the pubis (Fig. 29–11).

The *ilioinguinal nerve* (see Figs. 29–2, 29–5, 29–7, and 29–13B) follows a course similar to that of the iliohypogastric nerve but travels inferiorly and crosses the musculus quadratus lumborum and the musculus iliacus before pierc-

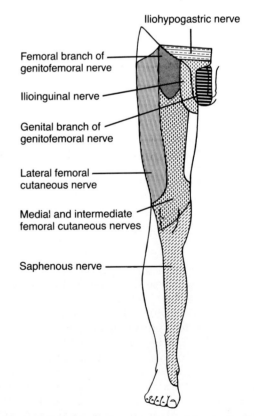

Iliohypogastric nerve

Femoral branch of genitofemoral nerve

Ilioinguinal nerve

Genital branch of genitofemoral nerve

Lateral femoral cutaneous nerve

Medial and intermediate femoral cutaneous nerves

Saphenous nerve

Figure 29–11. Areas of sensory innervation in the lower limb that are of relevant interest for the surgeon performing laparoscopic herniorraphy.

ing the musculus transversus abdominis just above the anterior portion of the iliac crest. After piercing the musculus obliquus internus abdominis, it runs along the inguinal canal over the musculus cremaster and finally exits through the external inguinal ring to innervate the skin of the superomedial portion of the thigh, the root of the penis, the pubic region, and the scrotum or labium majus (see Fig. 29–11).

The *genitofemoral nerve* (see Figs. 29–2, 29–5B, 29–7, 29–13B, and 29–14C) emerges from the fibers of the musculus psoas major at the level of the third or fourth lumbar vertebra and crosses behind the ureter to divide into the genital and femoral branches at a variable distance from the iliopubic tract. Occasionally, the division occurs within the fibers of the musculus psoas major (see Fig. 29–2). The *genital branch* is medial, traverses the iliac vessels to reach the internal inguinal ring, and runs along the inguinal canal together with the spermatic cord (see Figs. 29–2, 29–5, 29–7, 29–8A and B, 29–13B, and 29–14B and C). The genital branch of the genitofemoral nerve provides motor innervation to the musculus cremaster and sensory innervation to the skin of the penis and scrotum (see Fig. 29–11).[20, 30, 37] The *femoral branch* usually lies on the lateral edge of the musculus psoas beneath its fascia. It is not consistently a single trunk and may bifurcate before crossing the deep circumflex iliac artery to pass under

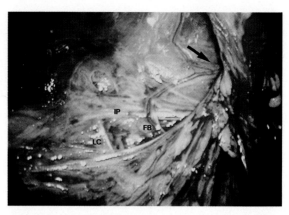

Figure 29–12. The femoral branch of the genitofemoral nerve and the lateral femoral cutaneous nerve as they approach and pass below the iliopubic tract, identified during laparoscopic hernia repair after precise dissection. The arrow indicates the enlarged deep inguinal ring, through which an indirect inguinal hernia found its outlet.

IP = iliopubic tract; LC = lateral femoral cutaneous nerve; FB = femoral branch of the genitofemoral nerve; IS = internal spermatic vessels.

the iliopubic tract lateral to the spermatic vessels (Figs. 29–12 through 29–14; see also Figs. 29–2, 29–5, 29–7, 29–8A and B, 29–12, 29–13B, and 29–14B and C). In the femoral sheath, it is sometimes also called the *lumboinguinal nerve* and lies lateral to the femoral artery. After piercing the anterior wall of the femoral sheath and the fascia lata, it reaches the superior por-

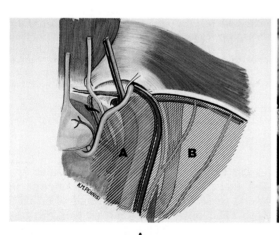

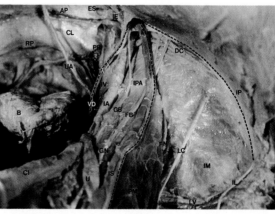

A   B

Figure 29–13. (A) Corresponds to the so-called triangle of doom (A). B is the area in which nerve injury due to entrapment may inadvertently take place. Staple placement in this area should be avoided. **(B)** Cadaver preparation *(right side)* that shows the structures included within the so-called triangle of doom (medial triangle) and the dangerous area beside it, bordered by the internal spermatic vessels inferomedially and the iliopubic tract superolaterally (lateral triangle).

B = bladder (reflected posteriorly); CI = common iliac artery; UA = umbilical artery; CL = Cooper's ligament; PB = anastomotic pubic branch; AP = anterior pubic branch and iliopubic vein; RP = retropubic vein; ES = external spermatic vessels; IE = inferior epigastric vessels; VD = vas deferens; IV = external iliac vein; IA = external iliac artery; GN = genitofemoral nerve; GB = genital branch of the genitofemoral nerve; FB = femoral branch of the genitofemoral nerve; IPA = iliopectineal arch; U = ureter; IS = internal spermatic vessels; DC = deep circumflex iliac vessels; IP = iliopubic tract; FN = femoral nerve; LC = lateral femoral cutaneous nerve; IL = ilioinguinal nerve; PM = musculus psoas major; IM = musculus iliacus; LV = iliolumbar vessels.

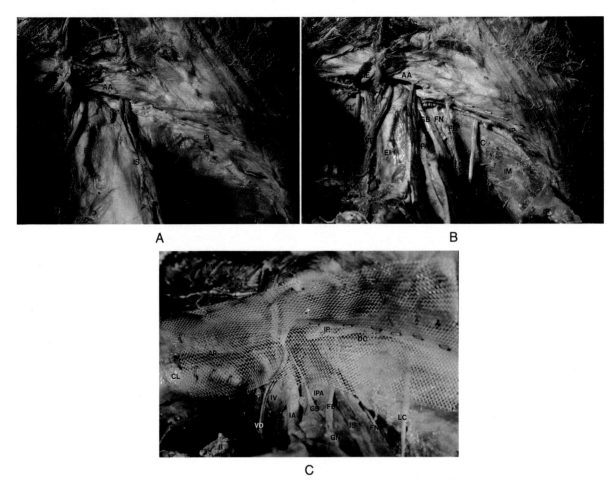

A   B

C

Figure 29–14. (A) Staples correctly placed above and parallel to the iliopubic tract. **(B)** Same view after removal of the psoas and iliac fascia. **(C)** Correct positioning of staples to tack the mesh into the preperitoneal space. (In **A** and **B** the internal spermatic vessels have been moved slightly laterally to better show the external iliac vessels on the floor of the so-called triangle of doom.)

VD = vas deferens; IS = internal spermatic vessels; EI = external iliac vessels; IV = external iliac vein; IA = external iliac artery; AA = aponeurotic arch of the musculus transversus abdominis; IP = iliopubic tract; IE = inferior epigastric vessels; RM = musculus rectus abdominis; TM = musculus transversus abdominis; IM = musculus iliacus; PM = musculus psoas major; PB = anastomotic pubic branch; LS = linea semicircularis; IPA = iliopectineal arch (partially removed); CL = Cooper's ligament; DC = deep circumflex iliac vessels; GN = genitofemoral nerve; GB = genital branch of the genitofemoral nerve; FB = femoral branch of the genitofemoral nerve; FN = femoral nerve; LC = lateral femoral cutaneous nerve; IF = iliac fascia (reflected); U = ureter; B = bladder (reflected posteriorly).

tion of the femoral triangle in the thigh. It provides sensory innervation to the anteromedial surface of the upper thigh (see Fig. 29–11).

The *lateral femoral cutaneous nerve* (also called the *lateral cutaneous nerve of the thigh*) emerges from the lateral margin of the musculus psoas major deep to the peritoneum and iliac fascia, through which it can often be seen (see Fig. 29–14; see also Figs. 29–2, 29–4, 29–5, 29–7, 29–12, 29–13*B*, and 29–14*B* and *C*). It crosses the musculus iliacus obliquely toward the anterior superior iliac spine. Medial to the latter, it passes below the iliopubic tract to reach the thigh and divides into two branches. The anterior branch becomes superficial approximately

10 cm below the anterior superior iliac spine and innervates the skin of the anterior and lateral surfaces of the upper thigh as far as the knee. The posterior branch pierces the fascia lata at a higher level and then runs posteriorly to reach the skin of the lateral aspect of the thigh. The innervated area extends from the greater trocanter to the midcalf level (see Fig. 29–11).

The *femoral nerve* is the largest nerve originating from the lumbar plexus (see Fig. 29–14; see also Figs. 29–2, 29–5, 29–7, 29–13*B*, and 29–14*B* and *C*). It emerges from the inferior aspect of the musculus psoas major, passes along the lateral border, and then runs between the musculi iliacus and pectineus, covered by a layer of fascia. It passes below the iliopubic tract, reaches the femoral triangle within the lacuna musculorum, and finally divides into anterior and posterior branches. The *anterior branch* originates approximately 8 cm distal to the inguinal ligament and provides the *intermediate femoral cutaneous* and the *medial femoral cutaneous nerves* to innervate the skin of the lower anteromedial thigh. The *saphenous nerve* is the largest sensory branch of the femoral nerve and continues to the leg to innervate the medial aspect of the leg and the great toe (see Fig. 29–11). The posterior branch contains the *muscular branches,* which provide motor innervation to the musculi pectineus, sartorius, and quadriceps.

Critical Areas for Laparoscopic Hernia Repair

The triangular area between the vas deferens medially and the spermatic vessels laterally is often referred to as the "triangle of doom" (see Fig. 29–13A and B).[27] The external iliac vessels lie in its floor, usually hidden by the peritoneum and the fascia transversalis. To avoid injury to these important structures, it has been strongly recommended that suturing or stapling only be done medial to the vas deferens or lateral to the spermatic vessels.[27] It is our opinion, however, that even these precautions are inadequate and that the borders of the "dangerous area" should be extended.

For laparoscopic inguinal herniorrhaphy, the iliopubic tract is another extremely important landmark for staple application. In fact, lateral to the spermatic vessels and immediately below (or, in some instances, directly through) the fibers of the iliopubic tract are the femoral branch of the genitofemoral nerve, the femoral nerve, and the lateral femoral cutaneous nerve. Consequently, staples placed caudal to the iliopubic tract and lateral to the testicular vessels can result in transient or permanent neuralgias involving one or more of the previously mentioned nerves or branches.

Pain in the groin or lower abdomen can be observed if the ilioinguinal or the iliohypogastric nerve is injured, whereas pain along the cord and scrotum is noted if the genital branch of the genitofemoral nerve has been damaged.[6] Injury of the iliohypogastric and ilioinguinal nerves, however, is much less frequent during laparoscopic hernia repair than with conventional anterior inguinal herniorrhaphy, since they lie in a plane superficial to the preperitoneal space.

On occasion, however, they can be compromised when staples are placed deeply, especially if a vigorous bimanual technique is used. The genital branch of the genitofemoral nerve is not commonly encountered in the area in which staples are applied. It may be damaged, however, by the maneuvers used to reduce the sac of an indirect hernia. Besides, it is not unusual to observe the genital branch passing below the iliopubic tract in the vicinities of the deep inguinal ring to enter the inguinal canal from below. This anatomic variation can occasionally expose the genital branch to the risk of damage.

The femoral branch of the genitofemoral nerve and the lateral femoral cutaneous nerve are at higher risk of being injured during laparoscopic herniorrhaphy, since they are more superficial (they lie on the anterior surfaces of the musculi psoas major and iliacus, respectively) and in the area where staples are usually applied to tack the inferolateral border of the mesh. The femoral nerve is medial and in a relatively deeper position: although less vulnerable, it may be injured by staples placed medially and close to the iliopectineal arch, with consequent possible sensory (usually pain in the anteromedial region of the thigh) or functional consequences (difficulty extending the leg, quadriceps atrophy), or both.

To prevent damage to the nerves, as well as to the external iliac and deep circumflex iliac vessels, we recommend that lateral to the vas deferens, staples be placed only above and parallel to the iliopubic tract (see Fig. 29–14).

Accordingly, it seems appropriate to introduce a new concept and include another triangular area besides the "triangle of doom" where no staples or sutures should be applied. The boundaries of this second dangerous zone include the internal spermatic vessels inferomedially and the iliopubic tract superolaterally (see Fig. 29–13). Medial to the vas deferens, staples should be applied on Cooper's ligament only, as staples placed too close to the deep inguinal ring and fascia transversalis sling could damage the terminal portion of the external iliac vein before it passes below the iliopubic tract (see Fig. 29–13B). Finally, when tacking the mesh to Cooper's ligament, care should be taken to avoid the anastomotic pubic branch, which usually lies on the lateral portion of the ligament itself (see Fig. 29–13B).

HISTORY

Just as hypotheses concerning the origins of inguinal herniation are thousands of years old, attempts to cure are also ancient.[60] Tight bandages were adopted by the Alexandrian school. Transillumination, taxis maneuvers (manual reduction), and rudimentary operations were first introduced during the Hippocratic era. They were also the basis for Roman practice under Galen's teaching. Celsus described in his *De Re Medicina* an operation performed through an incision in the scrotum and groin in which the sac was separated from the cord below the external ring and the wound closed.[6] Paul of Egina noted that ablation of the testicle was considered wise by Byzantine physicians when treating a large hernia.[61]

At the beginning of the Middle Ages, the practice of surgery was discouraged by the Church and relegated to barbers, executioners, and the so-called itinerant incisors.[60] Surgery survived, however, and in 1364, the Frenchman Guy de Chauliac recommended the use of laxatives and blood-letting, together with the avoidance of gas-producing foods and intense physical activities, for subjects with groin hernias. He also described an effective taxis maneuver to reduce incarcerated bowel, which was accomplished by suspending the individual by the feet. Patients were kept on bedrest for at least 50 days while poultice was applied to the inguinal region. In addition, he pointed out the difference between femoral and inguinal hernias and described an operation in which the sac was cauterized.[6, 61]

In the Middle Ages, hernias were treated mainly with trusses. In serious cases, however, castration together with tight ligature (usually with a gold stitch) of both the cord and the sac at the external ring was used, as described by the French authors Lanfranc and Paré.[23] This was called the Royal Operation, as it prevented the birth of new subjects for the king.[23]

In the 16th century, the Dane Heinrich Callisen treated a patient with a strangulated hernia with bloodletting until he fainted. The aim was to weaken him until the hernia became reducible.[61] At about the same time, William of Saliceto and Ruggero of Palermo excised the sac after double ligation.[23]

By the beginning of the 18th century, it had become apparent that the "itinerant incisors" had gained considerable skill in specific operations such as gallstone removal, cleft palate correction, and cataract and hernia repair. For example, Lorenz Heister from Frankfurt described one of them, called Eisenbart, who operated on a 9-year-old child with a hernia that no other famous physician in the city had been able to cure. Three weeks later the wound was perfectly healed.[61]

During the 18th and the beginning of the 19th centuries, valuable contributions to the understanding of the anatomy of the groin were made by Richter, Pott, Gimbernat, Scarpa, Cooper, Hesselbach, and Cloquet. They provided a rational approach to the surgical treatment of groin herniation.[21, 23, 60, 61]

In 1871, Henry Marcy of Boston, after visiting Lister in Edinburgh, began to realize the importance of adequate closure of the internal ring when repairing indirect inguinal hernias.[62, 63] He pointed out that failure to do so predisposed to recurrence. Andrews of Chicago, in 1924, also stressed the importance of internal ring closure. He pointed out the futility of performing a complicated herniorrhaphy if good tissue was not available for internal ring closure ("white fascia, a synonym for the fascia transversalis").[64] Adequate closure of the internal ring is of importance to the laparoscopic surgeon because this goal can be easily accomplished from an intraabdominal approach.

Perhaps the most important development in the history of groin hernia surgery came in 1884 when the Italian surgeon Edoardo Bassini developed a revolutionary method for groin herniorrhaphy. High ligation of the sac and physiologic reconstruction of the inguinal floor instead of obliterating it were the main features. [65, 66] After ligation of the sac, Bassini opened the fascia transversalis from the deep internal ring to the pubic tubercle and sutured what he called the "triple layer" (musculi obliquus internus abdominis and transversus abdominis and fascia transversalis) to the inguinal ligament. The result was a new oblique inguinal canal with a reinforced posterior wall. This innovation resulted in decreased morbidity and mortality for groin herniorrhaphy, as well as a reduction in the recurrence rate to one-fifth that commonly accepted at the time.[67]

Numerous modifications of Bassini's technique have been subsequently introduced. The goal was to further reduce recurrence rates and avoid testicular atrophy. For example, Bull and Ferguson decided to suture the musculus obliquus internus abdominis layer over the cord without opening the fascia transversalis.[68] Halsted's operation was basically the same as Bassini's, but the cord was transplanted above the aponeurosis of the musculus obliquus externus abdominis and covered by the skin only (Halsted I). Subsequently, he added a relaxation incision on the musculus rectus abdominis sheath (Halsted II).[69] A popular modification was described by McVay. He sutured the "triple layer" to Cooper's ligament instead of the inguinal ligament.[70] Despite these and other modifications, the average rate of recurrence recorded for all herniorrhaphies performed in the United States in 1981 was approximately 10%.[71]

In 1936, Shouldice in Toronto began to experiment with a modification of Bassini's technique. By 1952 he developed an operation with such good results that it has become the standard by which other repairs are judged. The principle of the operation is the apposition and overlapping of six layers of the abdominal wall with four lines of running stainless steel or monofilament sutures. It is usually performed under local anesthesia. Early mobilization and prompt return to work is the rule. Recurrence rates between 0.2% and 1% have been reported by Shouldice and others.[72–75]

Lichtenstein is credited with the development of the concept of tension-free hernia repair. He felt the major disadvantage of Bassini's technique (and its modifications) was that the tissue was approximated under tension, predisposing the procedure to failure. To avoid tension, he proposed the use of a prosthesis to bridge the defect.[13, 14, 47, 49, 76, 77] The prosthesis is sutured inferiorly to the inguinal ligament, medially to the fascia of the musculus rectus abdominis, and superiorly to the fascia of the musculus obliquus internus abdominis. A slit is made in the lateral side of the prothesis to encircle the cord and is then reapproximated. In addition to a lower recurrence rate, he felt that the avoidance of tension would result in less postoperative discomfort and an earlier return to normal activities. The technique is becoming increasingly popular. Whether the impressive results reported by Lichtenstein and other clinics specializing in the Lichtenstein approach can be reproduced by the general surgical community remains to be seen.

Another approach to inguinal herniorrhaphy using prosthetic material that has particular importance to the laparoscopic surgeon is to reinforce the abdominal wall with a prosthesis placed in the preperitoneal space. This method was initially described by Cheatle in 1920 and subsequently popularized by several renowned authors.[78–84]

The preperitoneal (Bogros') space may be entered through a variety of incisions. Stoppa and Warlaumont described the use of a lower midline abdominal incision, whereas Rignault preferred a transverse suprapubic (Pfannestiel) incision.[82, 84] Nyhus used a paramedian incision with medial displacement of the rectus muscle.[80] Once the preperitoneal space has been entered, the repair can be accomplished in several ways. Nyhus prefers formal repair of the hernia defect by approximating the aponeurotic arch of the musculus transversus abdominis with the iliopubic tract and closing the enlarged internal inguinal ring. Following this, a tailored piece of polypropylene mesh is fixed in place to "reinforce" the repair.[85]

Rignault closes the defect loosely to prevent a subsequent early postoperative bulge. He then places a piece of polypropylene mesh (considerably larger than the defect) in position. The mesh is not sutured, as in the author's opinion it should be kept in place by the endoabdominal pressure, in accordance with Laplace's law.[84] A keyhole is cut in the mesh to encircle the spermatic cord. In indirect hernias, the sac can be reduced and excised or otherwise divided at the internal ring, leaving the distal sac in situ. Rignault feels that a patch of polyester fibers (Mersilene, Dacron) is particularly useful for this repair because of its handling characteristics.

Stoppa's method is similar to Rignault's but employs a larger sheet of mesh (15 cm × 15 cm or greater). The hernia defect is not closed. One or two stitches are used to hold the mesh in place but, again, abdominal pressure is considered to be the major force in maintaining the mesh in its correct position. The cord structures may or may not be encircled by the mesh.[81, 82, 84] These methods have been associated with excellent results and are especially attractive for recurrent hernias after conventional herniorrhaphy because the preperitoneal space has not been previously dissected.[67] With the advent of preperitoneal techniques, recurrence rates have considerably improved, ranging between 0.4% and 2.2%.[80, 81, 84]

Early Laparoscopic Hernia Repairs and the Transabdominal Approach

I have the impression that the radical cure of herniae, other than umbilical, will bye-and-bye, be undertaken by abdominal section.[86]

L. TAIT, 1891

Marcy noted that closure of the abdominal internal ring is an important step in indirect hernia repair, emphasizing that failure to do so predisposed the patient to recurrence.[62, 63]

Andrews of Chicago, in 1924, also stressed the importance of closing the internal inguinal ring by placing sutures in the fascia around its borders.[64] He specifically pointed out the futility of performing a complicated herniorrhaphy if good tissue was not available for the repair of the enlarged orifice (white fascia).

In 1919, LaRoque described an intraabdominal approach for inguinal herniorrhaphy.[87, 88] His methods included a combined approach both from outside and inside the abdomen. The first step was equivalent to Bassini's operation— that is, dissection of the sac from the cord structures. Next, however, the hernia sac was removed and ligated from inside the peritoneal cavity after entering the abdomen through an incision above the internal inguinal ring. In doing so, LaRoque's aim was to ligate the sac as high as possible and have a clear view of both sides of the internal ring. LaRoque felt this approach offered several advantages to the surgeon in particular situations: if the hernia was of the sliding type, if the viability of hernia contents was in doubt, or if other concomitant intraabdominal problems needed to be evaluated or treated (ovarian cysts, appendicitis, and so on). Unfortunately, LaRoque did not provide follow-up data on the more than 1700 patients on whom he performed this procedure.

Ger, from Mineola, New York, in 1982 reported a series of 13 patients undergoing laparotomy for unrelated causes in whom a hernia was incidentally discovered.[89] In these cases he had simply closed the neck of the sac by approximating the peritoneal opening with a variable number (2 to 10) of interrupted stainless steel Michel's clips measuring 3 mm in width and 15 mm in length when opened.[90] These staples were applied with standard Kocher's forceps in the peritoneum and preperitoneal tissue, usually disappearing from view. The sac was left intact. A short follow-up (26 to 44 months) revealed a single recurrence in the case of a direct hernia. Some of these patients have now been followed for up to 10 years, and further recurrences have not been observed. In the last patient in the series (operated on in 1979) the staples were placed under laparoscopic guidance. This is thought to be the first laparoscopic herniorrhaphy performed in a human.

Encouraged by these results, Ger undertook an experimental study in which indirect hernias in 12 beagle dogs were treated by laparoscopic closure of the internal defect.[90] Through a second cannula, a specially designed instrument was introduced. It included forceps that gripped and immobilized the orifice of the hernia, allowing it to be closed by a stapling mechanism. All but one of these operations was successful. Twenty-four hernias in 20 human patients have been repaired with this laparoscopic approach: 12 indirect, 4 bilateral indirect, 2 direct, 1 femoral, and 1 recurrent.[91] Operations were accomplished on an outpatient basis and could be completed within 15 to 25 minutes. After a maximum follow-up of 14 months, two recurrences have been noted, both occurring as a result of technical errors. Postoperative complications included one case of thigh pain that persisted at 6 months. Among the advantages of laparoscopic herniorrhaphy listed by the author are smaller wounds, reduced chance of injury to the spermatic cord and testis, avoidance of ischemic orchitis and damage to nerves in the inguinal canal, high ligation of the sac, reduced postoperative discomfort, and the ability to treat bilateral hernias simultaneously with minimal dissection.

The first announcement of a laparoscopic herniorrhaphy at a scientific meeting was in 1989, when Bogojavlensky presented a videotape at the 1989 meeting of the American Association of Gynecological Laparoscopists in Washington, illustrating the treatment of indirect inguinal and femoral hernias by the laparoscopic introduction of a roll of polypropylene mesh into the sacs. The peritoneum was then closed over the defect using sutures.[92] Reich of Kingston, Pennsylvania used a similar technique.[93]

In 1990, Schultz of Minneapolis, Minnesota, presented the preliminary results of a clinical trial involving a series of 20 patients subjected to laparoscopic hernia repair.[94] His method consisted of incising the peritoneum adjacent to the musculofascial opening and filling the hernia defect with sheets of polypropylene mesh rolled into a cylinder resembling a cigarette. Two or three additional 1 in × 2 in pieces of mesh were placed over the defect and after partial decompression of the pneumoperitoneum, the peritoneum was closed. Schultz recommended the use of the neodymium-doped yttrium-aluminum-garnet laser for opening the peritoneum. He pointed out the importance of an angled (45°) laparoscope. The latter has proved to be very important in present laparoscopic hernia repair techniques.

Schultz initially reported a series of 22 patients, with 9 left, 9 right, and 2 bilateral hernias, with a follow-up of 3 to 11 months. He noted one failure identified at 2 weeks postoperatively, which was due to an unrecognized concomitant direct defect. This finding led Schultz to conclude that a wider piece of mesh covering both the direct and indirect spaces should be employed. The average length of time for patients to return to unrestricted activity following this repair has been 3.3 days.

In 1991, Corbitt of West Palm Beach, Florida, published an account of 20 patients with either indirect or direct hernias that were repaired using a modification of Schultz's technique. Corbitt inverted the sac into the abdomen and then opened it so that the polypropylene mesh plugs could be inserted into the hernia defect.[95] The sac itself was then excised with an endoscopic linear stapling device (Endo-GIA; U.S. Surgical Corp., Norwalk, CT). In his early report, Corbitt noted no recurrences with a maximum follow-up of 8 months. The patients were able to return to normal activities by the second postoperative day, with the procedure being performed on an outpatient basis.

Another modification was suggested by Seid and colleagues from Santa Monica, California. They described the use of a 4-cm flat, square piece of polypropylene being attached to a polypropylene mesh plug, with the idea that this would prevent migration of the plug into the hernia defect.[96] Two such rectangles of polypropylene mesh, each 4 cm × 6 cm, were used to reinforce both the direct and indirect spaces. Otherwise, the operation was similar to those of Schultz and Corbitt. His initial series consisted of 25 patients with 29 hernias with a maximum follow-up of 7 months. He reported no recurrences. All procedures were performed on an outpatient basis, and the average time to return to full employment was 5 days.

Katkhouda from Nice, France, also adopted the plug and mesh technique for his first 12 cases, but the observation of two recurrences persuaded him to suspend this method.[97]

These so-called plug and patch techniques have now been abandoned.[3] A longer term follow-up by all authors has revealed a high recurrence rate approaching 33%, with problems such as migration of the polypropylene mesh plugs and the development of palpable "meshomas." The failure of these procedures is not surprising because they do not incorporate the principles of an anatomic repair as described by Bassini,[65] McVay,[70] Nyhus,[5] and others.

Deep Inguinal Ring Closure

Rosin from London, England, simply inverts the indirect sac and ligates it high for indirect inguinal hernias.[98] If the defect is particularly large, he sutures the ring closed. With this method he has treated 57 cases (54 indirect, 2 femoral, and 1 spigelian hernia) in 51 patients. After an average follow-up of 12 months, one early recurrence due to technical failure has been reported, as has a postoperative hydrocele. Patients were allowed to return to full physical activity within 1 week.

For type II inguinal hernias (Nyhus' classification), Dion and Morin from Quebec, Canada, have performed 15 ring closures with a suture of 0 polypropylene. No recurrences or complications were observed. For all other types of hernia, the author follows the preperitoneal approach.[99]

Schlain from San Francisco also performs a repair by suturing the deep inguinal ring closed, without reducing the sac. Occasionally, he inserts a plug of mesh inside the hernia defect. He has reported no recurrences after treatment of 58 hernias with this technique. Patients are allowed to return to heavy manual work after 4 weeks.[100]

Transabdominal Preperitoneal Hernia Repair

The excellent results obtained with the classic preperitoneal approach by Stoppa, Rignault, Nyhus, and the others already mentioned encouraged laparoscopic surgeons to develop a repair that could employ these same principles and add the advantages of a minimally invasive procedure.

Laparoscopic procedures in which the preperitoneal space is opened by making an incision in the peritoneum from within the abdomen, with the placement of a prosthesis into the preperitoneal space, are grouped under the term transabdominal preperitoneal procedure (TAPP).

Our group recommends the TAPP approach for patients with extensive destruction of the inguinal floor. The procedure begins with an open laparoscopy at the inferior margin of the umbilicus, and the laparoscope is introduced through a Hasson cannula. Two additional cannulas are required on either side, lateral to each musculus rectus abdominis sheath (Fig. 29–15).

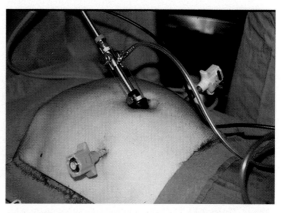

Figure 29–15. Port placement for laparoscopic inguinal hernia repair. Some surgeons prefer a larger cannula at the 5-mm site.

The peritoneum is opened from the anterior superior iliac spine to the medial umbilical ligament (Fig. 29–16*A* and *B*). The preperitoneal space is completely dissected using a combination of sharp and blunt dissection, with occasional use of electrocautery (Fig. 29–16*C* and *D*). The sac is reduced, and a large patch of polypropylene mesh (Prolene, 11 cm × 6 cm) is placed to cover the area from the symphysis pubis medially to the anterior superior iliac spine laterally, and from the anterior abdominal wall above the deep inguinal ring superiorly to

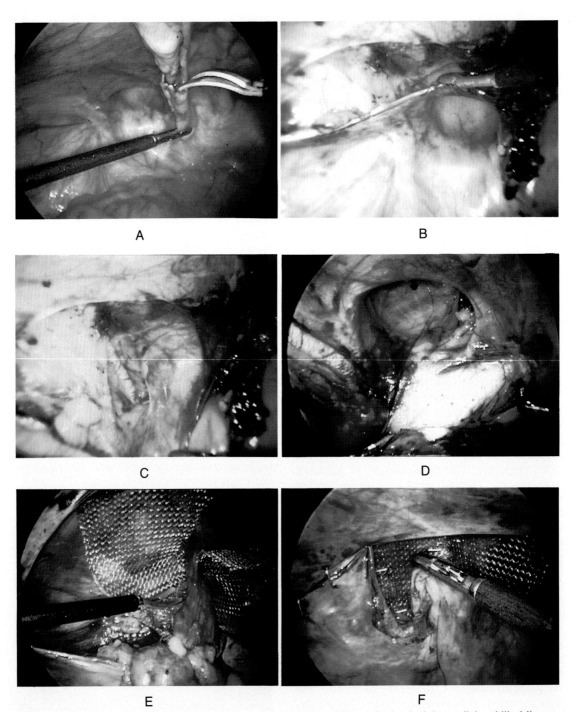

A

B

C

D

E

F

Figure 29–16. **(A)** The peritoneum of the abdominal wall is incised medially at the level of the medial umbilical ligament. **(B)** The incision is carried laterally toward the anterior superior iliac spine. **(C)** The peritoneum is reflected to expose the inferior epigastric vessels. **(D)** The dissection in the preperitoneal space is completed; the direct hernia defect is clearly exposed. **(E)** The mesh is placed to reinforce the defective area. **(F)** The peritoneum is reapproximated to cover the mesh.

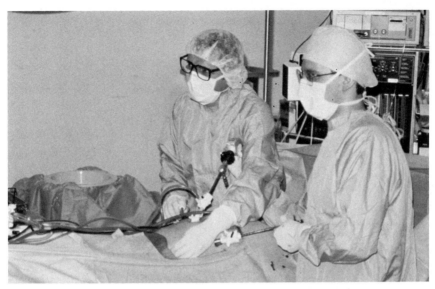

Figure 29–17. The bimanual technique is helpful to locate the area above the iliopubic tract, where staples can be safely applied.

Cooper's ligament inferiorly (Fig. 29–16*E* and *F*). The mesh is fixed in place with titanium staples. Care is taken not to staple below the level of the iliopubic tract when lateral to the internal spermatic vessels to avoid damage to the nerves innervating the groin, inguinal, and thigh regions. A helpful maneuver is to use a bimanual technique, as staples should not be applied in this area if one cannot palpate the head of the stapler through the anterior abdominal wall (Fig. 29–17). One must take care not to place staples too deeply when using the bimanual technique for fear of injuring the superficially located ilioinguinal and iliohypogastric nerves. The peritoneal flap is returned to its original position and closed with staples.

In the last 2 years, our group has performed 130 TAPP procedures in 100 patients (77 direct, 48 indirect, and 5 femoral hernias). Twenty-three hernias were recurrent. The mean operating time was 90 minutes. After a mean follow-up of 47 weeks, we have observed two recurrences. One occurred in a patient with a large indirect sliding hernia at the beginning of our experience. The other recurrent hernia was asymptomatic and was only detectable by physical examination. The patient has declined repair. Complications observed are listed in Table 29–3. We have observed that 8.5% of patients reported some kind of transient pain (testicular, groin, thigh). This confirms the importance of applying staples carefully during surgery. In the majority of cases, the procedure was performed on an outpatient basis and patients were allowed full physical activity within 1 week.

Arregui from Indianapolis has performed 97

Table 29–3. COMPLICATIONS OF LAPAROSCOPIC HERNIA REPAIR—PERSONAL SURVEY

Complications	TAPP		IPOM Repair		Total	%
	(No.)	*(%)*	*(No.)*	*(%)*		
Hematoma	0	0	2	3.38	2	1.05
Urinary dysfunction	2	1.53	2	3.38	4	2.11
Transient testicular pain	1	0.7	1	1.69	2	1.05
Transient groin pain	2	1.53	1	1.69	3	1.58
Persistent groin pain	1	0.7	0	0	1	0.5
Transient thigh pain	7	5.3	5	8.4	12	6.3
Persistent thigh pain	0	0	1	1.69	1	0.5
Seroma	0	0	1	1.69	1	0.5
Aspiration pneumonia	0	0	1	1.69	1	0.5
Infected prostheses	0	0	1	1.69	1	0.5
Postoperative bleeding	1	0.7	0	0	1	0.5
TOTAL	14	10.7	15	25.59	29	15.34

TAPP = transabdominal preperitoneal procedure; IPOM = intraperitoneal onlay mesh.

similar procedures in 94 patients (59 indirect, 10 direct, 1 femoral, 1 obturator, 14 recurrent, and 9 bilateral hernias).[101, 102] After incising the sac at its base with a wide circular incision in the peritoneum, and dissecting it from the surrounding structures, he entered the preperitoneal space. If an indirect hernia was encountered, he tightened the internal ring with sutures tied extracorporeally. For direct hernias, the redundant fascia transversalis was approximated with a pursestring or imbrication running suture. Prosthetic polypropylene mesh (Prolene, 10 cm × 15 cm) was then tailored to cover the deep inguinal ring, the inguinal (Hesselbach's) triangle, and the femoral canal. The prosthesis was fixed with three stitches applied to the musculus transversus abdominis aponeurotic arch, Cooper's ligament (or iliopubic tract), and the fascia transversalis lateral to the internal ring. One intraoperative and 14 postoperative complications have been recorded. The former consisted of a needle that was lost in the anterior abdominal wall while it was being pulled out through a laparoscopic cannula. Among the postoperative complications, there were four inguinal canal hematomas or seromas, six instances of transient testicular pain, one transient lateral femoral cutaneous nerve neuralgia, one case of epididymitis, one patient with hematuria, and one urinary tract infection. A single recurrence has been observed. Arregui feels it was related to the placement of a piece of mesh that was too small, as it was early in his experience.

Corbitt, who had initially recommended the plug and patch technique, has now adopted the TAPP approach. He has published a series of 75 such repairs with an approach similar to that of Fitzgibbons.[3] The incision, though, varies according to hernia type. In the case of an indirect hernia, the KTP/532 laser (Laserscope, San Jose, CA) or diathermy endoshears are employed to create a large defect in the peritoneum around the deep inguinal ring, leaving the sac in place. When treating a direct hernia, a transverse incision above the hernia defect is preferred. With either type of hernia, after creating a peritoneal flap, a large piece of polypropylene mesh (10 cm × 15 cm) is stapled in place to reinforce both the lateral and medial fossae. Preliminary results have been encouraging.

Schultz has also changed his method, converting to the TAPP operation.[3] Following a long transverse incision from the midline to a point inferolateral to the internal inguinal ring with a "hockey-stick" extension, a dissection of the preperitoneal space is carried out. An at-

tempt is made to reduce both direct and indirect hernias. If dissection of the latter from the cord is too difficult, the sac is severed at the neck and the distal portion is left in place. The hernia defect is then filled with a conical piece of mesh, and the whole area between the midline medially and the anterior superior iliac spine laterally is covered with a large, flat piece of polypropylene mesh. This is inserted beneath the epigastric vessels and kept in place by staples.

The German surgeon Popp has introduced a new technique to facilitate the dissection of the peritoneal flap: the introduction of 100 to 300 ml of saline solution into the peritoneal space under pressure (aquadissection).[103] The solution can be instilled either from inside the abdomen (endoscopic transperitoneal aquadissection) or through the skin (transcutaneous preperitoneal aquadissection). The latter is accomplished after the hernia sac has been visualized endoscopically and the musculofascial defect localized by palpation. The needle tip is then identified under the peritoneum of the hernia sac and aquadissection is performed. The water pillow in the area surrounding the opening enables the dissection to be performed easily with atraumatic grasping forceps. Popp recommends the use of an absorbable mesh for the repair, which he feels offers the advantage of no residual foreign material in the abdominal wall after scarring of the musculofascial defect has occurred. The biodegradable prosthesis is not fixed with staples or sutures.

At the University of Southern California, Peters isolates the spermatic cord preperitoneally, places a mesh with a slit around the cord, and leaves the sac within the cord structures.[67] No recurrences in the short-term follow-up have been observed in 35 patients operated on by this method.

The TAPP procedure is the most popular laparoscopic hernia repair performed to date. The approach is attractive because the preperitoneal space is easily approached laparoscopically (Table 29–4). Although the operation requires a considerable amount of dissection, patients have been reported to recover promptly and return to normal physical activity quickly. The TAPP procedure eliminates the need for large skin incisions when compared with the conventional preperitoneal repair. It is debatable whether this confers a significant enough advantage in terms of perioperative morbidity. A randomized prospective trial comparing the results of TAPP and conventional anterior hernia repair would be ideal.

Table 29–4. INDICATIONS AND CONTRAINDICATIONS FOR LAPAROSCOPIC TRANSABDOMINAL PREPERITONEAL INGUINAL HERNIA REPAIR

	Indications	Contraindications
Absolute	None	American Society of Anesthesiology Class IV
		Known adhesive peritoneal obliteration
		Uncorrected coagulopathy
		Previous peritonitis
		Obstruction or strangulation
Relative	Clinical evidence of groin hernia	Incarceration
		Previous preperitoneal dissection
		Existing preperitoneal prosthetic material
		"Huge" hernia
		Severe spinal deformity
		Synchronous intraabdominal pathologic condition
		Gross obesity
		Ascites

Intraperitoneal Onlay Mesh Repair

The excellent results obtained with TAPP raised the question whether the same results could have been obtained by simply fixing the prosthesis directly onto the peritoneum (intraperitoneal onlay mesh [IPOM] repair) using the same landmarks as with the TAPP operation. This would eliminate the need for dissection within the preperitoneal space, theoretically reducing perioperative morbidity.

To answer this question, a protocol was initiated in 1990 in the Laboratory for Experimental Laparoscopic Surgery at Creighton University to evaluate the feasibility of this approach. Twenty-six pigs with congenital unilateral or bilateral indirect inguinal hernias had repairs performed by the application of sheets of polypropylene mesh (approximately 5 cm × 5 cm) onto the peritoneum. In one half of the pigs, the prosthesis was applied laparoscopically and secured with staples. The other 13 pigs served as a control group, with the polypropylene patches being placed at laparotomy and secured with sutures. In none of these animals was the preperitoneal space actually entered. At 6 weeks, the pigs were sacrificed. All repairs were intact, and adhesion development, determined as the percentage of patch surface area covered by adhesions, showed a significantly reduced rate in the pigs who underwent the laparoscopic procedure when compared with those who underwent laparotomy. In the laparoscopic group, adhesions were reported primarily between the urinary bladder and the patch, and only 15% of the animals had adhesions to the small bowel. The significant decrease in adhesions when the patches were placed laparoscopically was theorized to be due to decreased manipulation of abdominal organs. A stapling device was developed to apply box-shaped staples with a 3-mm leg length in the closed configuration. It was felt that this short length would avoid deep penetration by the staples, thus decreasing the risk of blood vessel and nerve damage. Patch adherence was excellent, and revision of the prototype staples has resulted in a commercially available device (Fig. 29–18).

The results were presented to the Institutional Review Board at Creighton University and permission was obtained to begin performing the IPOM procedures in humans. The procedure was similar to that performed in the laboratory. A polypropylene mesh patch approximately 11 cm × 6 cm was positioned over the indirect inguinal hernia defect and stapled in place (Fig. 29–19). Landmarks for stapling were identical to those described previously for the TAPP procedure—that is, the fascia transversalis, musculus and posterior musculus rectus abdominis sheath superiorly, the transversus abdominis, the symphysis pubis and Cooper's ligament inferomedially, and the lateral abdominal wall medial to the anterior superior iliac spine laterally. The procedure was used routinely only for indirect hernias. It became obvious early that if staples were placed inferior to the iliopubic tract and lateral to the internal spermatic vessels, there would be an inordinately high incidence of neuralgias involving the lateral fem-

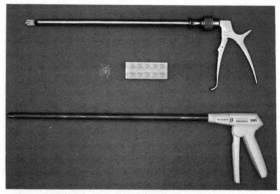

Figure 29–18. Prototype stapler *(top)*, skin-type staples and mounting tray *(middle)*, and Endopath EMS 30 (Ethicon, Inc., Cincinnati, OH) repeating disposable stapler *(bottom)*.

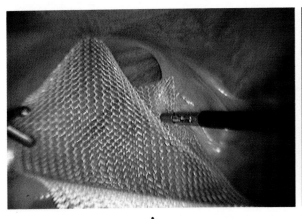
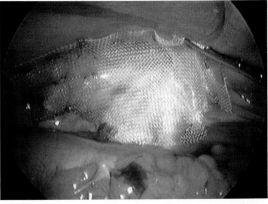

A   B

Figure 29–19. (A) Mesh placement over the indirect defect during an intraperitoneal onlay mesh (IPOM) repair. **(B)** The mesh is correctly positioned.

oral cutaneous nerve or the femoral branch of the genitofemoral nerve (see Fig. 29–14*A* and *B*). The same precautions as were described with the TAPP procedure are useful here. For patients with large indirect inguinal hernias, especially those extending into the scrotum, the sac was circumferentially divided at the internal ring to separate it from the parietal peritoneum (Fig. 29–20). This was felt to aid in fixation of the mesh at the internal ring, reducing the danger of the patch prolapsing into the hernia defect. This has been referred to as IPOM plus sac division.

Between June 16, 1991 and December 1, 1992, 59 IPOM operations were performed in 56 patients with indirect inguinal hernias (three hernias were bilateral), with a median follow-up of 45 weeks. One clinical recurrence has been noted. This patient has not been reoperated on, as the recurrence is asymptomatic and

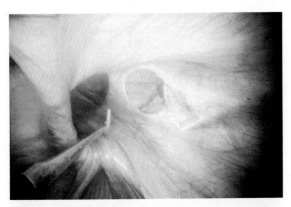

Figure 29–20. IPOM repair. For large indirect inguinal hernias, especially those extending into the scrotum, the sac is circumferentially divided at the internal ring to separate it from the parietal peritoneum.

only detectable by physical examination, so the cause of the failure is unclear. Postoperative complications have occurred in 14 patients (see Table 29–3). These were mostly minor, consisting of urinary retention, seroma formation, and one significant hematoma in a patient who required postoperative heparinization for a prosthetic heart valve. All of these complications resolved with supportive care. Once more, early in this series, thigh, groin, and testicular pain or numbness was reported by several patients. The majority of these neuralgias were transient and resolved spontaneously, but one patient required a second laparoscopy to remove the offending staple, with subsequent resolution of the neuralgia.

It is remarkable that transient groin and thigh pain has been observed in a procedure like the IPOM, which does not require dissection into the preperitoneal space. Before the introduction of this technique, it had been speculated that transient groin or leg pain observed after the TAPP operation was due to minor nerve irritation. Thus, it would have been the consequence of extensive traumatic dissection in the preperitoneal space lateral to the spermatic vessels and below the iliopubic tract, rather than direct stapling or entrapment of nerve fibers. This now seems unlikely, and staple placement is to be considered the major cause of both transient and persistent pain following a laparoscopic hernia repair. In our experience, this complication has been virtually eliminated with the appreciation that staples should not be placed in the area lateral to the spermatic vessels and caudad to the iliopubic tract.

The laboratory and clinical data presented here suggest that the intraperitoneal operation is effective in correcting indirect inguinal hernias. However, the most significant concern remains the placement of a foreign material on the peritoneum, which is potentially in contact with intraabdominal organs. The laboratory portion of this project suggested that adhesions are decreased with the laparoscopic approach but not completely eliminated. In this series of 59 patients, 4 patients have had their intraperitoneal mesh repairs inspected. One patient presented with a gunshot wound to the abdomen and required exploratory laparotomy. His polypropylene mesh was found to be completely occluding the hernia orifice without evidence of adhesions. The patient described earlier with the neuralgia treated by removing the offending staple underwent laparoscopy 3 weeks postoperatively and was found to have rather dense adhesions of the colon and small bowel to the prosthetic material. The third patient underwent laparoscopy when he presented with symptomatic gallbladder disease for cholecystectomy. Adhesions between the mesh prosthesis and both the omentum and bowel were observed. Finally, and most significantly, the fourth patient had a fluctuant mass in the groin (18 months after his IPOM procedure), which was incised and drained and was found to contain enteric organisms. The patient underwent repeat laparoscopy and was found to have dense adherence of the cecum to his prosthetic patch. His appendix could not be identified, and it was therefore unclear if the mesh had eroded into the cecum or if the patient had acquired appendicitis. A barium enema performed 6 weeks postoperatively failed to visualize the appendix. The abscess was drained extraperitoneally, and the mesh was easily removed laparoscopically, as the inflammatory process had caused the mesh and staples to separate from the peritoneum. An additional disturbing finding in this patient was that the medial side of the patient's left-sided indirect inguinal hernia repair had become separated from the parietal peritoneum, partially exposing the indirect inguinal hernia defect. It should be noted that the patient has no clinical evidence of a recurrent hernia on either side. This procedure was performed with a prototype stapling device, which has subsequently been modified and improved. This last complication has, in consultation with the Human Research Committee of Creighton University, resulted in suspension of the intraperitoneal operation until longer term follow-up of the rest of the group is obtained. To date, no further complications have been observed in any other patients.

Franklin of San Antonio, Texas, has noted one recurrence in a series of 65 hernias (32 direct and 33 indirect hernias) in 63 patients operated on using a technique similar to Fitzgibbons' after a mean follow-up of 11 months. Franklin stabilizes the mesh by placing three sutures through three small puncture wounds in the groin area. A straight needle is used to introduce the suture into the abdominal cavity. The stitch is then passed through the mesh and brought back out through the same skin incision using a hollow needle as a guide. The suture is then tied at the level of the fascia, and the skin is closed over. This allows full-thickness stabilization of the mesh over the abdominal wall. Among the complications were one intraoperative laceration of an inferior epigastric artery, one hematoma, two cases of thigh numbness, two cases of testicular pain, and three seromas. No significant complications related to the intraabdominal placement of a 12 cm × 15 cm piece of polypropylene mesh have been reported. This author also utilizes the IPOM approach for both direct and femoral hernias.[3]

In Seaford, Delaware, Toy and Smoot also use an IPOM technique but prefer polytetrafluoroethylene (PTFE) rather than polypropylene for the intraperitoneal prosthesis.[93] They attempt to reduce the sac from the indirect hernia defect to obtain a high ligation, utilizing a pretied loop or an endoscopic linear stapler. The technique is also used for direct hernias, but the sacs are only reduced if the hernia is large. The PTFE prosthesis is 5 cm long × 7 cm wide and 1 mm thick and is fixed in place with a specially designed spreader and newly designed stapling device. The authors open the peritoneum medially to expose Cooper's ligament, as they feel this is essential for adequate fixation and to protect against bladder injury. Ten patients have been followed for an average of 4.5 months without recurrence. Patients were allowed to return to normal activities after 2 days.

Spaw and associates of Nashville also prefer PTFE. They staple 5 cm × 10 cm sheets of expanded PTFE along Cooper's ligament inferomedially, the iliopubic tract inferiorly, and the fascia transversalis superiorly for large indirect or direct hernias.[27] They do not ligate the sac, nor do they enter the preperitoneal space. The prosthesis extends from Cooper's ligament inferiorly to a point lateral to the deep inguinal ring and from the lateral edge of the musculus rectus abdominis to the lateral border of the fascia transversalis superiorly. For small and medium indirect inguinal hernias, Spaw prefers to perform a ringplasty by approximating the fascia transversalis sling crura on the lateral side of the deep inguinal ring. He has treated 45 inguinal hernias (22 direct, 21 indirect, 1 femoral, and 1 incisional hernia) with these two methods: 19 of the procedures were performed with the intraperitoneal onlay technique. One recurrence medial to the intraperitoneal patch has been recorded. One laceration of an inferior epigastric vein and one scrotal edema have been observed as complications; in three cases a conversion to open surgery has been necessary.[104]

It would appear that the IPOM procedure is a quick and effective method to repair indirect inguinal hernias, and possibly direct hernias. Because of the lack of excessive dissection, it is associated with a very low operative morbidity rate. Nevertheless, the problem related to the intraperitoneal placement of prosthetic material, specifically the possibility of adhesion formation and erosion into intraabdominal organs, remains unsettled. Certainly, if there is going to be a significant incidence of complications related to either circumstance, this operation could not compete with conventional herniorrhaphy or the TAPP. We continue to feel that patients being offered IPOM repair should be informed of the experimental nature of the operation and should be placed in an experimental trial controlled by a human research committee. The future of this operation may be enhanced by the development of a less reactive prosthesis, at least on its peritoneal surface (see discussion of adhesion formation and mesh materials further on).

Totally Extraperitoneal Laparoscopic Hernia Repair

It is possible to perform a laparoscopically guided repair of a hernia defect without entering the peritoneal cavity. It is a contradiction to define it as a laparoscopic procedure because the abdominal cavity is not entered. Since laparoscopic instrumentation is used to dissect the preperitoneal space, however, the procedure is considered together with the other laparoscopic herniorraphies.

The technique has been most extensively used by McKernan and Laws.[105] They begin the procedure with an incision at the umbilicus, identical to that which would be used for open laparoscopy. The fascia at the umbilicus is opened but the peritoneum is left intact. An open laparoscopic cannula is placed in the incision and an operating laparoscope is used to create a working space between the peritoneum and the fascia transversalis.[105] As the dissection proceeds inferiorly, a space is developed that is large enough to accommodate additional laparoscopic cannulas. The operating laparoscope is then replaced with a standard 10-mm laparoscope. The "pneumoextraperitoneum" is maintained with CO_2 gas at pressures of approximately 8 to 10 mm Hg. As dissection continues, the preperitoneal space in the groin region is entered, and a dissection similar to that described earlier for the TAPP can be accomplished. If an indirect hernia is encountered and the sac is small, it is dissected away from the cord structures. For large indirect hernias, the sac is divided at the internal ring, leaving the distal portion in situ. For direct hernias, the sac is reduced and a 12.5-cm × 7.5-cm piece of polypropylene mesh is then introduced into the preperitoneal space after a slit and 1 cm defect is placed in the mesh to accommodate the cord structures. Staples are applied to tack the mesh inferomedially to Cooper's ligament, inferolaterally to the iliopubic tract, superiorly to the fascia transversalis well above the defect, medially to the musculus rectus abdominis and its investing sheath, and laterally to the abdominal wall just medial to the anterior superior iliac spine (these are the same landmarks used for the TAPP and IPOM procedures). If bilateral hernias are present, McKernan and Laws prefer two separate sheets of polypropylene mesh rather than a large one.

McKernan has performed 155 of these repairs on 106 patients—69 direct hernias, 85 indirect hernias (including 2 sliding), and 1 femoral hernia. The total number of recurrent hernias was 32, and 49 of the hernias were bilateral. They have seen no recurrences on short-term follow-up. Complications have included one case of postoperative orchitis, several cases of seromas in the preperitoneal space that responded to aspiration (n = 7) or observation only (n = 8), five transient testicular swellings, four genitofemoral and four lateral femoral cutaneous neuralgias, one hematoma, one wound infection, and two cases of urinary retention. Three procedures had to be converted to TAPP repair, two of them because of the creation of a small hole in the peritoneum and one in a patient who had a previous radical prostatectomy with radiation therapy, which obliterated the preperitoneal space. The average time reported for the operation is 55 minutes.[106]

Phillips from Los Angeles is also a proponent of the totally extraperitoneal procedure.[3] He prefers an initial diagnostic laparoscopy, however, so that he can carefully inspect both sides of the groin to assess the hernias from an intraabdominal viewpoint. He then introduces a Veress needle into the preperitoneal space and under direct vision creates the "pneumoextraperitoneum." A trocar is then placed directly into the preperitoneal space and the pneumoperitoneum is released. The procedure is then similar to McKernan and Laws'.[105] At the conclusion, the pneumoperitoneum can be reproduced and the hernia repair inspected again from an intraabdominal vantage point.

Arregui, one of the pioneers of the TAPP procedure, is now performing almost exclusively totally extraperitoneal laparoscopic hernia repairs. He also begins with an intraperitoneal inspection and has done 47 such operations.[102]

The totally extraperitoneal operation is attractive, as it has the advantage of avoiding the potential adhesive complications related to the incision in the peritoneum required to enter the preperitoneal space with the TAPP. The operating space is limited, however, and experience is required to become familiar with the anatomy from this perspective. In addition, care must be taken to avoid penetration of the peritoneum, as this will result in the creation of a pneumoperitoneum that will compromise the size of the extraperitoneal space. Because of its technical complexity, it is unclear whether this procedure will enjoy a wide acceptance among surgeons.

Adhesion Formation, Mesh Materials, and Adhesion Inhibitors

Mechanical trauma, infection, tissue ischemia, thermal injury, and foreign materials are the most important factors responsible for adhesion formation.[107] Trauma as a consequence of laparotomy causes adhesions in 67% of patients.[108] Adhesions are found in 88% of subjects who undergo laparotomy after previous abdominal surgery.[109] The mechanism by which peritonitis creates adhesion formation is not completely clear. It is known, however, that bacteria release substances that diminish tissue blood flow and attract inflammatory cells, with consequent production of exudates and tissue damage. Foreign bodies have been reported in 61% to 69% of postoperative adhesions. In 50% to 68% of cases, the foreign material was talc; other materials included sutures, lint, filaments of dressings, starch, extruded gut contents and, obviously, prosthetic grafts. A combination of different materials has also been noted (usually talc and thread).[108, 110] According to several authors, the presence of intraperitoneal blood associated with drying of the serosal surface dramatically increases subsequent adhesion development.[111, 112] However, large volumes of fresh and clotted blood, without the simultaneous presence of serosal injury, do not promote adhesion formation and are completely absorbed by normal peritoneum within 2 days.[112–114]

Whatever causative mechanism is involved, the common pathway leading to adhesion formation is inflammation that produces exudates containing high quantities of fibrinogen.[115–117] Fibrin clots develop, which cause adherence to surrounding structures. A healthy and well-vascularized peritoneum (even with a defect) has an effective fibrinolytic system due to a form of plasminogen activator that is able to completely absorb the newly developed fibrinous attachments.[107, 118] The fibrinolytic mechanism is considerably impaired if peritoneum is rendered ischemic—for example, by tight suturing or grafting. Moreover, ischemic tissues are potent stimuli to adhesion formation and actively inhibit fibrinolysis in adjacent peritoneal tissue.[115, 117–120]

In conclusion, retention of vascularization is essential for proper, adhesion-free peritoneal healing.[115, 121, 122] In open surgery, peritoneal defects should be left open to prevent tissue ischemia.[123] Laparoscopic surgery decreases the incidence of adhesion formation by reducing the length of incisions and the amount of blood loss, preventing talc from entering the abdominal cavity, allowing precise dissection with magnification, and eliminating traumatic microinjuries due to the use of abrasive materials such as sponges.

The use of electrocautery is felt by some to result in decreased adhesion formation, as the amount of loss is reduced.[124] Initial enthusiasm for laser use has been subsequently dampened by both animal and human studies.[107] No reduction in postoperative adhesion was observed when the CO_2 laser was compared with fine needle cautery in experimental animal studies.[125] In controlled human studies, no statistical difference in postoperative adhesion formation was found at the time of early second-look laparoscopy between two groups of women in whom lysis of periovarian and peritubal adhesions was performed at laparotomy with either the CO_2 laser or electromicrosurgery.[126–128] Titanium staples applied to close the peritoneal defect are highly inert but are nevertheless foreign bodies. Because of their box shape, however, they are less traumatic and induce less ischemia when compared with traditional sutures (see Fig. 29–18).

A number of experimental and clinical studies have been conducted to better understand the mechanism of adhesion formation and its prevention. In 1990, Luciano completed an experimental randomized study of laparoscopy versus laparotomy, comparing postoperative adhesions in rabbits subjected to laser incisions over one uterine horn and over the peritoneal surface of either lower quadrant.[129] He demonstrated that in the laparotomy group, postoperative adhesions were present not only on the tissues involved with initial injury but also at the laparotomy incision. In addition, adhesions were often found where no apparent injury had been inflicted. No adhesions were observed in the laparoscopy group. Filmar and associates, in contrast, reported no significant difference between the two procedures in postoperative adhesion formation in an animal model analogous to the one used by Luciano.[130] The difference may be explained by the fact that Filmar and coworkers inflicted the injury with sharp scissors, with subsequent bleeding that was not immediately controlled. These results support a number of clinical observations in which the incidence of adhesion formation was greater than 50% following open laparotomy for infertility (discovered at a second-look operation). When the procedure was accomplished laparoscopically, the incidence was considerably lower.[129]

Prosthetic materials used to replace abdominal wall defects are known to be associated with adhesions to intraabdominal organs. Adhesions will also form when protheses are grafted onto intact peritoneal surfaces, probably as a result of decreased fibrinolytic activity of the mesothelial layer. The relative importance of the type of prosthetic material is debated. Theoretically, the ideal prosthesis should be strong, durable, inert, hypoallergenic, sterilizable, stable in body fluids, and resistent to infections, and should stimulate fibrotic reaction to reinforce the repair. The prosthesis should not be associated with adhesions between its abdominal surface and intraabdominal organs.

Many prosthetic materials have been used in hernia repair, including polypropylene, PTFE, nylon net, polyglycolic acid, stainless steel, silver, and tantalum.[131]

Nonabsorbable *silver prostheses* were employed at the beginning of the century in Germany and came into use in the United States in 1903, but the metal was found to corrode when in contact with tissue fluids.[132]

Tantalum mesh, the use of which was first reported by Koontz in 1948, tended to fragment with repeated flexion within the tissues. Serious complications related to the fragments have been reported, such as erosion of the skin and peritoneum, ulcerations, and bowel fistulas.[133, 134]

Subsequently, synthetic meshes became available. The first inguinal hernia repair with prosthetic mesh was performed in 1958 by Usher and associates. They observed good results with the use of polypropylene mesh in a classic anterior hernioplasty.[135] The use of nonabsorbable prostheses gained popularity in Europe, especially in France.[82]

Polypropylene mesh (Marlex, Prolene) and *polyester fibers* (Dacron, Mersilene) have been the most widely used prosthetic patches in the repair of hernias.[132, 136, 137] They usually become incorporated by dense collagen fibers as a result of a mild foreign body reaction. They are strong and additional inguinal floor reinforcement occurs when fibrous ingrowth takes place. Observation for as long as 20 years in patients with conventional preperitoneal inguinal hernia repairs suggest that these materials are durable.[67] For these reasons, they have become the preferred prosthetic materials for hernia repair in the United States.[138]

Marked inflammatory reaction to the polypropylene mesh has proved to be responsible for dense scar formation. Secondary contraction sometimes can cause tension on the surrounding tissues, as well as distortion of the graft.[131] Occasionally, complications related to polypropylene mesh have been reported, including wound sepsis, mesh extrusion, erosion into intraabdominal organs, and bowel fistulas.[93, 132] These considerations have stimulated a search for other prosthetic materials.

The initial clinical experience with meshes woven from solid PTFE (Teflon, Gore-Tex) was unfavorable and discouraging.[139] The discovery in the 1970s of a new process to expand this material into a porous form *(expanded PTFE)* opened new possibilities.[140]

There are a number of studies comparing polypropylene and expanded PTFE in reinforcing the abdominal wall.[131, 136, 137, 141, 142] Wagner feels that polypropylene mesh (Marlex) is the least reactive based on his examination of several plastic prosthetic materials.[143] Usher found polypropylene (Marlex) to be intact at 4 years in an experimental study.[144] Amid and colleagues have shown that polypropylene mesh is very well tolerated, resists infection, has rapid host tissue fixation, and becomes completely incorporated into the host tissue, whereas the penetration of fibroblasts from the host tissue into the depth of expanded PTFE is only about 10% after 3 years (in case of a superimposed infection, this is further decreased).[142] Conversely, Elliott and Juler found polypropylene to be fragmented in some areas when studied with polarized light microscopy.[131] Others have reported a better fibrous tissue annexation of PTFE over polypropylene, with better imbedding in fibrous tissue and a more complete incorporation into a healing wound.[132, 137] Other advantages reported in favor of expanded PTFE include a lower infection rate and a lower rate of adhesion formation.[132, 138, 143] In other experimental studies, however, expanded PTFE increased postoperative peritoneal adhesion formation, possibly because it incited inflammatory and foreign body reactions.[145] One criticism about hernia repair with PTFE is that it is based entirely on the strength of the prosthesis, as fibrous ingrowth is reduced.[67]

Absorbable mesh has recently been introduced. In 1983, Lamb and associates reported that a *polyglactin mesh* (Vicryl) was not detectable 12 weeks after the implantation. At 3 weeks, the mesh showed peritoneal covering but there was no demonstrable fibrous tissue growth over the abdominal wall defect. The material was considered unsatisfactory for successful hernia repair by the authors.[137] *Polyglycolic acid mesh* (Dexon) did not induce a strong fibrous response, and consequently an adequate support, to the abdominal wall in a study conducted by Law and Ellis.[141]

The availability of many different types of prosthetic material probably indicates that the ideal one has yet to be found. Therefore, further investigation in this area is warranted.

Several types of adjuvants have been investigated to decrease adhesion formation. They belong to different classes. The *high-viscosity instillates* result in the osmotic influx of fluids into the peritoneal cavity, creating a sort of "hydroflotation bath." The aim is to reduce apposition of the serosal and peritoneal surfaces, thus decreasing adhesion formation during the period of epithelial regeneration.[125] They are also thought to prevent fibrin deposition. The most popular substance in this class is *32% Dextran 70* (molecular weight 70,000) (Hyskon). It proved to be effective at high dosages in animal studies.[146] Human studies, however, have had contradictory results. Both a prospective randomized multicenter trial and an additional retrospective study demonstrated beneficial effects of 32% Dextran 70, but two other human studies failed to reveal an advantage.[126, 147, 148] Moreover, various allergic reactions have been reported as side effects following peritoneal instillation of 32% Dextran 70, although they were not frequent.[125]

Another class of adjuvants is that of *mechanical barriers*. Various kinds of barriers have been employed: fascia, peritoneum, tunica vaginalis, vena cava, cellophane, nylon, and so on. Two of them have gained popularity. *Oxidized cellulose* (Surgicel; Johnson & Johnson Patient Care, Inc., New Brunswick, NJ) was first tested in laboratory animals and in two studies did not promote adhesions when left in the abdominal cavity after surgery.[149, 150] Hixon and associates, however, reported increased adhesion formation with the material.[151] Subsequent modifications in the degree of oxidation, porosity, and density led to the development of a new reabsorbable and biocompatible barrier called *Interceed* (TC7).[152, 153] A significant reduction of adhesion formation was achieved in two rabbit studies and subsequently confirmed in a human study conducted on 74 infertility patients treated for bilateral pelvic side wall adhesions with laparotomy adhesiolysis and follow-up second-look laparoscopy. The deperitonealized area of one side was covered with Interceed and the other served as a control. The covered area had a 90% improvement over control side walls in adhesion formation. In a study conducted at Creighton University, patches of polypropylene and composite patches of oxidized regenerated cellulose and polypropylene (Prolene, Interceed) were implanted in the groin areas of a swine model, one type of patch for each side. In one group of pigs the patches were implanted laparoscopically, while in another group an open laparotomy was performed. The average percentage of the surface area of prosthetic patches covered by adhesions did not vary significantly between patches of polypropylene alone and composite patches 6 weeks after implantation. The surface covered by adhesions was considerably less for both types of patches in the group of pigs operated on laparoscopically.[3] Other authors report an increase in de novo intraperitoneal adhesion formation caused by Interceed in a murine model.[154]

Pharmacologic substances have also been employed to try to reduce adhesion formation. *Calcium channel antagonists* such as nifedipine, verapamil, and diltiazem have been used based on the hypothesis that adhesion formation could be prevented by blocking the intracellular mechanisms of the cellular elements involved in the process of peritoneal repair (fibroblasts, platelets, phagocytes, and endothelial cells). Promising results have been noted in the rabbit model after treatment with verapamil.[155]

Tissue plasminogen activator (t-PA) converts plasminogen to plasmin and specifically acts on the fibrin surface without activating the liquid-phase plasminogen. Recombinant genetic technology has recently made t-PA available in pharmacologic quantities (rt-PA). It has been applied topically in a gel formulation in the rabbit uterine horn model and reduced both the incidence and density of adhesion formation and reformation.[156]

Intraperitoneal administration of *sodium tolmetin in a hyaluronic acid carrier* reduced adhesion formation in a study conducted on rabbits.[157] Tolmetin's action is due to an increased fibrinolytic activity obtained by reducing the levels of plasminogen activator inhibitor and the elastinolytic substance secreted by macrophages.

Carboxymethylcellulose (CMC) acts by coating the intraperitoneal surface to prevent direct apposition of injured structures. It is very slowly absorbed, and its action in decreasing postoperative adhesion formation is relatively prolonged.[125] In three studies in the rabbit model, CMC proved effective in significantly reducing adhesion formation and reformation.[148, 158–161] In two of these studies, CMC was more effective than 32% Dextran 70 in preventing adhesion reformation.[148, 158, 159] In another study, however, CMC not only increased adhesions in treated rats but also promoted anastomotic leaks and a high mortality rate in the treated group.[162]

Nonsteroidal antiinflammatory agents reduce vascular permeability and histamine release and stabilize lysosomes. Oxyphenbutazone and ibuprofen reduced the intensity of adhesion formation in animal studies.[163–167]

Iloprost, a prostacyclin analog, has proved effective in reducing postoperative primary posttraumatic adhesion formation in hamsters when administered perioperatively.[168]

The effectiveness of *steroids* in preventing adhesion formation is controversial. Some authors have demonstrated a beneficial effect of these drugs.[169, 170] Swolin and Jansen used hydrocortisone intraperitoneally before peritoneal closure and subsequently reported that all patients showed a considerable reduction in adhesion formation when laparoscopy was performed 3 months later.[171, 172] Others, however, have not confirmed the usefulness of glucocorticosteroids in preventing postoperative adhesions.[173–175] In addition, increased postoperative morbidity is possible because of the interference with immunologic defenses.[107]

The hypothesis that *antihistamines* decrease fibrin-rich inflammatory exudate in the abdominal cavity (and consequently limit adhesion formation) has been advanced.[169, 170, 176] However, in a recent randomized, controlled, and laparoscopically monitored study conducted by Jansen in 90 patients, no beneficial or deleterious effect on the extent of postoperative adhesions was demonstrated.[172]

Despite these promising data, a definitive solution to the problem of adhesion formation after intraperitoneal placement of synthetic prostheses has not yet been found. It is for this reason that most surgeons performing laparoscopic herniorrhaphy prefer the TAPP. Presumably, by covering the prosthesis with peritoneum, adhesions formed directly to the prosthesis and possible erosion into intraabdominal organs are avoided. Small bowel obstruction remains a possibility with this type of procedure, however, because of the peritoneal incision line used to enter the preperitoneal space. In fact, loops of bowel might migrate in through the opening of the peritoneum if the flaps are not closely reapproximated.

CONCLUSION

The number of techniques for laparoscopic hernia repair described in this chapter, as well as the differences in the materials and fixation techniques used, reflect a phase of evolution and research. The efforts are directed to devise the operation that could represent a viable alternative to conventional inguinal hernia repair. This procedure should result in a decreased recurrence rate and reduced postoperative morbidity, as well a short hospital stay and a prompt return to normal activity.

To better define the features of this ideal operation, our group has promoted a multicenter clinical trial for laparoscopic herniorrhaphy, which was initiated in the fall of 1991. Twenty institutions in North America and Europe were included. Preliminary results of 816 repairs in 636 patients have revealed an overall recurrence rate of 3.2% after a mean follow-up of 6 months. Considering the long learning curve for this procedure, these results seem satisfactory. Groin pain was present in 10.3%, and thigh pain in 5.3%, of patients. This confirms the need for a thorough understanding of the anatomy of the inguinal region as viewed laparoscopically before performing laparoscopic herniorrhaphy. Urinary retention was reported in 2.2%, and cord swelling in 1.8%, of patients. Laparoscopy itself did not cause any complication, and the mortality rate was 0.2% (a single postoperative myocardial infarction). A companion study to include international investigators outside of Europe and the United States is under way.

The individual centers have been left free to choose their preferred technique, but general guidelines have been given. These guidelines are presented in Table 29–5, according to Nyhus' classification. We hope that this investiga-

Table 29–5. GUIDELINES FOR LAPAROSCOPIC TREATMENT OF GROIN HERNIAS FOR A MULTICENTERED TRIAL

Hernia	Definition	Laparoscopic Treatment
Type I	Indirect inguinal hernia with normal internal inguinal ring (*i.e.*, pediatric hernia)	Simple herniotomy
Type II	Indirect inguinal hernia with dilated internal inguinal ring, anatomically intact	IPOM, TAPP, TEP
Type IIIA	Direct inguinal hernia	TAPP, TEP
Type IIIB	Indirect inguinal hernia with anatomic destruction of the ring	IPOM + sac division, TAPP, TEP
Type IIIC	Femoral hernia	TAPP, TEP
Type IV	Recurrent hernia	TAPP, TEP

IPOM = intraperitoneal onlay mesh; TAPP = transabdominal preperitoneal procedure; TEP = totally extraperitoneal.

tion provides an answer to the question of whether laparoscopic herniorrhaphy should become a valid alternative to conventional repair. This will be possible only if the complications of initial peritoneal cavity penetration, general anesthesia, and adhesions, both to sites of peritoneal penetration and to intraperitoneal prosthesis, are not excessive.

References

1. Ravitch MM. Repair of hernias. Chicago: Year Book Medical Publishers, 1969:9.
2. Filipi CJ, Fitzgibbons RJ Jr, Salerno GM. Historical review: diagnostic laparoscopy to laparoscopic cholecystectomy and beyond. In: Zucker KA, ed. Surgical laparoscopy. St. Louis: Quality Medical Publishing, 1991:3–21.
3. Salerno GM, Fitzgibbons RJ Jr, Corbitt RJ, et al. Laparoscopic inguinal hernia repair. In: Zucker KA, ed. Surgical laparoscopy update. St. Louis: Quality Medical Publishing, 1993:373–394.
4. Deysine M, Grimson RC, Soroff HS. Inguinal herniorraphy. Arch Surg 126:628–630, 1991.
5. Nyhus LM, Bombeck TC, Klein MS. Hernias. In: Sabiston DC Jr, ed. Textbook of surgery. Philadelphia: WB Saunders, 1991:1134–1147.
6. Gaster J. Hernia: one day repair. Darien, CT: Hafner Publishing, 1970:5–54.
7. Berliner SD. An approach to groin hernia. Surg Clin North Am 64:197–213, 1984.
8. Department of Health and Human Services, Public Health Service. National Health Survey: Utilization of short-stay hospitals, annual summary for the United States, 1980; 1982, Washington, DC: US Government Printing Office, Series 13, No. 64.
9. Department of Health, Education and Welfare. National health survey on hernias, 1960, Washington DC: US Government Printing Office, Series B, No. 25.
10. Abramson JH, Gofin J, Hopp C, et al. The epidemiology of inguinal hernia. A survey in western Jerusalem. J Epidemiol Community Health 32:59–67, 1978.
11. Harkins HN: Surgery, principles and practice. 2nd ed. Philadelphia: JB Lippincott, 1957.
12. Department of Health and Human Services, Public Health Service. National health survey: utilization of short-stay hospitals, annual summary for the United States, 1989; 1992, Washington, DC: US Government Printing Office, Series 13, No. 109.
13. Lichtenstein I, Shulman A, Amid P, et al. The pathophysiology of recurrent hernia. Contemp Surg 35:13–18, 1992.
14. Lichtenstein IL. The "one day" inguinal herniorraphy. Contemp Surg 20:17–36, 1982.
15. Nyhus LM, Klein MS, Rogers FB. Inguinal hernia. Curr Probl Surg 6:401–450, 1991.
16. Morton JH: Abdominal wall hernias. In: Schwartz S, Shires C, Spencer F, Storer E, ed. Principles of surgery. New York: McGraw Hill, 1984:1457–1474.
17. Heydorn WH, Velanovic V. A five-year U.S. experience with 36,250 abdominal hernia repairs. Am Surg 56:596–600, 1990.
18. Schneidmann DS. Selected data on hospitals and use services. In: Peebles RJ, Schneidmann DS, ed. Socioeconomic factbook for surgery 1991–1992. Chicago: American College of Surgeons, 1991:31–49.
19. Cooper A. The anatomy and surgical treatment of abdominal hernia. Vol I. London: Longman, 1804.
20. Condon RE. The anatomy of the inguinal region and its relationship to groin hernia. In: Nyhus L, Condon R, eds. Hernia. Philadelphia: JB Lippincott, 1978:14–78.
21. Zimmermann L, Anson B. Anatomy and surgery of hernia. 2nd ed. Baltimore: Williams & Wilkins, 1967:15.
22. Fruchaud H. Anatomie chirurgicale des hernies de l'aine. Paris: G. Doin, 1956.
23. Ponka J. Hernias of the abdominal wall. Philadelphia: WB Saunders, 1980:18–39.
24. Skandalakis J, Colborn G, Gray S, et al. The surgical anatomy of the inguinal area. Part I. Contemp Surg 38:20–34, 1991.
25. Lytle W. The internal inguinal ring. Br J Surg 32:441–446, 1944.
26. Thorek P. Anatomy surgery. 2nd ed. Philadelphia: JB Lippincott, 1962:375.
27. Spaw AT, Ennis BW, Spaw LP. Laparoscopic hernia repair: the anatomic basis. J Laparoendosc Surg 1:269–277, 1991.
28. Gullmö A, Broomé A, Smedberg S: Herniorraphy. Surg Clin North Am 64:229–244, 1984.
29. Skandalakis J, Colborn G, Gray S, et al. The surgical anatomy of the inguinal area. Part II. Contemp Surg 38:28–38, 1991.
30. Williams P, Warwick R, Dyson M, et al. Gray's anatomy. 37th ed. New York, Churchill-Livingstone, 1989:1123–1147.
31. Bouchet Y, Voilin C, Yver R. The peritoneum and its anatomy. In: Bengmark S, ed. The peritoneum and peritoneal access. London: Wright, 1989:1–13.
32. Nomina Anatomica. Revised by the International Anatomical Nomenclature Committee approved by the 11th Congress of Anatomy. Mexico City, 1980.
33. Pfitzer W. Uber die ursprungverhöltnisse der arteria oburatorie. Anat Anz 4:504–533, 1889.
34. Poynter C. Congenital anomalies of the arteries and veins of the human body with bibliography. University Studies XXII:33–35, 1922.
35. Edwards EA, Malone PD, MacArthur JD. Operative anatomy of abdomen and pelvis. Philadelphia: Lea & Febiger, 1975:44–47.

36. Bendavid R. The space of Bogros and the deep inguinal venous circulation. Surg Gynecol Obstet 174:355–358, 1992.

37. Esser M, Condon R. The surgical anatomy of the groin. Surg Rounds February, 1987:15–27.

38. Read RC. Cooper's posterior lamina of transversalis fascia. Surg Gynecol Obstet 174:426–434, 1992.

39. Cleland J, Mackay JY, Young BJ. The relations of the aponeurosis of the transversalis and internal oblique muscles to the deep epigastric artery and to the inguinal canal. In: Cleland J. Memoirs and memoranda in anatomy. London: Williams & Norgate, 1889:142–145.

40. Anson BJ, McVay CB. Inguinal hernia: the anatomy of the region. Surg Gynecol Obstet 66:186–191, 1938.

41. Lampe EW. Experiences with preperitoneal hernioplasty. In: Nyhus LM, Condon RE, ed. Hernia. Philadelphia: JB Lippincott, 1978:242–247.

42. Fowler R. The applied surgical anatomy of the peritoneal fascia of the groin and the "secondary" internal inguinal ring. Aust NZ J Surg 45:8–14, 1975.

43. Cooper AP. The anatomy and surgical treatment of abdominal hernia. Vol II. London: Longman, 1807.

44. Griffith CA. Inguinal hernia: an anatomic-surgical correlation. Surg Clin North Am 39:531–556, 1959.

45. McVay CB. The normal and pathologic anatomy of the transversus abdominis muscle in inguinal and femoral hernia. Surg Clin North Am 51:1251–1261, 1971.

46. Griffith CA. The Marcy repair of indirect inguinal hernia. In: Nyhus LM, Condon RE, eds. Hernia. Philadelphia: JB Lippincott, 1978:137–162.

47. Lichtenstein IL, Amid PK, Shulman AG. The iliopubic tract. Is it important in groin herniorraphy? Contemp Surg 40:22–24, 1992.

48. McVay CB. The anatomic basis for inguinal and femoral hernioplasty. Surg Gynecol Obstet 139:931–945, 1974.

49. Lichtenstein IL, Amid PK, Shulman AG. The iliopubic tract. The key to inguinal herniorraphy? Int Surg 75:244–246, 1990.

50. Gilroy AM, Marks SC Jr, Lei Q, et al. Anatomical characteristics of the iliopubic tract: implications for repair of inguinal hernias. Clin Anat 5:255–263, 1992.

51. Ellis H: Clinical anatomy: a revision and applied anatomy for clinical students. 6th ed. Oxford: Blackwell Scientific, 1977:257.

52. Hollinshead WH. The abdominal wall and inguinal region. Anatomy for surgeons: the thorax, abdomen and pelvis. New York: Paul B Hoeber, 1956:216–218.

53. Sorg J, Skandalakis JE, Gray SW. The emperor's new clothes or the myth of the conjoined tendon. Am Surg 45:588–589, 1979.

54. Skandalakis JE, Gray SW, Skandalakis LJ, et al. Surgical anatomy of the inguinal hernia. World J Surg 13:490–498, 1989.

55. Anson BJ, Morgan EH, McVay CB. Surgical anatomy of the inguinal region based upon a study of 500 body halves. Surg Gynecol Obstet 111:707–725, 1960.

56. Rizk NN. A new description of the anterior abdominal wall in man and mammals. J Anat 131:373–385, 1980.

57. Keith A. Human embryology and morphology. London: Arnold, 1923.

58. Russell RH. The saccular theory of hernia and the radical operation. Lancet 2:1197–1203, 1906.

59. Yeager VL. Intermediate inguinal ring. Clin Anat 5:289–295, 1992.

60. Read RC. The development of inguinal herniorraphy. Surg Clin North Am 64:185–196, 1984.

61. Haeger K. Illustrated history of surgery. Göteborg, Sweden: AB Nordbok, 1988.

62. Marcy HO. A new use of carbolized cat gut ligatures. Boston Med Surg J 85:315–316, 1871.

63. Marcy OH. The cure of hernia. JAMA 8:589–592, 1887.

64. Andrews E. A method of herniotomy utilizing only white fascia. Ann Surg 80:225–238, 1924.

65. Bassini E. Sulla cura radicale dell'ernia inguinale. Arch Soc Ital Chir 4:380, 1887.

66. Bassini E. Ueber die behandlung des leistenbruches. Arch Klin Chir 40:429–476, 1890.

67. Filipi CJ, Fitzgibbons RJ, Salerno GM, et al. Laparoscopic herniorraphy. Surg Clin North Am 72:1109–1124, 1992.

68. Bull WT. Notes on cases of hernia which have relapsed after various operations for radical cure. NY Med J 53:615–617, 1891.

69. Halsted WS. The radical cure of inguinal hernia in the male. John Hopkins Hosp Bull 4:17–24, 1893.

70. McVay CB, Chapp JD. Inguinal and femoral hernioplasty. The evaluation of a basic concept. Ann Surg 148:499–512, 1958.

71. Rubenstein RS, Beck S, Lohr KN, et al. Conceptualization and measurement of physiologic health for adults. Volume 15, Surgical Conditions. May 1983.

72. Glassow F. The Shouldice Hospital technique. Int Surg 71:148–153, 1986.

73. Shearburn EW, Myers RN. Shouldice repair for inguinal hernia. Surgery 66:450–459, 1969.

74. Alexander MAJ. How to select suitable procedures for outpatient surgery: the Shouldice Hospital experience. Am Coll Surg Bull 71:7–11, 1986.

75. Obney N. Application of Shouldice technique in large scrotal hernias and sliding hernias. Contemp Surg 24:11–16, 1984.

76. Lichtenstein IL. Hernia repair without disability. St. Louis: CV Mosby, 1970.

77. Lichtenstein IL, Shulman AG, Amid PK, et al. The tension-free hernioplasty. Am J Surg 157:188–193, 1989.

78. Cheatle GL. An operation for the radical cure of inguinal and femoral hernia. Br Med J 2:68, 1920.

79. Read RC. Preperitoneal herniorraphy: a historical review. World J Surg 13:532–540, 1989.

80. Nyhus LM, Pollack M, Bombeck T, et al. The preperitoneal approach and prosthetic buttress repair for recurrent hernia. Ann Surg 208:733–737, 1988.

81. Stoppa RE, Rives JL, Warlamount CR, et al. The use of Dacron in the repair of the hernias of the groin. Surg Clin North Am 64:269–285, 1984.

82. Stoppa RE, Warlaumont CR. The preperitoneal approach and prosthetic repair of groin hernia. In: Nyhus LM, Condon RE, ed. Hernia. Philadelphia: JB Lippincott, 1989:199–225.

83. Wantz GE. Giant prosthetic reinforcement of the visceral sac. Surg Gynecol Obstet 169:408–417, 1989.

84. Rignault DP. Properitoneal prosthetic inguinal hernioplasty through a Pfannestiel approach. Surg Gynecol Obstet 16(3):465–468, 1986.

85. Nyhus LM. The preperitoneal approach and iliopubic tract repair of inguinal hernia. In: Nyhus LM, Condon RE, eds. Hernia. Philadelphia: JB Lippincott, 1978:212–249.

86. Tait L. A discussion of treatment of hernia by median abdominal section. Br Med J 2:685–691, 1891.

87. LaRoque GP. The permanent cure of inguinal and femoral hernia. A modification of the standard operative procedures. Surg Gynecol Obstet 29:507–511, 1919.

88. LaRoque GP. The intra-abdominal method of removing inguinal and femoral hernia. Arch Surg 24:189–203, 1932.

89. Ger R. The management of certain abdominal herniae by intra-abdominal closure of the neck of the sac. Ann R Coll Surg Engl 64:342–344, 1982.

90. Ger R, Monroe K, Duvivier R, et al. Management of indirect inguinal hernias by laparoscopic closure of the neck of the sac. Am J Surg 159:370–373, 1990.

91. Ger R. The laparoscopic management of groin hernias. Contemp Surg 39:15–19, 1991.

92. Bogojavlenski S. Laparoscopic treatment of inguinal and femoral hernia (video presentation). Presented at the 18th Annual Meeting of the American Association of Gynecological Laparoscopists, Washington DC, 1989.

93. Toy FK, Smoot RT. Toy-Smoot laparoscopic hernioplasty. Surg Laparosc Endosc 1:151–155, 1991.

94. Schultz L, Graber J, Pietrafitta J, et al. Laser laparoscopic herniorraphy: a clinical trial. Preliminary results. J Laparoendosc Surg 1:41–45, 1990.

95. Corbitt JD. Laparoscopic herniorraphy. Surg Laparosc Endosc 1:23–25, 1991.

96. Seid AS, Deutsch H, Jacobson A. Laparoscopic herniorraphy. Surg Laparosc Endosc 2:59–60, 1992.

97. Katkhouda N. Personal communication, November 1992.

98. Rosin RD. Personal communication, November 1992.

99. Dion YM, Morin J. Laparoscopic inguinal herniorraphy. Can J Surg 35:209–212, 1992.

100. Schlain L. Personal communication, April 1992.

101. Arregui ME, Davis CJ, Yucel O, et al. Laparoscopic mesh repair of inguinal hernia using a preperitoneal approach: a preliminary report. Surg Laparosc Endosc 2:53–58, 1991.

102. Arregui ME. Personal communication, February 1993.

103. Popp LW. Improvement in endoscopic hernioplasty transcutaneous aquadissection of the musculofascial defect and preperitoneal endoscopic patch repair. J Laparoendosc Surg 1:83–90, 1991.

104. Spaw AT. Personal communication, April 1992.

105. McKernan JB, Laws HL. Laparoscopic repair of inguinal hernias using a totally extraperitoneal prosthetic approach. Surg Endosc 7:26–28, 1993.

106. McKernan JB. Personal communication, February 1993.

107. Breland U, Bengmark S. Peritoneum and adhesion formation. In: Bengmark S, ed. The peritoneum and peritoneal access. London: Wright, 1989:122–129.

108. Weibel M, Majno G. Peritoneal adhesions and their relation to abdominal surgery. Am J Surg 126:345–353, 1973.

109. Ellis H. The cause and prevention of intestinal adhesions. Br J Surg 69:241–243, 1982.

110. Myllarniemi H. Foreign material and adhesion formation after abdominal surgery. Acta Chir Scand (Suppl) 377:1–48, 1967.

111. Linsky CB, Diamond MP, Dizerega GS, et al. Effect of blood on the efficacy of barrier adhesion reduction in the rabbit uterine horn model. Infertility 11:273–280, 1988.

112. Ryan GB, Grobety J, Majno G. Post-operative peritoneal adhesions. A study of the mechanism. Am J Pathol 65:117–148, 1971.

113. Hertzler AE. The peritoneum. St. Louis: CV Mosby, 1919.

114. Nisell H, Larsson B. Role of blood and fibrinogen in the development of intraperitoneal adhesions in rats. Fertil Steril 30:470–473, 1978.

115. Ellis H. The aetiology of post-operative abdominal adhesions: an experimental study. Br J Surg 50:10–16, 1962.

116. Ellis H. The cause and prevention of postoperative intraperitoneal adhesions. Surg Gynecol Obstet 133:497–511, 1971.

117. Raftery AT. Regeneration of peritoneum. A fibrinolytic study. J Anat 129:659–664, 1979.

118. Buckmann RF, Buckmann PD, Hufnagel HW, et al. A physiologic basis for the adhesion-free healing of deperitonealized surfaces. J Surg Res 21:67–76, 1976.

119. Buckmann RF, Woods MC, Sargent L, et al. A unifying pathogenetic mechanism in the etiology of intraperitoneal adhesions. J Surg Res 20:1–5, 1976.

120. Gervin AS, Puckett CL, Silver D. Serosal hypofibrinolysis a cause of postoperative adhesions. Am J Surg 125:80–88, 1973.

121. Robbins GF, Brunschwig A, Fook FW. Deperitonealization: clinical and experimental observations. Ann Surg 130:266, 1949.

122. Ellis H, Harrison V, Hugh TB. The healing of peritoneum and normal and abnormal conditions. Br J Surg 52:471–476, 1965.

123. Ellis H. Intestinal adhesions. Ann Chir Gynecol 72:237–238, 1983.

124. Levinson CJ, Swollin K. Postoperative adhesions. Aetiology, preventions and therapy. Clin J Obstet Gynecol 23:213–220, 1980.

125. Diamond MP, Hershlag A. Adhesion formation/reformation. In: diZerega GS, Malinak LR, Diamond MP, Linsky CB, eds. Treatment of postsurgical adhesions. New York: Wiley-Liss, 1990:23–33.

126. Adhesion Study Group. Reduction of post-operative pelvic adhesions with intraperitoneal 32% Dextran 70: a prospective, randomized clinical trial. Fertil Steril 40:612–619, 1983.

127. Tulandi T. Salpingo-ovariolysis: a comparison between laser surgery and electrosurgery. Fertil Steril 45:489–491, 1986.

128. Barbot J, Parent B, Dubuisson JB, et al. A clinical study of the CO_2 laser and electrosurgery for adhesiolysis in 172 cases followed by early second-look laparoscopy. Fertil Steril 48:140–142, 1987.

129. Luciano AA. Laparotomy versus laparoscopy. In: diZerega GS, Malinak LR, Diamond MP, Linsky CB, eds. Treatment of postsurgical adhesions. New York: Wiley-Liss, 1990:35–44.

130. Filmar S, Gomel V, McComb PF. Operative laparoscopy versus open abdominal surgery: a comparative study on postoperative adhesion formation in the rat model. Fertil Steril 48:486–489, 1987.

131. Elliott MP, Juler GL. Comparison of Marlex mesh and microporous Teflon sheets when used for hernia repair in the experimental animal. Am J Surg 137:342–345, 1979.

132. Bauer JL, Salky BA, Gelernt IM, et al. Repair of large abdominal wall defects with expanded polytetrafluoroethylene (PTFE). Ann Surg 206:765–769, 1987.

133. Koontz AR. Preliminary report on the use of tantalum mesh in the repair of ventral hernias. Ann Surg 127:1079–1085, 1948.

134. Lam CR, Szilagy DE, Puppendahl M. Tantalum gauze in the repair of large postoperative ventral hernias. Arch Surg 57:234–244, 1948.

135. Usher FC, Fries JG, Oschner JL, et al. Marlex mesh—a new plastic mesh for replacing tissue defects. Arch Surg 78:138–145, 1959.

136. Brown GL, Richardson JD, Malangoni MA, et al. Comparison of prosthetic materials for abdominal wall reconstruction in the presence of contamination and infection. Ann Surg 201:705–711, 1985.

137. Lamb JP, Vitale T, Kaminski DL. Comparative evaluation of synthetic meshes used for abdominal wall replacement. Surgery 93:643–648, 1983.

138. Smith RS. The use of prosthetic materials in the repair of hernias. Surg Clin North Am 51:1387–1399, 1971.

139. Gibson LD, Stafford CE. Synthetic mesh repair of abdominal wall defects. Am Surg 30:481–486, 1964.

140. Soyer T, Lempinen M, Cooper P, et al. A new venous prosthesis. Surgery 72:864–872, 1972.

141. Law NH, Ellis H. Adhesion formation and peritoneal healing on prosthetic materials. Clin Materials 3:95–101, 1988.

142. Amid PK, Shulman AG, Lichtenstein IL. Selecting synthetic mesh for the repair of groin hernia. Postgrad Gen Surg 4:150–155, 1992.

143. Wagner MW. Evaluation of diverse plastic and cutis prostheses in a growing host. Surg Gynecol Obstet 130:1077–1088, 1970.

144. Usher FC. Hernia repair with Marlex mesh. In: Nyhus LM, Condon RE, eds. Hernia. Philadelphia: JB Lippincott, 1978:561–580.

145. Goldberg JM, Toledo AA, Mitchell DE. An evaluation of the Gore-Tex surgical membrane for the prevention of postoperative peritoneal adhesions. Obstet Gynecol 70:846–848, 1987.

146. Mazuji MK, Fadhi HA. Peritoneal adhesions. Arch Surg 91:872, 1965.

147. Rosenberg SM, Board JA. High-molecular weight Dextran in human infertility surgery. Am J Obstet Gynecol 148:380–385, 1984.

148. Diamond MP, De Cherney AH, Linsky CB, et al. Assessment of carboxymethylcellulose and 32% Dextran 70 for prevention of adhesions in a rabbit uterine horn model. Int J Fertil 33:278–282, 1988.

149. Larsson B, Nisell H, Granberg I. Surgicel—an absorbable hemostatic material—in prevention of peritoneal adhesions in rats. Acta Chir Scand 144:375–378, 1978.

150. Raftery A. Absorbable hemostatic materials and intraperitoneal adhesion formation. Br J Surg 67:57–58, 1980.

151. Hixson C, Swanson LA, Friedman CI. Oxidized cellulose for preventing adnexal adhesions. J Reprod Med 31:58–60, 1986.

152. Diamond MP, Linsky CB, Cunningham T, et al. A model for sidewall adhesions in the rabbit: reduction by an absorbable barrier. Microsurgery 8:197–200, 1987.

153. Interceed (TC7) Adhesion Barrier Study Group. Prevention of postsurgical adhesions by INTERCEED (TC7), an absorbable adhesion barrier: a prospective, randomized multicenter clinical study. Fertil Steril 51:933–938, 1989.

154. Hanney AF, Doty E. Murine peritoneal injury and de novo adhesion formation caused by oxidized-regenerated cellulose (Interceed* [TC7]) but not expanded polytetrafluoroethylene (Gore-Tex* Surgical Membrane). Fertil Steril 57:202–208, 1992.

155. Steinleitner A, Kozensky C, Lambert H. Calcium channel blockade prevents adhesion reformation following adhesiolysis (abstract). Presented at the 37th Annual Clinical Meeting of the American College of Surgeons, Atlanta, GA, 1989.

156. Doody KJ, Dunn RC, Buttram VC Jr. Recombinant tissue plasminogen activator reduces adhesion formation in a rabbit uterine horn model. Fertil Steril 51:509–512, 1989.

157. Abe H, Rodgers KE, Campeau JD, et al. The effect of intraperitoneal administration of sodium tolmetin–hyaluronic acid on the postsurgical cell infiltration in vivo. J Surg Res 49:322–327, 1990.

158. Elkins TE, Bury RJ, Ritter JL, et al. Adhesion prevention by solutions of sodium carboxymethylcellulose in the rat. I. Fertil Steril 41:926–928, 1984.

159. Elkins TE, Bury RJ, Ritter JL, et al. Adhesion prevention by solutions of sodium carboxymethylcellulose in the rat. II. Fertil Steril 41:929–932, 1984.

160. Diamond MP, De Cherney AH, Linsky CB, et al. Adhesion re-formation in the rabbit uterine horn model. I. Reduction with carboxymethylcellulose. Int J Fertil 33:372–375, 1988.

161. Fredericks CM, Kotry I, Holtz G, et al. Adhesion prevention in the rabbit with sodium carboxymethylcellulose solutions. Am J Obstet Gynecol 155:667–670, 1986.

162. Felton RJ, Tuggle DW, Milewicz AL, et al. High mortality with an intraperitoneal adhesive in the rat. Curr Surg 47:444–446, November–December 1990.

163. Kapur BML, Gulati SM, Talwar JR. Prevention of reformation of peritoneal adhesions: effect of oxyphenbutazone, proteolytic enzymes from carica papaya, and dextrose 40. Arch Surg 105:761–766, 1972.

164. Larsson B, Svanberg SG, Swolin K. Oxybutazone—an adjuvant to be used in the prevention of adhesions in operations for fertility. Fertil Steril 28:807–808, 1977.

165. Nishimura K, Nakamura RM, diZerega GS. Biochemical evaluation of postsurgical wound repair: prevention of intraperitoneal adhesion formation with ibuprofen. J Surg Res 34:219–226, 1983.

166. Siegler AM, Kontopoulos V, Wang CE. Prevention of postoperative adhesions in rabbits with ibuprofen, a non-steroidal anti-inflammatory agent. Fertil Steril 34:46–49, 1980.

167. Bateman BG, Nunley WC, Kitchen JD. Prevention of postoperative peritoneal adhesion: an assessment of ibuprofen. Fertil Steril 38:107–115, 1982.

168. Steinleitner AS, Lambert H, Suarez M, et al. Reduction of primary posttraumatic adhesion formation with the prostacyclin analog iloprost in a rodent model. Am J Obstet Gynecol 165:1817–1820, 1991.

169. Horne RW, Clyman M, Debrovner C, et al. The prevention of postoperative adhesions following conservative operative treatment for human infertility. Int J Fertil 18:109–115, 1973.

170. Replogue RL, Johnson R, Gross RE. Prevention of postoperative intestinal adhesions with combined promethazine and dexamethasone therapy: experimental and clinical studies. Ann Surg 163:580–588, 1966.

171. Swolin K. Die einwirkung von grossen, intraperitonealen dosen glukokortikoid auf die bildung von postoperativen adhaesionen. Acta Obstet Gynecol Scand 46:1–15, 1967.

172. Jansen RPS. Clinical approach to prevention. In: diZerega GS, Malinak LR, Diamond MP, Linsky CB, eds. Treatment of post-surgical adhesions. New York: Wiley-Liss Publishers, 1990:177–192.

173. Gomel V. Recent advances in surgical correction of tubal disease producing infertility. Curr Probl Obstet Gynecol 1:28–29, 1978.

174. Seitz HM Jr, Schenker JG, Epstein S, et al. Postoperative intraperitoneal adhesions: a double blind assessment of their prevention in the monkey. Fertil Steril 24:935–940, 1973.

175. Punnonon R, Vinamaki O. Polyethylene glycol 4000 in the prevention of peritoneal adhesion. Fertil Steril 38:491–492, 1982.

176. Berman JK, Habegger ED, Berman EJ. The effect of antihistamine drugs on fibroplasia. Am Surg 19:1152–1161, 1953.

30

Minimal Access Approaches for the Treatment of Peptic Ulcer Disease

Alfred Cuschieri

Currently, the surgical treatment of ulcer disease worldwide is limited to patients who experience acute or chronic complications, as well as a few patients who prove refractory to medical treatment or are non-compliant with medication.[1] The advent of laparoscopic surgical treatment of duodenal ulcer disease is expected by some surgeons to reverse the existing practice whereby the vast majority of patients with duodenal ulcer disease are treated medically. There is now the potential for definitive surgical therapy with minimum inconvenience to the patient and early return to full activity.[2] Before the case for laparoscopic surgery can be established, however, two considerations have to be taken into account. The first concerns the relative efficacy and morbidity of laparoscopic surgery versus medical therapy for ulcer disease. Adjudication of this question is impossible at present, as the results of laparoscopic antiulcer surgery are preliminary. Furthermore, medical therapy itself is changing from the H_2-receptor antagonist era to reversible inhibition of the acid proton pump and, more recently, eradication of *Helicobacter pylori* infection.

The second consideration relates to the cost-efficacy and cost-benefit issues that will henceforth influence patient management and disease therapy in a significant fashion. On a priori grounds, laparoscopic antiulcer surgery should provide a more cost-effective option than long-term medical treatment, although this premise may not be valid if the early results of triple-agent therapy for the eradication of *H. pylori* infection are confirmed by longer follow-up.

MEDICAL THERAPY FOR DUODENAL ULCER DISEASE

Currently, there are three options used in the medical treatment of patients with duodenal ulcer disease. The problems with medical therapy designed to achieve acid suppression either by blocking the H_2-receptors or by inhibiting the acid proton pump include the need for expensive long-term maintenance therapy, as well as drug tolerance, non-compliance, and side effects. The aim of triple-agent therapy is different from these two approaches. This treatment is designed to eradicate the underlying *H. pylori* infection. When achieved, ulcer healing follows, and there is a low recurrence rate after cessation of therapy.

H_2-receptor Antagonists

The vast majority of ulcers can be healed by these acid-reducing drugs, but long-term, continuous maintenance therapy is needed to prevent recurrence and reduce the risk of complications.[3] The reduction in the incidence of serious complications, such as hemorrhage and perforation, by long-term H_2-receptor antagonists appears to be on the same order as that achieved by ulcer surgery.[3] Some 10% to 15% of patients prove refractory (non-healing ulcers after 2 months of therapy) to medication with H_2-receptor antagonists. Although a small minority of these patients have the Zollinger-

387

Ellison syndrome, the majority of cases are "idiopathic" and exhibit either acid hypersecretion or inadequate acid suppression. Included in this group are patients with prepyloric ulcers that are not controlled by this medication and often require surgical treatment.[4, 5]

Reversible Proton Pump Inhibitors

Omeprazole and lansoprazole exemplify the reversible proton pump inhibitors, which produce covalent (reversible) inhibition of the acid proton pump. Acid secretion is therefore suppressed so that the pH of the gastric contents remains above 3 for at least 16 hours of every 24-hour period while the patient is on the drug. A meta-analysis of 17 controlled studies has clearly indicated that healing of ulcers occurs faster with proton pump inhibitors than with H_2-receptor antagonists, although the overall healing rates are similar at 8 weeks.[6] In addition, proton pump inhibitors achieve healing in the majority of patients with H_2-receptor antagonists–refractory duodenal ulcers.[7] As in H_2-receptor antagonist management, maintenance therapy is necessary to prevent recurrence and reduce complications.

There are justifiable fears concerning long-term therapy with proton pump inhibitors. Some side effects are the result of profound acid inhibition and include persistent hypergastrinemia with hyperplasia of the enterochromaffin cells, bacterial overgrowth of the upper gastrointestinal tract, and the risk of infections. Others result from its metabolic consequences. Although protein homeostasis and calcium metabolism seem to be unaffected by long-term omeprazole therapy, the absorption of vitamin B_{12} is impaired, and for this reason the body stores of this vitamin decrease steadily and reach a clinically relevant deficit after 4 years of therapy.[8] Slightly decreased serum iron levels have been observed in some patients on omeprazole therapy,[8] although the serum ferritin (iron stores) remains normal during the first 4 years of therapy. There is, therefore, the distinct probability that patients with an increased iron demand (menstruating females) may develop iron deficiency anemia.

Treatment of *Helicobacter pylori* Infection

The indication for triple-agent therapy for duodenal ulcer disease was reviewed by the Working Party convened during the World Congress of Gastroenterology in Sydney[9]. The recommendations from this Working Party have important implications. In the first instance, the treatment has been standardized and consists of a triple combination of bismuth subsalicylate (one tablet every day), tetracycline hydrochloride (500 mg every day), and metronidazole, (400 mg twice daily) administered for 2 weeks. Amoxicillin, 500 mg, every day may be substituted for tetracycline, but more patients are intolerant to this drug. Triple-agent therapy is advocated only in patients with duodenal ulceration in whom the condition presents a serious management problem requiring either continuous medication or consideration of surgery. It is also indicated in patients with a history of complications. Thus, in essence, the Working Party recommends triple-agent therapy as a substitute for surgery in patients who do not respond to acid-reducing measures. If this recommendation is followed, fewer patients than ever before will be referred for surgical treatment, despite the advent of laparoscopic vagotomy procedures. Awareness by gastroenterologists of the limitations of triple-agent therapy is therefore important, since in its current form, this treatment approach has several problems. In the first instance, there is a high non-compliance rate because of the side effects of therapy and persistence of ulcer symptoms during the treatment. Resistance to antibiotics develops in some patients, and therapy fails to eradicate the infection in 20% of patients. Serious side effects, including fungal infections, diarrhea, and pseudomembranous colitis, occur in 30% of patients. Although permanent cure is being suggested as the outcome following successful eradication of the *H. pylori* infection, much longer follow-up is needed before this assertion can be confirmed.

ENDOSCOPIC VAGOTOMY PROCEDURES

There is little doubt that endoscopic vagotomy for duodenal ulcer disease has not been introduced in a coordinated fashion by the surgical community. First, procedures are being performed that are either known to be unsatisfactory (from past experience and prospective clinical trials on equivalent procedures performed by the open approach) or have never been validated in the long term. In addition, there have been no prospective studies (comparative or otherwise), outcome audits of the reported procedures, and long-term results reported.

Types of Endoscopic Vagotomy Procedures

The currently performed endoscopic vagotomy procedures are shown in Table 30–1. These operations can be classified as (1) *validated*, including truncal vagotomy and drainage, truncal vagotomy and antrectomy, highly selective vagotomy (HSV), and posterior truncal vagotomy and anterior seromyotomy, and (2) *untested*, including posterior truncal vagotomy and anterior HSV, truncal vagotomy and pyloric stretch, and posterior truncal vagotomy and anterior linear gastrectomy. Validated operations are those that have been subjected to clinical trials and long-term usage such that the efficacy, ulcer recurrence rate, morbidity, and sequelae are known. By contrast, information on these parameters of outcome is not available for the untested procedures.

It would seem prudent that the surgical effort in establishing laparoscopic antiulcer surgery should concentrate on validated operations. In addition, prospective multicenter studies are needed to establish morbidity, recovery, efficacy, and ulcer recurrence rates.

Selective Policy

As in open surgery, the procedure used varies with the pathophysiology and altered pathologic anatomy in the individual case. In open surgery for most patients, a parietal cell denervation gives the overall best results and can be performed laparoscopically either by the classic HSV technique[10, 11] or by the Taylor procedure of posterior truncal vagotomy and anterior seromyotomy.[12–15] It is the author's view that this type of vagotomy should be the standard laparoscopic antiulcer treatment. Currently, the laparoscopic Taylor procedure[16] is easier than laparoscopic HSV and is, for this reason, more widely practiced. In the author's institution, the laparoscopic Taylor procedure is the routine operation performed for otherwise uncomplicated disease, HSV being reserved for those patients who have documented severe reflux disease and who require an additional antireflux procedure. Instead of a sutured seromyotomy, Gómez-Ferrer and colleagues[17, 18] perform a linear gastrectomy of the anterior wall of the stomach using the Endo-GIA stapler (U.S. Surgical, Norwalk, CT). Although the preliminary results of this modification are encouraging, it does require long-term validation. The Hill operation[19] can also be performed laparoscopically.[20] Although theoretically sound, this operation has never been subjected to long-term evaluation, and the reported experience with its use in open surgery is very limited.

Bilateral truncal vagotomy and drainage are still widely practiced. In our institution, this procedure is performed laparoscopically in patients with pyloric stenosis when the bilateral truncal vagotomy is combined with an anterior gastroenterostomy (stapled or sutured). In elderly patients, the stenosis is not usually associated with hyperchlorhydria, and indeed these patients often exhibit low gastric acid secretion. A gastroenterostomy or pyloroplasty (if the duodenum is not extensively deformed or scarred) without a vagotomy is carried out in these patients.

All the preceding operations are accompanied by unacceptably high non-healing and recurrence rates in patients with prepyloric ulcers,[3] for which the only effective surgical management is bilateral truncal vagotomy and antrectomy.

Table 30–1. VAGOTOMY PROCEDURES PERFORMED ENDOSCOPICALLY

- Thoracoscopic bilateral vagotomy and pyloric stretch
- Laparoscopic bilateral truncal vagotomy and pyloric stretch
- Bilateral truncal vagotomy and drainage
- Highly selective vagotomy
- Posterior truncal vagotomy and anterior seromyotomy
- Posterior truncal vagotomy and anterior linear gastrectomy
- Posterior truncal vagotomy and anterior highly selective vagotomy
- Bilateral truncal vagotomy and antrectomy

GENERAL CONSIDERATIONS FOR LAPAROSCOPIC ULCER SURGERY

Preoperative Preparation

All the operations are conducted under antibiotic prophylaxis, with cefuroxime administered at the time of induction. Chemoprophylaxis against deep vein thrombosis by subcutaneous heparin is used in elderly and obese patients and in patients with varicose veins or a history of deep vein thrombosis. In addition, all patients wear graduated antithrombosis stockings. Complete deflation of the stomach by a No. 16 French Salem sump nasogastric tube attached to continuous low suction is essential for all gastric laparoscopic procedures.

Patient Position

We prefer to place the anesthetized patient in the supine position with a head-up tilt. French surgeons use the lithotomy position, which is indeed more comfortable for the surgeon, as he or she operates standing or sitting between the patient's thighs. However, this position is attended by increased compression trauma on the calf veins, which becomes an important consideration in prolonged operations.

The skin of the entire abdomen is washed with medicated soap and is then disinfected with the disinfectant of choice. The operating field left exposed by the sterile drapes extends from the costal margins to the suprapubic region.

During laparoscopic gastric surgery, the surgeon operates mainly from the left side of the operating table, with the camera person by his or her side and the first assistant and the scrub nurse on the opposite side. A two-monitor visual display is essential. The electrosurgical unit (preferably of the microprocessor automated type [ICC-350; Erbe, Tubingen, Germany]), suction irrigation, insufflator, light source, and camera unit are stacked behind the surgeon.

Instrumentation and Consumables

The vagotomy operations discussed in this chapter are facilitated by the use of the curved coaxial and bayonet instruments introduced through flexible metal cannulas (Fig. 30–1). Other requirements include a 30° forward oblique good-quality 10-mm telescope, an atraumatic retractor for the left lobe of the liver, a

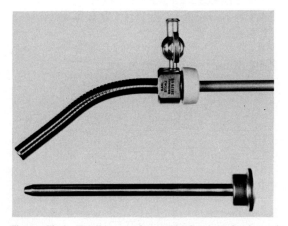

Figure 30–1. Flexible metal cannula for introduction of coaxially curved and bayonet instruments (Storz, Tuttlingen, Germany).

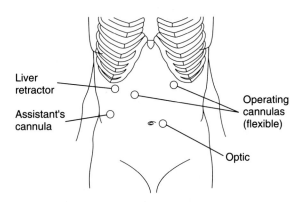

Figure 30–2. Basic disposition of ports for laparoscopic vagotomy procedures.

clip applicator, a pair of 5-mm needle holders, and rubber-shod suture graspers. Suturing is done with atraumatic 3–0 sutures mounted on ski-shaped needles; either absorbable or nonabsorbable sutures can be used. Other consumables include Endoloops (Ethicon Endosurgery, Cincinnati, OH) and the Endo-GIA staplers (United States Surgical Corp., Norwalk, CT) with the blue cartridges.

Definition of the anatomy is considerably improved by the use of a digital enhancement system (Storz, Tuttlingen, Germany) coupled to either a good single-chip or three-chip camera.

Trocar and Cannula Sites

The basic disposition of the ports for vagotomy procedures is shown in Figure 30–2, although there are differences in the exact positions, types, and number of trocars and cannulas used, depending on the nature of the procedure being performed (see further on). The optical (11-mm) cannula is always placed just to the left of the umbilicus. The cannula for the liver retractor is positioned below the right costal margin in the midclavicular line. The left operating cannula (preferably of the flexible type) is placed along the lower end of the left costal margin, whereas the right operating port is situated a few inches to the right of the midline, midway between the xiphoid and the umbilicus. A 12.5-mm cannula is inserted low down in the right upper quadrant along the anterior axillary line. This cannula (with the appropriate reducer) is used by the assistant mainly for retraction. It also provides a convenient port for the introduction of the Endo-GIA stapler. Whenever the 6-cm stapler is used, this cannula is

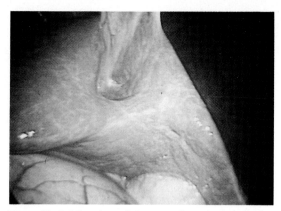

Figure 30–3. Elevation of the central portion of the liver achieved by the falciform lift.

replaced by an appropriate one to accommodate the larger stapler.

Falciform Lift

Exposure of the stomach and the subdiaphragmatic region is considerably enhanced by the employment of the round ligament lift.[21] After insertion of the tube, the external ends are tied and attached to a hook and chain assembly, which is used to lift the central portion of the liver by traction on the falciform and round ligaments, together with the anterior abdominal wall (Fig. 30–3).

PROCEDURES

Posterior Truncal Vagotomy and Anterior Seromyotomy

The posterior truncal vagotomy is performed first and is followed by the anterior seromyotomy, which is sutured. The sites of the ports are as outlined previously.

Exposure of the Subdiaphragmatic Region

The left lobe of the liver is retracted upward without division of the left triangular portion of the liver. We have found the 10.5-mm plastic rod to be the best liver retractor, although the plastic inflatable retractors introduced recently are also effective and are atraumatic to the liver parenchyma. The anterior wall of the stomach is grasped to the left of the esophagogastric junction by a Babcock type of forceps and is pulled downward. This combined maneuver ex-

poses the hiatal region and, unless the patient is obese, the hiatal pillars, which are covered at this stage by intact peritoneum, can be identified. The dissection is limited to the right side of the hiatus and the adjacent transparent section of the lesser omentum (pars flaccida). Not infrequently, an accessory hepatic artery arising from the left gastric artery is encountered running from the esophagogastric junction to the liver. In most instances, this can be preserved, but if it limits the exposure it should be dissected, doubly clipped, and then divided. Otherwise, the dissection starts high with scissors division of the peritoneum at the upper margin of the hiatus. This is extended downward along the right side of the arch and then laterally across the medial part of the transparent portion of the lesser omentum (Fig. 30–4). The division of the pars flaccida exposes the caudate lobe and the fat pad overlying the right crus. Care must be taken to avoid extensive division of the lesser omentum, as this results in disruption of the hepatic vagal fibers that traverse this structure. The next step consists of the detachment of the fat pad overlying the right crus. This is achieved by the electrosurgical hook, using both soft coagulation and the electrocutting mode. Upon excision of the fat pad, the groove between the right crus and the esophagus is identified, as is the lower margin of the anterior leaf of the phrenoesophageal membrane. The latter is gently teased upward, and the areolar tissue plane between the right margin of the esophagus and the crus is deepened by blunt dissection using two curved coaxial duckbill graspers.

Exposure and Resection of the Posterior Vagal Trunk

The posterior vagal trunk is located between the lower margin of the right crus and the esophagus. It is lifted up with a curved coaxial grasper or hook and is then dissected away from the esophagus (Fig. 30–5). The telescope is advanced for close-up viewing when the main vagal trunk is scrutinized until its posterior branch to the left side of the esophagogastric junction and fundus is identified. A 1-cm segment of the posterior vagal trunk, including the posterior branch, is resected between clips. No further esophageal dissection is performed.

Anterior Seromyotomy

The anterior seromyotomy achieves denervation of the branches of the anterior vagal trunk to the parietal cell mass. For this reason, it must extend from the fundus to the antrum.

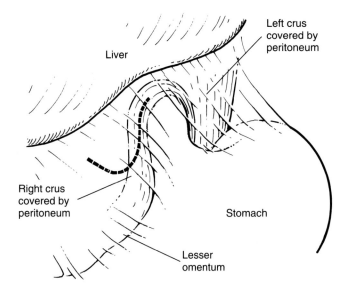

Figure 30–4. The dissection starts high with division of the peritoneum at the upper margin of the hiatus. This is extended downward along the right side of the arch and then laterally across the medial part of the transparent portion of the lesser omentum.

Proximally, the myotomy is commenced well up on the fundus at the level of the greater curvature to ensure total denervation. This may necessitate some mobilization of the gastrophrenic peritoneum. Distally, the myotomy is extended to include the first branch of the "crow's foot," sparing the terminal two branches of the nerve of Latarget to the antrum. Another important practical consideration is to ensure that the stomach is not completely collapsed, although obvious gastric distention with air is to be avoided, as this not only limits the exposure and work space but also results in stretching and thinning of the muscular walls of the stomach, thereby increasing the risk of mucosal perforation. The seromyotomy is conducted some 1.5 cm from the lesser curve to avoid the gastroepiploic vessels, some of which may be quite large. The line of the myotomy should skirt away from these vessels. Alternatively, the larger vessels can be underrun and suture-ligated before the start of the myotomy.

A combined electrocutting-distraction technique is undoubtedly the most expeditious and safest method for effecting a seromyotomy. There is also benefit in the use of automated microprocessor-controlled bipolar cutting and coagulation using the Erbe ICC-350 system in the autocut and autocoagulation modes (Fig. 30–6). The advantage of this system is uniform depth of cut, abolition of charring, and limitation of the spread of collateral damage.[22]

The first stage consists of electrocutting the serosa and the superficial layers of the gastric musculature over the entire length of the seromyotomy (Fig. 30–7). Thereafter, the two edges are grasped by two curved coaxial graspers, and with gentle distraction the deeper tissues are split, exposing the mucosa without damage to

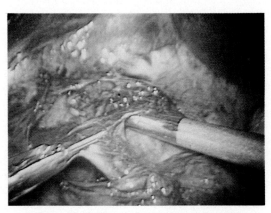

Figure 30–5. Dissected posterior vagal trunk.

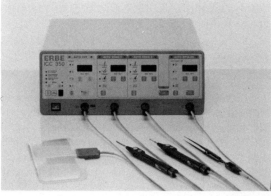

Figure 30–6. Automated microprocessor-controlled intelligent cutting coagulation (ICC) system (Erbe, Tubingen, Germany).

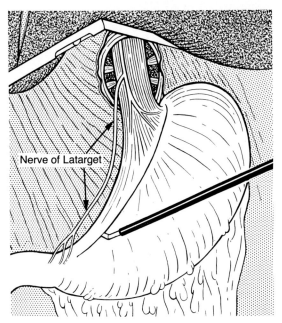

Figure 30–7. Cutting-distraction technique of seromyotomy. The first stage consists of electrocutting the serosa and the superficial layers of the gastric musculature over the entire length of the seromyotomy.

the submucosal vessels. There is virtually no bleeding (Fig. 30–8). Once the seromyotomy is completed, the integrity of the gastric mucosa is checked by distending the stomach with air.

Suture of the Seromyotomy With Overlap

The suture closure of the seromyotomy achieves two purposes. First, it protects against leakage from a missed perforation of the gastric mucosa. Second, because the suturing is carried out with an overlapping technique, it prevents possible regeneration of the severed nerves. Continuous suturing of the seromyotomy is performed with 3–0 coated polyglactin mesh mounted on ski-shaped needles. Starting at the proximal end, the lateral gastric wall is penetrated by the needle down to the seromuscular layer, and the tip of the needle is then exteriorized (by supination of the wrist) about 0.5 cm from the laterally cut muscular layer. The needle is then made to pick the medial cut edge of the seromyotomy. The starter knot is usually of the surgeon's type and is tied with two needle holders. During the continuous suturing by the surgeon, the assistant maintains tension on the suture line by holding the suture with a suture holder that does not damage it. The suturing is terminated either with an Aberdeen knot or by

tying it to an anchor knot at the distal end of the myotomy. The sutured seromyotomy is illustrated in Figure 30–9.

Highly Selective Vagotomy

Laparoscopic HSV is the preferred operation in some centers in Europe.[23] It is a technically exacting operation when conducted by the laparoscopic route, and in our experience the procedure takes significantly longer to perform than the Taylor operation, which in prospective clinical trials in open surgery has been shown to give similar results. Our policy therefore is to limit laparoscopic HSV to those patients who have significant reflux disease documented preoperatively and who require a vagotomy and an antireflux procedure. In these patients, we perform a partial (270°) posterior, crurally fixed fundoplication.

The sites of the access ports are identical to those used in posterior truncal vagotomy and anterior seromyotomy. We use a specially designed hook to assist in the detachment of the lesser omentum from the greater curvatures (Fig. 30–10).

Exposure of the Hiatus and Mobilization of the Esophagus and Esophagogastric Junction With Preservation of the Vagal Trunks and Nerves of Latarget

The procedure starts by retraction of the left lobe of the liver upward and downward traction on the stomach to expose the hiatal region. The dissection of the esophagus from the crura is identical to that used for bilateral truncal vagotomy (see further on). Careful mobilization is needed, and the dissection is kept high and close to the esophagus so that the main nerves are not damaged. A sling is passed around the mobilized gullet and is used to lift this organ and the esophagogastric junction from the crura and the mediastinum.

Opening of the Gastrocolic Omentum

Two vessels adjacent to the greater curvature arising from the gastroepiploic arcade are ligated in continuity and are then divided. The resulting gap is widened to enable entry into the lesser sac. Any adhesions between the posterior wall of the stomach and the pancreas are divided (Fig. 30–11). A coaxial curved atraumatic grasp-

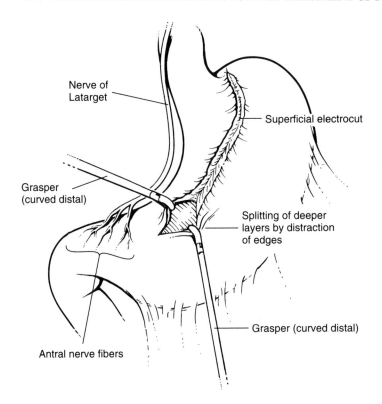

Nerve of Latarget

Superficial electrocut

Grasper (curved distal)

Splitting of deeper layers by distraction of edges

Grasper (curved distal)

Antral nerve fibers

Figure 30–8. The two edges are grasped by two curved coaxial graspers, and with gentle distraction the deeper tissues are split, exposing the mucosa to the submucosal vessels without damage and with an almost virtual lack of bleeding.

er is then applied close to the posterior aspect of the lesser curvature near the antrum. Gentle traction on this grasper greatly facilitates the detachment of the lesser omentum from the lesser curvature of the stomach.

Detachment of the Lesser Omentum From the Greater Curvature and Insertion of Sling Around Stomach

The antral fibers of the anterior nerve of Latarget are identified, and the terminal two fibers are preserved. The dissection starts at this level. The vessels (and accompanying nerves) are gently lifted with the special hook, and after a sufficient window is cleared, the proximal end is clipped (Fig. 30–12). A curved forceps inserted through an endoloop is used to grasp the vessel close to the stomach wall. The vessel is divided between the forceps and the clip. The endoloop is then placed behind the forceps and is tightened with the push rod, after which the forceps is released. The detachment of the lesser omentum proceeds in this way in a cephalad direction and is extended deeply to divide the posterior nerves. After a sufficient separation of lesser omentum from stomach is achieved, it

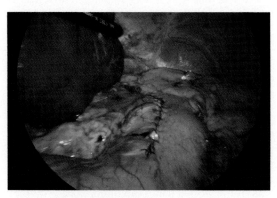

Figure 30–9. Sutured seromyotomy.

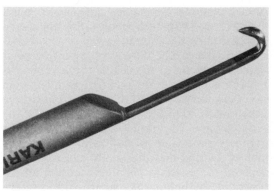

Figure 30–10. Hook for dissection of the lesser curve vessels and nerves during highly selective vagotomy.

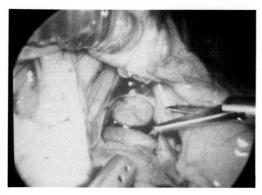

Figure 30–11. The lesser sac is opened and the stomach is retracted upward.

is usually possible to identify a posterior clear window of peritoneum. This peritoneum is penetrated by the curved coaxial posterior grasper as close to the stomach as possible. Once negotiated in this fashion, the grasper is used to pass a silicone sling around the stomach. Traction on this sling greatly simplifies and expedites the detachment of the lesser omentum, which is continued upward until the esophagogastric junction is reached.

Clearance of the Abdominal Esophagus

The anterior aspects of the esophagogastric junction and lower esophagus are then cleared of all nerve fibers using the electrosurgical hook-knife. This is followed by denervation of the lateral and posterior walls of the abdominal esophagus using the same technique.

Bilateral Truncal Vagotomy and Drainage

In our institution, bilateral truncal vagotomy and drainage are performed in patients who have pyloric obstruction or evidence of delay in the gastric emptying by radiolabeled meal studies. As in open surgery, the vagotomy is conducted first.

In general, we prefer laparoscopic gastroenterostomy to pyloroplasty in patients with pyloric obstruction from stenosis. In elderly or hypochlorhydric patients, the bilateral truncal vagotomy is omitted. The easiest procedure to perform laparoscopically is the anterior (antecolic) gastrojejunostomy in which the upper jejunal loop is anastomosed to the stomach near the greater curvature in front of the transverse

colon and greater omentum. However, a posterior anastomosis (retrogastric) can be performed laparoscopically, although it is undoubtedly more difficult.

A Heineke-Mikulicz operation can be performed laparoscopically without much difficulty provided that the surgeon has mastered the technique of interrupted suturing with internal knotting. The procedure is carried out either as a component of bilateral truncal vagotomy for duodenal ulcer disease or as a drainage operation in patients with gastroparesis from any cause. Gastroparesis is encountered in a few patients with reflux disease (before and after fundoplication) and in diabetic patients. In addition to the appropriate symptomatology, the diagnosis of gastroparesis must be confirmed by emptying studies after the ingestion of isotope-labeled standardized meals. In patients with confirmed delayed emptying, a truncal vagotomy is not performed, but if the patient is not hypochlorhydric, the procedure is followed by long-term therapy with H_2-receptor antagonists. In patients with associated symptomatic gastroesophageal reflux, the pyloroplasty is performed at the same time as the laparoscopic antireflux operation.

A Finney pyloroplasty is difficult to perform laparoscopically, as it requires complete mobilization of the second and proximal parts of the third portion of the duodenum. This procedure

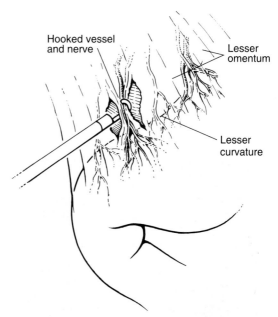

Figure 30–12. The vessels and accompanying nerves are gently lifted with the special hook, and after a sufficient window is cleared, the proximal end is clipped.

is seldom performed in open surgery nowadays and to the author's knowledge has not been attempted by the laparoscopic route.

Bilateral Truncal Vagotomy

The first step of the operation consists of the insertion of the falciform-round ligament lift to elevate the central portion of the liver. The hiatal region is exposed by retraction of the left lobe of the liver upward and downward traction of the stomach. A complete mobilization of the abdominal esophagus and esophagogastric junction is necessary. The peritoneum over the hiatal margin is divided from the left to the right side. The phrenoesophageal membrane is identified and teased up with blunt pledget dissection. The mobilization of the right crus and right margin of the esophagus is carried out as previously described. The left margin of the esophagus is mobilized from the left crus. This requires division of some of the attachments of the phrenoesophageal membrane and often entails dissection, clipping, and ligature of a branch of the left inferior phrenic artery. Thereafter, the areolar tissue of the mediastinum is exposed, and by blunt dissection the left side of the esophagus is mobilized from the hiatal canal. At this stage, a curved coaxial duckbill grasper is passed from the left side behind the esophagus to emerge on the right side of the esophagus between this organ and the posterior vagal trunk. A sling is passed around the esophagus and is used to pull the organ away from the crura and the mediastinum.

The posterior vagal trunk is resected first. This is followed by identification of the anterior vagal trunk, which is lifted from the anterior wall of the esophagus by a curved coaxial grasper or hook and is mobilized over a distance of about 3 cm (Fig. 30–13). A 1-cm section is resected between clips.

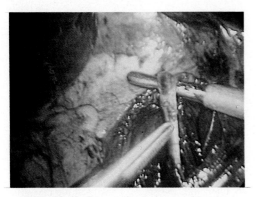

Figure 30–13. Dissected anterior vagal trunk.

Clearance of the Abdominal Esophagus of Accessory Nerve Fibers

It is essential to clear the abdominal esophagus of accessory nerve fibers when performing a bilateral truncal vagotomy. Good camera work is also essential. The entire circumference of the mobilized abdominal esophagus is cleared of any nerve fibers using the electrosurgical hook-knife. This step of the operation is greatly facilitated by use of the digital enhancement system, as this allows easy identification of any nerve fibers.

Anterior Stapled Gastrojejunostomy

The ideal site for the anastomosis of the jejunal loop is with the antrum along its greater curvature. A loop of upper jejunum some 40 to 50 cm from the duodenojejunal junction is selected. This step requires elevation of the left half of the transverse colon by the assistant as the surgeon follows the upper jejunal loops to the ligament of Trietz. The selected loop is marked by a serosal suture.

Next, attention is paid to the stomach. Two adjacent vessels supplying the greater curvature from the gastroepiploic arcade at the proposed site of the anastomosis are ligated and divided. The next step consists of the alignment of the stomach and the selected jejunal loop by the insertion of two corner deep seromuscular sutures that are approximately 6 cm apart. The left extremity suture is inserted first. The needle picks the jejunum on the medial side of the antimesenteric border and then the adjacent stomach. The suture is tied internally using a standard microsurgical knot and is then cut long. Traction is kept on this suture as the right corner suture is inserted though the two organs and is tied and left uncut. This suture is subsequently used to close the defect created for the insertion of the stapler (see further on). As traction is held on the tail of the right extremity suture, appropriate-size openings are made in the jejunum and stomach (medial to the suture) for the insertion of the limbs of the Endo-GIA stapler. The two limbs of the opened Endo-GIA stapler are introduced, respectively, into the stomach and the jejunum. Once inside the lumen of the stomach and jejunum, the stapler limbs are elevated to tent the two organs and are then closed before the instrument is fired. Thereafter, the stapler heads are released and withdrawn from the anastomosis. Following reloading, the 3-cm stapler is reintroduced, and a second application is made beyond, but overlap-

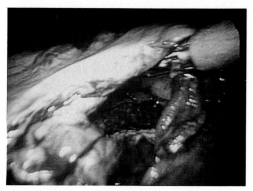

Figure 30–14. Gastrojejunostomy. Interior view of anastomatic stapled line.

ping by 0.5 to 1 cm, the left extremity of the first stapled anastomotic line. If a 6-cm stapler is available, only one application is used to effect the anastomosis. The anterior wall of the gastrojejunostomy is then lifted up to inspect the stapled anastomotic line (Fig. 30–14) and to ensure that there are no mucosal bridges (encountered in 10% of cases in our experience). If present, these mucosal bridges are cut with scissors.

The final stage of the procedure consists of the suture closure of the defect. The right corner suture is used to approximate the two edges with a continuous seromuscular technique. The suture line is ended either by an Aberdeen knot or by being tied to a separate anchor knot. At the end of the procedure, air is injected through the nasogastric tube to distend the stomach and test the integrity of the anastomosis, after which the stomach is deflated.

Posterior Stapled Gastrojejunostomy

The instruments, sites of access ports, and consumables are the same as those used for anterior gastroenterostomy. Likewise, the stomach is kept deflated by low suction applied to a Salem sump nasogastric tube, and a falciform-round ligament lift is inserted.

The procedure commences with the opening of the lesser sac opposite the middle third of the stomach by ligature and division of the vessels supplying the greater curvature from the gastroepiploic arcade.

The left half of the transverse colon is lifted up by the assistant, and the middle colic vessels are identified. A 3-cm opening is cut by scissors in the transverse mesocolon just to the left of the middle colic vessels. An upper jejunal loop some 20 cm from the ligament of Trietz is

grasped by an atraumatic forceps and inserted through the defect into the lesser sac. At this stage, the transverse colon and greater omentum are released and allowed to drop over the grasper holding the bowel. A coaxially curved Babcock grasper is applied to the anterior wall of the mobilized greater curvature, which is then pulled up to expose the lesser sac, the posterior surface of the stomach, and the transposed jejunal loop held by the infracolic grasper.

After the assistant grasps the jejunal loop with an atraumatic forceps inserted into the lesser sac between the transverse colon and the stomach, the infracolic grasper is released. The transposed jejunal loop is secured to the posterior surface of the stomach by the right corner suture, which is left uncut after it is tied. The assistant then releases the hold on the jejunal loop. The left corner suture is then inserted some 6 cm proximally and is tied and cut. The anastomosis is fashioned using the Endo-GIA stapler as described previously, and the defect is closed using a running suture. On completion, the edges of the mesocolic defect are attached to the stomach by a few interrupted sutures above the anastomosis.

Heineke-Mikulicz Pyloroplasty

The two working cannulas (preferably flexible) are placed along the linea semilunaris at the level of the umbilicus. The assistant's cannula is inserted in the right subcostal region along the anterior axillary line. The quadrate lobe and fifth segment of the right side of the liver are elevated by the insertion of the falciform-round ligament lift. Excessive leakage of bile through the antroduodenotomy, which can obscure the field during the suturing of the pyloroplasty, can be controlled by the temporary insertion of a Foley balloon catheter into the second portion of the duodenum. Throughout the entire procedure, it is essential that the stomach is kept empty and collapsed by continuous low suction through a No. 16 French Salem sump nasogastric tube.

The exact position of the pylorus is then identified by reference to the prepyloric veins of Mayo. A stay suture is inserted at its lower border, tied internally, and then cut some 3 cm from the knot. The proposed pyloroplasty incision is mapped with soft electrocoagulation. The coagulated line runs horizontally in the center of the antropyloroduodenal segment and extends from the duodenal bulb across the pyloric sphincter to the adjacent antrum over a distance of 4 cm. The incision is deepened, preferably using microprocessor-controlled bipolar electrocutting in the autocut and autocoagulation modes. During this step, an insulated forceps is held in the left hand and is used to grasp and coagulate bleeding submucosal vessels as they are encountered. On completion, traction is applied to the suture previously attached to the lower border of the pylorus, converting the horizontal incision to a vertically disposed rhomboid defect.

Interrupted full-thickness inverting sutures are used to fashion the pyloroplasty. As traction is maintained on the stay suture, the first stitch, approximating the margins of the proximal end of the rhomboid, is inserted, tied internally, and cut long. The assistant then grasps the long ends of the tied first suture to facilitate the insertion of the second suture, and the process is repeated until the lower 1 cm of the defect is reached. The last two sutures are inserted first before being tied. If a Foley balloon catheter has been placed in the second part of the duodenum, the balloon is deflated and the catheter removed before the last two sutures are tied. Once the suturing of the pyloroplasty has been completed, the suction on the nasogastric tube is disconnected and air is injected using a 50-ml syringe to test the integrity of the suture line.

Vagotomy and Antrectomy for Prepyloric Ulcer Disease

The author reserves vagotomy and antrectomy for patients with prepyloric ulcers and for patients who require long-term steroids for medical disorders such as asthma. Bilateral truncal vagotomy and antrectomy is both tedious and protracted if straight laparoscopic instruments are employed. The use of the curved coaxial instruments greatly expedites the procedure.

The two operating cannulas (flexible) are placed along the linea semilunaris at the level of the umbilicus. One 12.5-mm cannula is inserted in each subcostal region. These cannulas are used for the introduction of the Endo-GIA stapler. In addition, the right subcostal cannula is employed to retract the left lobe of the liver and is used as the assistant's grasping-holding cannula (with 5.5-mm reducer).

Exposure of the Hiatus and Truncal Vagotomy

The first step of the procedure is exposure of the hiatus and truncal vagotomy, which is carried out as previously described. Complete dissection of the esophagus and division of all accessory vagal branches, including the nerves of Grassi, are important to ensure a complete vagotomy.

Identification and Marking of the Pylorus

The identification of the pylorus is essential and should be the next step. It is marked by a suture on its anterior surface. If the surgeon overlooks this measure, he or she will encounter problems during the antrectomy when, as a result of oozing, determination of the distal limit of the resection becomes difficult and a real risk is incurred of either leaving antral tissue behind or resecting an excessive segment of the first part of the duodenum, rendering the anastomosis difficult.

Antral Mobilization

The mobilization of the stomach is commenced at the junction of the upper and the lower thirds of the organ by ligature and division of one or two vessels supplying the greater curvature from the gastroepiploic arcade. These vessels are surrounded by fat and therefore cannot be secured safely by clips. The author's technique for securing these vessels before their division entails ligation of the distal end in continuity with chromic catgut using a Roeder or Melzer knot. A curved grasper is then passed inside a preformed chronic catgut endoloop and is applied to the vessel close to its origin from the gastroepiploic arcade. The vessel is then divided between the grasper and the proximal tie. The endoloop is positioned and tightened on the vessel behind the grasper before it is released.

The stomach is then elevated with the curved coaxial grasper, and any adhesions between its posterior surface and the pancreas are divided by the curved coaxial scissors. As the stomach is held tented upward, the Endo-GIA stapler (loaded with the white cartridge) is introduced through the left subcostal cannula; the open limbs of the stapler are placed on either side of the greater omentum and are then approximated close to the greater curvature before the device is fired. The process is repeated until the right gastroepiploic artery and its accompanying vein are reached. The proximal end of these vessels is best ligated in continuity with polyester using an external slip knot of the Melzer type (Fig. 30–15). The distal end is secured by an endoloop inside a curved grasper as described previously.

The curved duckbill forceps is then passed behind the stomach and is used to push and tent

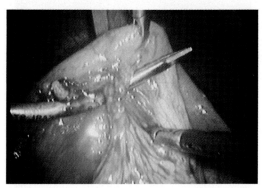

Figure 30–15. Ligature of right gastroepiploic vessels.

the lesser omentum forward. The lesser omentum is divided with scissors through its avascular section from the duodenum to the esophagogastric junction. The left gastric vessels are suture-ligated close to the mobilized lesser curvature 1 cm proximal to the proposed proximal transection line. For this purpose, a 3–0 silk suture mounted on a ski-shaped needle is passed through the serosa of the lesser curvature and is then tied over the vessels using a standard microsurgical knot. The right gastric artery is also suture-ligated in continuity with 3–0 black silk at the proximal end using a similar technique. A clip is placed on the vessel close to the antrum before the artery is divided. This completes the mobilization of the distal stomach.

Transection and Stapling

The extent of the stapling of the proximal end depends on the type of reconstruction intended. For Billroth I procedures, the Endo-GIA stapler (using blue cartridges) introduced through the left subcostal cannula is applied from the lesser curvature side slightly obliquely and with the ends of the stapler limbs some 2.5 to 3 cm from the lesser curvature, the exact distance depending on the width of the first part of the duodenum. The stapler is then fired. Sometimes two overlapping applications are needed to reach the appropriate distance. If a Polya type of reconstruction is intended, the proximal stapling is continued until the stomach is stapled and transected in a slightly oblique fashion from the lesser to the greater curvature. This can be accomplished in most instances by a single application of the 6-cm stapler. Thereafter, the left lobe of the liver is allowed to drop down on the proximal stomach, and the plastic rod is used to elevate the right lobe of the liver to expose the antroduodenal segment.

The technique of duodenal transection also varies with the type of anastomosis that is intended. For a Polya or end-to-side Billroth I anastomosis, the duodenum is completely stapled and transected with the Endo-GIA stapler (using blue cartridges) just distal to the pylorus.

For gastroduodenal reconstructions (end-to-end or end-to-side), the proximal gastric resection line extends from the stapled proximal part of the stomach vertically down to the greater curvature. This division of the stomach walls is performed with the L-shaped electrosurgical hook-knife using cutting current. Often, bleeding submucosal vessels are encountered. They are grasped by an insulated duckbill forceps and electrocoagulated. If an end-to-end gastroduodenal anastomosis is intended, both distal and proximal resection lines are effected with electrosurgical cutting.

A Laparobag (United States Surgical Corp., Norwalk, CT) is introduced through the left 12-mm subcostal cannula, and the detached antrum is placed inside the bag. Extraction of the antrum is best delayed until the continuity of the gastrointestinal tract has been restored.

Anastomosis

Polya Antecolic Anastomosis. This procedure is easiest and is performed using the Endo-GIA stapler (with blue cartridges). An upper jejunal loop some 40 to 50 cm from the ligament of Trietz is selected and is brought up by the assistant with an atraumatic grasper to the stapled body of the stomach so that the efferent loop lies near the lesser curvature. A 3–0 deep seromuscular suture is passed through the upper antimesenteric corner of the jejunum and then through the anterior wall of the stomach just proximal to the stapled line and close to the lesser curvature. The suture is tied using an internal microsurgical knot and is cut. A corresponding suture is placed at the opposite end close to the greater curvature. After tying, this suture is left uncut. As traction is maintained on the tail of the lower corner suture, an opening is made with the electrosurgical hook-knife in the lower end of the aligned jejunal loop and in the adjacent stomach proximal to the corner knot. The stapler limbs are introduced, respectively, into the jejunal and gastric lumens; their ends are lifted anteriorly and are then approximated. If the position of the opposed limbs of the stapler is judged to be correct, the instrument is fired and then released. The second application of the stapler overlaps the first by about 1 cm. Alternatively, a single application of the 6-cm stapler is used. On completion, the anterior wall of the anastomosis is lifted up to inspect the interior and exclude mucosal bridges. The defect at the lower end is closed with a running deep seromuscular suture using the lower corner suture, which is carried upward until the stapler line is reached. The suturing is terminated by an Aberdeen knot or is tied to a separate anchor knot.

End-to-Side Billroth Gastroduodenal Anastomosis. This anastomosis is fashioned along an oblique line running from the top stapled corner of the duodenal stump to the upper aspect of the anterior wall of the second part of this organ. A hand suturing technique is used. The upper corner seromuscular suture is passed through the stomach and then the duodenum medial to the upper end of the stapled line and tied. A corresponding corner suture is placed at the lower end and after it is tied, the tail is grasped by the assistant to align and steady the anastomosis. The posterior suture line is effected in a continuous fashion using deep seromuscular bites until the lower corner is reached, at which point the suture is tied to the tail held by the assistant. The duodenum and the stomach are then opened on either side of the completed posterior suture line using the electrosurgical hook-knife. Often, bile flow from the second part of the duodenum obscures the field. In this situation, a No. 12 French Foley catheter is introduced through a stab wound in the right hypochondrium and is placed inside the second part of the duodenum before the balloon is inflated with air. The anterior wall of the anastomosis is sutured, either with a continuous or interrupted technique using inverting sutures.

End-to-End Billroth I Anastomosis. This procedure requires the insertion of a No. 12 French Foley catheter to control bile flow and stretch the posterior wall of the duodenum. A full-thickness suturing technique is used. The upper corner suture is inserted and tied externally. A corresponding suture is placed at the lower corner of the anastomosis and tied, and the tail is kept on traction by the assistant. The needle of the upper suture is then passed through the stomach into its lumen so that the suturing of the posterior wall of the anastomosis is performed from the mucosal aspect. Even tension on the suture line must be kept by the assistant using a rubber-shod suture holder. Once the opposite corner is reached, the suture is exteriorized through the stomach side and is then tied to the lower corner suture. The anterior wall of the anastomosis is closed with a continuous or interrupted suture. The balloon catheter

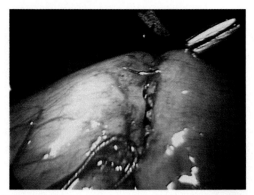
Figure 30–16. Completed gastroduodenal anastomosis.

is deflated and removed as the approximation of the anterior walls of the gastroduodenostomy is nearing completion (Fig. 30–16).

Extraction of the Antrum and Toilet of the Peritoneal Gutters

Irrespective of the restoration of continuity that is performed, on completion air is injected through the nasogastric tube to test the integrity of the anastomosis. Thereafter, the stomach is deflated, and the nasogastric tube is left in situ. The antrum is extracted inside the Laparobag through one of the subcostal cannulas after the placement of a speculum-type retractor to distract the wound edges. The gutters are thoroughly irrigated with saline and aspirated dry. Any clots or tissue debris is removed, the cannulas are withdrawn under vision, and the pneumoperitoneum is desufflated. No drain is inserted.

POSTOPERATIVE CARE

It is our practice to remove the nasogastric tube early, after recovery of consciousness. A second dose of antibiotic is administered 12 hours after the operation. Analgesia with opiates is usually required during the first 24 hours. All patients in whom a gastroenterostomy, gastroduodenal anastomosis, or pyloroplasty has been performed undergo examination with a meglumine diatrizoate swallow on the third postoperative day to establish that there is no anastomotic leakage. During this period, the patients receive nothing by mouth except for hourly sips of water.

Fluids are started orally within 24 hours after the Taylor procedure or HSV, and soft food is begun on the second postoperative day. In procedures with an upper gastrointestinal anastomosis, fluids are started on the third postoperative day if the contrast study is satisfactory. The median duration of the postoperative stay after the Taylor procedure or HSV is 3 days as compared with 6 days after vagotomy and antrectomy or vagotomy and drainage.

CONCLUSION

Laparoscopic antiulcer surgery is still in the early phase of clinical evaluation. All the established and validated operations can be performed laparoscopically, and the early experience with these procedures has been favorable in terms of safety and accelerated recovery. The long-term results including recurrent ulcer rates are not known. Prospective well-audited studies on established validated operations should precede newer approaches and data accumulated on outcome parameters such as overall efficacy, morbidity, and cost benefit of the various operations. Procedures that are known to yield inferior results should not be attempted laparoscopically simply because they are quick and easy to execute by this approach. Comparisons with medical therapy are also required to establish whether the surgical laparoscopic approach provides a cost-benefit advantage for all or for specific groups of patients with ulcer disease.

References

1. Alexandre-Williams J. A requiem for vagotomy. Br Med J 302:547, 1991.
2. Cuschieri A. Laparoscopic vagotomy. Surg Clin North Am 72:357, 1992.
3. Penston JG, Wormsley KG. Maintenance treatment with H₂-receptor antagonists for peptic ulcer disease. Alimentary Pharmacol 6:3, 1992.
4. Strom M, Berstad A, Bodemar G, Walan A. Results of short and long-term cimetidine treatment in patients with juxtapyloric ulcers, with special reference to gastric acid and pepsin secretion. Scand J Gastroenterol 21:521, 1986.
5. Andersen D. Prevention of ulcer recurrence—medical versus surgical treatment. The surgeon's view. Scand J Gastroenterol 20(Suppl 110):89, 1985.
6. Bader JP, Walan A, eds: Proceedings of the International Symposium on Omeprazole. Scand J Gastroenterol 24(Suppl 166), 1986.
7. Delle-Fave G, Annibale B, Helander H, et al. Omeprazole versus high dose ranitidine in H₂ blocker resistant duodenal ulcer patients. Eur J Gastroenterol Hepatol 3:337, 1991.
8. Koop H. Metabolic consequences of long-term inhibition of acid secretion by omeprazole. Alimentary Pharmacol Ther 6:399, 1992.
9. Tytgat GJN, Axon AT, Dixon MF, et al. *Helicobacter pylori*: causal agent in peptic ulcer disease? Working Party Reports: World Congress of Gastroenterology, Sydney, Australia, 1990. Oxford: Blackwell Scientific Publications: 1990:36–45.
10. Amdrup E, Andersen D, Hostrup H. The Aarhus county vagotomy trial. An interim report on primary results and incidence of sequelae following parietal cell vagotomy and selective gastric vagotomy in 748 patients. World J Surg 2:85, 1978.
11. Stoddard CJ, Vassilakis JS, Duthie HL: Highly selective vagotomy or truncal vagotomy and pyloroplasty for chronic duodenal ulceration: a randomised, prospective clinical study. Br J Surg 65:793, 1978.
12. Taylor TV, Gunn AA, MacLeod DAD. Anterior lesser curve seromyotomy and posterior truncal vagotomy in the treatment of chronic duodenal ulcer. Lancet 2:846, 1982.
13. Taylor TV, Holt S, Heading RC. Gastric emptying after lesser curve myotomy and posterior truncal vagotomy. Br J Surg 72:620, 1985.
14. Taylor TV, Lythgoe JP, McFarland JB, et al. Anterior lesser curve seromyotomy and posterior truncal vagotomy versus truncal vagotomy and pyloroplasty in the treatment of chronic duodenal ulcer disease. Br J Surg 77:1007, 1990.
15. Oostvogel HJM, van Vroonhoven TJMV. Anterior lesser curve seromyotomy with posterior truncal vagotomy versus proximal gastric vagotomy. Br J Surg 75:121, 1988.
16. Katkhouda N, Mouiel J. A new surgical technique of treatment of chronic duodenal ulcer without laparotomy by videocoelioscopy. Am J Surg 161:361, 1991.
17. Gómez-Ferrer F, Arena J, Pardo J, et al: Gastrectomia lineal anterior + vagotomia troncular laparoscópica. Nueva técnica para el tratamiento de la úlcera duodenal crónica. Acta Chir Catal 13:117, 1992.
18. Gómez-Ferrer F. Gastrectomie lineaire anterieure et vagotomie tronculaire posterieure. Une nouvelle technique laparoscopique dans le traitement de l'ulcere duodenal. J Coel Chir 4:35.
19. Hill GL, Barker CJ. Anterior highly selective vagotomy with posterior truncal vagotomy: a simple technique for denervating the parietal cell mass. Br J Surg 65:702, 1978.
20. Bailey RW, Flowers JL, Graham SM. Combined laparoscopic cholecystectomy and selective vagotomy. Surg Laparosc Endosc, 1991.
21. Banting S, Shimi S, Vander Velpen G, Cuschieri A. Abdominal wall lift: low pressure pneumoperitoneum laparoscopic surgery. Surg Endosc 7:57, 1993.
22. Haag R, Cuschieri A. Recent advances in H-F electrosurgery: development of automatic microprocessor-controlled systems, in press.
23. Dallemagne B. Laparoscopic highly selective vagotomy. Third World Congress of Endoscopic Surgery. Bordeaux, France, June 1992.

31

Laparoscopic Surgery of the Gastrointestinal Tract

Daniel T. Martin and Karl A. Zucker

The innovative nature of surgeons, coupled with their desire to improve clinical results, continues to manifest itself in the application and acceptance of new surgical techniques. It was only logical, therefore, that after practicing various endoscopic surgical techniques while performing laparoscopic biliary tract surgery, surgeons would begin expanding the number of operations performed using this novel approach. One of the most exciting potential applications of this minimally invasive form of surgery is laparoscopic intestinal surgery. Operations involving the intestinal tract, especially the colon, are among the most common procedures performed by many general surgeons. Although many of these procedures are still in the earliest stages of development, the preliminary data are quite encouraging.

It is the intent of this chapter to briefly describe the indications, basic operative techniques, and current results regarding laparoscopic surgery of the small bowel and colon. As new and ever more innovative instrumentation emerges and the limitations of fixed two-dimensional visualization are overcome, this early experience will undoubtedly serve as a catalyst for the development and furtherance of even more complicated laparoscopic procedures.

SPECIAL INSTRUMENTATION FOR LAPAROSCOPIC INTESTINAL SURGERY

In order to safely perform laparoscopic intestinal surgery, a number of specific instruments

are recommended. In our experience a side-viewing (30° to 50°) laparoscope is essential to adequately visualize the necessary intestinal and mesenteric landmarks. By simply rotating the shaft of the laparoscope, the surgeon can view left, right, up, and down and therefore visualize areas of the peritoneal cavity that are impossible to see with conventional forward-viewing laparoscopes (Fig. 31–1). Specially designed atraumatic grasping instruments are also important to avoid injuring the small and large intestines. Recently, laparoscopic Babcock and Allis clamps, as well as flat nontraumatic bowel-grasping forceps, have become available (Fig. 31–2). Dissection of the mesenteric vessels is facilitated by the use of curved forceps (with angled tips ranging from 45° to 90°) and dissecting scissors with monopolar electric current. Some of these instruments have recently been modified to work with bipolar electrocautery, which is believed to be safer in the closed abdomen.[1] Some of the disposable versions of these instruments also incorporate a flexible or roticulating shaft that makes it easier to guide them into areas of the peritoneal cavity that are normally difficult to work in (i.e., deep in the pelvis). Both reuseable and disposable fan-like retractors are available and are often used to retract the small bowel, colon, and other structures to improve exposure during laparoscopic surgery. Neither the small bowel nor the colon can be safely eviscerated through the lumen of a standard 5- to 11-mm laparoscopic cannula. Therefore larger sheathes have been developed by several companies, with diameters ranging from 18 to 50 mm. A reducer sleeve allows the introduction of standard (5- or 10-mm) instru-

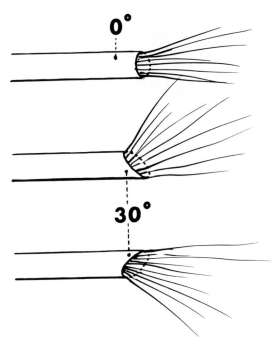

Figure 31–1. Rotating the angled laparoscope allows the surgeon to look left, right, up, or down. (From Talamini MA, Gadacz TR. Equipment and instrumentation. In: Zucker KA, Bailey RW, Reddick EJ, eds. Surgical laparoscopy update. St. Louis: Quality Medical Publishing, Inc., 1993, p. 17.)

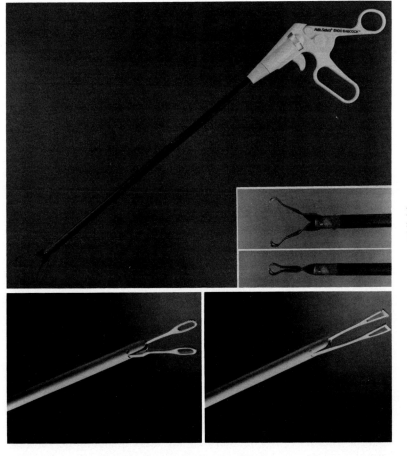

Figure 31–2. An assortment of instruments used for laparoscopic bowel surgery.

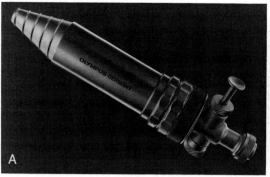
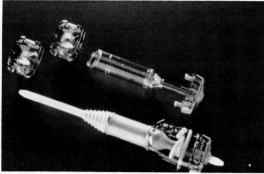

Figure 31–3. A reusable (**A**) and disposable (**B**) cannula designed for laparoscopic intestinal surgery.

ments while maintaining the pneumoperitoneum. In addition to being wider, many of these devices are also designed with much shorter cannulas to allow the bowel to be pulled out of the peritoneal cavity with less tension on the underlying mesentery (Fig. 31–3).

The recent introduction of endoscopic linear staplers has clearly played an important role in the development of laparoscopic intestinal surgery. These instruments have already been used successfully to ligate and divide both bowel and mesentery within the closed abdomen. The use of these stapling instruments is rapidly increasing, and it is therefore important that surgeons become familiar not only with their potential applications but also with their limitations. Although these stapling devices, as well as those that are anticipated in the near future, will be used frequently during laparoscopic surgery, it is still essential that surgeons become skilled at endoscopic suturing and knot tying. Several laparoscopic needle holders-drivers are now available, and each surgeon should become adept at using the particular model he or she prefers. In addition, surgeons need to become proficient with several different suturing techniques, as each has advantages and disadvantages.[2]

PREOPERATIVE EVALUATION AND PREPARATION

Patients must be prepared for laparoscopic surgery in the same manner they would be if laparotomy was the planned approach. This includes a thorough discussion regarding the diagnosis, therapeutic options, and limitations of the laparoscopic approach, as well as the possibility of conversion to an open procedure should the need present itself. In addition, the

potential complications peculiar to laparoscopy must be discussed and the appropriate informed consent obtained. We also emphasize that conversion to laparotomy in itself must *not* be considered a complication but instead a decision made by the surgeon in the best interest of the patient. Absolute contraindications to attempting intestinal laparoscopic surgery are essentially the same as those for biliary tract surgery: irreversible coagulopathy and generalized peritonitis (*i.e.,* board-like abdomen). Relative contraindications include previous surgery, partial or complete bowel obstruction, massive obesity, pregnancy, a large intraabdominal mass and preoperative evidence of fixation of either a benign or malignant lesion to any adjacent viscera (*e.g.,* ureter, bladder). This latter group of patients should be evaluated on a case-by-case basis to determine the appropriateness of laparoscopic surgery.

Accurate localization of the intestinal pathologic lesion is critical with the laparoscopic approach because the surgeon is deprived of the tactile sensation normally relied on to palpate intraluminal lesions during open laparotomy.[3] Radiographic contrast procedures (*i.e.,* barium enema) may provide useful information about the location of the lesion; however, many patients are now being operated on based solely on the information obtained at colonoscopy or upper gastrointestinal tract endoscopy. Often it can be difficult to precisely identify the location of such lesions at the time of flexible endoscopy, especially colonoscopy. Therefore some surgeons prefer to inject methylene blue or India ink beneath the submucosa at the time of the endoscopic examination to mark the lesion. Unfortunately, many times the dye is infused only into the lumen or completely through the bowel wall and into the peritoneal cavity. Some dyes are quickly absorbed or may be difficult to see if there is an accompanying hematoma. Alternative methods of preoperative localization that have been proposed include the use of a prototype endoscopic stapling device that can be introduced through the working channel of a colonoscope.[4] The endoscopist can then place metallic clips near the site of the pathologic lesion, which are easily seen with a scout film or fluoroscopy. Our preferred method at present is to perform intraoperative flexible endoscopy at the time of laparoscopic surgery (Fig. 31–4). The flexible scope can then be used to identify the area of abnormality as well as other significant gastrointestinal tract landmarks.

General endotracheal anesthesia with continuous monitoring of end tidal $PaCO_2$ is strongly advised when performing laparoscopic intestinal surgery. Nitrous oxide should be avoided, as its use may result in luminal distention, which can complicate any laparoscopic procedure. Other monitoring devices such as arterial lines and central venous or pulmonary artery catheters should be used as clinically indicated. The bladder is decompressed with a urinary catheter to minimize its risk of injury and to facilitate the exposure of the lower abdomen and pelvis. A nasogastric tube is also inserted for similar reasons. Although there are no data to suggest that there is an increased risk of deep venous thrombosis or pulmonary emboli when performing laparoscopic surgery, many surgeons (ourselves included) use intermittent compression stockings as a preventive measure. In our opinion, the use of this device is preferable to the potential deleterious effects of subcutaneous heparin administration.

Positioning of the patient, surgeon, first assistant, and video monitors will depend on the site of the pathologic lesion, as well as on the preference of the surgeon. All patients, however, are routinely prepared and draped for both laparoscopy and open laparotomy. Initial access to the peritoneal cavity may be accom-

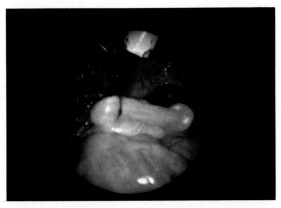

Figure 31–4. Laparoscopic image of the colonoscope being advanced to the site of the lesion intended to be resected.

plished with a percutaneously inserted insufflation needle or the open (Hassan) approach, depending on the patient's history of prior surgery and the preference of the surgeon.[5, 6]

LAPAROSCOPIC SMALL BOWEL SURGERY

The smaller diameter, longer mesentery, and greater mobility of the small bowel make it ideally suited for laparoscopic surgery. However, the indications for operative intervention on the small bowel are infrequent. Aside from various enteral access procedures, little has been done or reported in the area of laparoscopic resection of the ileum or jejunum. Laparoscopically assisted Roux-en-Y enterocutaneous jejunostomy and placement of jejunal feeding tubes, however, appear to be attractive options for patients who are not candidates for flexible endoscopic methods of placing feeding gastrostomy or duodenal tubes (*i.e.,* patients with esophageal or gastric outlet obstruction). These same individuals are generally at poor risk for major surgery, and a minimally invasive procedure for establishing enteral access would appear to be an appealing concept.

Laparoscopic Jejunostomy Tube Placement

The patient is placed in a supine position with the surgeon standing on the right for laparoscopic jejunostomy tube placement. The first assistant is positioned directly across from the surgeon, and both video monitors are placed at the head of the operating room table. A general anesthetic is administered along with controlled mechanical ventilation, and the patient is prepared and draped. If clinically indicated, this procedure can be accomplished with a regional epidural anesthetic using less insufflation pressure (<10 mm Hg). In patients who have not previously had a midline incision, the primary cannula site is generally just below the umbilicus. The abdomen is distended with 3 to 4 L of CO_2 (maximum pressure 14 mm Hg) and a side-viewing (30° to 50°) 10-mm laparoscope is introduced. The patient is placed in a 30° to 40° reverse Trendelenburg position, and the abdominal cavity is surveyed. If extensive adhesions are found and the jejunum cannot be safely mobilized, conversion to minilaparotomy and open jejunostomy may be necessary. If no contraindications to proceeding are noted, three

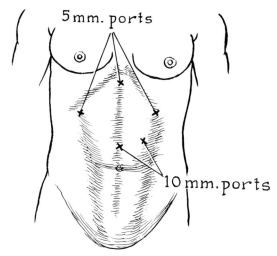

Figure 31–5. Suggested cannula insertion sites for laparoscopic jejunostomy tube placement.

accessory cannulas are inserted under direct videoscopic vision (Fig. 31–5). One is placed subcostal in the right midclavicular line, the second is placed approximately 5 cm below the xiphoid, and the third sheath is placed in the left side of the midabdomen and is the intended exit site for the jejunostomy tube. The diameters of the cannulas used in these accessary sites will depend on the type of laparoscopic instru-

mentation available and the surgeon's preference. We now prefer to use all 10/11-mm sheaths to allow greater flexibility in inserting specialized bowel instruments and moving the laparoscope to various positions during the course of the operative procedure.

The transverse colon is identified, grasped with an atraumatic bowel-grasping forceps or Babcock clamp, and lifted anterior and cephalad (Fig. 31–6). The jejunum is retracted caudad and to the patient's right side with an atraumatic fan-like device. This maneuver facilitates the identification of the ligament of Treitz and the proximal jejunum. The proximal jejunum is grasped and followed for a length of 25 to 50 cm by manipulating it with blunt probes and atraumatic bowel-grasping forceps. The jejunum is then brought to the anterior abdominal wall, and the 10-mm infraumbilical cannula is replaced with a larger (18- to 40-mm) cannula by extending the skin incision and dilating the fascial opening. This maneuver has been demonstrated to be a satisfactory method of widening the access to the peritoneal cavity and carries with it a minimum of morbidity, postoperative discomfort, or cosmetic disfiguration.[7] Care is taken to avoid overenlarging the incision to prevent persistent leakage of pneumoperitoneum. If leaks occur, a pursestring suture care-

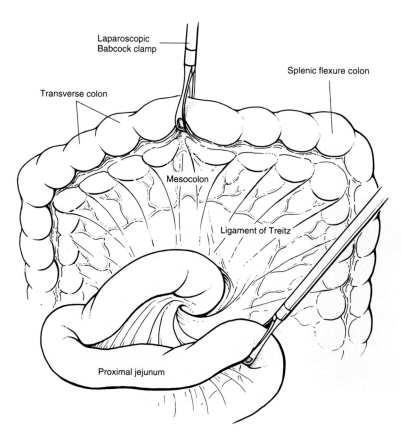

Figure 31–6. The splenic flexure is retracted anterior and cephalad to expose the ligament of Treitz.

fully placed in the fascia, snug to the larger cannula, will generally halt most desufflation. The laparoscope is moved to the right subcostal cannula, and the appropriate segment of jejunum is grasped and exteriorized through the large umbilical cannula. As the jejunum is pulled into the cannula, the reducer sleeve is removed and the bowel is eviscerated (Fig. 31–7). An alternative method of eviscerating the jejunum is through a minilaparotomy (3- to 4-cm) created within the lower folds of the umbilicus (Fig. 31–8).[8, 9] The advantage of the latter technique may be easier access to the bowel, but the disadvantage is that the incision must be securely closed to allow reinsufflation.

Once outside the abdomen, a small enterotomy is made and an appropriate feeding catheter is guided into the lumen of the jejunum. The enterotomy is closed in either a Stamm- or Witzel-like fashion.[10, 11] We prefer the latter, as in our experience it allows a more secure closure of the enterotomy and is associated with fewer problems of inadvertent tube removal. The jejunostomy tube may be introduced into the peritoneal cavity by first passing it through the left midabdominal cannula and then bringing the distal tip out alongside the eviscerated bowel, or the tube may be dropped into the abdomen through the enlarged umbilical opening after securing it within the bowel. With the latter technique, the external portion of the tube is brought out through the left abdominal trocar puncture before the operative procedure is completed. With either method, two or three sutures must be placed through the seromuscular layer of the jejunum in preparation for fixation to the anterior abdominal fascia. These sutures are positioned in the jejunum while it is still outside of the abdomen. The sutures are cut short (10 to 12 cm), with the needle still attached to minimize problems with tangling. The jejunum

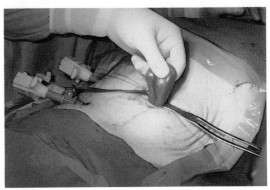

Figure 31–8. Evisceration of the small bowel through a widened fascial opening (approximately 3 cm) made just below the umbilicus.

is dropped back into the abdomen and the pneumoperitoneum is reestablished. The balloon at the tip of the jejunostomy tube is inflated and then pulled up to the anterior abdominal wall as the cannula is removed. Visualization of the jejunum lying against the anterior abdominal wall for suture placement is best accomplished with a 30° laparoscope. A laparoscopic needle driver is then used to complete the suturing of the jejunum to the abdominal wall. An alternative method of securing the jejunum to the undersurface of the abdominal wall employs several T-fasteners, which are inserted percutaneously into the bowel lumen.[12] Use of these fasteners avoids the need to suture intracorporeally. The tube is then secured to the skin, the fascial defect in the umbilicus is closed, and a final survey of the abdomen is carried out with the video laparoscope before closing the small port sites with skin sutures or staples.

Roux-en-Y Enterocutaneous Jejunostomy

More permanent access for prolonged enteral feeding can be accomplished by a Roux-en-Y enterocutaneous jejunostomy. This method of enteral access effectively eliminates many of the problems encountered with tubes emanating from the anterior abdominal wall, such as inadvertent removal, leakage around the catheter, tract infections, and so on. The same technique of four puncture sites is used as described for tube jejunostomy placement. After identifying an acceptable site 60 to 100 cm distal to the ligament of Treitz, the umbilical fascia is enlarged and the skin incision is extended to accept a 30-mm or larger cannula and sheath. As mentioned previously, an alternative method is

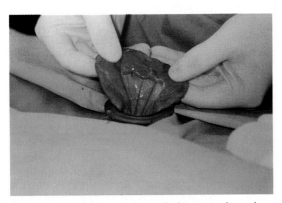

Figure 31–7. Operative photograph demonstrating evisceration of a segment of the jejunum through a larger, specially designed laparoscopic cannula.

simply to enlarge the umbilical fascial defect until it is large enough to allow evisceration of the intended segment of small bowel. The jejunum is brought out through this port and the pneumoperitoneum is allowed to escape. A gastrointestinal stapling and dividing device is used to divide the bowel. A jejunojejunostomy is performed, leaving an isoperistaltic limb of jejunum approximately 30 cm in length (Fig. 31–9). The distal portion of the isoperistaltic limb is prepared for stoma creation by removing the mesenteric fat from the end while taking care not to devascularize the small bowel.

Since the stoma will be placed at the left-sided midabdominal port, sutures are placed (leaving needles attached) in the limb to facilitate closure of the space along the lateral abdominal wall. The small bowel is then returned to the abdominal cavity and the abdomen is reinsufflated. The end of the jejunal limb is then pulled through the 10-mm fascial opening in the left side of the midabdomen, removing the cannula as the bowel is pulled through the abdominal wall. This maneuver may require dilating the fascial defect and tract of the cannula to accommodate the small bowel. The jejunal limb is then secured in place to the fascia, permitting about 1 cm to protrude above the level of the skin (Fig. 31–10). The lateral abdominal wall sutures are placed and tied to prevent internal herniation, and the stoma is matured. The stoma can be intubated and feedings started after a reasonable time has passed to allow sealing of the fascial tract.

Clinical Experience

Morris and coworkers published their results in three patients who underwent laparoscopically assisted jejunostomy tube placement in

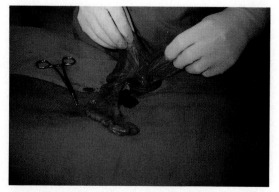

Figure 31–9. A jejunal segment of intestine is eviscerated, and a Roux-en-Y isoperistaltic limb is created.

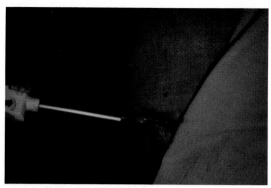

Figure 31–10. View of the jejunal stoma.

1992.[9] There were no complications, and feedings were started as early as the second postoperative day. A total of 17 patients from both the Baltimore and Albuquerque Veterans' Hospitals (from 1990 through 1992) underwent laparoscopically assisted enteral access procedures.[13] Fourteen procedures were for jejunostomy tube placement and the remainder were Roux-en-Y enterocutaneous fistula procedures. There was one death at 5 weeks from progressive esophageal cancer in a patient who underwent laparoscopically assisted jejunostomy tube placement. There were no operative complications, and feeding was initiated in all patients within 24 hours of surgery.

LAPAROSCOPIC SURGERY OF THE LARGE INTESTINE

The first reported series of laparoscopically assisted colectomies was that of Jacobs and colleagues in 1991.[14] After progressing from laparoscopic biliary surgery to difficult appendectomies, they proceeded to the animal laboratory and began their endeavors in bowel resection. They then elected to use this technique on a patient with intermittent cecal volvulus, performing a laparoscopically assisted right hemicolectomy. The patient's postoperative course was remarkably pain-free, with bowel function returning within a few hours after surgery. This spurred further work in this field, and the indications for laparoscopic intervention have rapidly expanded to include patients with many other colon disorders, including malignancy. The latter indication for laparoscopic surgery has generated considerable debate regarding the appropriateness of minimally invasive surgery in patients with localized intestinal cancers. Limited follow-up at this time allows only speculation as to the end results, but the early results are promising.

Regardless of one's stand on minimally invasive surgery for malignancy, there is little debate about the advantages of this method with regard to segmental colon resection for benign or even pre-malignant lesions (*i.e.,* broad-based sessile polyps). Laparoscopic surgery has also been used in the management of diseases such as rectal prolapse, intermittent volvulus, complicated diverticular disease, and resection of ischemic strictures.[15–21] Exclusive of operations for malignancy, the myriad other indications for colon resection should allow ample use of the described techniques, and therefore a brief explanation and illustration of techniques is warranted.

Two techniques of laparoscopic colon resection have thus far been described, and they differ mainly in the methods used to remove the specimen and to reestablish gastrointestinal tract continuity. The most common technique at this time is the extracorporeal method, whereby a small fascial opening is made to remove the specimen and to eviscerate both the proximal and distal limbs of bowel. The anastomosis is then performed outside the peritoneal cavity using conventional hand-sewn or stapling techniques. In some instances, this opening may simply be an extension of the umbilical cannula site, or it may be a separate counterincision made over the abdominal wall at the point at which the proximal and distal limbs of the colon can be brought up in the most facile manner. Since a small laparotomy incision is made, the term laparoscopically assisted colectomy is perhaps the most descriptive term.

Laparoscopic stapling devices have recently been developed that allow the surgeon to resect and perform a colon anastomosis entirely within the confines of the abdomen (intracorporeal anastomosis). If the entire resection and anastomosis are to be done inside a body cavity, specimen extraction must be carefully planned. Several methods have been described. The specimen may be brought out transrectally through an open rectal stump, particularly when a laparoscopic low anterior resection is performed. In females, the specimen may be removed through the posterior cul-de-sac and extracted transvaginally. Other options include the use of an enlarged umbilical port site or a small (3- to 4-cm) muscle-splitting counterincision. However, if an enlarged fascial opening is needed, extracorporeal resection and anastomosis might be more prudent.

One of the concerns that has been raised by medical and surgical oncologists relates to the possibility of tumor seeding as the specimen is extracted through either a small fascial opening or by one of the alternative routes mentioned previously. One case of gallbladder cancer being seeded after laparoscopic cholecystectomy has been reported, as has a case of gastric adenocarcinoma that spread to the umbilicus after diagnostic laparoscopy and biopsy.[22, 23] If such concerns are to be circumvented, the specimen can be placed in a sterile specimen bag prior to extraction. Commercial reservoirs are available, but they are generally too small to remove large segments of the colon. We have found that gas-sterilized "zipper" freezer bags are useful for this purpose.

Patient Preparation

The preparation for large bowel surgery includes appropriate mechanical cleansing of the colon and antibiotic coverage. In this era of same-day surgery, this is routinely carried out by the patient at home on the day preceding surgery. A general anesthetic with controlled mechanical ventilation is advised, as is the use of compression leg stockings. As mentioned earlier, patients must be advised of the innovative nature of laparoscopic colon surgery and the complications associated with this approach. In addition, patients must be aware of the possibility of conversion to open laparotomy. Positioning of the patient and the operating room setup will vary according to the surgeon's preference and the location of the pathologic lesion.

Right Hemicolectomy

The patient undergoing right hemicolectomy is placed supine on the operating room table and is prepared and draped in a conventional manner. The surgeon stands on the patient's left side with the first assistant directly across from the surgeon. Video monitors are placed on both sides of the anesthesiologist. Often the surgeon may relocate to various positions around the operating room table as the operative dissection moves from the right lower quadrant to the upper abdomen. An alternative position popular in Europe is a modified lithotomy position with the surgeon standing between the patient's legs.

The pneumoperitoneum is established using either a percutaneous or an open method. A minimum of four laparoscopic cannulas are used, and their placement will also vary among different surgeons. The configuration of the port placement must also take into consideration the lengths of the instruments used, as poor positioning will make the operation very difficult. One must also be careful not to place the cannulas too close together, as this will make it difficult to manipulate the various instruments. Suggested locations of trocar puncture sites for a laparoscopically assisted right hemicolectomy are (1) umbilical, (2) suprapubic, (3) subxiphoid, and (4) right subcostal–midclavicular line (Fig. 31–11). We generally use larger diameter cannulas (10/11 mm) so that the laparoscope, bowel-grasping forceps, clip applier, and so on may be moved to various locations without difficulty. If a laparoscopic linear stapling device is to be used, an appropriate-sized sheath (12 to 18 mm) must be placed in the anticipated site of its use. Occasionally, a fifth or even sixth cannula may be necessary to provide adequate exposure. The locations of these additional cannulas will depend on the operative findings.

The patient is placed in a reverse Trendelenburg position with the left side lowered 15° to 20°. This maneuver allows the small bowel to fall away from the ascending colon. The cecum is then grasped with atraumatic, laparoscopic, bowel-grasping forceps and is retracted medially and toward the left shoulder of the patient. This will expose the avascular white line of Toldt, which is then divided with curved scissors connected to a monopolar electrocautery generator (Fig. 31–12). Other means of accomplishing this

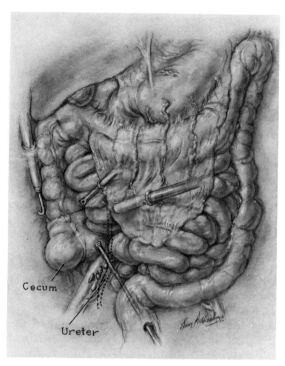

Figure 31–12. The cecum and ascending colon are retracted medially, and the lateral peritoneal attachments are divided. (From Jacobs M, Verdja J-C, Plasencia G. Laparoscopic colonic surgery. In: Zucker KA, Bailey RW, Reddick EJ, eds. Surgical laparoscopy update. St. Louis: Quality Medical Publishing, Inc., 1993, p. 333.)

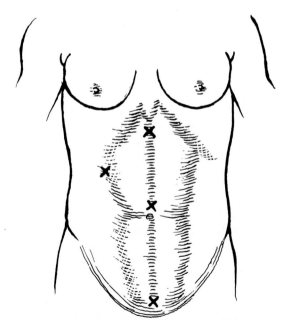

Figure 31–11. Suggested cannula placement sites for laparoscopic-assisted right hemicolectomy. (From Jacobs M, Verdja J-C, Plasencia G. Laparoscopic colonic surgery. In: Zucker KA, Bailey RW, Reddick EJ, eds. Surgical laparoscopy update. St. Louis: Quality Medical Publishing, Inc., 1993, p. 331.)

dissection include the use of a hook/spatula or a laser energy probe. Using the surgical principle of retraction and countertraction, the ascending colon is mobilized medially, exposing the right ureter and common iliac vessels (Fig. 31–13). The dissection is then continued proximally toward the hepatic flexure, at which point the direction of traction on the ascending colon is aimed toward the left hip of the patient. The gastrocolic ligament often contains blood vessels that are too large to be safely cauterized. These modest-size arteries and veins may be controlled with titanium surgical clips, individual suture ligatures, or a hemostatic linear stapler.

Most surgeons use a side-viewing (30° to 45°) laparoscope inserted through the umbilical port for better visualization of the lateral peritoneal attachments and hepatic flexure. If a 0° scope must be used, the laparoscope can be inserted through the upper abdominal cannulas to provide adequate exposure. Any vessels encountered in mobilizing the colon must be carefully controlled with clips, suture ligatures, or cautery.

Following mobilization and dissection, the colon generally will reach the anterior abdomi-

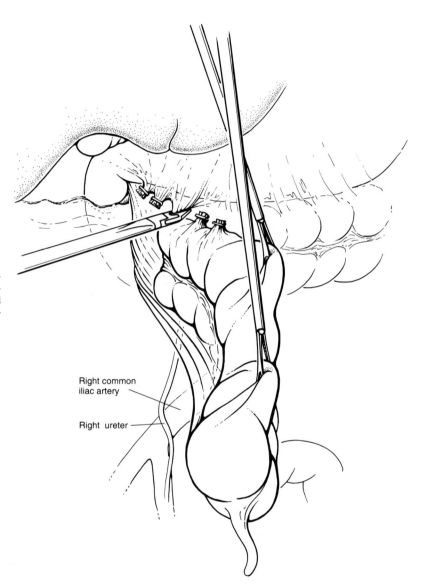

Figure 31–13. Operative photograph demonstrates the right ureter. (Redrawn from art provided by Ethicon Endosurgery, Cincinnati, OH.)

Right common iliac artery

Right ureter

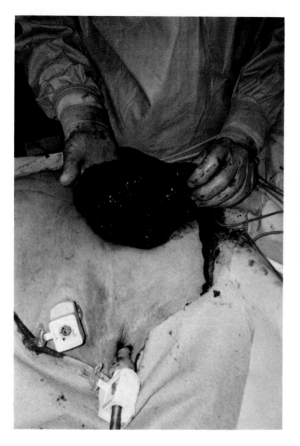

Figure 31–14. The ascending colon is eviscerated through an enlarged umbilical fascial opening, at which point the mesentery and bowel are divided between conventional clamps and sutures. (From Jacobs M, Verdja J-C, Plasencia G. Laparoscopic colonic surgery. In: Zucker KA, Bailey RW, Reddick EJ, eds. Surgical laparoscopy update. St. Louis: Quality Medical Publishing, Inc., 1993, p. 337.)

nal wall and be easily eviscerated through an enlarged umbilical fascial opening (Fig. 31–14). The umbilical puncture site is gradually dilated, and if the adjacent musculi recti are not incised, there is very little additional pain or cosmetic disfigurement. If the bowel cannot be exteriorized satisfactorily through the umbilicus, a separate muscle-splitting incision can be made in the right upper quadrant. As the pneumoperitoneum is released, the bowel usually reaches the skin without difficulty. The mesenteric vessels are then ligated and divided between conventional clamps and sutures. The bowel is divided proximally and distally, and an extracorporeal anastomosis (stapled or sewn) is performed in a standard fashion (Fig. 31–15). The resulting mesenteric defect is then closed with interrupted sutures.

Although easily accomplished, this method of extracorporeal right hemicolectomy is no longer recommended for patients with localized malignancies because the mesenteric vessels are ligated too close to the bowel wall. If a more extensive en bloc resection of the regional lymph nodes is desired, the mesentery must be divided close to the juncture with the retroperitoneum under laparoscopic guidance. The colon is re-

tracted up toward the anterior abdominal wall, and the peritoneum is scored close to the root of the mesentery. The mesenteric vessels are then identified, dissected free, and divided between surgical clips (Fig. 31–16). Laparoscopic Doppler probes are now available that may be used to identify these blood vessels during laparoscopic surgery.[24] Alternatively, some surgeons advocate the use of a second laparoscope and light source, which can be used to transilluminate the mesentery. If surgical clips are used to control the mesenteric vessels, they should be long enough (*i.e.,* 9 to 11 mm) to encompass the vessels securely. Most surgeons also prefer to apply a pretied looped suture on the mesenteric side of the vessel. Alternatively, the mesentery may be divided totally using a linear stapler. If this instrument is used, small windows are created in the mesentery and the jaws of the stapler are then placed through the window. The jaws are then closed and fired (Fig. 31–17). These instruments apply multiple rows of staples with a knife blade simultaneously dividing the tissues. Different sizes and configurations of staples are available, depending on the thickness of the tissue being divided. This same linear stapling instrument can also be used

Figure 31–15. The eviscerated ascending colon is divided, and an extracorporeal anastomosis is performed. (From Jacobs M, Verdja J-C, Plasencia G. Laparoscopic colonic surgery. In: Zucker KA, Bailey RW, Reddick EJ, eds. Surgical laparoscopy update. St. Louis: Quality Medical Publishing, Inc., 1993, p. 338.)

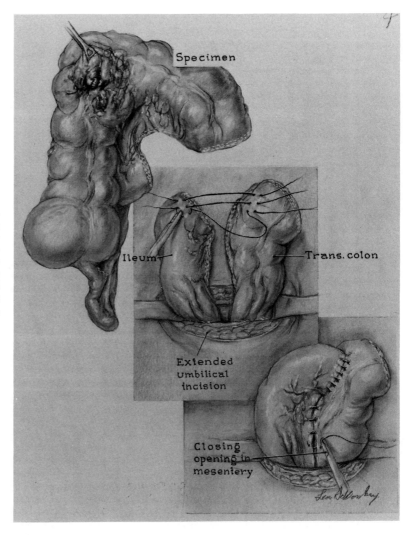

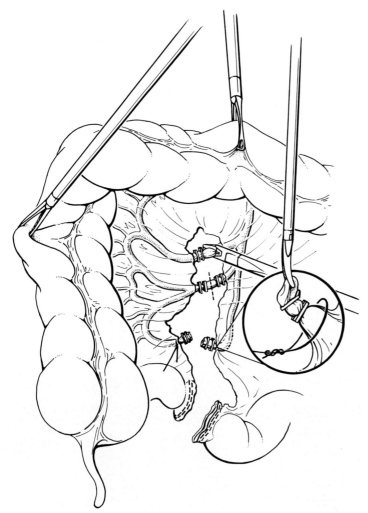

Figure 31–16. Dissection of the individual mesenteric vessels and ligation with surgical clips or sutures. (Redrawn from art provided by Ethicon Endosurgery, Cincinnati, OH.)

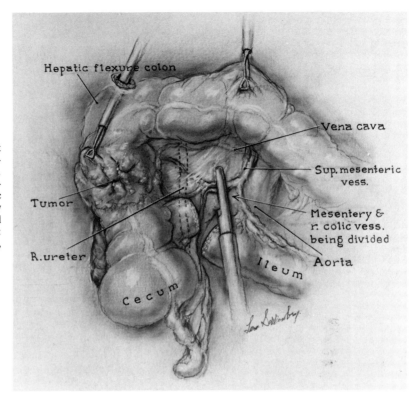

Figure 31–17. Ligation of the right colonic mesentery with a laparoscopic linear stapling device. (From Jacobs M, Verdja J-C, Plasencia G. Laparoscopic colonic surgery. In: Zucker KA, Bailey RW, Reddick EJ, eds. Surgical laparoscopy update. St. Louis: Quality Medical Publishing, Inc., 1993, p. 335.)

to divide the proximal and distal portions of the specimen, making it easier to extract from the peritoneal cavity. With either technique, a wide en bloc resection of the mesenteric vessels and lymph nodes can be performed.

Once the specimen is removed and the anastomosis completed, the bowel is returned to the abdominal cavity, and the pneumoperitoneum is reestablished after closing the fascia. Any remaining mesenteric defect is reapproximated using laparoscopic suturing techniques. If irrigation is desired, it is done at this time and then completely evacuated. If desired, drains are placed, and the catheters are brought out through one of the puncture sites. Fascial wounds are closed and skin is reapproximated as described previously.

Left Hemicolectomy and Anterior Resection

An extended left hemicolectomy, sigmoid colectomy, or low anterior resection can also be performed under laparoscopic guidance. Benign disorders such as rectal prolapse, large polyps, or volvulus of the sigmoid require a less extensive resection, but operations for malignancy *can* also be accomplished provided that care is taken to adequately mobilize and dissect the appropriate structures as necessary.

Patients are usually placed in a modified lithotomy position to allow easy access to the anus (for intraoperative colonoscopy, insertion of a circular end-to-end anastomotic (EEA) stapler, and so on). The surgeon and assistant stand on the right side of the patient with both video monitors placed near the foot of the bed. Nasogastric and urinary catheters are routinely inserted. Four and usually five laparoscopic cannulas are necessary to perform these procedures. The positioning of these sheaths will also vary depending on the location of the colonic lesion and the surgeon's preference, but a suggested scheme is shown in Figure 31–18.

After the laparoscopic cannulas are inserted, the patient is placed in a reverse Trendelenburg position with the table tilted right side down. Laparoscopic Babcock clamps or bowel-grasping forceps are then used to grasp the sigmoid colon and retract it medially and cephalad to visualize the lateral peritoneal attachments. Dissection of the white line of Toldt can be done in a similar fashion to that described for resection of the ascending colon. Again, the ureter is identified in the retroperitoneum, as are the iliac and gonadal vessels (Fig. 31–19). If the splenic flexure is to be mobilized, care must be taken in controlling the vessels coursing through the lienocolic attachments. Caution is exercised to avoid avulsing these vessels by placing too

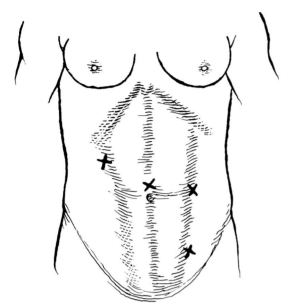

Figure 31–18. Suggested sites for cannula placement for laparoscopic-assisted left-sided hemicolectomy. (Modified from Jacobs M, Verdja J-C, Plasencia G. Laparoscopic colonic surgery. In: Zucker KA, Bailey RW, Reddick EJ, eds. Surgical laparoscopy update. St. Louis: Quality Medical Publishing, Inc., 1993, p. 340.)

much caudad traction on the colon (Fig. 31–20). After dissecting the vessels, surgical clips or suture ligatures are applied and the vessels divided. The lienocolic ligament is also amenable to division using a laparoscopic linear stapler.

After full mobilization of the colon to the midline, the bowel is brought up to the anterior abdominal wall and eviscerated as described for the ascending colon. Usually it is not possible to extract an adequate length of the descending colon through the umbilicus, and instead a 5- to 8-cm left lower quadrant muscle-splitting incision is made at a site from which both the proximal and distal margins can be easily brought out of the abdomen (Fig. 31–21). The mesentery and bowel are divided and a conventional hand-sewn or stapled anastomosis is performed. If a more extensive resection of the mesentery is desired, these vessels can be ligated and divided intracorporeally as described for the ascending colon (Fig. 31–22).

When performing a low anterior resection, it is usually not possible to eviscerate the distal limb for an extracorporeal anastomosis. In this situation, a conventional circular EEA stapler is often used to complete the anastomosis. A 4- to 6-cm incision is made in the left lower quadrant over the intended site of the anastomosis.

The proximal and distal margins of the specimen are divided with a laparoscopic linear stapler, and the specimen is removed. The proximal limb is eviscerated, and the anvil of the circular EEA stapler is inserted and a pursestring suture placed around the the bowel and anvil. If a side-to-end (Baker) anastomosis is preferred, the anvil and pursestring suture are placed accordingly. The shaft of the stapler is inserted into the anus and maneuvered proximal to the staple line (Fig. 31–23). The anvil is inserted into the shaft under direct vision and the device is closed and fired. After firing, the doughnuts of tissue are inspected for completeness. Air or methylene blue can be gently instilled into the "neorectum" to check anastomotic integrity. If air is used, the pelvis is filled with saline and inspected for bubbling. After irrigation and evacuation, the mesocolon is reapproximated, the pneumoperitoneum is decompressed, and the wounds are closed.

Alternatively, the anastomosis can be performed without making a separate fascial opening. The specimen can be brought out through an open rectal stump or the posterior cul-de-sac in females. The bowel ends in this technique are left open to allow for transanal passage of the EEA stapler. The anvil is advanced into the proximal bowel and tied down with a pursestring suture using endoscopic suturing techniques. The rectal stump is closed around the shaft in a similar manner. The device is closed and fired. If this is the method used, it is especially important to control the proximal bowel to avoid spillage because the end must remain open to receive the anvil of the stapler. The pelvis is then irrigated, the mesenteric defect closed, and the integrity of the anastomosis checked as described previously.

Clinical Experience

The largest published experience with laparoscopic colon resection is from Jacobs and colleagues.[3] Seventy-six selected patients underwent either laparoscopically assisted right or left hemicolectomy. Indications for laparoscopic intervention included both benign and malignant disease. The vast majority of patients were able to leave the hospital within 72 to 96 hours after surgery and were able to return to normal activity within 14 days. There were no operative deaths, and significant complications that were felt to delay the patient's discharge from the hospital occurred in only 7% of cases. These complications included postoperative intraab-

(Continued on page 420)

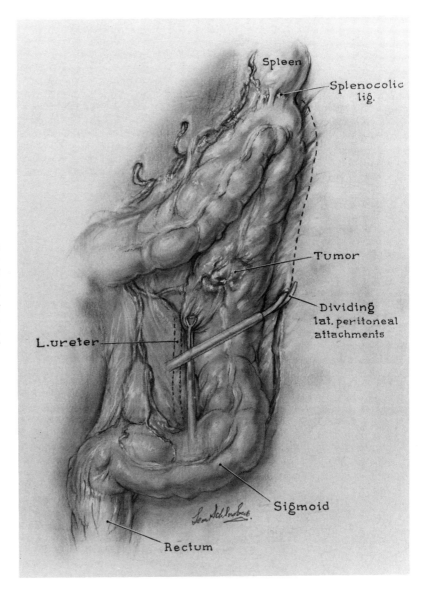

Figure 31–19. Lateral retraction and dissection of the sigmoid colon demonstrates the left ureter and iliac vessels. (From Jacobs M, Verdja J-C, Plasencia G. Laparoscopic colonic surgery. In: Zucker KA, Bailey RW, Reddick EJ, eds. Surgical laparoscopy update. St. Louis: Quality Medical Publishing, Inc., 1993, p. 341.)

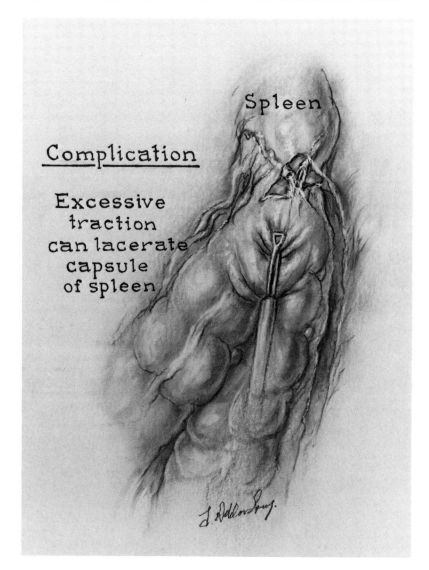

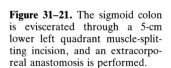

Figure 31–20. Excessive traction on the descending colon and splenic flexure may result in avulsion of the lower pole of the spleen. (From Jacobs M, Verdja J-C, Plasencia G. Laparoscopic colonic surgery. In: Zucker KA, Bailey RW, Reddick EJ, eds. Surgical laparoscopy update. St. Louis: Quality Medical Publishing, Inc., 1993, p. 342.)

Figure 31–21. The sigmoid colon is eviscerated through a 5-cm lower left quadrant muscle-splitting incision, and an extracorporeal anastomosis is performed.

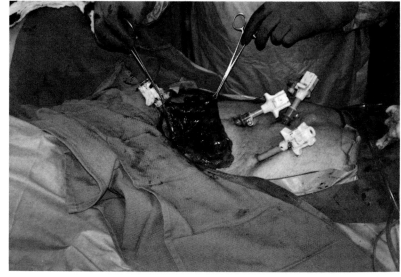

Figure 31–22. A laparoscopic linear stapling device may be used to ligate and divide the mesentery of the descending and sigmoid colons. (From Jacobs M, Verdja J-C, Plasencia G. Laparoscopic colonic surgery. In: Zucker KA, Bailey RW, Reddick EJ, eds. Surgical laparoscopy update. St. Louis: Quality Medical Publishing, Inc., 1993, p. 343.)

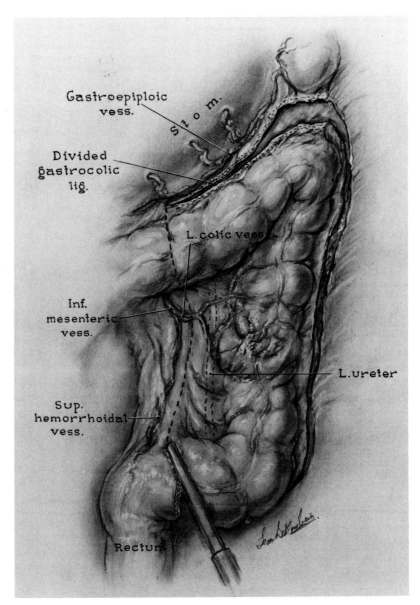

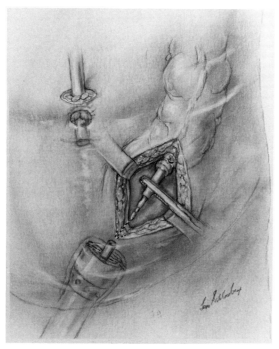

Figure 31–23. After the specimen is removed, the anvil of the circular stapler is positioned with the proximal limb. The shaft of the instrument is guided through the anus and rectum. The two portions of the stapler are joined, and the stapled anastomosis is completed under direct vision. (From Jacobs M, Verdja J-C, Plasencia G. Laparoscopic colonic surgery. In: Zucker KA, Bailey RW, Reddick EJ, eds. Surgical laparoscopy update. St. Louis: Quality Medical Publishing, Inc., 1993, p. 347.)

dominal bleeding, bowel obstruction, prolonged ileus, and urinary retention. A combined series from the University of Maryland and New Mexico Medical Center reported 65 patients who underwent laparoscopically assisted intestinal surgery.[25] Indications also included both benign (26) and malignant (39) disorders. There were no operation-related deaths and only one major complication, a subfascial abscess that required percutaneous drainage. Minor complications occured in three patients and included urinary tract infection, atelectasis, and prolonged ileus (>96 hours). The mean postoperative hospital stay was 4.1 days.

OTHER LAPAROSCOPIC COLORECTAL PROCEDURES

Abdominal-Perineal Resection

Laparoscopy may also be used in selected patients undergoing abdominal-perineal resec-

tion (Miles' procedure). As most surgeons will attest, during open procedures (especially in android pelves), the abdominal dissection on the middle third of the rectum can be difficult or tedious at best. A number of surgeons have reported that laparoscopic dissection of the rectum is technically possible and, in fact, may be easier than that during conventional surgery.[21, 26] The patient is positioned in a manner similar to that described for a low anterior resection. The left midabdominal cannula site will be the eventual colostomy location, so care is taken to choose this location judiciously. The pelvic dissection is facilitated by a slight alteration in port sites, with a cannula inserted in the left side of the midabdomen rather than in a right subcostal location. The five cannula sites are then (1) umbilical, (2) suprapubic, (3) left lower quadrant, (4) right lower quadrant, and (5) the eventual left-sided colostomy site.

Mobilization of the sigmoid and descending colon is carried out as necessary, again with great care to avoid injury to the iliac vessels, ureters, and the bowel itself. The peritoneal reflection anterior to the rectum is incised and Denonvilliers' fascia is identified as the plane of dissection anteriorly. This anterior separation can be accomplished by blunt dissection or with curved scissors aided by cautery. The lateral and posterior attachments are then identified and divided using surgical clips and cautery to maintain hemostasis as needed. The middle rectal vessels are identified and securely controlled with clips or suture ligatures prior to being divided. The superior rectal vessels are controlled during dissection of the mesorectum. After circumferential mobilization of the rectum, it may be helpful to identify the proximal extent of resection and divide the bowel with the laparoscopic linear stapler. The mesentery is scored up to the base of the inferior mesenteric artery, and windows are created in the mesentery for the jaws of the stapler to pass through. The vessels are then progressively ligated and divided across the entire mesorectum. After completely mobilizing the sigmoid colon and rectum, the remainder of the pelvic dissection is completed before the final stages of the perineal portion of the procedure. This is because opening the peritoneum from the perineal dissection will result in an immediate loss of the pneumoperitoneum. The specimen is then recovered through the perineum, and after achieving hemostasis, closed suction drains can be guided into position, the perineum closed, and reinsufflation commenced after clamping the drainage catheters. The pelvis is irrigated thoroughly and aspirated dry. The peritoneum is approximated across the pelvis, and the distal colon is brought up through the colostomy site. It will usually be necessary to enlarge this puncture site to accommodate the stoma. The colon is tacked to the anterior abdominal wall, and the lateral defect is closed using endoscopic suturing skills. All of the cannulas are removed, the wounds are closed, and the stoma is matured in the normal manner.

Rectal Prolapse

Rectal procidentia is a well-described phenomenon in several groups of patients, many of whom are debilitated or poor surgical candidates because of concurrent medical problems. The treatment of this condition has varied, with numerous procedures described and accepted as appropriate surgical intervention when necessary.[20] In the expanding field of surgical endoscopy, reports are emerging that describe the management of this problem with minimally invasive surgical techniques.

Laparoscopic fixation of the rectosigmoid colon (i.e., the Ripstein procedure) with prosthetic mesh has recently been reported by Kusminsky and associates.[20] The patient is placed in the low lithotomy position with the head of the table lowered 20° to 30°. Four or five laparoscopic cannulas (10 mm or larger in diameter) are inserted as described for low anterior resection. Laparoscopically guided dissection mobilizes the descending colon, the rectosigmoid junction, and the rectum, as for anterior resection. Retraction is accomplished by endoscopic atraumatic graspers applied to the bowel as necessary. A sling is fashioned from a 4- × 20-cm strip of mersilene mesh. One end of the sling is then secured to the sacrum with endoscopic staples. The rectum is then wrapped and the remainder of the sling is stapled to the sacrum, reangulating the rectosigmoid junction and suspending it as much as possible. Some surgeons have described securing the mesh to the rectum with the same staples,[20] but conceivably this can be more safely accomplished with endoscopic suturing techniques.

Other surgeons have advocated laparoscopic low anterior resection as an effective method of managing individuals with rectal prolapse, either alone or in combination with rectopexy.[19]

Creation and Takedown of Colostomies

Colostomy creation and takedown may also be accomplished using laparoscopic skills. In the event that a colostomy is necessary (either end or loop), the pneumoperitoneum is established with the open method because of accompanying intestinal distention. With the video laparoscope in the umbilicus, the abdomen is surveyed, and the most accessible portion of the colon is mobilized to the abdominal wall. The placement of the accessory cannulas will be dependent on the section of bowel to be brought up. The critical factor to keep in mind is that with careful placement of the ports, a cannula site in the left side of the midabdomen can ultimately become the colostomy site, although it may need to be enlarged slightly to accommodate the colon being brought out.

Although the possibility of adhesions from previous surgery must be entertained when considering a patient for takedown of colostomy, there will be a significant number of patients who can be approached through open laparoscopy, with the procedure of reanastomosing the bowel being completed as a laparoscopically assisted procedure. The advantages of proceeding with these operations in the most minimally invasive fashion is that the patient should have a remarkably shortened recovery period, and bowel function may return more rapidly.

POTENTIAL COMPLICATIONS OF LAPAROSCOPIC INTESTINAL SURGERY

As has been widely published, some of the risks of laparoscopy include injuries from insufflation needles or trocars, visceral organ injuries from instruments used in the procedures, burns from electrocautery or other energy modalities, and iatrogenic injuries from failure to clearly identify specific structures.[27, 28] Coupled with the known risks of intestinal surgery (i.e., bleeding, infection, anastomotic leakage, ureteral injury), the endeavor becomes rather challenging in the current climate. In addition to the cumulative risks of the approach and the procedure itself, one must take into consideration the fact that unless a great deal of attention is given to each step of the operation, errors may be made that lead to complications. Excessive instrumentation of the organs must be avoided to prevent undue tissue injury and edema. The rules of anastomosing segments of bowel together must be strictly adhered to, especially with regard to closing mesenteric defects and avoiding rotation or undue tension on the staple or suture line. Attention must be given to blood supply, localization of the lesion to be removed, and caution to avoid injuring structures in the vicinity of the task being performed.

CONCLUSION

Despite the limited data thus far available, laparoscopy appears to have a promising role in many aspects of intestinal surgery. Although acceptance by patients has been rapid, many surgeons remain somewhat skeptical of the long-term consequences of these minimally invasive procedures. Whether the results will substantiate the enthusiasm with which some surgeons have embraced these new methods remains to be seen, but few can argue that in the early stages of development, the prospects are intriguing. The current emphasis must be placed on careful study of ongoing work, as well as planning prospective clinical studies to answer the many questions at hand.

References

1. Hertzmann P. Thermal instrumentation. In: Zucker KA. Bailey RW, Reddick EJ, eds. Surgical laparoscopy. St. Louis: Quality Medical Publishing, 1991:57–76.
2. Dorsey JH, Tabb R. Laparoscopic suturing and knot tying. In: Zucker KA, ed. Surgical laparoscopy update. St. Louis: Quality Medical Publishing, 1993:84–105.
3. Jacobs M, Verdeja JC, Goldstein HS. Laparoscopic assisted colonic surgery. In: Zucker KA, ed. Surgical laparoscopy update. St. Louis: Quality Medical Publishing, 1993:327–356.
4. Corbitt JD. Preliminary experience with laparoscopic-guided colectomy. Surg Laparosc Endosc 2(1):79–81, 1992.
5. Hassan HM. Open laparoscopy versus closed laparoscopy. Adv Planned Parenthood 13:41–50, 1978.
6. Fitzgibbons RJ, Salerno GM, Filipi CJ. Open laparoscopy. In: Zucker KA, ed. Surgical laparoscopy. St. Louis: Quality Medical Publishing, 1991:87–97.
7. Zucker KA. Laparoscopic guided cholecystectomy with electrocautery dissection. In: Zucker KA, ed. Surgical laparoscopy. St. Louis: Quality Medical Publishing, 1991:143–182.
8. Cooperman AM, Zucker KA. Laparoscopic guided intestinal surgery. In: Zucker KA, ed. Surgical laparos-

copy. St. Louis: Quality Medical Publishing, 1991:295–310.
9. Morris JB, Mullen JL, Yu JC, Rosato EF. Laparoscopic-guided jejunostomy. Surgery 112(1):96–99, 1992.
10. Stamm M. Gastrostomy: a new method. Med News 65:324, 1894.
11. Witzel O. Zur technik der magenfistelanlegung. Zentralbl Chir 18:601, 1891.
12. Duh QY, Way LW. Laparoscopic jejunostomy using T-fasteners as retractors and anchors. Arch Surg 128:105–108, 1993.
13. Zucker KA, Pitcher DA, Martin DT. Laparoscopic assisted enteral access procedures. Submitted for publication, Am J Surg 1993.
14. Jacobs M, Verdeja JC, Goldstein HS. Minimally invasive colon resection. Surg Laparosc Endosc 1(3):144–150, 1991.
15. Coller JA. Laparoscopic assisted right hemi-colectomy. Dis Colon Rectum 34(11):1030–1031, 1991.
16. Brune IB, Schonleben K. Laparoskopische sigmaresektion. Der Chir 63:342–344, 1992.
17. Kockerling F, Gastinger I, Schneider B, et al. Laparoskopiche abdino-perineale rectumexstirpation mit hoher durchtrennung der arteria mesenterica inferior. Der Chir 63:345–348, 1992.
18. Fowler DL, White SA. Laparoscopic-assisted sigmoid resection. Surg Laparosc Endosc 1(3):183–188, 1991.
19. Ballantyne GH. Laparoscopic-assisted anterior resection for rectal prolapse. Surg Laparosc Endosc 2(3):230–236, 1992.
20. Kusminsky RE, Tiley EH, Boland JP. Laparoscopic Ripstein procedure. Surg Laparosc Endosc 2(4):346–347, 1993.
21. Sundin JA, Wasson D, McMillen MM, Ballantyne GH. Laparoscopic-assisted sigmoid colectomy for sigmoid volvulus. Surg Laparosc Endosc 2(4):353–358, 1993.
22. Pezet D, Fondrinier E, Rotman N, et al. Parietal seeding of carcinoma of the gallbladder after laparoscopic cholecystectomy. Br J Surg 79:230, 1992.
23. Cava A, Roman J, Gonzalez QA, Martin F, Arambuco P. Subcutaneous metastasis following laparoscopy in gastric adenocarcinoma. Eur J Surg Oncol 16:63–67, 1990.
24. Fowler DL, White SA. The use of a Doppler probe for identifying the cystic artery during a laparoscopic cholecystectomy: a pilot study. Surg Laparosc Endosc 2(2):117–119, 1992.
25. Zucker KA, Pitcher DA, Martin DT, et al. Laparoscopic assisted colon resection. In press. Surg Endosc 1994.
26. Larach SW, Salomon MC, Williamson PR, Goldstein E. Laparoscopic assisted abdominoperineal resection. Surg Laparosc Endosc 3(2):115–118, 1993.
27. Phillips JM. Complications in laparoscopy. Int J Gynecol Obstet 15:157–162, 1977.
28. Bailey RW. Complications of laparoscopic general surgery. In: Zucker KA, ed. Surgical laparoscopy. St. Louis: Quality Medical Publishing, 1991:311–341.

32

Laparoscopic Cholangiography

Mohan C. Airan and Sung-Tao Ko

Langenbuch introduced open cholecystectomy as a procedure of choice in the treatment of chronic cholecystitis in 1882.[1] Mirizzi[2] of Cordoba, Argentina started performing routine operative cholangiograms in 1931 using iodized oil (Lipiodal) solution through the cystic duct or gallbladder or by the direct puncture of the common bile duct (CBD). The rationale for performing these procedures was to study the CBD with the intention of reducing unnecessary CBD explorations and limiting choledochotomy to those cases in which it was indicated. However, routine use of cholangiography has not been widely practiced in open cholecystectomy, even though Hickens and associates[3] advocated its use as early as 1936.

Laparoscopic cholecystectomy (LC) has supplanted open cholecystectomy as the procedure of choice for the treatment of chronic cholecystitis since its introduction in 1989.[4, 5] The Intraoperative cholangiogram (IOC) has become crucial in laparoscopic cholecystectomy because of the loss of tactile sense and binocular vision. IOCs can be performed during LC without any increase in morbidity or mortality.[5, 6] Successful cannulation of the cystic duct with an IOC can be performed in 90% of all cases.[7] As Moossa and associates[8] have pointed out, injuries to the bile ducts are not rare even in open cholecystectomies, and the lack of an IOC probably has contributed to some of these injuries (Fig. 32–1).

There are four reasons for performing a routine IOC during LC: (1) to identify the cystic duct–CBD junction,[6] (2) to detect inadvertent injury,[8] (3) to find unsuspected CBD stones,[5] and (4) to detect abnormal anatomy (*e.g.,* cystic duct opening into right hepatic duct).[9]

ANATOMY OF CYSTIC DUCT

The cystic duct can be short, long, wide, or spiral-shaped and can open into the right hepatic duct or run parallel with the CBD (Figs. 32–2 through 32–8). The spiral cystic duct may wrap around the CBD either anteriorly or posteriorly and will run parallel with the CBD. The cystic duct may be accompanied by variations of the anterior or posterior segmental branches of the hepatic ducts (Fig. 32–9).

The so-called valve of Heister is a formation of loose mucosal folds in the cystic duct and is not a valve in the true anatomic sense. Physiologically, it permits the bile to go back and forth into the gallbladder. This valve-like structure inside the cystic duct can usually be identified

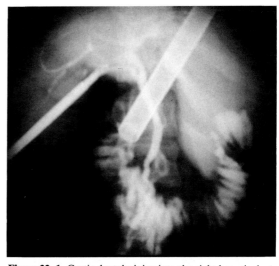

Figure 32–1. Cystic duct draining into the right hepatic duct.

423

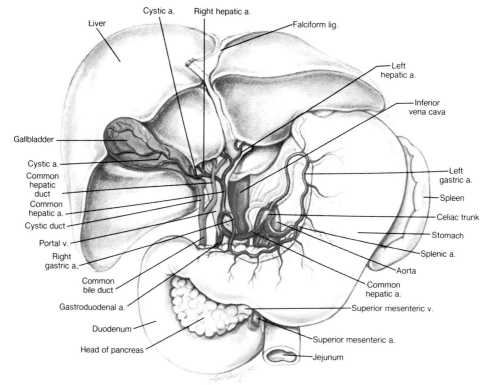

Figure 32–2. Anatomy of a cystic duct. (From Gray SW, Skandalakis JE. Atlas of surgical anatomy for general surgeons. Baltimore: Williams & Wilkins, 1985.)

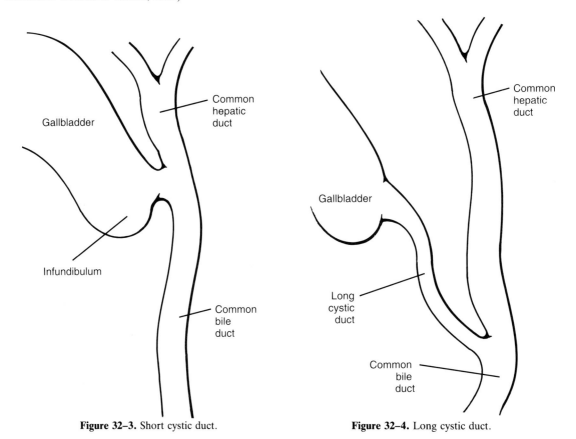

Figure 32–3. Short cystic duct.

Figure 32–4. Long cystic duct.

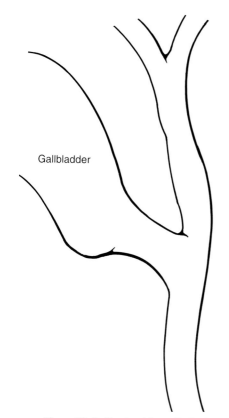

Figure 32–5. Short, wide cystic duct.

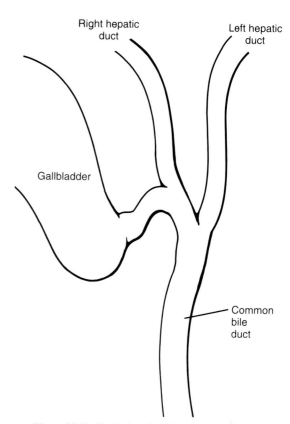

Figure 32–7. Cystic duct into the right hepatic duct.

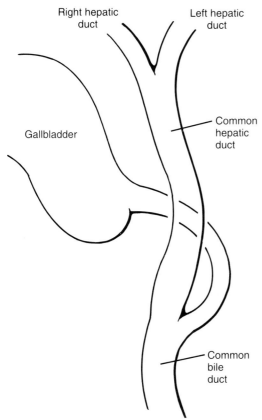

Figure 32–6. Spiral cystic duct.

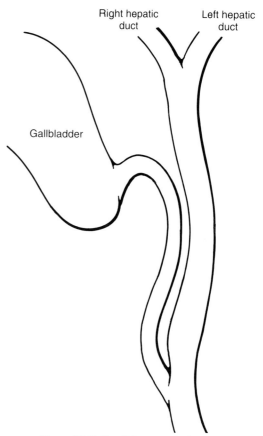

Figure 32–8. Parallel run cystic duct.

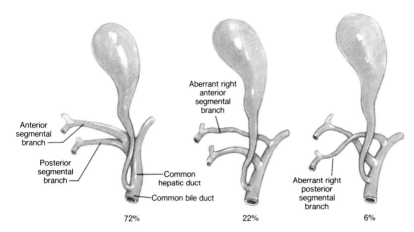

Anterior
segmental
branch

Posterior
segmental
branch

Aberrant right
anterior
segmental
branch

Common
hepatic duct

Common bile duct

Aberrant right
posterior
segmental
branch

72%   22%   6%

Figure 32–9. Variations of anterior or posterior segmental branches of hepatic ducts. (From Gray SW. Skandalakis JE. Atlas of surgical anatomy for general surgeons. Baltimore: Williams & Wilkins, 1985.)

as a mild bulge in the cystic duct close to the infundibulum of the gallbladder.

The microanatomy of the cystic duct is depicted in Figures 32–10 and 32–11. The anatomy depicted is from the observation of Calot's triangle in 500 cases of LC. The inferior antimesenteric border of the cystic duct has a very small arteriole that runs parallel to the duct until it disappears into the infundibulum. Very small capillaries go into the cystic duct from this branch of the 9 o'clock artery of the CBD.[10] There is also a parallel arteriole located on the superior border of the cystic duct, and its course is generally variable. However, it has a rich arcade of capillaries that supply the junction of the cystic duct and the CBD. This arteriolar arcade usually originates from the cystic artery but occasionally can be the continuation of the 9 o'clock artery.

TECHNIQUES OF LAPAROSCOPIC CHOLANGIOGRAPHY

Cannulation of Cystic Duct

Wire-Guided Catheter Technique (Technique No. 1). This technique, developed by the author in 1989,[4] requires a surgeon and a cosurgeon. The cosurgeon performs the cholangiogram from the right side of the patient. He or she uses the midclavicular port to make an incision into the cystic duct using a microscissors. The operating surgeon grasps Hartmann's pouch and retracts the pouch toward the free peritoneal cavity, thereby opening Calot's triangle and facilitating the positioning of the cystic duct at an obtuse angle for the cosurgeon to make the

incision into the cystic duct (Fig. 32–12). *The incision should always be placed distal to the last bulge in the cystic duct if it can be visualized.* Care should be taken not to go close to the junction of the cystic duct and the CBD. In many cases this may not be possible, and additional careful dissection may be necessary using very small amounts of current (18 to 20 W) with a thin wire L-shaped dissector to provide additional length of cystic duct toward the infundibulum of the gallbladder. In this situation, the incision in the cystic duct almost invariably is placed distal to the spiral valve of Heister (Fig. 32–13), which results in difficulty in placing the catheter in the true lumen of the cystic duct. Therefore, we developed the technique of using a 0.038-mm flexible-tip guidewire through a No. 5 ureteric catheter. One to 2 mm of the flexible tip can be protruded through the ureteric catheter to stiffen the wire and direct it into the true opening of the cystic duct. If the guidewire gets obstructed at the mucosal folds (Fig. 32–13), the cystic duct opening can be increased proximally toward the CBD until the true opening can be seen.

A microscissors is best for this extension of the incision into the cystic duct. The opening in the cystic duct can be widened by dilation with the microscissors. Once the guidewire is placed in the cystic duct, it is carefully advanced into the CBD, and the No. 5 ureteric catheter is threaded over the wire into the cystic duct. Only 1 cm of the marked catheter is used to obtain a satisfactory watertight closure around the cystic duct. A cholangioclamp is normally used to secure the catheter in the cystic duct. If a cholangioclamp is not available, a Wisap atraumatic grasper (Wisap USA, Tomball, TX) can be used to hold the catheter in the cystic duct. The Wisap clamp has to be inserted through the operating port, resulting in a radiopaque shadow

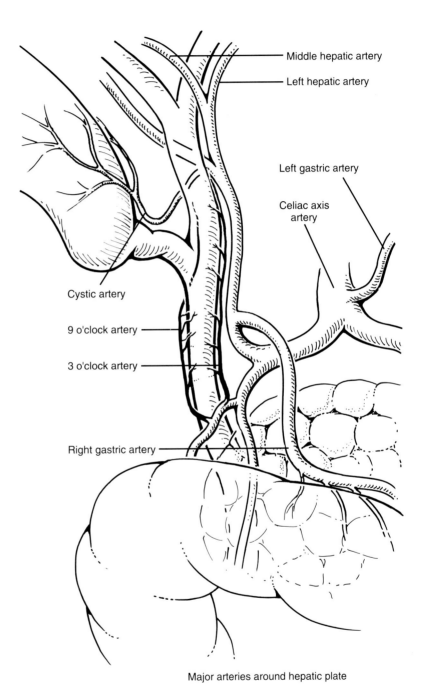

Middle hepatic artery

Left hepatic artery

Left gastric artery

Celiac axis artery

Cystic artery

9 o'clock artery

3 o'clock artery

Right gastric artery

Major arteries around hepatic plate

Figure 32–10. Microanatomy of a cystic duct. (Adapted from Northover JMA, Terblanche J. A new look at the arterial supply of the bile duct in man and its surgical implications. Br J Surg 66:379–384, 1979. By permission of the publisher, Butterworth-Heinemann Ltd.)

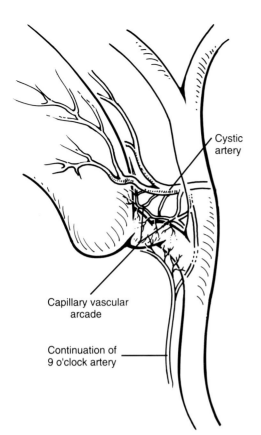

Figure 32–11. Arterial supply of a cystic duct.

Cystic
artery

Capillary vascular
arcade

Continuation of
9 o'clock artery

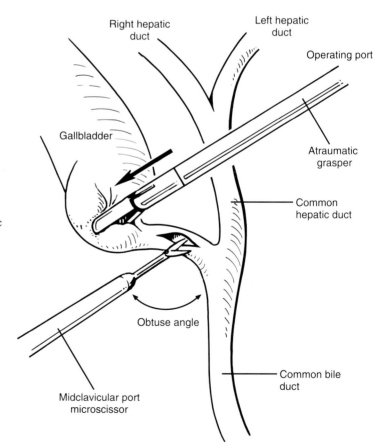

Figure 32–12. Precise incision into a cystic
duct.

Right hepatic
duct

Left hepatic
duct

Operating port

Gallbladder

Atraumatic
grasper

Common
hepatic duct

Obtuse angle

Common bile
duct

Midclavicular port
microscissor

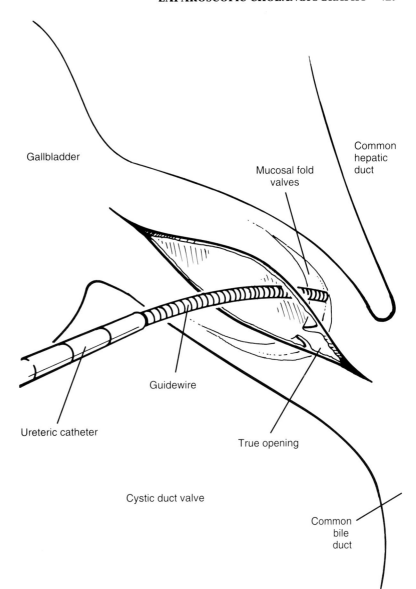

Figure 32–13. Technique for placing a catheter in the true opening of a cystic duct.

across the CBD. This is unavoidable if a Wisap clamp is used. Sometimes the angle of the catheter is not optimal for insertion into the opening of the cystic duct. To obtain a proper catheter angle, the cholangioclamp can be used to flex the catheter guidewire set-up at a gentle 15° angle by closing the jaws of the clamp behind the set-up. This angle facilitates placement of the guidewire tip into the cystic duct opening. Once the guidewire is mated to the opening, it is gently advanced into the cystic duct. Care should be taken not to push the guidewire when resistance is felt. The guidewire will negotiate small bends in the cystic duct without difficulty. Once it has passed into the CBD, the No. 5 ureteric catheter can be advanced over the

guidewire into the CBD. To date we have used this technique in 500 LCs without any complications and with a 93% success rate (Table 32–1). There have been no perforations of the cystic duct or the CBD. Failures of cannulation have

Table 32–1. FIVE HUNDRED CONSECUTIVE INTRAOPERATIVE CHOLANGIOGRAMS PERFORMED DURING LAPAROSCOPIC CHOLECYSTECTOMY

Attempted	480
Successful	446
Success rate	93%
Not attempted	20
Unsuspected CBD stones	25 (5%)

occurred in cases in which there was a lot of inflammation around the cystic duct, making it friable, as well as in very small cystic ducts in which the lumen was smaller than 1 mm. In such cases, the cystic duct may be transected accidentally during attempts to cannulate it. If this happens, an Endoloop (Ethicon Endosurgery, Cincinnati, OH) should be used to occlude the lumen of the duct. Division of the cystic artery prior to cannulation of the cystic duct should be avoided because an intact cystic artery prevents retraction of the cystic duct if it is accidentally transected or avulsed. Once the cystic duct is securely cannulated, the cholangiogram can be performed.

Percutaneous Puncture Technique (Technique No. 2). This technique can be performed by a single surgeon. In the event the surgeon does not wish to give up the midclavicular port and wants to perform the cannulation of the cystic duct alone, it is possible to accomplish this by using an 18-gauge intra-cath placed percutaneously into the abdomen near the midclavicular port in the right upper quadrant. A No. 4 ureteric catheter with an end hole is then passed into the abdomen through this intra-cath. The surgeon makes the opening in the cystic duct from the operating port and then grasps the catheter with a grasper or a needle holder and pushes it into the cystic duct. The catheter is then secured with a clip, and a cholangiogram is performed. Balloon catheter tips to facilitate secure retention in the cystic duct have been developed and can be used. However, there are disadvantages to the balloon catheters. They are sometimes difficult to place in a tortuous cystic duct, and when placed in short cystic ducts, they have a tendency to migrate into the CBD and occlude the common hepatic duct, resulting in an inaccurate cholangiogram (Tables 32–2 and 32–3).

Table 32–2. ADVANTAGES AND DISADVANTAGES OF THE TWO TECHNIQUES OF INTRAOPERATIVE CHOLANGIOGRAMS IN LAPAROSCOPIC CHOLECYSTECTOMY

Technique No. 1	Technique No. 2
Advantages	
Precise dissection and opening into cystic duct can be achieved.	Single surgeon can stand on the operating side (*i.e.,* the left side) of patient and perform the opening into cystic duct and cannulate the duct.
Spiral valve can be dissected to advance the guidewire and catheter.	
Tactile sensations are preserved in the insertion of the guidewire. Chance of perforation is minimized, and the force necessary to cannulate is reduced and well modulated.	There is no need for the surgeon to change position to the opposite side of patient.
	No problems with air bubbles in the system.
Disadvantages	
Needs cholangioclamp. Cosurgeon must be present or single surgeon must change position to the right side of patient to perform ductotomy and cannulation.	Precise dissection of cystic duct difficult or impossible because of operating angles.
Head-down lithotomy position necessary, as is irrigation to eliminate air bubbles prior to cholangiogram.	Insertion of catheter into cystic duct is performed with a grasper or needle holder and there is loss of tactile feel, which increases chances of perforation or avulsion, or both.
	Catheter needs to be clipped into cystic duct to secure watertight closure or balloon catheters must be used.
	Possibility of accidental transection of the catheter because of clip.
	Sometimes too much clip pressure leads to occlusion of the lumen of the catheter.

ELIMINATION OF AIR BUBBLES FOR A SUCCESSFUL CHOLANGIOGRAM

When a wire guide is used through a ureteric catheter, there is always a small amount of air in the catheter. To eliminate these air bubbles, the operating table is adjusted so that the patient is in the Trendelenburg position, and then 30 to 40 ml of warm saline is injected into the CBD. Invariably the air is flushed into the duodenum. In the 500 consecutive IOCs we have performed, there were air bubbles in three cases, all of which were early in our experience. Since we began tilting the table and then irrigating the CBD, air bubbles have not been a problem.

STATE OF THE ART CHOLANGIOGRAM

The cholangiogram is performed under fluoroscopic guidance with aimed multiple film exposures. An image amplifier with a television monitor and an x-ray camera opposite the x-ray tube are placed on a C-arm table (Fig. 32–14).

Table 32–3. ESSENTIAL EQUIPMENT FOR INTRAOPERATIVE CHOLANGIOGRAM DURING LAPAROSCOPIC CHOLECYSTECTOMY

Technique No. 1
1. Cholangioclamp (Storz)
2. Wisap grasper
3. 0.038-mm flexible-tip guidewire (Cook or Microvasive, Boston Scientific, Watertown, MA)
4. No. 5 ureteric catheter
5. Microscissors
6. L-shaped wire electrode dissector

Technique No. 2
1. 18-gauge intra-cath
2. No. 4 ureteric catheter or balloon tip cholangiocatheter
3. Clip applicator to secure catheter in CD
4. Microscissors

Fluoroscopy gives an immediate picture of the area of interest. Modern machines use a three-phase generator, which requires a short exposure time, and 8 to 10 films of high quality are obtained in 5 to 7 minutes. The filling phase, filled phase, and emptying phase into the duodenum can be captured on films or stored in video memory for later reproduction.

STANDARD CHOLANGIOGRAM

In our experience, 90% of the hospitals in our area use a portable x-ray machine. We have developed a single-film technique that is quite satisfactory. It does not prolong operating time and the results in 500 consecutive LCs have been excellent. A description follows:

The head of the patient is lowered in the Trendelenburg position. This facilitates filling of the intrahepatic and common hepatic ducts.

The head of the portable x-ray unit is positioned so that it is parallel to the table.

Full-strength dye (Renografin-60, Bristol-Myers Squibb Co., Princeton, NJ), 10 to 15 ml, is used.

One exposure is obtained.

When the cholangioclamp is used, the pictures are excellent with no obstruction of view. The only disadvantage of this technique is that one does not get to see the filling phase and the filled phase of the CBD. The function of the sphincter is not observed. We believe this is a minor problem in elective LCs.

SPECIAL PROBLEMS OF INTRAOPERATIVE CHOLANGIOGRAMS PERFORMED DURING LAPAROSCOPIC CHOLECYSTECTOMY

Visualizing Calot's Triangle

The majority of surgeons performing LC use 0° telescopes. This limits the ability to see around the CBD or look into Calot's triangle. A proper IOC would allow the surgeon to gauge the distance to the common hepatic duct and the CBD. This may prevent thermal or mechanical injuries to the common hepatic duct and the CBD in the event of a small amount of bleeding in this area, which may be electrocoagulated or clipped electively. We recommend the use of 25° to 30° telescopes as an aid to visualizing Calot's triangle. Inadvertent clipping or injury to the CBD can be detected by the IOC. This information may prevent further damage to the ductal system and will result in immediate repair of the injured duct.[9]

Dissection of the Cystic Duct

The best technique for dissecting and dividing the small capillaries of the cystic duct is to use an L-shaped hook. The diameter of the hook electrode should not exceed 0.8 mm. The current should be set at 18 to 20 W and the

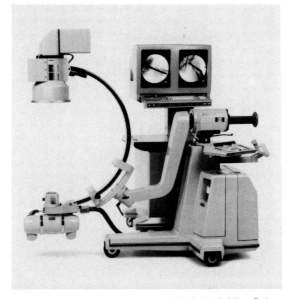

Figure 32–14. High-performance Digital Mobile C-Arm (OEC Medical Systems, Inc.: Larry E. Harrawood).

electrosurgical unit should be switched to the coagulation mode. The burn time should consist of no more than a "tap" on the foot control. The capillary should be encircled, held away from the CBD, and put on gentle tension. Too much tension will result in avulsion of the vessels, and too little tension will desiccate the vessel without cutting it. If the vessel is desiccated, it will have to be divided with a microscissors. One should never tear these capillaries. When this maneuver is used, the surgeon should make sure of the following:

1. There are no conducting clips in the vicinity of the L-shaped hook dissector.

2. The entire uninsulated shaft of the hook electrode is visible and not in contact with the CBD or any other adjacent tissue.

3. The actual activation time of the electrode does not exceed a tap on the foot or hand control.

4. There is no fluid in Morrison's pouch (right prerenal space).

5. The capillary to be divided is clearly visible and not submerged in a clot.

6. All clots in the vicinity are irrigated and aspirated prior to trying this maneuver.

One should note that this maneuver is dangerous if not properly managed and could result in unintentional, unrecognized CBD injury. If properly performed, the junction of the cystic duct and the CBD can be visualized very clearly. To prevent CBD injuries one should stay close to the junction of Hartmann's pouch and the cystic duct.

Control of Bleeding in Calot's Triangle

If these capillaries are accidentally avulsed and cannot be controlled with a fine grasper, the procedure should be converted to open surgery rather than persisting in using electrosurgical means to control the bleeding. When irrigated with heparinized saline solution, small capillaries will stop bleeding naturally. However, if there is accidental injury to the cystic artery or its branches, the so-called Ko-Airan[5] maneuver can be performed to control the bleeding. An additional 5-mm port is inserted approximately 4 cm below the operating port, and appropriate instrumentation is used to obtain precise pinpoint ligation of the bleeding artery. If the maneuver is not successful, the procedure should be converted to open surgery to prevent further injury to the structures.

Filling of Hepatic Ducts

We have been successful in filling the hepatic ducts by simply lowering the head of the table (Trendelenburg position). Occasionally, however, there may be a patulous ampulla that allows the dye to go into the duodenum rather freely. In this situation, 5 mg of morphine sulfate is given intravenously, and the IOC is repeated in 2 to 3 minutes. Usually this results in satisfactory filling of the intra-hepatic ductal system.

Spasm of the Sphincter of Oddi

Occasionally, the dye does not flow into the duodenum and there may be a suspicion of a stone in the terminal CBD. In this case, 1 to 2 mg of glucagon is given. The IOC is repeated in 4 minutes, which usually results in a satisfactory opening of the ampulla, unless there is an impacted stone there.

Small Filling Defects: Questionable Air Bubbles Versus Small Stones

When an IOC suggests questionable small air bubbles or small stones, the CBD is gently irrigated with 200 to 300 ml of warm saline with the patient in the Trendelenburg position. If these filling defects are caused by small air bubbles, these bubbles will be flushed down into the duodenum. However, small stones will stay in the CBD unless the ampulla is dilated. If there are stones in the CBD, the flow of saline suddenly stops because of the *ball-valve* action of the stones against the ampulla. This is usually an indication of a stone in the CBD. Gently releasing pressure will cause the flow to restart.

RADIATION EXPOSURE

Because all radiation exposure is additive, it is recommended that proper shielding be used to protect the surgeon, anesthesiologist, and nurses. This is probably the single most important reason for opting to buy the more expensive, state of the art C-arm–dependent x-ray machines (see Fig. 32–14). Our single-exposure technique also reduces the amount of radiation patients and surgeons receive.

CONCLUSION

1. The IOC is vital in LC.

2. Many avoidable duct injuries can be prevented by routine use of IOCs.

3. The surgeon and cosurgeon technique is preferred because of the ability to perform precise dissection of the spiral valve of Heister to facilitate placement of a wire-guided catheter.

4. State of the art fluoroscopic equipment is not mandatory for performance of excellent IOCs, but if available it should be used to visualize the early filling phase of the CBD.

References

1. Langenbuch C. Ein fal von exstirpation der gallenblase wegen chronischer cholelithiasis. Heilung Berlin Klin Wochenschr 19:725–727, 1882.

2. Mirizzi PL. Operative cholangiography. Lancet 1:366–369, 1938.

3. Hickens NF, Best RR, Hunt HB. Cholangiography. Ann Surg 103:210–216, 1936.

4. Dubois F, Berthelot G, Levard H. Cholecystectomy par coelioscopie. Presse Med 18:980–982, 1989.

5. Ko ST, Airan MC. Review of 300 consecutive laparoscopic cholecystectomies: development, evolution and results. Surg Endosc 5:103–108, 1991.

6. Sackier JM, Berci G, Phillips E, et al. The role of cholangiography in laparoscopic cholecystectomy. Arch Surg 126:1021–1026, 1991.

7. Berci G, Sackier JM, Paz-Partlow M. Routine or selected intraoperative cholangiography during laparoscopic cholecystectomy? Am J Surg 161:355–360, 1991.

8. Moossa AR, Mayer AD, Stabile B. Iatrogenic injury to the bile duct. Arch Surg 125:1028–1030, 1990.

9. Berci G, Hamlin JA. Biliary ductal anomalies. In: Berci G, Hamlin JA, eds. Operative Biliary Radiology. Baltimore: Williams & Wilkins, 1981:109–141.

10. Terblanche J, Northover JMA. A new look at the arterial supply of the bile duct in man and its surgical implications. Br J Surg 66:379–384, 1979.

33

Complications of Flexible Endoscopy

Frederick W. Ackroyd

Flexible endoscopy has revolutionized the diagnosis and treatment of gastrointestinal diseases. As techniques are refined and expanded, they are at times applied to situations beyond the usual indications—that is, in the setting of a challenging disease process. Under these circumstances, complications can occur, which are defined as an unexpected event or concurrent disease that aggravates the original disease process. They occur because of the technical difficulties of the procedure, as well as the circumstances of an advanced pathologic process, or perhaps because of lack of experience of the operator or overly aggressive application of the technique in hazardous circumstances. Occasionally the endoscopic procedure, performed at the limits of the technique to avoid abdominal surgery, results in the urgent need for laparotomy, for example, to repair perforation of the bowel or stop hemorrhage in the pedicle of the large polyp.

Being ill places patients at risk, however small, for injury and death, which is quantified as part of hospital-based risk management and quality assurance activities.[1, 2] The patient consent process implies a discussion with the patient of the risks of the intervention. These risks must be compared with doing nothing or considering other options. These other options may be less invasive and therefore less accurate at defining the pathologic condition for diagnosis and less therapeutically effective in terms of interventions.

In a recent survey of accidental injuries taken from a sample of 30,195 randomly selected records of patients admitted to acute care hospitals in New York state, 3.7% of patients were

identified as incurring disabling injuries caused by medical treatment, and of this group, 28% of cases were due to negligent care. In summary, then, 1% of patients in this sample of admissions to acute care hospitals in New York state suffered an adverse event that was preventable or attributable to negligence.[3, 4]

Complications occur unexpectedly and can aggravate the original disease, require surgical intervention, prolong hospitalization, and increase the monetary and personal costs of care. This review of the more commonly encountered complications of flexible endoscopy is designed to raise the level of awareness of the surgeon so that these complications might be avoided or recognized promptly to reduce morbidity and mortality and the overall cost to the health care system.

TRAINING AND EXPERIENCE OF THE ENDOSCOPIST AND THE ENDOSCOPY UNIT

High-caliber flexible endoscopy requires that the indications and contraindications for the application of these techniques are intelligently applied and requires skillful and atraumatic introduction and manipulation of the scopes and instruments through rather tortuous angulations of the upper and lower gastrointestinal (GI) tracts. It further requires a fund of pathophysiologic knowledge to aid in the intelligent interpretation of what the operator sees so that the correct conclusions are drawn, diagnoses made, and appropriate interventions carried out.

There are many ways to acquire these skills. The early generations of endoscopists were generally self-taught or learned from one-on-one instruction with teachers who were scarcely more experienced than the students. The logarithmic growth of endoscopy has required more formalized training opportunities in response to increasing numbers of physicians and surgeons who recognize the value of these techniques in patient care and the clamor for improved standards of practice. Training fellowships of 6 months or a year for those desiring superior skills in the diagnostic and interventional areas of endoscopy, as well as segments of formal training in residency programs, are now provided for those interested in routine diagnostic endoscopic procedures. More recently, minicourses with hands-on training sessions and "how to do it" videotapes have been added to the instructional armamentarium. Sharing of graduated clinical experience and proctored courses, as well as national meetings of societies and endoscopic journals have all enhanced the development of skills of those doing endoscopy.[5, 6]

There is, however, no substitute for common sense, an informed, cautious approach, and a willingness to stop procedures not progressing as well as might be expected, recognizing the possibility of an adverse event with all the attendant dangers to the patient.

The endoscopy unit needs nurses, or individuals with their equivalent in training and experience, who are skilled in administering intravenous medication and in monitoring vital signs, the electrocardiogram, and oxygen saturations, and who are competent to carry out cardiopulmonary resuscitation should the patient experience an arrest. Advanced cardiac life support training is one way to achieve this skill for both endoscopists and their staffs. A crash cart should be available nearby. A second technician or assistant should be available to assist the endoscopist with abdominal compression, instrumentation, collecting and labeling specimens, operating the laser and cautery machines, and providing any other assistance required by the endoscopist.[7–11]

Generalized seizures occasionally occur after overly generous use of local anesthetics for numbing the hypopharynx and esophagus in preparation for upper endoscopy. These seizures can be avoided by small doses of premedication with sedatives such as diazepam (Valium), midazolam (Versed), or barbiturates.

The equipment should be maintained in good working condition and thoroughly cleaned between procedures to protect patients from cross-contamination. The instruments are scrubbed and irrigated in a sterilizing machine with warm bactericidal solution after each case.[12, 13]

All patients who have had conscious sedation should be accompanied on the trip home after the procedure by a friend or relative. Patients often receive a phone call the next day to inquire about how they fared, and a letter is sent summarizing the pathology report on polyps and the diagnostic findings of the procedure when that information is available.

In summary, the professional demeanor and close attention to the patient by the professional staff of the endoscopy unit, who provide emotional support and reassurance as well as close monitoring and resuscitation when necessary for respiratory or cardiovascular arrest, are absolutely essential to the conduct of the patient through endoscopy under conscious sedation.

Experience is universally regarded as an essential ingredient for safe, effective flexible endoscopy, since the learning curves associated with these procedures indicate that the rate of complications drops off rapidly after the endoscopist passes the first 40 to 50 procedures.

SELECTION AND PREPARATION OF THE PATIENT

Candidates for endoscopy present with a wide spectrum of diseases, from the dangerously ill patient with GI bleeding to the asymptomatic patient with a polyp that was picked up on barium enema for occult rectal bleeding. The principles of good patient care apply to those patients who appear healthy, as well as to those who are acutely ill. A good history and physical examination, screening laboratory tests to achieve a careful appraisal of cardiopulmonary status, and a review of the patient's problem to clarify the strategy and goals of the undertaking are all essential to safe endoscopy.

A thorough review of the risks and benefits of the procedure, including the possibility of a cardiovascular complication from conscious sedation, of perforation and bleeding, of a failed polyp removal, or of inability to determine whether a cancer is present, are all possible outcomes and should be discussed with the patient before commencing the procedure. Abdominal exploration may be required if these adverse events occur and must be accepted by the patient prior to proceeding with the endoscopy.

DIAGNOSTIC AND THERAPEUTIC UPPER ENDOSCOPY

Diagnostic Upper Endoscopy

Esophagogastroduodenoscopy for diagnosis had a complication rate of 1.3/1000 cases according to an American Society for Gastrointestinal Endoscopy survey that included 211,410 examinations.[14] The major complications of upper endoscopy include (1) the patient experiencing a seizure while the pharynx is being anesthetized; (2) respiratory arrest; (3) aspiration of teeth and dentures, blood, or gastric contents into the tracheobronchial tree; (4) perforation of the esophagus and stomach; (5) bleeding; and (6) failure to diagnose cancer in a non-healing ulcer.

Seizure. Overdose of local anesthetics should be watched for, particularly if generous amounts are swallowed in preparing for passage of the scope, as seizures will result. A small premedicating dose of diazepam will usually protect against this possibility. If seizure activity does occur, protection of the airway is the first priority. Additional incremental doses of diazepam or barbiturates will usually control the seizures.

Respiratory Arrest. Compromise of the upper airway must be guarded against, particularly in patients with chronic obstructive pulmonary disease. Forty-five percent of patients undergoing endoscopic procedures (both upper and lower) were noted to have oxygen saturations less than 90% without clinical signs or symptoms. The presence of the scope in the pharynx causing a degree of mechanical obstruction, combined with some intravenous sedation, analgesics, and local anesthetics in patients who ordinarily have a high PCO_2, creates a potentially dangerous situation that can lead to respiratory arrest. When respiratory arrest occurs, patients will usually respond to prompt reversal of all drugs and vigorous bag-mask ventilation. However, endotracheal intubation should be carried out promptly if necessary for protection of the airway.[10]

Aspiration. Loose teeth in elderly patients can be a hazard. They may be dislodged and aspirated secondary to placement of the mouthguard or passage of the scope through the oropharynx. If loose teeth are noted prior to the endoscopy, it may be necessary to remove them before proceeding. The patient should be consulted about this beforehand whenever possible.

In patients with brisk GI bleeding, particularly those bleeding from esophageal varices, it is wise to intubate the trachea before proceeding with passage of the endoscope. This guarantees protection of the airway and avoids aspiration of blood and gastric contents into the tracheobronchial tree, which could then produce aspiration pneumonia. If the patient is bleeding actively, it is necessary to thoroughly irrigate and empty the clots from the stomach using a large Ewald tube and iced saline before passing the scope. The clots will obscure the view, preventing accurate assessment of the cause of bleeding, and will not pass through the suction channel, thereby blocking it and preventing suction of insufflated air and blood and possibly leading to overdistention of the stomach and small bowel.

If aspiration of teeth or dentures occurs, they should be removed by bronchoscopy during the same procedure. If aspiration of blood and gastric contents occurs, bronchoscopy and thorough irrigation of the tracheobronchial tree may reduce the severity of the aspiration pneumonia.

Perforation. The esophagus can readily become perforated just beyond the cricopharyngeus muscle, where the esophagus is fixed and sits on a rigid vertebral column offering no opportunity for flexibility (particularly in the kyphotic patient) when the scope is passed. Unsuspected esophageal diverticula may lie in wait for the passing scope and cause perforation. Peptic esophagitis and stricture in the lower third of the esophagus, particularly when the distal esophagus is inflamed and stiff, will not permit the esophagogastric junction to accommodate to a fairly rigid advancing scope at its natural anterior curve, thus producing another common cause of perforation. Overdistention of the stomach, combined with weakened areas at biopsy sites, ulcerations, or previously sealed-off microperforations will result in blowouts and soilage of the peritoneum by erosive gastric and duodenal contents. Laparotomy, closure of the perforation, irrigation of the peritoneal cavity and, when appropriate, gastric resection may all be necessary in these circumstances.

Bleeding. The identification of the source of bleeding in the upper GI tract is critical to the formulation of strategies for its control. The surgical management of a bleeding duodenal ulcer, a bleeding gastric cancer, gastritis, a Mallory-Weiss tear of the cardioesophageal junction, or varices is different in each condition. Success or failure of the outcome depends on accurate observations and interpretations of the procedure. Errors in diagnosis are common, particularly in the presence of brisk bleeding.

Failure to Diagnose Cancer. Non-healing gastric or distal esophageal ulcers require aggressive attempts at diagnosis with multiple biopsies, brushings, and washings. Sampling errors occur, and if the results are negative, the procedure should be repeated in 3 to 6 weeks. If healing has still not taken place, surgical treatment must be entertained.

Small cell carcinoma and lymphoma of the stomach are notoriously difficult to diagnose histologically and distinguish from chronic inflammation, particularly in the small biopsy specimens obtained through the endoscope.

Upper endoscopy by skilled, well-trained professionals is a safe and minimally uncomfortable procedure. It is, however, invasive and requires the cooperation of a relaxed patient. It helps greatly if the patient is well informed, knows what to expect, and has confidence in the endoscopist.

Therapeutic Upper Endoscopy

Therapeutic upper endoscopy has a much higher complication rate because of the more complicated techniques on much sicker patients (compare endoscopic retrograde cholangiopancreatography [ERCP] 21.6 complications/1000 procedures in 3884 examinations and esophageal dilation for achalasia, 18.4 complications/1000 procedures in 1224 patients). The most common complications are bleeding and perforation (see previous discussion).

Therapeutic interventions include (1) sclerotherapy or banding of varices, (2) control of gastric and duodenal hemorrhage, (3) ERCP and papillotomy for cholangitis with placement of a nasobiliary catheter, (4) removal of common duct stones, (5) transduodenal stent placement for common duct obstruction that is usually secondary to cholangiocarcinoma of the common duct or carcinoma of the head of the pancreas, and (6) percutaneous endoscopic gastrostomy.

Control of Bleeding. It is difficult to separate bleeding from the pathologic process, such as an ulcer, gastritis, or varices from bleeding produced secondary to biopsy, sclerotherapy, or banding of varices. Moderate bleeding from ulcers can usually be controlled, first with irrigation using 1:1000 epinephrine solution and then with injection around the base of the ulcers with epinephrine followed by alcohol or with applications of a heater probe or neodymium-doped yttrium-aluminum-garnet laser.

Briskly bleeding varices may need compression with a Sengstaken tube for 8 hours to staunch the torrential hemorrhage and correct the clotting factors. This then permits a return under more favorable conditions so that the bleeding point can be visualized and either banded or thrombosed with sclerotherapy more safely. Sclerotherapy of gastric varices has been discontinued because of the high incidence of full-thickness necrosis of the stomach wall from the sclerosant, with resulting perforation. Usually, if the endoscopist can visualize the bleeding point it can be controlled. When the bleeding is torrential, open surgery is the only alternative to exsanguination, as with gastroduodenal artery erosion by an ulcer.

Endoscopic Retrograde Cholangiopancreatography and Papillotomy. The most common complications of ERCP and papillotomy are the inability to cannulate a tight ampullary orifice, pancreatitis, bleeding, perforation, the inability to remove an elusive stone that floats up and down in a large common duct, and removal of a stone that is too large even for the papillotomized ampullary sphincter.

Non-cannulation of the Ampulla of Vater. Often, patients with chronic cholecystitis or cholelithiasis with choledocholithiasis and a mild degree of pancreatitis have scarring of the ampullary orifice from chronic inflammation, which makes the cannulation of the tight, scarred ampulla extremely difficult or impossible. Preliminary papillotomy with a sharkfin or needle knife papillotome may be the only means of cannulating the ampulla, but this is very hazardous and should be undertaken only by the most experienced operators.

Pancreatitis. The injection of contrast medium for the ERCP under pressure will occasionally produce an episode of pancreatitis, which usually clears in several days. If the bile is infected, injection of dye under pressure may produce an episode of severe cholangitis with bacteremia, gram-negative sepsis, and hypotension. This will require, above all, relief of the biliary obstruction, by (1) papillotomy and further decompression by placement of a nasobiliary catheter or (2) decompression from above using the percutaneous transhepatic biliary decompression technique in the interventional radiology suite, or even (3) open surgery with common duct exploration, stone extractions, and T-tube placement.

Bleeding at the Papillotomy Site. The papillotomy, when carried out, must not go beyond the transverse hood or fold over the ampulla of Vater. A small artery is fairly constantly present there and will produce brisk bleeding that is difficult to control. It usually stops in response to epinephrine injections and washes but can be avoided by not carrying the papillotomy beyond the transverse fold.

Perforation of the Duodenum. When the papillotomy is carried beyond the transverse fold, there is also the risk of going outside the duodenal wall, since the intramural portion of the common duct stops at the transverse fold. The temptation to extend the papillotomy to accommodate large stones will lead to perforation and must be avoided. If perforation occurs, it can occasionally be managed conservatively with nasogastric suction and antibiotics. If there is any question of generalized peritonitis, or if deterioration of the patient's condition is obvious, laparotomy, repair, and even diverticularization of the duodenum with an absorbable suture in the pylorus and gastrojejunostomy bypass may be necessary.

Non-removal of Common Duct Stones. The stone that floats up and down in the common duct, eluding the Dormier basket or Fogarty balloon, may pass on its own. In the event that the stone cannot be removed during the procedure, it is often possible for the patient to pass the stone once the ampulla has been papillotomized. Stones that are very large, on the order of 2 cm and more, may require external shock wave lithotripsy or direct application of laser shock wave lithotripsy using a fiber passed through the side-viewing endoscope into the ampulla and common duct. A Dormier basket with stone crushing capability may also be employed in these circumstances.

If the stone still cannot be crushed, and the basket cannot be removed because the stone is impacted in the crusher, the basket should be removed with open surgery.

Stent Placement. The placement of common duct stents to relieve common duct obstruction from primary common duct tumors or tumors of the head of the pancreas is a demanding and complex technique. It can result in perforation of the common duct through its side wall at the site of the tumor, since the tumor makes the common duct very rigid and unaccommodating to the rigid stent. Duodenal perforation and periduodenal bile collections usually require surgical treatment. This is most unfortunate in this group of patients who are usually near death and in whom the stent placement was undertaken to avoid surgical intervention.

Ampullary, Common Duct, and Pancreatic Duct Pressure Studies. These studies often result in episodes of pancreatitis that can be very severe. When pancreatitis occurs, it requires vigorous management—that is, putting the GI tract at rest and treating with antibiotics if there is secondary infection (characterized by a high white cell count and fever). Waiting and observing are best; often the episode will subside.

Percutaneous Endoscopic Gastrostomy. Patients who are candidates for percutaneous endoscopic gastrostomy usually are unable to swallow because of advanced head and neck cancers, neurologic disability secondary to a cerebrovascular accident, or esophageal cancers or strictures. They are thus debilitated, nutritionally deprived, and prone to complications. The passage of the gastroscope into the stomach is necessary to select the location in the stomach for the gastrostomy tube and later to ensure that the tube is placed firmly against the anterior wall, which protects against leakage. Thus, bulky tumors of the hypopharynx, surgical strictures of the cricopharyngeus muscle, tumors, strictures of the esophagus or the esophagogastric junction, some types of gastric resection, or abnormal displacement of the transverse colon between a low-lying stomach and the abdominal wall may all make percutaneous endoscopic gastrostomy difficult or impossible. In such cases, open gastrostomy under local anesthesia is preferred. Complications can occur, such as perforation of the esophagus, respiratory impairment from obstruction of a narrowed hypopharynx by tumor and the presence of the endoscope, passage of the tube through an overlying colon or small bowel, or premature removal of the gastrostomy tube before a tract has formed and the stomach is firmly fixed to the anterior wall; these complications may require surgical exploration for repair.

DIAGNOSTIC AND THERAPEUTIC LOWER ENDOSCOPY

Diagnostic Lower Endoscopy

The successful intubation of the colon to the cecum is a complex and demanding technique that requires a cooperative patient, a good colonic preparation, a skillful endoscopist, and anatomic conditions that lend themselves to passage of the scope. Lack of any one of these conditions means that the procedure should not be attempted. Complications include (1) poor colonic preparation and a dehydrated patient, (2) respiratory arrest with conscious sedation, (3) failure to reach the cecum, (4) perforation, (5) transient bacteremia, and (6) bleeding.

Poor Colonic Preparation and a Dehydrated Patient with Excessive Fecal Material in Bowel Lumen. Bowel preparation with either an isoosmotic solution in large volume (4 L) or thorough purging with laxatives and cleansing enemas ensures that the colon will be cleaned out well, which is essential if small lesions are not to be missed. Some patients become dehydrated and hypovolemic after the purges and require rehydration lest they become hypotensive after the sedation. Polyethylene glycol electrolyte solutions avoid this problem. A purge is contraindicated if obstruction is suspected, since perforation may occur. These patients must be cleaned out with enemas and medicated suppositories. Prophylactic antibiotics must be given if the patient has any indwelling foreign bodies, including artificial orthopedic joints and hardware.[13] Coagulation factors and red blood cell volume should be restored if bleeding has been a problem and polypectomy is a possibility.

If large amounts of fecal material are in the bowel, the procedure should be terminated and the procedure rescheduled. Lesions will be missed under these circumstances, and the suction channel of the scope will become blocked, resulting in excessive amounts of air being retained in the colon, with its attendant risks. Elderly patients, patients with extensive diverticulosis, "burned-out" colitis patients, and those who chronically use laxatives and have "lazy" colons may require a 3- to 4-day liquid diet and additional medicated suppositories to obtain a satisfactorily cleaned out colon, permitting adequate inspection of its entirety.

Conscious Sedation and Respiratory Arrest. Colonoscopy is an inherently unpleasant experience, and conscious sedation is employed to make this procedure tolerable because a cooperative patient is essential. Meperidine (Demerol) is used to control pain and diazepam or midazolam is used to provide euphoria and amnesia. Small test doses should be given initially, since older patients, hypovolemic patients, and those who are critically ill may become profoundly hypotensive and apneic after even small doses.

The drugs are given incrementally during the procedure while monitoring for hypotension, patient unresponsiveness, or apnea. If respiratory depression, apnea, or unresponsiveness occurs, the patient should undergo drug reversal therapy at once, with bag-mask ventilation if needed. Usually, this will be sufficient, but endotracheal intubation and full cardiopulmonary resuscitation should be initiated immediately, before it is too late, if it appears that the patient remains unresponsive and in ventilatory arrest. Marked vagal stimulation from heavy manipulation of the bowel with the scope will produce bradycardia, but the moderate stimu-

lation of the procedure will usually be enough to compensate for this and counteract the sedatives' effects on respiratory drive.

Remember, if in doubt, the patient must undergo drug reversal therapy immediately with naloxone (Narcan) for opiates and flumazenil (Mazicon [Rocke Laboratories, Nutley, NJ]) for benzodiazepines. Fragile, elderly, dehydrated, or chronically ill patients are extremely sensitive to even small doses of sedatives and analgesics, so great care must be taken in administering these agents. It should be the sole responsibility of the nurse monitoring the patient to be aware of the patient's reactions; he or she should not be distracted with other duties during conscious sedation.

General anesthesia is generally to be avoided, as it deprives the endoscopist of the valuable symptom of pain caused by severe traction on the mesentery and distention of the bowel.

All patients should undergo drug reversal with naloxone before leaving the endoscopy suite to prevent sleepiness or unsteadiness on the way home after the procedure. A thorough discussion of the procedure with the patient beforehand as to what to expect in terms of the mechanics of the procedure and the discomfort entailed will often result in a more confident, less frightened patient who can cooperate fully, is more at ease, and requires less medication.

Failure to Reach the Cecum. There are a number of patients with severe diverticulosis or adhesions from previous surgery or radiotherapy who have stenoses of the bowel lumen or sharp angulations of the bowel with kinks that simply will not permit the safe passage of the scope. To attempt passage under these circumstances poses a significant risk of perforation. Similarly, the anatomy in many patients with very large sigmoid loops and pendulous, long transverse colons, coupled with a very acutely angulated splenic flexure, makes intubation to the cecum very difficult. Abdominal compression, internal stiffening devices, and a sigmoid overtube have been employed to overcome these problems. However, these maneuvers carry risks as well and must be used in moderation by endoscopists familiar with their application. In experienced hands, these techniques, in addition to repositioning the patient on the table, make it very rare that the cecum cannot be reached (as long as there are no obstructing lesions and no sharp angulations in the sigmoid colon). If what the examiner is doing does not work, something different must be tried.

When failure to reach the cecum occurs, a barium enema should be given to establish the lack of any lesions in the unexplored colon. If the colonoscopy attempt was vigorous, involving extensive manipulation of the bowel, the barium enema can be deferred for 6 weeks until weaknesses produced in the bowel by the colonoscopy attempt can heal completely.

When the passage of the scope cannot proceed because of excessive pain, either from formation of a loop and traction on the mesentery or spasm of the bowel, which then grips the scope so that movement is difficult and painful, intravenous glucagon may release the spasm and permit the scope to advance easily. Withdrawal of the scope, straightening out the loops, and shortening the course within the colon often result in eventual advancement. One often has to pull back to get ahead.

Flexible Sigmoidoscopy. This procedure is analagous to full colonoscopy with all of the same caveats and complications. The important difference is that many operators who perform flexible sigmoidoscopy may not have had formal training or much experience, so problems are more frequent in this group of patients, all other things being equal.

Perforation. The incidence of perforation associated with simple diagnostic colonoscopy varies according to the survey, but it is on the order of 1/300 to 1/700 colonoscopies.[14–16] The perforation can result from penetration of the tip of the scope into the bowel wall or elbow-type splitting of the tinea of the bowel from side pressure exerted by a loop of the scope against a loop of the colon. Pressure blowout may occur through a diverticulum or in an area of weakness caused by a biopsy or electrocautery polypectomy burn.

Free air in the peritoneal cavity, abdominal pain and tenderness, subcutaneous emphysema, and fever indicate peritonitis, and in most cases, exploratory laparotomy, segmental resection of the perforated segment, and primary anastomosis if soilage of the peritoneal cavity is minimal are the recommended treatments, along with a vigorous washing out of the abdominal cavity.

There is a group of patients with limited or partial-thickness burns of the bowel wall or retroperitoneal perforation with very minimal injury to the bowel wall and little or no contamination who are being treated expectantly without laparotomy but with antibiotics, nasogastric suction, and nothing by mouth for bowel rest; these patients will often do well. If there is deterioration in their condition, such as increasing signs of peritoneal irritation, laparotomy is carried out immediately and repair of the bowel wall is performed.

Therapeutic Lower Endoscopy

Polypectomy, relief of colonic overdistention (Ogilvie's syndrome), and coagulation of angiodysplasia are indications for therapeutic lower endoscopy.

The advent of colonoscopic polypectomy, popularized by Wolff and Shinya[20] in the early 1970s, has prevented literally thousands of laparotomies and colon resections, which were previously the standard treatment for newly discovered polyps. The downside of colonoscopic polypectomy is bleeding, perforation, and inadequately excised cancer invading the base of the polyp.

In therapeutic colonoscopy, the complication rate after polypectomy includes a 2% incidence of hemorrhage, a 0.3% incidence of perforation, and a 0.1% mortality rate. This complication rate, while significant, is acceptable considering the greater morbidity and mortality of open colon surgery for the same lesions for which colonoscopic polypectomy is performed.[17, 18]

Bleeding. Hemorrhage following polypectomy is also rare, occurring in about 1/500 to 600 polyps.[12] It almost always stops, and one must guard against recoagulating the stalk unless absolutely necessary because perforation may result. The preferred way of dealing with a bleeding polypectomy site is to regrasp the pedicle and apply light, intermittent, coagulating current in short bursts with ample intervals to allow the heat to dissipate. The snare is left on and 10 to 15 minutes is allowed to pass. The snare is then released and the situation reassessed. Irrigation with 1:10,000 or 1:1000 epinephrine solution will reduce bleeding, permitting accurate replacement of the snare. Bleeding almost always stops, and it is important not to overreact to it and risk perforation of the bowel with overapplication of cautery.

Perforation. Electrocautery snare polypectomy may result in a partial- or full-thickness burn through the bowel wall, producing pain with no signs of peritonitis. When applying coagulating current to the snare, it is important to use short bursts with intervals in between to permit the heat to dissipate, thus avoiding a wider coagulation of tissue than necessary or desired. A mixed cutting and coagulating current is then used to sever the polyp from the bowel wall. Care must be taken to inflate the bowel so that the polyp does not touch the opposite wall and thereby conduct coagulating current to the other parts of the colon, injuring the wall at that point of contact as well.

The incidence of perforation following polypectomy on different series runs from 3/1000 to 2/100 polypectomies.[12]

Pedunculated polyps lend themselves to the lassoing technique with the electrocautery snare. Care must be taken not to close the snare completely before the coagulating current is applied. The polyp should be recovered for histologic analysis. If the polyp is mislaid in the colon, 300 or 400 ml of saline is infused into the lumen and irrigation is performed to flush the polyp out. Usually, it can be recovered by readvancing the scope and carefully searching the lumen in both directions, keeping in mind gravity's effect and the patient's position on the table. The snare or polyp grasper may facilitate the recovery of the excised lesion as well. Accurate location of each and every polyp removed is essential in case a polyp is later discovered to be malignant with involvement of the stalk, making segmental resection of the colon necessary. On occasion, clinical suspicion or frozen section of a suspicious polyp indicates that segmental resection should be done. In these cases, injection of the polyp site with sterile India ink facilitates identification of the site. Resection should then be done before the India ink spreads out too widely in the bowel mesentery.

Sessile polyps, particularly those greater than 1 cm, are a real challenge. They usually cannot be excised without risk of tenting up the full thickness of the bowel wall, which would produce a perforation. Therefore, piecemeal resection—first one end, then the other end, then the middle—is carried out, taking care not to overcoagulate the polyp site and burn through the bowel wall. Large, sessile, villous polyps have a significant incidence of adenocarcinoma, and the distance to the lamina propria is therefore shorter, making colon resection more of a possibility in these polyps than in the pedunculated variety. Because of sampling errors, colonoscopic biopsy of large villous adenomas may fail to diagnose an adenocarcinoma even though it is there; therefore, plenty of biopsy specimens should be taken. Decisions about resection may have to be made on clinical grounds. It is important to review the pathology slides personally with the pathologist, since chronic inflammation is very hard to distinguish from lymphomas, and clinical input is helpful to the pathologist in interpreting the relationship of the coagulation resection burn to the pedicle and the focus of cancer.

Ogilvie's Syndrome. Colonoscopic decompression of idiopathic colonic distention (Ogilvie's syndrome) is often effective in relieving the distention. It may have to be repeated two or three times, and care must be taken to avoid overdistention of the bowel with air in the process of passing the scope. Blowouts are most often seen in the cecum, since the cecum experiences the greatest pressure in accordance with Laplace's law. An overtube is helpful and at the end of the procedure may be left in place for several days.

Angiodysplasia. Multiple episodes of brisk colonic bleeding in patients with normal results on barium enema suggest angiodysplasia as the cause of bleeding. Electrocoagulation or laser photocoagulation is effective in controlling these arteriovenous malformations, but these treatments may have to be performed in stages, since overapplication of heat by either method of current will result in full-thickness necrosis of the bowel wall and perforation. Multiple site coagulation increases this risk of perforation and, under these circumstances, multiple colonoscopies with staged coagulation of the lesions is recommended; even segmental resection of the colon in severe cases may be advisable.

CONCLUSION

If a patient is ill enough to require an invasive procedure, it makes the procedure inherently risky. Complications are a way of life for the busy surgeon who cares for seriously ill patients, if for no other reason than the law of random chance. Good surgeons are obsessed with reducing the incidence and severity of these complications and always consider the risks of everything they do, balancing those risks in the equation of necessity and measurable benefit to the patient. When complications occur, early recognition and appropriate damage control will reduce the morbidity of the adverse event.

As in most cases in medicine, the alert, well-informed, and attentive surgeon with a generous amount of common sense is the best prevention for complications and the best solution for them if they occur.[19]

References

1. Sapienza PC, Levine GM, Pomerantz S, et al. Impact of a quality assurance program on gastrointestinal endoscopy. Gastroenterology 102:387–393, 1992.
2. Fleischer DE, Al-Kawas F, Benjamin S, et al. Prospective evaluation of complications in an endoscopy unit: use of the A/S/G/E quality care guidelines. Gastrointest Endosc 38:411–414, 1992.
3. Brennan TA, Leape LL, Laird NM, et al. Incidence of adverse events and negligence in hospitalized patients. Results from the Harvard Medical Practice Study. I. N Engl J Med 324:370–376, 1991.
4. Leape LL, Brennan TA, Laird N, et al. The nature of

adverse events in hospitalized patients. N Engl J Med 324:377–384, 1991.

5. Morrissey JF, Reichelderfer M. Gastrointestinal endoscopy. N Engl J Med 325:1142–1149, 1991.

6. Morrissey JF, Reichelderfer M. Gastrointestinal endoscopy. N Engl J Med 325:1214–1222, 1991.

7. Simon IB, Lewis RJ, Satava RM. A safe method for sedating and monitoring patients for upper and lower gastrointestinal endoscopy. Surg Endosc 4:58, 1990.

8. Barkin JS, Krieger B, Binder M, et al. Oxygen desaturation and changes in breathing patterns in patients undergoing colonoscopy and gastroscopy. Gastrointest Endosc 35:526–530, 1989.

9. Gross JB, Long WB. Nasal oxygen alleviates hypoxemia in colonoscopy patients sedated with midazolam and meperidine. Gastrointest Endosc 36:26–29, 1990.

10. Lieberman DA, Wuerker CK, Katon RM. Cardiopulmonary risk of esophagogastroduodenoscopy: role of endoscopic diameter and systemic sedation. Gastroenterology 88:468–472, 1985.

11. Fleischer DE. Monitoring for conscious sedation: perspective of the gastrointestinal endoscopist. Gastrointest Endosc 36(Suppl):S19, 1990.

12. Vennes JA. Infectious complications of gastrointestinal endoscopy. Dig Dis Sci 26(Suppl):60S–64S, 1981.

13. Stray N, Midtvedt T, Valnes K, et al. Endoscopy related bacteremia. Scand J Gastroenterol 13:345–347, 1978.

14. Silvis SE, Nebel O, Rogers G, et al. Endoscopic complications. Results of the 1974 American Society for Gastrointestinal Endoscopy Survey. JAMA 235:928–930, 1976.

15. Ghazi A, Grossman M. Complications of colonoscopy and polypectomy. Surg Clin North Am 62:889–896, 1982.

16. Macrae FA, Tan KG, Williams CB. Towards safer colonoscopy: a report on the complications of 5000 diagnostic or therapeutic colonoscopies. Gut 24:376–383, 1983.

17. Fruhmorgen P, Demling L. Complications of diagnostic and therapeutic colonoscopy in the Federal Republic of Germany. Results of an inquiry. Endoscopy 11:146–150, 1979.

18. Brynitz S, Kjaergard H, Struckmann J. Perforations from colonoscopy during diagnosis and treatment of polyps. Ann Chir Gynecol 75:142–145, 1986.

19. Hunt R. Towards safer colonoscopy. Gut 24:371–375, 1983.

20. Wolff WI, Shinya H. Polypectomy via the fiberoptic colonoscope—removal of neoplasms beyond the reach of the sigmoidoscope. N Engl J Med 288:329–333, 1973.

34

Complications of Laparoscopy

Bruce D. Schirmer

Laparoscopy has commonly been incorporated into gynecologic practice for more than 2 decades. In rapidly increasing numbers in the last 3 years, general surgeons have begun to use laparoscopy in their practices as well. Initially, laparoscopic cholecystectomy was the only procedure performed by most general surgeons, but now the general surgeon is beginning to use laparoscopic techniques for various other abdominal conditions. Meanwhile, laparoscopic techniques for gynecologic procedures have also continued to evolve and have found further applications during this time. Finally, urologists, pediatric surgeons, and cardiothoracic surgeons are also using video telescopic techniques in their practices. As the use of minimal access surgery expands, continued monitoring of the safety and efficacy of adapting the technology to a wider range of procedures is necessary to foster optimal care of the surgical patient.

This discussion addresses the complications and their incidence in those general surgical laparoscopic procedures, including diagnostic laparoscopy, now being commonly practiced. Some attention is also devoted to the potential complications, whose incidence is not yet clearly established, in those general surgical procedures whose laparoscopic applications are still in the early stages.

COMPLICATIONS OF DIAGNOSTIC LAPAROSCOPY

Diagnostic laparoscopy is associated with a low incidence of morbidity and mortality. In the gynecologic literature, the reported complication rate for laparoscopy has been from 0.3% to 2.3% for major complications and 1.1% to 5.1% for minor complications, with a mortality rate of 0.005% to 0.05%.[1-4] Complications can be divided into those associated with the establishment of the pneumoperitoneum and those associated with further diagnostic manipulations, such as liver biopsy or other diagnostic procedures. The addition of such additional invasive diagnostic procedures increases the incidence and seriousness of the complications.

Complications of Veress Needle Insertion

Insertion of the Veress needle is associated with the potential for its misplacement and insufflation of gas into a space other than the free peritoneal cavity. In such circumstances, the complications can vary from insignificant to life-threatening.

Use of proper technique in Veress needle insertion minimizes the incidence of such complications. Insertion of the needle in the umbilical or infraumbilical skin fold is associated with the least difficulty in entering the peritoneal cavity, since the abdominal wall is at its thinnest in this location. Decompression of the bladder, with a urethral catheter, and the stomach, with a nasogastric tube, prior to Veress needle insertion minimizes the possibility of perforating these organs with the needle.

Aspiration is performed through the needle after insertion in an effort to recognize promptly if perforation of a blood vessel or hollow viscus has occurred. If there is evidence on aspiration of blood or intestinal fluid, it is assumed that injury from Veress needle insertion has occurred until proved otherwise. Laparoscopic examination of the injury is then indicated, if possible. The injury should be treated appropriately based on its size and the patient's clinical course. Observation alone may suffice for small direct needle punctures of a viscus or vessel if no significant peritoneal contamination or bleeding results. The surgeon should, however, follow a conservative course in the management of such incidents, ensuring that patient safety is never compromised. Conversion to laparotomy and repair of the injury is always indicated if peritoneal contamination or bleeding is confirmed by laparoscopy. The same course should be followed if there is any doubt as to the extent of injury. Surgeons who are laparoscopic novices should be extremely cautious and aware that the extent of such an injury might not be fully appreciated because of the inability to visualize it laparoscopically. Any postoperative signs of incompletely treated injury that suggest either intraabdominal blood loss or peritonitis should be followed by immediate laparotomy to fully define the extent of the missed injury.

Careful attention must be paid to the intraabdominal pressure registered through the Veress needle as it is attached to the automatic insufflation device. The needle's baseline pressure when it is exposed to the atmosphere should be known and used as a basis for comparison. Excess pressure (usually in the range of 8 mm Hg or greater) suggests the needle is not in the free peritoneal space. Shifting the position and direction of the needle tip may often reduce the pressure if it is resting against a viscus or the omentum or is in a preperitoneal location. Insufflation should never proceed unless the measured pressure is at an acceptably low level.

The patient's abdominal wall may present special difficulties that must be considered before attempting to place a Veress needle for creation of a pneumoperitoneum. The presence of a previous abdominal incision, particularly one involving the midline near the umbilicus, is a contraindication to direct blind Veress needle placement in the umbilical area. Instead, two different techniques should be considered. The safest is to use an open laparoscopy approach in which a small 1.5- to 2-cm incision is made in the infraumbilical area. Direct dissection of the abdominal wall layers, allowing entry into the peritoneal cavity under direct visualization, is performed. Open laparoscopy has its advocates as the procedure of choice for initiating all laparoscopic procedures. Selective use of this technique in patients with previous abdominal incisions can result in a complication rate for laparoscopic procedures that is not significantly different from that in patients without such incisions.[5] Alternatively, the Veress needle can be placed in a secondary entrance location—an abdominal quadrant that is least likely to have intraabdominal adhesions—and insufflation performed. This latter technique is slightly less safe than open laparoscopy, since there is still the chance that previous intraperitoneal adhesions could be present despite a location distant from the scar.

Obesity adds difficulty to infraumbilical Veress needle insertion. When an insertion technique is used with the needle in a 45° angle toward the pelvis, the severely obese patient's abdominal wall is less likely to be penetrated with the needle tip, and preperitoneal insufflation is instead performed (Fig. 34–1).

Direct insertion of the trocar into the abdominal cavity through a small infraumbilical incision, using a technique similar to Veress needle insertion, has also been shown to be a safe method of initiating laparoscopy in patients who have not had previous abdominal incisions. Complications using this method are comparable in frequency to those of Veress needle insertion in the gynecologic literature.[6] It has been our observation, however, that the most severe complications associated with general surgical laparoscopic procedures are a result of trocar insertion injuries rather than Veress needle insertion (see further on). Most gynecologists and general surgeons use a Veress needle approach to create a pneumoperitoneum prior to trocar insertion.[7]

Complications Associated With Pneumoperitoneum

Insufflation of gas into the improper space is a common cause of complications associated with diagnostic laparoscopy. Subcutaneous emphysema is the most common such problem and occurs at a rate of approximately 0.43% to 2% in laparoscopy.[8] However, the potential for gas insufflation to result in pneumomediastinum, pneumothorax, pneumopericardium, and omental and mesenteric emphysema is also well known.

Carbon dioxide is the gas commonly employed for all therapeutic and many diagnostic laparoscopic procedures, whereas some groups use compressed air or nitrous oxide instead for diagnostic laparoscopy.[9] Small amounts of sub-

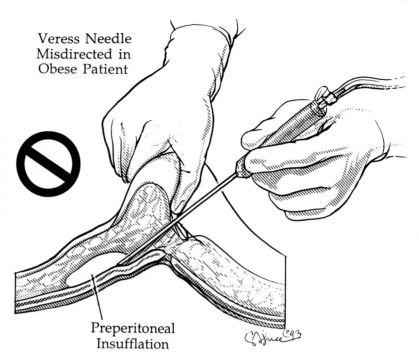

Veress Needle
Misdirected in
Obese Patient

Figure 34–1. Illustration of the potential difficulty of inserting a Veress needle correctly through the wall of an obese patient if the standard 45° angle of penetration is used. The thickness of the abdominal wall predisposes to inadvertent preperitoneal insufflation.

Preperitoneal
Insufflation

cutaneous emphysema from carbon dioxide are usually well tolerated. The anesthesiologist must be aware of the need for increased ventilation to increase the exchange of carbon dioxide. Since an end tidal carbon dioxide monitor is standard equipment in modern anesthesiology, the sudden increase in this parameter without other obvious explanation should lead to the immediate suspicion of subcutaneous emphysema. Its presence is easily confirmed with examination of the abdominal and chest wall and neck, the usual sites of gas dissemination. We have observed that subcutaneous emphysema is more common in thin elderly patients, in whom the subcutaneous tissues are relatively loose. This finding may allow easier dissection of the gas through the subcutaneous tissue planes.

Once subcutaneous emphysema is recognized, its treatment may take several forms based on its severity. If the amount of subcutaneous emphysema is small, the patient's cardiovascular system is sound, the patient's plasma pH is not excessively lowered (from tissue production of carbonic acid caused by absorption of the carbon dioxide gas), and the operation is near its termination, the procedure may proceed to its timely conclusion before the pneumoperitoneum is deflated. However, if any of these factors suggest patient safety will be compromised by worsening of the subcutaneous emphysema, the pneumoperitoneum should be immediately deflated, the carbon dioxide insufflation stopped, and the operation converted to

an open laparotomy for its safe completion. Rapid absorption of subcutaneous emphysema is the rule; patients will usually have few signs remaining on physical examination after only several hours in the postoperative recovery suite.

In addition to stopping carbon dioxide insufflation, increasing the ventilatory rate to maintain pH is indicated for treating significant subcutaneous emphysema. Administration of sodium bicarbonate as a measure to correct the pH instead is to be avoided, as excessive alkalosis will easily result once the carbon dioxide is absorbed.

Although subcutaneous emphysema is the most common complication of misdirected carbon dioxide insufflation, gas embolism is a far less common but much more serious complication. The incidence is approximately 0.016%[10] and can be rapidly fatal if not immediately detected or if the bolus of gas is too large. Small amounts of carbon dioxide are better tolerated than other gases, such as compressed air or nitrous oxide. A gas embolus theoretically occurs only when a vascular laceration allows entrance of gas into the venous space. In some reported cases, however, the site of such entry is never found. Treatment of gas embolism involves immediate cessation of gas insufflation, placing the patient in the right-side-down position, and passing a central venous catheter into the right side of the heart to aspirate the gas if possible. Hyperbaric oxygen treatment may also be of benefit if available,[11] and treatment using cardiopulmonary bypass has also been reported.[12]

Cardiac arrest can rarely occur following the establishment of a pneumoperitoneum. The incidence is about 1 in 2500 cases.[13] The causes leading to cardiac arrest include air embolism, decreased venous return to the heart secondary to elevated intraabdominal pressure, hypercapnia or anoxia from hypoventilation during anesthesia, and a profound vagal response to peritoneal distention. Treatment is prompt deflation of the pneumoperitoneum, as well as cardiovascular resuscitative and supportive measures.

Cardiac arrhythmias can also result as a consequence of the creation of the pneumoperitoneum. The mechanism of such arrhythmias is felt to be secondary to the same cardiovascular consequences that may result in cardiac arrest, but on a lesser scale. Patients with a history of cardiac arrhythmias are at increased risk for complications during laparoscopy. Arrhythmias are usually self-limited but may on occasion lead to serious hemodynamic consequences. The incidence of such events is less than 1%. In patients at increased risk, the use of careful perioperative monitoring of cardiovascular and pulmonary parameters is indicated to assess and immediately treat any arrhythmias that might arise.

Complications of Trocar Insertion

Trocar insertion during diagnostic or therapeutic laparoscopy can result in the complication of hemorrhage. The most serious, immediately life-threatening complication of laparoscopy, other than cardiac arrest, is trocar injury to one of the great vessels of the abdomen. This occurs in approximately 0.1% of cases or less. Because of the severity of this complication, however, its immediate recognition and prompt treatment are essential if mortality is to be avoided. Emergent open laparotomy with appropriate surgical treatment of the vascular injury is indicated.

Less severe hemorrhagic complications may result from trocar insertion, the most common of which is bleeding from the abdominal wall. Such bleeding may be immediately apparent or may present in the postoperative period as an abdominal wall hematoma. The loss of blood from such an event can be significant, requiring blood transfusion and resulting in considerable pain and discomfort for the patient. Surveillance for such bleeding at trocar sites should accom-

pany both the insertion of the trocar and its removal at the end of the procedure. Peritoneal surface as well as skin inspection should be performed.

Trocar site bleeding can be treated in a variety of ways. Enlarging the incision for better exposure of the vessel is one option. Another is use of a full-thickness abdominal wall suture externally tied over a pledget to prevent skin injury. Direct pressure using the inflated balloon of a Foley catheter may also achieve effective tamponade of the bleeding site.

Visceral injury from laparoscopy occurs at a low but recognized rate. In a recent large survey of nearly 37,000 gynecologic laparoscopic procedures performed in the United States, the rate of unintended laparotomy to manage intraabdominal injuries to bowel or urinary tract was 0.16%. The rate of laparotomy for hemorrhage was 0.26%.[3] A large survey of gynecologists in the United Kingdom showed a bowel injury rate of 0.18%, a urinary tract injury rate of 0.02%, and a bowel mesentery injury rate of 0.11%.[7] Such injuries were correlated to the difficulty of trocar insertion, as well as to the training of the surgeon.

The consequences of unrecognized visceral injury are major contributors to the morbidity and mortality of both diagnostic and therapeutic laparoscopy. Following laparoscopy, postoperative signs of fever, abdominal tenderness, sepsis, or other untoward and unexpected findings should initiate the concern that an unrecognized visceral injury has occurred.

Electrocautery Injury

Included in the injuries that were unrecognized at the time of laparoscopy are those attributed to electrocautery. Because of a low but appreciable incidence of intestinal injury involving cases in which monopolar electrocautery was used in gynecologic procedures (estimated at 0.05% to 0.28%), there arose the theory that such injuries resulted from conduction of electric current to the bowel without direct contact.[14] Because of concern over such incidents, gynecologists began to use alternative methods for hemostasis, such as bipolar cautery forceps and cautery forceps based on strictly thermal heat. The latter still carried a significant risk of visceral injury if the hot tip of the instrument were to touch an organ while the instrument was momentarily out of the field of visualization of the telescope. Although in theory, monopolar cautery arc injuries may certainly have resulted, the subsequent proliferation of laparoscopic use by general surgeons has failed to substantiate this rate of suspected conduction injuries from electrocautery. In addition, laboratory studies in animals suggest such a mechanism to be unlikely.[15]

Since laparoscopic cholecystectomy and other therapeutic general surgical procedures have become popular, there is no evidence in reports on large numbers of such procedures that the use of monopolar electrocautery carries excess risk or results in an increased number of complications. Studies have reviewed the efficacy of monopolar cautery versus laser in performing laparoscopic cholecystectomy, with no significant advantage or increased complication rate with either method.[16] However, laser use is associated with significantly increased cost.[17]

Other Postoperative Complications of Laparoscopic Procedures

Bowel obstruction and infection are late complications of laparoscopic procedures. Many of the infections may result as a consequence of unrecognized visceral injury during laparoscopic surgery. Specific intraabdominal procedures are associated with an increased risk of local intraabdominal abscess or infection, such as an increased risk of subhepatic contamination and infection following laparoscopic cholecystectomy or pelvic abscess following laparoscopic appendectomy. The incidence of such complications is usually similar to that seen after the procedure is performed via celiotomy.

The incidence of wound infections following laparoscopic surgery is generally low, consistent with that expected after clean or clean-contaminated–type operations. In addition, management of trocar site wound infection is easier than that of traditional wound infection because of the size of the wound. Common causes for wound infection include wound site contamination with infected tissue, such as in improper extraction of a resected appendix. Omphalitis at the umbilical trocar site can be an annoying problem, but its incidence can be virtually eliminated with careful cleansing of the umbilicus before the start of the procedure.[18]

Bowel incarcerations through the laparoscopic wound site have been reported in the literature.[19] The incidence of such events is much less than 1%. The incidence of bowel obstruction after laparoscopic surgery is poorly reported in the literture, but it is felt to be extremely low.

COMPLICATIONS OF LAPAROSCOPIC CHOLECYSTECTOMY

Laparoscopic cholecystectomy is now the most commonly performed procedure for surgical treatment of cholelithiasis. Its adoption as the treatment of choice for this condition occurred in just 4 years after its introduction in 1987.[20, 21] This revolution in biliary surgery has occurred largely because the new procedure is associated with considerable benefits for the patient, including less pain, shorter hospitalization, and a more rapid return to work.[16, 17, 20–27] Laparoscopic cholecystectomy is now the most commonly performed laparoscopic general surgical procedure.

During the past year, however, there has been increasing concern and attention in both the medical literature[28–32] and the lay press regarding the increased incidence of serious complications resulting from laparoscopic cholecystectomy, the most prevalent of which have been bile duct injuries. In addition, the State Board of Health of New York,[33] in response to what was considered an unusually high number of such complications, issued a set of guidelines for appropriate training and monitoring of surgeons performing laparoscopic cholecystectomy. It includes guidelines for suspension of a surgeon's privileges as a result of bile duct injuries.

Complications of laparoscopic cholecystectomy can be divided into two groups: (1) those that involve the specific laparoscopic aspects of the operation, including biliary tract injuries, and (2) those that are common to all surgical procedures. The latter have already been described to some extent earlier.

Bile Duct Injuries

The main source of significant morbidity arising from laparoscopic cholecystectomy that is somewhat specific for this procedure is bile duct injury. The incidence of injuries to the common bile duct during open cholecystectomy is controversial. Based on large series in the literature,[34, 35] the incidence can be estimated at approximately 0.1% to 0.4%. The incidence may be as high as 0.5% in actuality, since published series probably underestimated the true incidence of ductal injuries in general practice.[36]

In the published literature, the incidence of bile duct injuries related to laparoscopic cholecystectomy is higher than that of open cholecystectomy. In the experience of the Southern

Table 34-1. COMPLICATIONS FOLLOWING LAPAROSCOPIC CHOLECYSTECTOMY—SELECTED SERIES FROM THE LITERATURE

Reference	No. of Patients	Complications (%)	Bile Duct Injuries (%)
Deziel et al[32]	77,604	2	0.6
Scott et al[27]	8016	3	0.7
SAGES group[24]	2671	9	0.2
Larson et al[16]	1983	2.1	0.2
Southern Surgeons Club[23]	1518	3	0.7
Cushieri et al[25]	1236	1.6	0.3
Graffis[22]	900	2	0.1
Baird et al[38]	800	3.1	0.0
Davis et al[39]	622	3.8	0.2
Spaw et al[40]	500	1	0.2
Sigman et al[41]	500	5	0.4
Wolfe et al[42]	381	6	0
Nottle[43]	265	5.5	0
Dashaw et al[44]	250	3.6	0

Surgeons Club,[37] the incidence of bile duct injuries was 1.7% for surgeons in their initial cases but dropped to 0.17% after their first 13 cases. Other large published series have estimated the series of bile duct injury to be between 0% and 0.7% (Table 34–1).[38–44]

In New York, where reporting of surgical complications is mandatory by law, the New York State Health Authority cited 35 cases of ligation or severance of the common bile duct in a period of less than 2 years. Unfortunately, the total number of laparoscopic cholecystectomies from which these cases were derived is unknown. This same memorandum also cited another 53 cases of bile leak following laparoscopic cholecystectomy.

Bile duct injuries occurring during laparoscopic cholecystectomy may be due to several differences between laparoscopic and open cholecystectomy. Primary among these is the adaptation by the surgeon to the differences in visualization of the relevant biliary anatomy. Video imaging used to perform laparoscopic cholecystectomy substitutes two-dimensional visual perception for the three-dimensional perception to which surgeons are accustomed. Inexperience in performing dissection of the relevant biliary structures using laparoscopic techniques, combined with the known variability in biliary anatomy, is likely responsible for the intraoperative misidentification of structures and subsequent biliary injury that occurs in many of these reported cases. However, videotapes of some cases of bile duct injury that are available for review have simply shown that factors not unique to laparoscopic surgery, such as poor surgical technique, can be important in contributing to these complications. In particular, a lack of proper laparoscopic technique, including the surgeon's accepting limited or poor visualization of the operative field through the telescope during dissection, was often evident.[45] Such errors negate the only advantage of laparoscopic surgery over open surgery: enhanced visualization.

Reported series of bile duct injuries following laparoscopic cholecystectomy have shown that they can be broken down into several commonly occurring types (Table 34–2). The most common type, numerically, is the mistaken removal of a portion of the common hepatic duct when that structure is misidentified as the cystic duct (Fig. 34–2). Unfortunately, this misidentification is frequently coupled with division of the ductal structure just at its junction with another bile duct—in this case the bifurcation of the left and right hepatic ducts. This injury is now becoming known in the surgical literature on this topic as the "classic" injury, and it necessitates performance of a hepaticojejunostomy for biliary reconstruction.

Table 34-2. BILIARY COMPLICATIONS RESULTING FROM LAPAROSCOPIC CHOLECYSTECTOMY

Bile Duct Injuries
Classic injury: resection of a portion of the common hepatic and common bile duct
Occlusion of common bile duct, common hepatic duct, or branch of biliary tree secondary to clips
Injury to bile ducts from cautery or laser, producing stricture or postoperative necrosis and leakage
Injury to common bile duct or common hepatic duct from cholangiocatheter insertion
Lacerations of biliary tree from dissection or traction

Other Causes of Bile Leakage
Incomplete occlusion of cystic duct and leakage
Incomplete removal of gallbladder and leakage
Failure to recognize and ligate duct of Luschka in hepatic bed

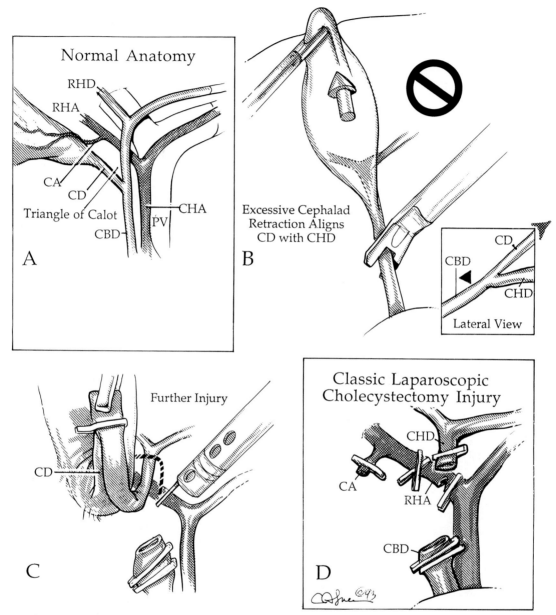

Figure 34–2. The "classic injury" to the biliary tree during laparoscopic cholecystectomy. **(A)** Diagram of the "normal" or most common anatomic configuration of the hilar structures. **(B)** Excessive cephalad retraction of the gallbladder tends to align the cystic duct, particularly when it is short, with the underlying common hepatic duct. The common bile duct is mistaken for the distal cystic duct and is clipped. **(C)** Division of the common bile duct is followed by dissection along the common hepatic duct, mistaken for the cystic duct, until a bile duct division occurs. The bifurcation of the common hepatic duct can be mistaken for the cystic duct–common duct intersection. Frequent simultaneous injury to the right hepatic artery may occur, obscuring the visualization with hemorrhage. **(D)** The resulting anatomy once the gallbladder and resected portion of the biliary tree are removed. CA = cystic artery; CD = cystic duct; CHA = common hepatic artery; CHD = common hepatic duct; PV = portal vein; RHA = right hepatic artery; RHD = right hepatic duct.

Factors Involved in Bile Duct Injury

Improper exposure of the cystic duct and the triangle of Calot can predispose to bile duct injury. Retraction of the cystic duct anteriorly and upward will distort the relationship between the cystic duct and the common bile duct so that the surgeon may mistake the common bile duct for the cystic duct (Fig. 34–2B). This is particularly true if the cystic duct is short. Failure to identify the infundibular end of the gallbladder and the takeoff of the cystic duct is a common error in cases of injury to the biliary tree. Once such identification has been performed, the dissection down the cystic duct can proceed safely; a short cystic duct and its intersection with the common hepatic duct are easily recognized.

Steps that can assist the surgeon in clear identification of the biliary anatomy include retraction of the gallbladder anteriorly away from the liver bed by the assistant (Fig. 34–3), allowing maximum exposure of the structures within the triangle of Calot. Removal of the peritoneum covering this area should always be performed, with clear identification of the structures in the area. Another helpful step in identifying structures in this area, including the cystic duct, is dissection of the peritoneum away from the base of the gallbladder on the lateral side (Fig. 34–4). This exposes the triangle of Calot

from the lateral underside, further helping to identify the biliary anatomy. Dissection of the cystic duct is more safely performed by beginning on the lateral side of the gallbladder and proceeding medially. The potential misidentification of the common bile duct for the cystic duct can occur when these two structures lie in close approximation and dissection is initiated on the medial side of the gallbladder.

Dissection from the infundibulum of the gallbladder down to the cystic duct is the safest method for delineating the necessary anatomy for performing laparoscopic cholecystectomy. Clear identification of the takeoff of the cystic duct is probably the most important step in preventing bile duct injury. This can be accomplished only with adequate visualization of the anatomy and adequate exposure provided by the assistant.

The role of the first assistant in exposing the triangle of Calot and the infundibular area of the gallbladder is extremely important in the prevention of bile duct injuries and is not to be underemphasized. The commonly taught method of using a fixed retraction of the gallbladder fundus by the right anterior axillary trocar, at times securing it to the drapes with a towel clip, is to be condemned. The first assistant should instead use a two-handed technique, using the grasping forceps from the right axillary and right midclavicular trocars in the right and left hands, respectively. This prevents the automatic cephalad retraction of the gallbladder mandated by

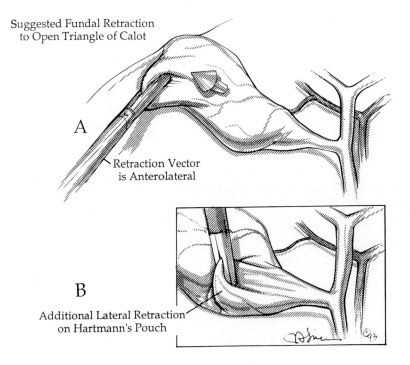

Suggested Fundal Retraction to Open Triangle of Calot

A — Retraction Vector is Anterolateral

B — Additional Lateral Retraction on Hartmann's Pouch

Figure 34–3. Recommended retraction of the gallbladder by the first assistant during laparoscopic cholecystectomy. **(A)** Retraction vector of the fundus of the gallbladder, once cephalad exposure is adequate, is in the anterolateral direction to maximally expose the triangle of Calot. **(B)** Additional lateral retraction of Hartmann's pouch will allow further visualization of the cystic duct takeoff, especially in cases in which there is a stone impacted in the distal gallbladder or the cystic duct is short.

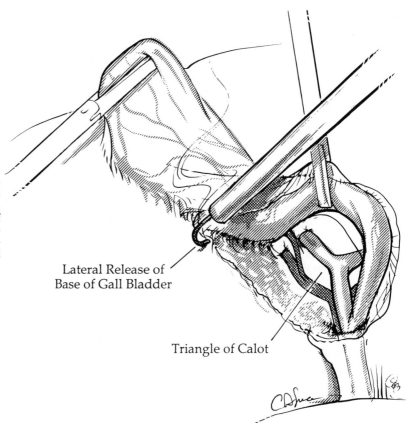

Figure 34–4. By incising the lateral peritoneal attachments of the infundibulum of the gallbladder, safe exposure of the triangle of Calot is obtained and maximal visualization is achieved before dissecting the more variable medial side of the infundibulum.

Lateral Release of
Base of Gall Bladder

Triangle of Calot

fixed retraction. Such cephalad retraction can predispose the bile duct to injuries because the common bile duct is aligned longitudinally in a cephalad direction with the cystic duct, whereas the common hepatic duct is in a posterior position and is not appreciated (see Fig. 34–2B). In contrast, the two-handed retraction technique allows the first assistant to retract the gallbladder more laterally, and the infundibulum of the gallbladder can be turned and rotated so that both sides of the triangle of Calot are visible

and appreciated by the surgeon as he or she dissects and identifies structures adjacent to the gallbladder (see Fig. 34–3B).

Inadvertent traction at the junction of the cystic and common bile ducts during cystic duct division can predispose to placement of a clip or tie on the tented-up portion of the common bile duct (Fig. 34–5), which has been a cause of bile duct injury during open cholecystectomy in the past.

Another factor that has been cited as contrib-

Figure 34–5. Traction at the junction of the cystic and common bile ducts produces distortion of the common bile duct, predisposing to partial occlusion of the duct from clips placed across what is perceived as the base of the cystic duct.

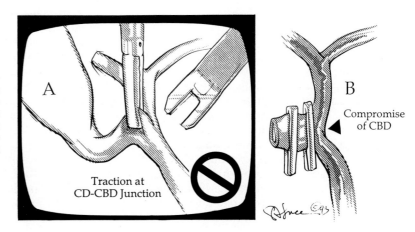

A

Traction at
CD-CBD Junction

B

Compromise
of CBD

uting to the increased incidence of common bile duct injuries is the practice of not performing intraoperative cholangiography, which can frequently alert the surgeon to anatomic irregularities or anatomic misidentification errors already committed. However, review of series of common bile duct injuries shows that clear identification and dissection of the biliary tree is probably more important than intraoperative cholangiography for preventing bile duct injuries. In several series, there have been cases documented in which bile duct injury occurred despite the performance of an intraoperative cholangiogram.[16] At times, intraoperative cholangiography has revealed no filling of the proximal biliary tree because of the presence of the catheter in the common bile duct, yet surgeons have persisted in dividing the common bile duct in such a situation, despite lack of documentation by the radiograph that the hepatic duct had been identified. In defense of routine cholangiography, however, it is true that the procedure will clarify in the surgeons's mind the biliary anatomy in all cases in which it is properly performed and interpreted. In addition, under these circumstances it will lessen the severity of bile duct injuries if they have already occurred and will prevent resection of portions of the biliary tree. In addition, it should serve to limit the number of unrecognized bile duct injuries.

Other injuries to the biliary tree that have occurred during laparoscopic cholecystectomy have resulted from placement of clips across the common bile duct; incomplete removal of the gallbladder, with leakage from the remaining infundibular portion; and lack of secure closure of the cystic duct, with postoperative cystic duct stump leakage. The incidence of these complications approximates those of the classic injury, with the exception that improper or incomplete closure of the cystic duct occurs more frequently.

Management of Bile Duct Injuries

The incidence of biliary duct injury during laparoscopic cholecystectomy appears increased in the setting of previous inflammation or acute cholelithiasis. In such situations, accurate identification of biliary anatomy is more difficult than in the elective setting with minimal scarring. Surgeons should always adhere to the dictum that open cholecystectomy should be performed whenever laparoscopic visualization is unclear. Failure to do so has undoubtedly contributed to some cases of bile duct injury.

It is just as likely that bile duct injuries will go unrecognized at the time of operation as it is that they will be identified. Reports to date have shown that only 25% to 50% of injuries are recognized at the time of operation. Through a large survey, Deziel and associates found that 49% of major bile duct injuries were recognized at the time of operation.[32] When they are recognized, there is an improved chance for appropriate definitive repair, which should be performed immediately if the surgeon is experienced with such procedures. Inexperienced surgeons would probably best serve their patient's needs by referral at this point to someone experienced with biliary reconstruction, since reports are appearing from tertiary care centers in which a significant percentage of the patients referred for bile duct injuries are seen after a previous biliary reconstruction at the referring hospital. Stricture formation after such procedures can be common, necessitating further treatment with either surgical reconstruction or biliary stenting and dilation.

Patients whose bile duct injuries go unrecognized intraoperatively generally present with symptoms soon after surgery. Retrospective review of the records of such patients frequently reveals that complaints of abdominal pain and tenderness were present within 24 hours after surgery, which often corresponded to the time of discharge. The exception to this finding are patients with cystic stump leakage, who may not present for several days to even a week postoperatively. Upper abdominal pain and tenderness are the most common complaints of patients with bile duct injury, but jaundice and fever can also be present.

Evaluation of patients who present postoperatively with possible bile duct leakage should include ultrasound of the abdomen to assess for fluid collection. If a bile fluid collection is documented by ultrasound and subsequent aspiration, patients should undergo either open surgery (especially when any sign of peritonitis is present) or further diagnostic evaluation. Patients with jaundice in whom ultrasound shows biliary ductal dilation should undergo percutaneous transhepatic cholangiography to accurately diagnose and define the proximal extent of biliary tract injury and obstruction. Patients with bile leakage who present with pain and fever but no sign of jaundice or extrahepatic bile duct obstruction should undergo endoscopic retrograde cholangiography (ERC) to identify the source of the bile leak and biliary tree injury.

Some authorities have recommended the use of radionuclide scans to determine if bile leakage is occurring. Although this test may confirm that suspicion, ultrasound and fluid aspiration should confirm it as well. Scans are not nearly as helpful as ERC in identifying the location of the bile leak. In addition, when ERC is accomplished, immediate endoscopic sphincterotomy, with or without stent placement into the biliary tree or nasobiliary tube drainage, can be adequate therapy for small bile duct leaks. After such treatment, small leaks may subsequently close spontaneously.

Repair of a bile duct injury is based on the location and type of injury. Reconstruction using biliary-enteric anastomosis is necessary for all injuries that have involved removal of a portion of the bile duct. Such procedures are best performed by surgeons with considerable experience in biliary reconstruction, since in inexperienced hands, the stricture rate after such repairs is generally high.

Simple laceration of the bile duct, especially if not complete, can be repaired with primary reanastomosis and stenting with a T tube. The amount of time that the tube should be left in place is not clear, but the significant incidence of stricture following such procedures suggests that a conservative approach is indicated.

Leakage from an incompletely secured cystic duct can be corrected by suture ligation or reocclusion of the cystic duct lumen with clips. Depending on the time elapsed since the laparoscopic cholecystectomy, as well as the laparoscopic experience and skill of the surgeon, this procedure also may potentially be done laparoscopically. As with all laparoscopic procedures, however, when there is any doubt as to the anatomy or success of the case under laparoscopic vision, conversion to celiotomy is indicated.

Prevention of injuries to the common bile duct should be of paramount importance to the surgeon performing laparoscopic cholecystectomy. This is especially true because the morbidity of such injuries can be significant. Restenosis, reobstruction, and a requirement for reoperation are not uncommon in patients who have had biliary reconstruction because of iatrogenic injuries to the common bile duct. The surgeon who follows the principles of careful identification of structures, use of intraoperative cholangiography, clear identification of the junction of the cystic duct and the gallbladder, and conversion to open cholecystectomy in any instance in which the preceding cannot be accomplished will minimize the chances for bile duct injury.

Other Laparoscopic Injuries That Occur During Laparoscopic Cholecystectomy

Other complications arising from laparoscopic cholecystectomy include injury to intraabdominal structures from the trocars or instruments. Laceration of major blood vessels during trocar insertion is the most immediately life-threatening complication that can occur. Although the incidence of such injuries is low, it is not exceedingly rare. The New York State Department of Health memorandum listed 13 major vascular perforations reported during the same period as the 35 major bile duct injuries.[34] This suggests the incidence of major vascular injuries during laparoscopic cholecystectomy may be in the 0.2% range, higher than that reported in previous gynecologic laparoscopic literature. The occurrence of such events is particularly serious because their immediate recognition is necessary if appropriate conversion to open laparotomy and lifesaving repair of the vascular injury is to be performed. A significant proportion of the mortality related to laparoscopic cholecystectomy reported to date is secondary to this complication.

The other complication that has led to a significant percentage of the reported mortality for laparoscopic cholecystectomy is unrecognized intestinal perforation during the operation. This can initially occur secondary to trocar injury or from inadvertent cautery or laser injury during the course of dissecting the gallbladder and hilar structures. The duodenum is the structure most frequently injured by cautery (Fig. 34–6A), whereas the remainder of the small intestine is most frequently injured from trocar perforation (Fig. 34–6C). Such injuries can be minimized with appropriate technique, in particular by using an open laparoscopic approach when performing this procedure in patients who have had previous intraabdominal surgery.

Minimization of morbidity from intestinal injury can occur only if the injury is recognized. Unrecognized injury leads to postoperative sepsis, intraabdominal abscess formation and, not infrequently, death. Immediate recognition requires conversion to open laparotomy for repair of the intestine with appropriate suturing techniques.

Cautery injury can be unrecognized and will frequently present as delayed perforations following surgery if the bowel is the organ involved. The incidence of such injuries is prob-

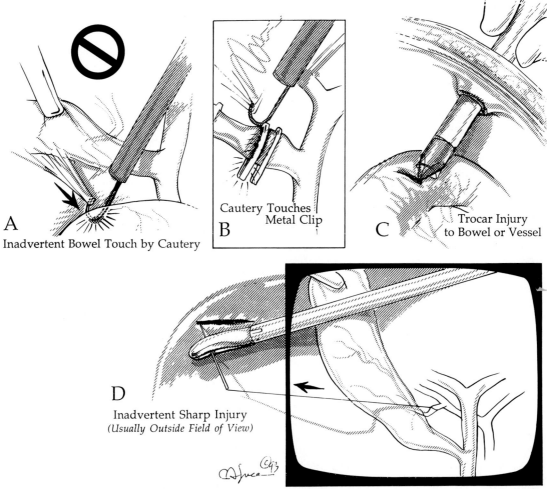

A   Inadvertent Bowel Touch by Cautery

B   Cautery Touches Metal Clip

C   Trocar Injury to Bowel or Vessel

D   Inadvertent Sharp Injury
(Usually Outside Field of View)

Figure 34–6. Other injuries that may occur during laparoscopic cholecystectomy. **(A)** Inadvertent cautery injury of the duodenum during dissection of the hilar structures. This is particularly likely to occur with dense adhesions in the area of the infundibulum of the gallbladder. Unrecognized injury can result in postoperative perforation, peritonitis, and life-threatening sepsis. **(B)** Touching the cystic duct clips with the electrocautery can result in postoperative necrosis of the duct, clip dislodgement, and bile leak. **(C)** Trocar injury to the jejunum, the ileum, or a vascular structure is possible on initial insertion. **(D)** Failure to keep the working instruments in the field of view of the video telescope can result in injury, such as this laceration of the liver with a needle.

ably on the order of 0.1% to 0.5%. Cautery injury to other hilar structures is also known. Stricture of the common bile duct can result from cautery or laser injury. Touching the metal clips that have been applied to the divided cystic duct with the cautery can result in transmission of a burn injury to the bile duct (Fig. 34–6B). If the cystic duct alone is injured, postoperative tissue necrosis may lead to cystic duct stump leakage, which is often blamed on poorly placed clips or clips that "fell off."

Inadvertent injury to other organs can result whenever the laparoscopic telescope is not focused on the surgeon's instruments. An example of such an injury is shown in Figure 34–6D, in which suture ligation of the cystic duct is being performed and the needle, off the video telescopic screen, has lacerated the undersurface of the liver.

It is unclear whether the use of laser has been responsible for a higher percentage of inadvertent intraabdominal organ injuries than has monopolar cautery. Contact lasers probably were not responsible for any higher percentage injury than cautery was, but free beam lasers may have been. Fortunately, the popularity of the use of laser as part of laparoscopic cholecystectomy is declining after studies have shown it has no significant advantage and is costly.[17]

A less common, but still reported, complication of laparoscopic cholecystectomy is abscess formation from retained gallstones not removed at the time of laparoscopic cholecystectomy for acute cholecystitis.[46] Other complications of laparoscopic cholecystectomy are those related to the performance of any surgical extirpative procedure. They include wound infection, a missed diagnosis with the return of the patient for readmission to the hospital because of abdominal pain of other cause, postoperative fever, atelectasis, and urinary tract infection or urinary retention. Cardiovascular complications compose a significant percentage of the life-threatening complications in the elderly population.[35]

The overall complication rate for laparoscopic cholecystectomy has been documented as being between 1% and 9% (see Table 34–1). A recent National Institutes of Health consensus conference on laparoscopic cholecystectomy showed the aggregate complication rate of a review of data based on more than 100,000 cases to be between 2% and 5%.[47] The conference noted, however, that these numbers were more a reflection of the characteristics of the patients in the reports and how complications were defined than they were a reflection of the procedure.

COMPLICATIONS FOLLOWING OTHER LAPAROSCOPIC PROCEDURES

Although cholecystectomy is now the most commonly performed procedure using a laparoscopic rather than traditional open surgical technique, most other general surgical procedures are in the early phase of assessment regarding the feasibility or the advisability of performing them using a laparoscopic approach. As such, the limited number of surgeons performing these operations are more likely to be accomplished laparoscopic surgeons. Similarly, the collective experiences in these procedures are still too small to reflect the likely complication rates that will be experienced with more widespread application. The preliminary information that is available is based on personal experience and communication as well as on published reports.

Inguinal Herniorrhaphy

Laparoscopic inguinal herniorrhaphy has evolved over the past few years to incorporate the principles advocated by Stoppa[48] and the preperitoneal approach first widely popularized by Nyhus.[49] A laparoscopic repair method using a prosthetic plug inserted into the inguinal canal, advocated by Corbitt,[50] has now been generally abandoned because of reported high recurrence rates of more than 20% in 2 years (unpublished reports). Repair using a large sheet of prosthetic mesh stapled over the inguinal floor in the preperitoneal space is now the most commonly advocated method of laparoscopic repair. Recurrence rates with this method are reportedly low. In a large multicenter trial, preliminary results of either preperitoneal or intraabdominal prosthetic mesh placement have shown a recurrence rate of 2% to 3%,[51] although long-term follow-up is limited to 2 years at most. Complications related to laparoscopic inguinal hernia repair are reportedly low, with the sole exception of entrapment or injury to inguinal nerve structures. Injury or entrapment to either the lateral femoral cutaneous nerve or the femoral branch of the genitofemoral nerve has been reported in up to 9% of cases in the multicenter trial.[51] In our own experience, the lateral femoral cutaneous nerve has been entrapped in 2 of 35 cases. In both instances, reoperation after 1 week to laparoscopically remove lateral staples provided prompt resolution of symptoms. Based on these experiences, it has now been recommended that no staples be placed laterally below the level of the iliopubic tract.[52] Modification of laparoscopic herniorrhaphy to include this guideline should limit the number of nerve entrapments and thereby significantly reduce the overall complication rate currently seen with this procedure.

The potential for other, as yet unreported, complications with laparoscopic inguinal herniorrhaphy also exists, particularly intraperitoneal ones in which mesh is secured in an intraperitoneal location as a repair. This latter technique may predispose to complications resulting from adherence of intraabdominal organs to the mesh.

Appendectomy

Laparoscopic appendectomy is currently being practiced in a large number of medical centers in the United States. However, reports of the results of significant series are few. The most extensive experience with the procedure has been reported by Gotz and his German colleagues.[53] They report a low complication rate: only one case of appendiceal stump leakage in a series of more than 400 patients. Our initial experience has shown laparoscopic appendectomy to have a low incidence of postoperative wound infections if appropriate techniques for correctly extracting the appendix are followed.[54] Another group has reported little difference in the complication rates between open and laparoscopic appendectomy.[55] Laparoscopy has been shown to decrease the incidence of unnecessary appendectomy.[56] This may be especially important in patient populations in whom the incidence of misdiagnosis of appendicitis is common, such as in menstruating women.

It is likely that laparoscopic appendectomy will produce a spectrum of complications that is no wider than has been associated with open appendectomy. The use of laparoscopy to define the cause of suspected acute appendicitis may lessen the number of missed diagnoses for this problem, which, in turn, may lessen some of the severe morbidity associated with a perforated appendix and peritonitis. The wound infection rate may be decreased with laparoscopic appendectomy once the learning curve and errors in technique are overcome. The complications inherent in laparoscopy itself should be anticipated with laparoscopic appendectomy. The potential also exists that improper performance of the ligation of the appendiceal stump could lead to a higher than expected incidence of stump leakage, with resultant fistula or abscess complications.

Laparoscopic Colon Resection

Laparoscopic colon resection and laparoscopic-assisted colon resection (in which the anastomosis is performed extracorporeally) are currently being initiated in a number of medical centers. Caution has been urged in the widespread application of this procedure in patients with resectable adenocarcinoma of the colon, since data to confirm that as an oncologic treatment, the technique is as therapeutic as celiotomy and colon resection are as yet unavailable. The number of lymph nodes in the surgical specimens appear to be comparable for the two procedures when the laparoscopic colon resection is performed by an experienced laparoscopic surgeon.[57, 58] Reports regarding the operative results of such procedures have been relatively few. However, the morbidity and mortality rates appear to be in the range similar to or lower than those seen for open colon resections.[57-62] Complications include wound infections, cardiovascular events, small bowel obstruction, ileus, anastomotic bleeding, and other complications as seen with celiotomy and colon resection. As yet, there appear to be no specific complications related to laparoscopic colon resection that have been documented as occurring in excessive frequency.

Other Procedures

Other general surgical procedures are also being performed using a laparoscopic approach. They include laparoscopic vagotomy, Nissen fundoplication, splenectomy, gastrojejunostomy, and small bowel resection. However, the data regarding the outcome of these procedures is still scanty. Reports to date have simply demonstrated the ability to accomplish these procedures using a laparoscopic approach with relative safety. These preliminary results also suggest no significant increase in the complication rates when performing such procedures using a laparoscopic approach, nor significant incidence of any particular complication specific to any of these procedures. Some reports also suggest that the benefits of more rapid recovery and shorter hospitalization, as was seen in cholecystectomy, may extend to these procedures. However, it must be emphasized that the number of such procedures being performed is still relatively low, and the reporting of results, including complication rates, is very limited and of such a preliminary nature to prevent significant conclusions. In addition, preliminary reports on such procedures are from skilled laparoscopic surgeons. It is therefore possible that potentially higher complication rates may be seen if there is widespread application of a laparoscopic approach to such procedures by less skilled surgeons. The community of general surgeons appears less compelled to embrace a laparoscopic approach for these other procedures than for cholecystectomy, probably in part because of the more advanced laparoscopic skills required to perform them. The acquisition of such skills in a methodical and thorough fashion will hopefully prevent any future significant increase in complications related to the laparoscopic performance of these other general surgical procedures.

References

1. Bruhl W. Complications of laparoscopy and liver biopsy under vision: the results of a survey. German Med Monthly 12:31–32, 1967.
2. Kane MG, Krejs GJ. Complications of diagnostic laparoscopy in Dallas: a 7-year prospective study. Gastrointest Endosc 30:237, 1984.
3. Peterson HB, Hulka JF, Phillips JM. American Association of Gynecologic Laparoscopists' 1988 membership survey on operative laparoscopy. J Reprod Med 35:587–589, 1990.

4. Phillips J, Keith D, Hulka J, Keith L. Gynaecological laparoscopy in 1975. J Reprod Med 16:205–217, 1976.
5. Schirmer BD, Dix J, Schmieg RE, Aguilar M. Laparoscopic cholecystectomy in patients with previous abdominal surgery. Surg Endosc 6:107, 1992.
6. Borgatta L, Gruss L, Barad D, Kaali SG. Direct trocar insertion vs. Veress needle use for laparoscopic sterilization. J Reprod Med 35:891–894, 1990.
7. Yuzpe AA. Pneumoperitoneum needle and trocar injuries in laparoscopy. A survey on possible contributing factors and prevention. J Reprod Med 35:485–490, 1990.
8. Kalhan SB, Reaney JA, Collins RL. Pneumomediastinum and subcutaneous emphysema during laparoscopy. Cleve Clin J Med 57:639–642, 1990.
9. Nord HJ, Boyd WP. Diagnostic laparoscopy. Endoscopy 24:133–137, 1992.
10. Phillips J, Keith D, Hulka J, Keith L. Gynaecological laparoscopy in 1975. J Reprod Med 16:205–217, 1976.
11. McGrath BJ, Zimmerman JE, Williams JF, Parmet J. Carbon dioxide embolism treated with hyperbaric oxygen. Can J Anaesth 36:586–589, 1989.
12. Diakun TA. Carbon dioxide embolism: successful resuscitation with cardiopulmonary bypass. Anesthesiology 74:1151–1153, 1991.
13. Shifren JL, Adlestein L, Finkler NJ. Asystolic cardiac arrest: a rare complication of laparoscopy. Obstet Gynecol 79:840–841, 1992.
14. Thompson BH, Wheeless CR. Gastrointestinal complications of laparoscopy sterilization. Obstet Gynecol 41:669, 1973.
15. DiGiovanni M, Vasilenko P, Belsky D. Laparoscopic tubal sterilization. The potential for thermal bowel injury. J Reprod Med 35:951–954, 1990.
16. Larson GM, Vitale GC, Casey J, et al. Multipractice analysis of laparoscopic cholecystectomy in 1983 patients. Am J Surg 163:221–226, 1992.
17. Voyles CR, Petro AB, Meena AL, et al. A practical approach to laparoscopic cholecystectomy. Am J Surg 161:365–370, 1991.
18. Gotz F, Pier A, Bacher C. Modified laparoscopic appendectomy in surgery. A report of 388 operations. Surg Endosc 4:6–9, 1990.
19. Thomas AG, Mclymont F, Moshipur J. Incarcerated hernia after laparoscopic sterilization. A case report. J Reprod Med 35:639–640, 1990.
20. Schirmer BD, Edge SB, Dix J, et al. Laparoscopic cholecystectomy: treatment of choice for symptomatic cholelithiasis. Ann Surg 213:665–677, 1991.
21. Soper NJ, Stockmann PT, Dunnigan DL, Ashley SW. Laparoscopic cholecystectomy. The new "gold standard"? Arch Surg 127:917–923, 1992.
22. Graffis R. Laparoscopic cholecystectomy: the Methodist Hospital experience. J Laparoendosc Surg 1:69–73, 1992.
23. The Southern Surgeons Club. A prospective analysis of 1,518 laparoscopic cholecystectomies performed by Southern U.S. surgeons. N Engl J Med 324:1073–1078, 1991.
24. Airan M, Appel M, Berci G, et al. Retrospective and prospective multi-institutional laparoscopic cholecystectomy study organized by the Society of American Gastrointestinal Endoscopic Surgeons. Surg Endosc 6:169–176, 1992.
25. Cushieri A, Dubois F, Mouiel J, et al. The European experience with laparoscopic cholecystectomy. Am J Surg 161:385–387, 1991.
26. Meakins JL, Barkun JS, Sampalis JS, et al. Open versus laparoscopic cholecystectomy: a randomized controlled clinical trial. Presented at 3rd World Congress of Endoscopic Surgery, Bordeaux, France, June 1992.

27. Scott TR, Zucker KA, Bailey RM. Laparoscopic cholecystectomy: a review of 8,016 patients. Presented at 3rd World Congress of Endoscopic Surgery, Bordeaux, June 1992.
28. Davidoff AM, Pappas TN, Murray EA, et al. Mechanisms of major biliary injury during laparoscopic cholecystectomy. Ann Surg 215:196–202, 1992.
29. Moosa AR, Easter DW, Vansonnenberg E, et al. Laparoscopic injuries to the bile duct: a cause for concern. Ann Surg 215:203–208, 1992.
30. Ferguson CM, Rattner DW, Warshaw AL. Bile duct injury in laparoscopic cholecystectomy. Surg Laparosc Endosc 1:1–7, 1992.
31. Wootton FT, Hoffman BJ, Marsh WH, Cunningham JT. Biliary complications following laparoscopic cholecystectomy. Gastrointest Endosc 38:183–185, 1992.
32. Deziel DJ, Millikan KW, Airan MC, et al. Complications of laparoscopic cholecystectomy: results of a national survey of 4,292 hospitals and analysis of 77,604 cases. Presented at the Society for Surgery of the Alimentary Tract meeting, May 1992.
33. Hartman TW. Laparoscopic cholecystectomy. State of New York Department of Health Memorandum, 1992.
34. McSherry CK. Cholecystectomy: the gold standard. Am J Surg 158:174–178, 1989.
35. Gilliland TM, Traverso LW. Modern standards for comparison of cholecystectomy with alternative treatments for symptomatic cholelithiasis with emphasis on long term relief of symptoms. Surg Gynecol Obstet 170:39–44, 1990.
36. Hermann RE. A plea for safer technique of cholecystectomy. Surgery 79:609–611, 1976.
37. Meyers WC, Saperstein LA, Moore MJ, et al. The relation between physician experience and bile duct injury for laparoscopic cholecystectomy: results from 8,839 cases. Presented at NIH Consensus Conference, Gallstones and Laparoscopic Cholecystectomy, Bethesda, MD, September 1992.
38. Baird DR, Wilson JP, Mason EM, et al. An early review of 800 laparoscopic cholecystectomies at a university-affiliated community teaching hospital. Am Surg 58:206–210, 1992.
39. Davis CJ, Arregui ME, Nagan RF, Shaar C. Laparoscopic cholecystectomy: the St. Vincent experience. Surg Laparosc Endosc 2:64–68, 1992.
40. Spaw AT, Reddick EJ, Olsen DO. Laparoscopic laser cholecystectomy: analysis of 500 procedures. Surg Laparosc Endosc 1:2–7, 1991.
41. Sigman HH, Fried GM, Hinchey EJ, et al. Role of the teaching hospital in the development of a laparoscopic cholecystectomy program. Can J Surg 35:49–54, 1992.
42. Wolfe BM, Gardiner BN, Leary BF, Frey CF. Endoscopic cholecystectomy. An analysis of complications. Arch Surg 126:1192–1198, 1991.
43. Nottle PD. Percutaneous laparoscopic cholecystectomy: indications, contraindications, and complications. Aust NZ J Surg 62:188–192, 1992.
44. Dashaw L, Friedman I, Kempner R, et al. Initial experience with laparoscopic cholecystectomy at the Beth Israel Medical Center. Surg Gynecol Obstet 175:25–30, 1992.
45. Branum G, Schmitt C, Baille J, et al. Management of major biliary complications after laparoscopic cholecystectomy. Ann Surg 217:532–541, 1993.
46. Campbell WB, McGarity WC. An unusual complication of laparoscopic cholecystectomy. Am Surg 54:641–642, 1992.
47. NIH Consensus Conference: Gallstones and laparoscopic cholecystectomy. JAMA 269:1018–1024, 1993.

48. Stoppa RE. The treatment of complicated groin and incisional hernias. World J Surg 13:545–554, 1989.
49. Nyhus LM. The preperitoneal approach and iliopubic tract repair of inguinal hernia. In: Nyhus LM, Condon RE, eds. Hernia. 2nd ed. Philadelphia: JB Lippincott, 1978:212–232.
50. Corbitt JD. Laparoscopic herniorrhaphy. Surg Laparosc Endosc 1:23–25, 1991.
51. Fitzgibbons R Jr, Annibali R, Litke B, et al. A multicentered clinical trial on laparoscopic inguinal hernia repair: preliminary results. Presented at 1993 Scientific Session, Society of American Gastrointestinal Endoscopic Surgeons, Phoenix AZ, April 1993.
52. Rosser JC Jr, Evans D. Anatomic review in order to avoid nerve injuries associated with laparoscopic inguinal hernia repair. Presented at 1993 Scientific Session, Society of American Gastrointestinal Endoscopic Surgeons, Phoenix, AZ, April 1993.
53. Pier A, Gotz F, Bacher C. Laparoscopic appendectomy in 625 cases: from innovation to routine. Surg Laparosc Endosc 1:8–13, 1991.
54. Schirmer BD, Schmieg RE Jr, Dix J, et al. Laparoscopic versus traditional appendectomy for suspected appendicitis. Am J Surg 165:670–675, 1993.
55. Molnar RG, Apelgren KN, Kisala JM. Open versus laparoscopic appendectomy: an update. Presented at 1993 Scientific Session, Society of American Gastrointestinal Endoscopic Surgeons, Phoenix, AZ, April 1993.
56. Leape LL, Ramenofsky MI. Laparoscopy for questionable appendicitis. Ann Surg 191:410–413, 1980.
57. Schirmer BD, Schmieg RE Jr, Minasi JS, Dix J. Laparoscopic colon surgery in the high-risk patient population. Presented at 1993 Scientific Session, Society of American Gastrointestinal Endoscopic Surgeons, Phoenix, AZ, April 1993.
58. Jacobs M, Verdeja JC, Goldstein HS. Minimally invasive colon resection (laparoscopic colectomy). Surg Laparosc Endosc 1:144–150, 1991.
59. Wexner SD, Johansen OB, Nogueras JJ, Jagelman DG. Laparoscopic total abdominal colectomy. A prospective trial. Dis Colon Rectum 35:651–655, 1992.
60. Zucker KA, Martin D, Pitcher D, Ford S. Laparoscopic assisted colon resection. Presented at 1993 Scientific Session, Society of American Gastrointestinal Endoscopic Surgeons, Phoenix, AZ, April 1993.
61. Fowler DL, White SA. Laparoscopic colon surgery for benign disease. Presented at 1993 Scientific Session, Society of American Gastrointestinal Endoscopic Surgeons, Phoenix, AZ, April 1993.
62. Phillips EH, Franklin M, Carroll BJ, et al. Laparoscopic colectomy. Ann Surg 216:703–707, 1992.

35

Angioscopy in Peripheral Vascular Disease

Timothy R. S. Harward and James M. Seeger

Contrast arteriography has long been the "gold standard" for the detection of arterial pathologic conditions. However, studies have shown that despite excellent specificity, the sensitivity of this technique for accurately defining significant intraluminal vascular lesions is suboptimal.[1] In an effort to rectify this situation, angioscopy—the direct visualization of vascular structures using small fiberoptic catheters—is being used with increasing frequency. Recent reports have demonstrated the utility of angioscopy in the management of patients with peripheral vascular disease and have answered the question posed by Towne and Bernhard in their article Vascular Endoscopy: Useful Tool or Interesting Toy.[2] This chapter reviews these data to provide a critical assessment of the indications, efficacy, and safety of this new diagnostic technique.

TECHNICAL ADVANCES IN ANGIOSCOPY

Technical advances in fiberoptic catheter construction and better systems for clearing blood from the field of view have allowed widespread use of angioscopy in patients with peripheral and, more recently, coronary arterial disease. Fiberoptic angioscopes range in diameter from 0.85 to 2.9 mm. Small vessels (<2 mm in diameter) are viewed with the smallest angioscopes (0.85 to 1.5 mm OD). These angioscopes contain 4000 to 8000 imaging fibers surrounded by a concentric ring of illuminating fibers. Irrigation fluid to clear the visual field of blood is injected through a separate arterial catheter

when these small angioscopes are used. Medium-size vessels are viewed with 1.4 to 2.5 mm OD angioscopes of similar design containing 10,000 to 15,000 imaging fibers (Fig. 35–1). In contrast to the smallest angioscopes, these angioscopes contain channels that allow irrigation at the working end of the scope for improved clearance of blood from the field of view. Larger vessels are viewed with angioscopes having an outside diameter greater than 2.5 OD, with similar fiber construction. These large scopes have working channels for passage of guidewires, laser fibers, or other instruments in addition to irrigation channels (Fig. 35–2). Some of these larger angioscopes also have systems that allow angulation of the tip of the scope. Minimal focal lengths in all angioscopes range from 2 to 6.5 mm, the shorter focal lengths

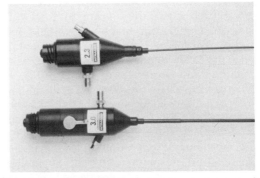

Figure 35–1. Disposable intraoperative angioscopes (Intramed Laboratories, Inc., San Diego, CA). One angioscope is approximately 2.3 mm in diameter, and the other is 3.0 mm in diameter. Both angioscopes have separate irrigation and working channels.

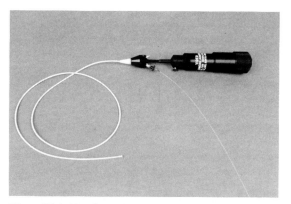

Figure 35–2. Nondisposable angioscope designed for use in peripheral vascular therapy (Courtesy of Trimedyne, Inc., Irvine CA). The angioscope is 2.8 mm in diameter and has separate irrigation and working channels. A laser fiber has been inserted through the working channel.

being used mostly in the smaller vessels. The spatial resolution at a focal length of 5 mm is greater than 20 μ.[3, 4]

Clearing the intraluminal field of blood is essential in obtaining optimal results. Dedicated pumps for the irrigation of heparinized saline are now available (Fig. 35–3). Unlike the pressurized blood bags used previously, these pumps are able to clear the field of blood more quickly, maintain this clear field longer, and limit the amount of infused fluid to an average of less than 500 ml for each procedure.[5, 6] Use of computer processing units and pulsatile fluid infusion, which produces an intermittent freeze-frame image, reduces the amount of fluid used in clearing the fields even further.[7]

Another potential advance in obtaining an optimal viewing field was reported by Silverman and associates.[8] Using a canine model, CO_2 gas was used to displace blood from the arterial lumen during simulated percutaneous angioscopy. This method resulted in a shorter time interval from onset of infusion to total field clearance, a longer duration of a clear field once blood was displaced, and a greater percentage of viewing fields totally cleared of blood when compared with heparinized saline (80% vs. 14%, respectively, $p < .0001$). These findings have since been confirmed by Mladinich and colleagues[9] and Smits and associates.[10] In addition, Mladinich and colleagues[9] showed that in dogs, upstream visualization of the iliac and even renal arteries with retrograde angioscopy could be done using power-injected CO_2 gas (Fig. 35–4), whereas Smits and associates[10] showed that in dogs and pigs, coronary angioscopy with CO_2 gas was also possible. Unfortunately, coronary angioscopy using CO_2 gas pro-

duced mechanical heart failure in all instances and was lethal in 80% of animals. Thus, these studies document the safety and efficacy of CO_2 gas when used to clear the visual field for angioscopy of the peripheral circulation in animals while demonstrating that its use in the coronary circulation appears quite risky. However, the use of CO_2 gas infusion to displace blood during angioscopy in the peripheral circulation in humans is still experimental and its safety has not been established.

INDICATIONS FOR ANGIOSCOPY

Initially, the projected uses of intraluminal angioscopy were unlimited. These uses included both intraoperative and percutaneous passage of the angioscope. However, percutaneous angioscopy in the large vessels of the peripheral vascular system is frequently suboptimal because of an inability to completely clear the viewing field of flowing blood. Because of this, essentially all reported series of angioscopy of peripheral vessels have used angioscopy during surgical procedures in which the inflow artery to the vessel being examined could be occluded. In contrast, percutaneous coronary angioscopy during coronary angiography has usually been successful, and preliminary studies suggest that this procedure may provide significant insights into the pathophysiology of coronary artery disease.[11, 12] Regardless, because angioscopy of the peripheral vascular system is the focus of this chapter, the remainder of this discussion will relate only to the intraoperative use of angioscopy during peripheral arterial reconstruction procedures.

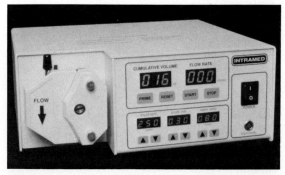

Figure 35–3. Irrigation pump specifically designed for angioscopy (Intramed Laboratories, Inc., San Diego, CA). This is a peristaltic pump that can achieve various flush rates and allow clear visualization of most peripheral vessels.

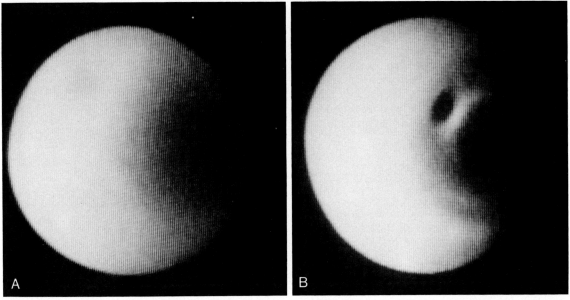

Figure 35–4. Angioscopic images produced using saline **(A)** or CO_2 **(B)** to clear the visual field during retrograde percutaneous angioscopy. The take-off of the right renal artery can be seen. The improved visual clarity of the image obtained using CO_2 gas is evident.

At present, the potential uses of angioscopy in patients with peripheral vascular disease can be grouped into three broad categories: (1) angioscopy as an adjunct to arterial thrombectomy-embolectomy, (2) angioscopy as an adjunct to infrainguinal arterial reconstruction, and (3) angioscopy as an adjunct to endovascular therapy.

EFFICACY OF ANGIOSCOPY

Adjunct to Thromboembolectomy Procedures

Angioscopic inspection of arterial or bypass graft lumens following attempted thrombectomy-embolectomy allows assessment of the adequacy of clot removal. Grundfest and coworkers[4] initially used the angioscope to demonstrate retained clot after standard Fogarty catheter thrombectomy. These findings were reiterated by Mehigan and Olcott.[13] White and colleagues subsequently reported that 80% to 90% of arterial lumens retain copious amounts of clot following standard blind thrombectomy-embolectomy and completion arteriography (Fig. 35–5).[14, 15] This thrombus could be removed by repeated passage of the Fogarty catheter or by the use of flexible biopsy forceps.[14, 15] However, use of biopsy forceps required contin-

ued direct visual inspection of the site of the retained thrombus through the angioscope to prevent vessel injury. Miller and associates[5] went one step beyond assessment of the com-

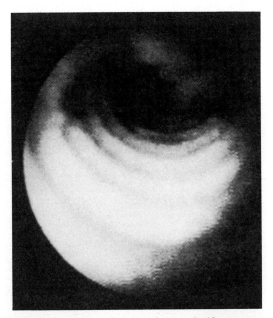

Figure 35–5. Angioscopic image shows a significant amount of retained thrombus adherent to the wall of an aortobifemoral bypass graft after multiple passes with a balloon catheter. (From White GH, White RA, Kopchok GE, et al. Endoscopic intravascular surgery removes intraluminal flaps, dissections, and thrombus. J Vasc Surg 11:280–288, 1990.)

pleteness of clot removal and used the angioscope to attempt to determine the cause of graft thrombosis. In 3 of their 17 cases, they were able to identify and repair an anastomotic stenosis, a residual competent valve leaflet, and a distal posterior wall atherosclerotic plaque. Thus, angioscopy is of significant value in thrombectomy-embolectomy and probably should be considered a standard part of this procedure.

Adjunct to Infrainguinal Reconstructions

The uses of angioscopy as an adjunct to infrainguinal arterial reconstruction includes (1) intraluminal visualization of in situ or nonreversed vein grafts during valvulotomy to prevent vein injury and to ensure complete valve disruption; (2) inspection of postreconstruction anastomoses for technical defects such as intimal flaps, suture line stenoses, platelet deposition, or thrombus formation; (3) evaluation of distal arterial runoff vessels for occlusive atherosclerotic disease; and (4) assessment of venous conduits for sites of fibrosis or areas of previous thrombosis and recanalization before bypass surgery.

Simultaneously, Mehigan and Olcott,[13] Seeger and Abela,[16] and Fleisher and coworkers[17] described the use of angioscopy to directly visualize the disruption of valve cusps in in situ and nonreversed vein bypass grafts (Fig. 35–6). Subsequently, many other authors[3-5, 14] reported

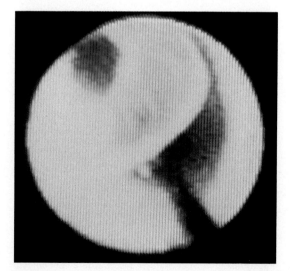

Figure 35–6. Angioscopic monitoring of a valvulotomy. The shaft of the modified Mills' valvulotome is seen adjacent to the valve cusp prior to valvulotomy.

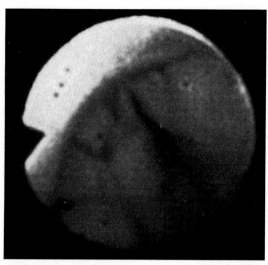

Figure 35–7. Angioscopic image of the distal anastomosis and narrowed outflow tract of a patient with rest pain who underwent a femoropopliteal bypass using using a saphenous cephalic vein composite graft. Significant narrowing of the outflow tract can be seen. (From Grundfest WS, Litvack F, Glick D, et al. Intraoperative decisions based on angioscopy in peripheral vascular surgery. Circulation 78: I13–I17, 1988, by permission of the American Heart Association, Inc.)

inspecting vein conduits with angioscopes after blind attempts at valvulotomy to ensure completeness of valve disruption. Typical of the findings of these studies is the report by Grundfest and colleagues[4] in which 8 of 17 (47%) in situ vein grafts were found to possess competent valves after initial valvulotomy.

Inspection of the distal anastomosis of peripheral bypass grafts using angioscopy was initially reported by Grundfest and associates.[3] They identified 7 (15%) anastomotic abnormalities in 46 patients, including one intimal flap, two suture line stenoses, and four areas of intimal irregularity. The former three defects required surgical revision. In a later report, Grundfest and associates[4] reported revising 5 of 37 (14%) anastomoses because of abnormalities seen on angioscopy. Anastomotic defects were from misplaced sutures, redundant graft material, and atheromatous flaps incorporated into the suture line. All of the defects resulted in partial stenosis of the anastomotic lumen and were readily identified by angioscopy (Fig. 35–7).

Baxter and associates[6] went one step further and prospectively compared the findings seen on completion arteriography with the findings of angioscopy in 49 patients undergoing infrainguinal arterial reconstructions. Of eight defects seen on arteriography, six were verified by angioscopy and repaired. More importantly, three grafts thought to be normal by arteriography were found to have significant defects (fresh thrombus in the perianastomotic region in one graft [Fig. 35–8] and significant intimal flaps at or just distal to the anastomosis in two other grafts). All three abnormalities required surgical repair. Similar results were reported in a study by White and colleagues,[18] in which arteriography produced a false-negative rate of 12.5% and a false-positive rate of 8% when compared with intraoperative angioscopy.

More recently, Miller and coworkers[19] further demonstrated the value of angioscopy as an adjunct to arterial reconstruction, reporting the results of intraoperative angioscopy during 259 infrainguinal bypass procedures (63 femoropopliteal, 196 femorotibial). The distal artery was visualized in 79.9% of cases, the distal anastomosis was seen in 92.1% of cases, and the entire vein graft was visible in 97.5% of cases. Defects requiring repair or a change in the bypass procedure were found during 124 procedures (47.9%). Defects at the anastomosis or in the artery just distal to the anastomosis were seen in 15 procedures (5.8%), including technically inadequate anastomoses in 2 cases, postanastomotic stenosis in 1 procedure; and intimal flaps in 3 instances. In addition, defects in the vein graft after in situ or nonreversed saphenous vein bypass were seen in more than one half of these procedures. The vein graft defects included incomplete valvulotomy in 33 cases, unligated tributaries in 58 cases, and graft torsion in 2 instances. Unfortunately, completion arteriog-

raphy was not done in most of the patients in this series, which might explain the high incidence of unligated venous tributaries. However, continuous wave Doppler examination of the exposed vein was routinely performed prior to angioscopy, and this commonly used intraoperative method of bypass graft evaluation did not detect either retained valve leaflets or patent vein tributaries seen with angioscopy.

Finally, Miller and coworkers[19] also used angioscopy to identify areas of sclerosis or recanalization of previous thrombi in 12 veins thought, on the basis of intraoperative inspection and palpation, to be adequate for use as a bypass conduit. Similar findings have been reported by Mehigan and Olcott.[13] These results appear to be of particular importance in view of the recent findings of Panetta and colleagues,[20] who reported a 14% early failure rate in bypass grafts that contained diseased vein segments; therefore, the detection of these vein graft luminal abnormalities becomes even more significant.

These studies clearly demonstrate that angioscopy is more sensitive than arteriography for detecting anastomotic and vein graft abnormalities that could lead to early graft failure. Also, angioscopic monitoring of vein graft valvulotomy appears to be necessary if complete valve lysis without vein injury is to be achieved during in situ or nonreversed vein bypass procedures. However, angioscopy is time-consuming and expensive; therefore, if angioscopy is to be accepted as a necessary adjunct to infrain-

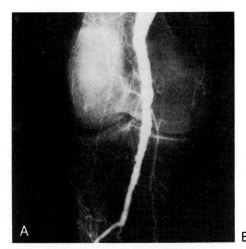
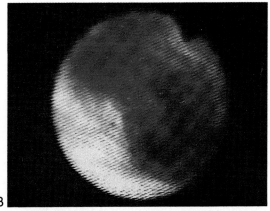

Figure 35–8. Completion arteriogram **(A)** and angioscopic view **(B)** of the distal anastomosis of a polytetrafluoroethylene femoropopliteal bypass graft. The completion arteriogram was interpreted as showing no technical problems, but angioscopy revealed significant thrombus at and just beyond the distal anastomosis. (From Baxter BP, Rizzo RJ, Flinn WR, et al. A comparative study of intraoperative angioscopy and completion arteriography following femoral distal bypass. Arch Surg 125:997–1002, 1990. Copyright 1990, American Medical Association.)

guinal bypass procedures, its use must be shown to improve graft patency. This improved patency after the use of angioscopy remains to be established, but Miller and associates[21] reviewed retrospectively the intraoperative angioscopic videotapes of 25 failed infrainguinal bypass procedures. Nineteen of the operations were classified as early failures (<30 days after surgery) and six of the procedures were classified as late failures (>3 months after surgery). In the early failure group, angioscopy findings that potentially were the cause of graft failure were seen in 13 of 19 cases. These findings were severe atherosclerosis distal to the anastomosis in 3 cases, distal arterial disease and concomitant anastomotic disease in 3 cases, and a vein of poor quality or improper placement of the vein conduit in 7 cases. In the patients with late graft failure, angioscopic findings that potentially caused graft failure were seen in all 6 cases, these findings being severe distal atherosclerotic disease in the outflow artery in 3 cases, multiple valvulotomy-induced vein injuries in 2 cases, and a large, partially occluding flap in the apex of the distal anastomosis in 1 case. This last defect had not been seen during the initial angioscopic examination but was evident on review of the videotape of the study. Also, Miller and associates[22] recently presented results of a randomized trial of angioscopy compared with angiography to monitor peripheral bypass procedures and demonstrated improved 30-day and 18-month graft patency in patients undergoing angioscopy. The statistical methods used in this study have been questioned, however. Regardless, these findings strongly suggest that angioscopy done at the time of the bypass procedure can identify significant pathologic conditions. When these conditions are repaired, graft patency will improve. Preliminary results of a study currently under way at the University of Florida College of Medicine support this conclusion: a statistically significant improvement in early infrainguinal graft patency has been demonstrated in patients who received both angioscopy and completion arteriography when compared with patients undergoing completion arteriography alone.

Adjunct to Endovascular Surgery

The use of angioscopy in association with various endovascular procedures is still not well defined. Seeger and Abela[16] initially attempted to use angioscopy during laser angioplasty to visualize and position the metallic tip of a fiberoptic laser probe in contact with the area of arterial occlusion. The use of angioscopy during laser angioplasty did allow observation of the lazing process (Fig. 35–9) but did not prevent complications, particularly perforation, which occurred in 5 of the 11 patients studied (45%).

White and coworkers[23] reported the use of angioscopy as an adjunct to laser angioplasty in 30 patients. They found that angioscopy was of little value in 24 patients with long or multisegmental occlusions. Significant proximal disease, which had not been identified by the arteriogram performed before the procedure, prevented passage of the angioscope in 18 of these 24 patients. In addition, in the 6 patients in whom the angioscope could be passed to the desired site, angioscopy was no longer of value once the laser probe entered the area of obstruction, and fluoroscopic monitoring was needed. Overall, arterial wall perforation occurred in 5 of 24 patients (20%). In contrast, in 6 patients who had a focal tight stenosis or occlusion less than 3 cm in length, laser angioplasty was easily performed under direct angioscopic visualization. Thorough inspection of the lesion before and after angioplasty was also possible in 88% of these patients. This allowed identification and assessment of thermal damage, wall charring, intimal fragmentation, mural thrombus formation, and development of false channels or intimal flaps. Four patients seen to have severe wall damage experienced occlusion within 48 hours, and 3 patients seen to have a small lumen diameter after passage of the laser probe required balloon angioplasty.

Recently, Diethrich and coworkers[24] used angioscopy in 23 patients to characterize intraarterial pathologic features and to select the optimal recanalization technique in patients undergoing endovascular therapy using multiple types of devices. Angioscopy was done successfully without complication. Concentric stenotic lesions were visualized in 12 patients and treated with the transluminal endarterectomy catheter (TEC) atherectomy device. Of this group, 3 patients required further balloon angioplasty, and 1 patient underwent a concomitant laser-assisted angioplasty to achieve a satisfactory outcome. Total arterial occlusion was identified and characterized in 8 patients. In 3 patients, an atherosclerotic occlusion (Fig. 35–10A) was opened successfully with laser-assisted balloon angioplasty, and recent thrombosis (Fig. 35–10B) was successfully lysed with urokinase in 5 patients. Reevaluation with angioscopy after thrombolysis identified severe popliteal artery stenosis in 2 patients, which was successfully

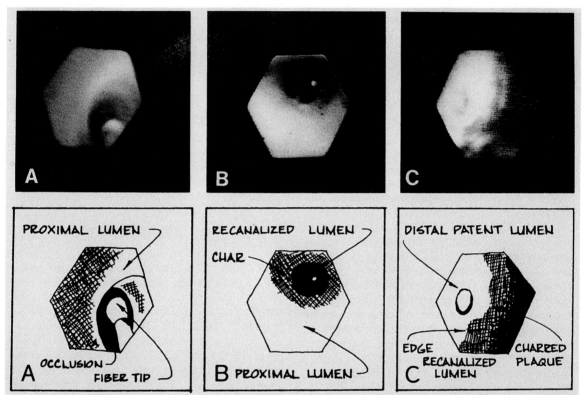

Figure 35–9. (A) Angioscopic view of a 2-mm laser probe seen in the center of the artery just proximal to an area of total occlusion. The angioscope has been rotated, showing the laser probe at the 5 o'clock position. **(B)** Angioscopic view of the lumen created by laser angioplasty. The new channel is seen as a dark tunnel in the right upper quadrant. The bright spot in the center of the new lumen is due to light reflection from saline profusate. Charring can be seen around the edges of the lumen from the lasing process. **(C)** Angioscopic view of the communication between the charred, recannulized vascular segment and the patent distal artery at the 9 o'clock position. Charring within the newly created vascular lumen is seen. (From Abela GS, Seeger JM, Barbieri E, et al. Laser angioplasty with angioscopic guidance in humans. Reprinted with permission from the American College of Cardiology, Journal of the American College of Cardiology, 8:184–192, 1986.)

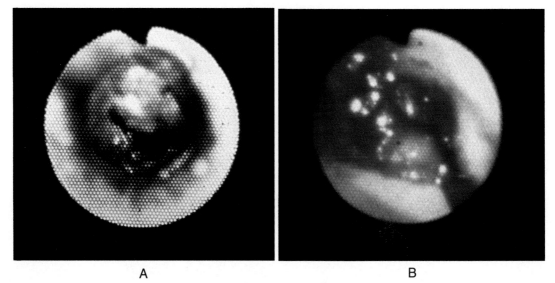

Figure 35–10. Angioscopic view of two types of total peripheral arterial occlusion. The atherosclerotic occlusion **(A)** is easily differentiated from the thrombotic occlusion **(B)**, which can be treated using thrombolysis.

dilated with balloon angioplasty. Finally, 1 patient underwent balloon angioplasty alone, whereas 2 patients were discharged without further therapy.

On the basis of these findings, angioscopy appears to be of value during endovascular therapy. However, it has a restricted role in guiding laser probes during their passage through occluded arterial segments and does not prevent arterial wall perforation during laser recanalization. Along with other endovascular techniques, angioscopy would seem to have an important role in selecting and guiding therapy. However, supporting data are scant, and further investigation of this area will be needed before the precise role and value of angioscopy in endovascular therapy can be determined.

MISCELLANEOUS USES

Other applications of angioscopy not grouped in the three categories already discussed include its use to inspect and treat traumatic vascular injuries and to treat anastomotic intimal hyperplasia. White and colleagues[15] visualized arterial intimal flaps or dissection planes created by external trauma or iatrogenic cannulation in 11 patients. Long, flexible biopsy forceps guided by direct visualization through the angioscope were used to successfully remove nine of these intimal defects and to avoid open arterial repair. Angioscopy-directed treatment of anastomotic stenoses by removal of intimal hyperplasia has also been reported. However, this has proved unsuccessful, as the stenosis recurs rapidly.[15]

SAFETY OF ANGIOSCOPY

Lee and colleagues[25] evaluated the histologic effects of passing various-sized angioscopes through in vivo canine arteries. Few gross injuries were seen with less than 10 passes, although minor intimal damage with early sloughing of the endothelial layer and occasional small intimal flaps were observed. However, when the angioscope fit tightly, extensive intimal flap formation and intimal damage occurred, and the endothelial cell layer and underlying internal elastic membrane were frequently lacking. With an increased number of passes, the medial layer was also damaged, although no actual dissections were seen.

Hashizume and associates[26] examined canine veins after passage of a polyethylene tube, which simulates an angioscope. Using 6-keto-prostaglandin $F_{1\alpha}$ and electron microscopy as markers of venous endothelial cell injury, they demonstrated intimal injury after a single passage of the angioscope. However, by 3 to 4 weeks, the endothelial lining had been repaired and 6-keto-prostaglandin $F_{1\alpha}$ levels had returned to normal. It was their conclusion that the intraluminal venous trauma created by angioscopy would not have a negative effect on early bypass graft patency.

These findings have been verified by multiple

clinical studies. The publications of Miller and colleagues,[5] Baxter and associates,[6] Mehigan and Olcott,[13] and Seeger and Abela[16] report no major arterial complications due to the use of the angioscope. Only Grundfest and coworkers[3] have reported an arterial injury from angioscopy, a single intimal flap that required surgical repair.

Volume overload from the irrigating fluid infused to provide a clear field of view during angioscopy has also been raised as a potential problem. In the early reports, volumes greater than 1 L were infused. With the development of dedicated infusion pumps, the average volume of fluid infused is now less than 500 ml.[5, 6] The reported rate of cardiac events after angioscopy is also low,[3, 5, 15] although Baxter and colleagues[6] reported an 8.2% incidence of early postoperative myocardial infarction, two cases of which were fatal. However, these cardiac events were not associated with volume overload. In addition, Kwolek and colleagues[27] recently reported 110 patients who underwent arterial reconstruction and were randomized to either angioscopy or angiography after bypass grafting. There were no differences between these groups in total administered intraoperative fluid, intraoperative use of vasodilators and diuretics, postoperative cardiac morbidity, and less-than-30-day mortality rates.

CONCLUSION

In a short time, angioscopy has become a technique that greatly aids vascular surgeons in evaluating their work. The procedure can be performed quickly with little risk. It has greater sensitivity than the intraoperative arteriogram in the visualization of retained thrombus after thrombectomy and in the detection of vein graft and anastomotic defects during arterial bypass surgery. Bypass graft failure appears to be associated with defects seen on angioscopy, strongly suggesting that correction of these defects will improve graft patency. This remains to be established, however. Finally, angioscopy may have a role in the control and evaluation of endovascular procedures, but its use as a guidance device for laser probes appears very limited. The use of angioscopy will likely increase as the technique and equipment improve, as better methods of clearing the field of view (e.g., displacement of blood with CO_2 gas) are developed, and as technical advances are made in catheter manufacture, such as smaller, steerable catheters with working channels. Thus an-

gioscopy is a valuable tool in the treatment of peripheral vascular disease and probably should be available to all vascular surgeons.

References

1. Stept LL, Flinn WR, McCarthy WJ, et al. Technical defects as a cause of early graft failure after femorodistal bypass. Arch Surg 122:599–604, 1987.
2. Towne JB, Bernhard VM. Vascular endoscopy: useful tool or interesting toy. Surgery 82:415–419, 1977.
3. Grundfest WS, Litvack F, Sherman T, et al. Delineation of peripheral and coronary detail by intraoperative angioscopy. Ann Surg 202:394–400, 1985.
4. Grundfest WS, Litvack F, Glick D, et al. Intraoperative decisions based on angioscopy in peripheral vascular surgery. Circulation 78(Suppl I):I13–I17, 1988.
5. Miller A, Campbell DR, Gibbons GW, et al. Routine intraoperative angioscopy in lower extremity revascularization. Arch Surg 124:604–608, 1989.
6. Baxter BT, Rizzo RJ, Flinn WR, et al. A comparative study of intraoperative angioscopy and completion arteriography following femorodistal bypass. Arch Surg 125:997–1022, 1990.
7. Chin AK, Nobles AA, Lai AK: Digital angioscopy. In: Moore WS, Ahn SS, eds. Endovascular Surgery. Philadelphia: WB Saunders, 1992:111–116.
8. Silverman SH, Mladinich CJ, Hawkins IF, et al. The use of carbon dioxide gas to displace flowing blood during angioscopy. J Vasc Surg 10:313–317, 1980.
9. Mladinich CRJ, Akins EW, Weingarten KE, Hawkins IF. Carbon dioxide as an angioscopic medium: comparison to various methods of saline delivery. Invest Radiol 26:874–878, 1991.
10. Smits PC, Post MJ, Velema E, et al. Percutaneous coronary and peripheral angioscopy with saline solution and carbon dioxide gas in porcine and canine arteries. Am Heart J 122:1315–1322, 1991.
11. Mizuno K, Satomura K, Miyamoto A, et al. Angioscopic evaluation of coronary-artery thrombi in acute coronary syndromes. N Engl J Med 326:287–291, 1992.
12. Sherman CT, Litvack F, Grundfest W, et al. Coronary angioscopy in patients with unstable angina pectoris. N Engl J Med 315:913–919, 1986.
13. Mehigan JT, Olcott C. Video angioscopy as an alternative to intraoperative arteriography. Am J Surg 152:139–145, 1986.
14. White GH, White RA, Kopchok GE, Wilson SE. Angioscopic thromboembolectomy: preliminary observations with a recent technique. J Vasc Surg 7:318–325, 1988.
15. White GH, White RA, Kopchok GE, et al. Endoscopic intravascular surgery removes intraluminal flaps, dissections, and thrombus. J Vasc Surg 11:280–288, 1990.
16. Seeger JM, Abela GS. Angioscopy as an adjunct to arterial reconstructive surgery: a preliminary report. J Vasc Surg 4:315–320, 1986.
17. Fleisher HL, Thompson BW, McCowan TC, et al. Angioscopically monitored saphenous vein valvulotomy. J Vasc Surg 4:360–364, 1986.
18. White GH, White RA, Kopchok GE, Klein SR. Intraoperative video angioscopy compared with arteriography during peripheral vascular operations. J Vasc Surg 6:488–495, 1987.
19. Miller A, Stonebridge PA, Jepsen SJ, et al. Continued experience with intraoperative angioscopy for monitoring infrainguinal bypass grafting. Surgery 109:286–293, 1991.

20. Panetta TF, Marin ML, Veith FJ, et al. Unsuspected preexisting saphenous vein disease: an unrecognized cause of vein bypass failure. J Vasc Surg 15:102–112, 1991.
21. Miller A, Jepsen SJ, Stonebridge PA, et al. New angioscopic findings in graft failure after infrainguinal bypass. Arch Surg 125:749–755, 1990.
22. Miller A, Marcaccio E, Tannenbaum G, et al. Comparison of angioscopy and angiography for monitoring infrainguinal bypass vein grafts: results of a prospective randomized trial. Presented at the 40th scientific meeting of the International Society For Cardiovascular Surgery, Chicago, 1992.
23. White GH, White RA, Colman PD, Kopchock GE. Experimental and clinical applications of angioscopic guidance for laser angioplasty. Am J Surg 158:495–501, 1989.
24. Diethrich EB, Yoffe B, Kiessling JJ, et al. Angioscopy in endovascular surgery: recent technical advances to enhance intervention selection and failure analysis. Angiology 43:1–10, 1991.
25. Lee G, Beerline D, Lee MH, et al. Hazards of angioscopic examination: documentation of damage to the arterial intima. Am Heart J 116:1530–1536, 1988.
26. Hashizume M, Yang Y, Galt S, et al. Intimal response of saphenous vein to intraluminal trauma by simulated angioscopic insertion. J Vasc Surg 5:862–868, 1987.
27. Kwolek CJ, Miller A, Stonebridge PA, et al. Safety of saline irrigation for angioscopy: results of a prospective randomized trial. Ann Vasc Surg 6:62–68, 1992.

36

Bronchoscopy and Mediastinoscopy

Darryl S. Weiman, Joe W. R. Bolton, Francis D. Ferdinand, and Glenn J. R. Whitman

BRONCHOSCOPY

History

In 1879, Killian performed what is felt to be the first bronchoscopy when he used a direct laryngoscope to inspect the trachea and remove a piece of pork bone from the right main stem bronchus.[1] In 1898, Collidge removed a portion of a displaced tracheal cannula from the right main stem bronchus, becoming the first American to perform a bronchoscopy.[1] Credit for developing modern bronchoscopy goes to Jackson. During Jackson's renowned career, he served on the faculty of each of the five Philadelphia medical schools. "All the laryngologists who had been doing bronchoscopy and esophagoscopy gave up the work and referred such cases to me. The rivalries of medical colleges and hospitals had been so keen that this was unheard of . . . I do not think that this would have been possible in any city other than Philadelphia."[1]

Indications

Bronchoscopy allows the surgeon to look into the lungs via the tracheobronchial tree. This view can be used for both diagnostic and therapeutic reasons. Bronchoscopy can be performed on an elective basis in a stable patient or in an emergency situation in the operating room for lifesaving treatment in critically ill patients. Bronchoscopy is also used as a modern research tool in the study of pulmonary pathophysiology.

The indications for performing bronchoscopy are continually being expanded. Perhaps the most common reason to perform diagnostic bronchoscopy is to determine whether or not a patient has a bronchogenic carcinoma. Bronchoscopy can aid in making the initial diagnosis, help determine resectability, and detect recurrences.

Bronchoscopy can be performed with either rigid or flexible scopes. The advantage of the flexible bronchoscope is that it can be advanced further out in the tracheobronchial tree, thus allowing visualization of, and ultimately the obtainment of a biopsy specimen from, smaller and more peripherally located lesions. Ikeda and colleagues were able to diagnose 60% to 70% more lesions with the flexible bronchoscope when compared with the rigid bronchoscope.[2] The trend toward smaller bronchoscopes to diagnose smaller and more peripheral lesions is ongoing, but the significance remains to be determined.[3]

In addition to identifying mass lesions in the lung, careful inspection for subtle changes in the bronchi may be required to select appropriate areas for biopsy.[4] The bronchoscopist must be meticulous in sampling tissue for the diagnosis of neoplasia. More than one biopsy—and the combination of biopsy, brushings, and washings—should be used to gain the maximum yield. Biopsy, however, remains the most accurate sampling technique owing to the amount of tissue obtained for review by the pathologist. Lesions not visualized at bronchoscopy but seen on x-ray film may require a fluoroscopically guided biopsy procedure. It is important to keep the jaws of the biopsy forceps closed during this procedure so that passage into the distal airway is not impeded. Another technique for sampling more peripheral lesions is with transbronchial needle aspiration.[5] This technique has also been used to aid in the staging of bronchogenic carcinoma by sampling the subcarinal nodes of the mediastinum. This is essentially done by passing the needle through the carina.[6]

Hemoptysis is one of the more common indications for performing bronchoscopy. Factors to be considered in this setting include a history of smoking, acute or chronic infection, associated physical findings, the presence of cough, sputum production, and the quantity of blood produced. It is also important to distinguish between an isolated event and a repetitive occurrence. Mild to moderate hemoptysis is considered to be less than 500 ml in 24 hours. Under these circumstances, either the rigid or the flexible bronchoscope may be used to locate the source of bleeding. Massive hemoptysis, which is defined as greater than 500 ml of blood in 24 hours, is considered a surgical emergency. Under these circumstances, the rigid bronchoscope is required so that the airways can be cleared of blood, and various treatment modalities can be achieved through the bronchoscope.

The diagnosis of infectious processes can be separated into two clinical settings. In the immunocompromised patient with diffuse pulmonary infiltrates, an accurate diagnosis could be elusive without examination of bronchopulmonary secretions and tissue.[7] Bronchoalveolar lavage is a useful technique whereby aliquots of sterile 0.9N saline at 37°C are instilled with the flexible bronchoscope wedged into the subsegmental bronchus and are then aspirated. The aspirated saline, of which 50% is considered an adequate recovery, is then sent for special staining, for example with hematoxylin and eosin, silver, and periodic acid–Schiff stains. Culture and sensitivity testing are also performed. This technique can significantly increase the yield when recovering opportunistic organisms such as *Pneumocystis carinii* and cytomegalovirus in patients with acquired immunodeficiency syndrome and those with other immunocompromised states.[8]

In immune competent patients with segmental or lobar infiltrates due to a partially occluded bronchus, tumors or mucus plugs can be diagnosed with the bronchoscope. In a patient with a tumor of the airways that has not responded to other forms of therapy, such as radiation or chemotherapy, the bronchoscope can be used to apply laser energy for tumor ablation. Special bronchoscopes have been developed for this setting; they have a separate channel to pass the laser fiber, as well as another channel so that a suction catheter can be placed without obstructing the bronchoscopist's view. Attachments can be placed at the end of these bronchoscopes so that a video system can be used to observe the entire field of view on a television monitor. Tumors that are in the more distal airways can be approached with the laser, using the flexible bronchoscope. In experienced hands, the risk from laser bronchoscopy is low. Significant risks include bleeding and perforation of a major airway or an airway fire. Major bleeding can be handled by local pressure through the rigid scope. An airway fire can be avoided by using a low FIO_2 during the procedure. Also, it is important to use a nonflammable endotracheal tube so that a tube fire is avoided. If an airway fire were to occur, the treatment of the patient would be supportive: complications such as pneumonia, airway sloughing, or stenoses are treated as they arise.

Equipment

Laryngoscopes were the first tools used to view the upper airways. Since then, modern bronchoscopes have evolved. Two significant milestones were the introduction of a flexible fiberoptic bronchoscope by Ikeda and associates[2] and the development of the rod-lens optical telescope by Hopkins for use in rigid bronchoscopes.

Standard Jackson bronchoscopes are rigid bronchoscopes that range in size from 3 mm in diameter × 20 cm in length, for use in pediatric patients, to 7 mm in diameter × 40 cm in length, for use in adults. In these bronchoscopes, light is transmitted within a channel in the wall to the tip. The bronchoscope is usually connected by way of a flexible fiberoptic cable to a halogen light source. There are also one or more channels for ventilation and suction. The large diameter of these scopes offers their primary advantage—that is, a large, controlled airway that allows ventilation—especially for pediatric patients in whom this is the preferred technique. Other major advantages are its use in massive hemoptysis for the removal of foreign bodies[9] and for endobronchial operations.

In patients with massive hemoptysis, the bronchoscope can be used to clear the airways of bloody material so that the site of bleeding can be found. The rigid scope allows various therapeutic maneuvers to be performed, such as applying local pressure to the site of the bleeding, and it can also allow cautery devices to be placed on the area of bleeding so that hemostasis can be obtained. Lasers can also be used to help stop the bleeding.

Biopsy forceps that can pass through the rigid scopes can be manipulated to remove large foreign bodies. In exceptional cases in which standard biopsy forceps are not able to grasp a large foreign body, laparoscopic biopsy instruments can be used to grasp it and remove it in its entirety along with the scope, since in some instances the foreign body is larger than the diameter of the scope.

The flexible bronchoscope allows the observation of more distal airways than is possible with the rigid scope. Modern fiberoptic flexible bronchoscopes range in size from a 3.5-mm outside diameter, with a 1.2-mm diameter inner channel for use in pediatric patients, to a 6-mm diameter, with a 2.6-mm inner channel for use in adults. Smaller outside diameters are available but have the disadvantage of not having an inner channel. In addition to the inner channel, these scopes have a fiberoptic bundle to transmit light, providing illumination at the tip. Transmitted images come back through a series of lenses in the handpiece. There are several fine cables running from the tip to the lever wheel that provide steering and maneuverability. Small size and flexibility provide the major advantages of these instruments—they are well tolerated in the awake patient and they can be passed farther within the tracheobronchial tree. In general, the flexible scopes are too small for dealing with copious secretions or blood and are not useful in extracting many foreign bodies that are too large to be grasped with the standard biopsy forceps that come through the flexible scope.

Preparation of the Patient

The first step in preparing the patient for bronchoscopy is to establish an appropriate physician-patient relationship. The physician should explain the entire procedure, including the sequence of events, what the patient can expect to feel, and why various maneuvers will be undertaken. This discussion not only will help prevent fears and relieve anxiety[10] but also will make pharmacologic control easier. The patient will tend to be more cooperative and willing to put up with the minor discomforts of the procedure, making the examination smoother and faster.

All patients undergoing bronchoscopy should be monitored with a blood pressure cuff, a pulse oximeter, and electrocardiographic monitoring.

An intravenous line should be placed. The most frequent adverse effects occurring during bronchoscopy are related to the premedication agents and hypoxia. Signs of these adverse effects are readily picked up with these basic monitoring measures and include altered vital signs, arrhythmias, and hypoxia.[11, 12] In general, supplemental oxygen should also be given.

It takes a brave patient and physician to undergo and perform, respectively, a rigid bronchoscopy while the patient is awake but sedated. It can be done but, in general, patients undergoing rigid bronchoscopy are fully anesthetized.

In awake patients undergoing flexible bronchoscopy, it is sometimes necessary to administer an antisialagogue. This will decrease the amount of tracheobronchial secretions, which would have a tendency to obscure visual inspection of the airways. Also, it will decrease the amount of suction needed to remove the secretions. Too much suctioning can induce hypoxia. As much as 2 L/minute of air can be aspirated through a 2-mm channel, resulting in a loss of both administered and alveolar oxygen.[13] In addition, a topical anesthetic must be used to anesthetize the upper airways. Such an agent would be ineffective if the presence of secretions prevented it from acting on the underlying mucosa. Atropine or glycopyrrolate may be used, according to one's preference.

The next consideration is to sedate the patient sufficiently to relieve anxiety while maintaining adequate ventilation, oxygenation, and cooperation. The benzodiazepines (midazolam and diazepam) have a rapid onset of action, a relatively short half-life, and produce antegrade amnesia, making them ideal agents. The addition of a narcotic such as morphine or fentanyl will produce an analgesic effect. In addition, these narcotics will suppress upper airway reflexes somewhat, thereby facilitating passage and manipulation of the bronchoscope.

Anesthetizing the upper airways requires a topical agent. A 4% solution of lidocaine administered through an atomizer, or a combination of benzocaine and tetracaine given by way of a spray is commonly employed and well tolerated. The bronchoscopist must be diligent to ensure that the entire upper airway is treated, as the sensory innervation starting at the mouth or nose and progressing to the trachea involves three cranial nerves (V, IX, and X), making it easy to miss an area, causing the patient unnecessary discomfort.

In general, prophylactic antibiotics are not required for most patients undergoing bronchoscopy. Patients at risk for endocarditis who undergo rigid bronchoscopy should receive prophylactic antibiotics according to the American Heart Association's recommendations. In addition, patients with prior history of endocarditis, prosthetic heart valves, or surgical systemic to pulmonary shunts may also benefit from receiving prophylactic antibiotics.[14]

Technique

Rigid Bronchoscopy

During rigid bronchoscopy, the patient should be positioned supine on the operating table. The head may or may not be lowered depending on one's preference. Using gauze pads or plastic "teeth protectors" to protect the surgeon's fingers and the patient's teeth, the bronchoscope is inserted into the patient's mouth with the surgeon in a standing position. The bevel of the bronchoscope is pointed up and the direction of the scope is horizontal to the patient's tracheal axis. The scope is passed over the thumb, proximal to the distal interphalangeal joint, while the index and middle fingers of the operator gently pull the patient's incisors cephalad. With the patient's head rotated slightly to the left, the operator approaches the oropharynx. Next, the viewing end is gently rotated down to approach the orientation parallel to the patient's trachea. This rotation should occur around an axis created by the operator's thumb upon which the scope rests. At no time should the scope be pushed against the patient's teeth. The view should now approach the hypopharynx and the epiglottis.

At this point, the operator should be sitting with the bronchoscope in line with the patient's trachea. The tip of the scope can then be used to elevate the epiglottis, much like the straight blade of the laryngoscope used for intubation. As one performs these introductory maneuvers, inspection of the pertinent anatomy is carried out.

To facilitate passage through the vocal cords, the bronchoscope is rotated 90° to the right and advanced. Once through the vocal cords, the bronchoscope is rotated back to its original position and advanced toward the carina. When going through the vocal cords, they are examined for orientation, movement, and lesions. As the carina is approached, it is inspected for sharpness and subtle movements with respiration. The trachea should be examined for mucosal appearance, intraluminal masses, and signs of extraluminal compression.

The left main stem bronchus is slightly more difficult to enter than the right main stem bronchus because of its more acute angle relative to the trachea. By rotating the patient's head to the contralateral side, the bronchoscope may be advanced into the main stem bronchus and the lobar orifices may be visualized. In particular, it should be noted if there are any luminal irregularities, masses, foreign bodies, bleeding, or excess secretions. Access to the right tracheobronchial tree is gained with rotation of the patient's head to the left. Oblique and right-angle telescopes can be used to better visualize the lobar orifices, such as the upper lobe bronchus and the middle lobe bronchus.

Flexible Bronchoscopy

Although positioning and technique are not as critical in flexible bronchoscopy as in rigid bronchoscopy, certain principles are fundamental to both types of instruments. First, a routine should always be employed so that a systematic inspection can be performed. Second, although most patients examined with the flexible bronchoscope will be awake, the bronchoscopist must be aware of ventilation and oxygenation. If the patient is not intubated, supplemental oxygen can be administered by way of nasal prongs or with an aerosol mask. For intubated patients, the bronchoscope can be passed through a special connector that allows the anesthesia circuit to remain closed while the bronchoscope advances through a soft plastic seal. The relative diameters of the bronchoscope and the endotracheal tube must be kept in mind from a physiologic point of view. The residual cross-sectional area is the area remaining for ventilation once the bronchoscope is within the endotracheal tube. Practically speaking, if a 6-mm bronchoscope is passed within a 7.5-mm endotracheal tube, the residual cross-sectional area would be equivalent to a 4-mm endotracheal tube. This could be inadequate for ensuring adequate ventilation while preventing elevated airway pressure. High airway pressures during bronchoscopy could lead to barotrauma or pneumothorax, especially if a biopsy is required.

The flexible bronchoscope may be passed transnasally or transorally through a bite block. The tip can be flexed ventrally to gain access to the larynx and ultimately the vocal cords. Having the patient phonate prior to going through the vocal cords will demonstrate cord function. Once through the vocal cords, the tracheobronchial tree is examined. If performing bronchoscopy on an intubated patient, the examination starts at the level of the tip of the endotracheal tube. Proximal structures are blocked from view by the endotracheal tube. Maneuverability of the flexible bronchoscope is facilitated by rotation of the entire scope along its long axis and by flexing the tip. The carina is always used as a landmark for orientation purposes.

Complications

During bronchoscopy, complications can occur because of preoperative medications, technical difficulties with the scope, complications of the biopsy procedure, or the patient's cardiac or pulmonary disease. The rigid scope can cause injury to the larynx or the upper airways. The complications seen with the rigid scope include broken teeth and lacerations to the lip, pharynx, and larynx. By keeping a finger between the patient's teeth and the bronchoscope, the endoscopist can be sure that he or she is not causing any undue pressure that may lead to injury in these areas. Injury to the arytenoid cartilage can occur if the bronchoscopist fails to rotate the scope 90° when passing it through the vocal cords. If the endoscopist is not careful, the scope can be passed unintentionally into the esophagus with, of course, the possible risk of esophageal perforation. It is important to be gentle in manipulating the bronchoscope so that injury to the airway does not occur. Even with the appropriate manipulations, the patient can experience some subglotic or glottic edema, which may lead to airway compromise. If the patient experiences any sort of airway obstruction, the procedure should be terminated and the patient treated with some racemic epinephrine, humidified oxygen, and possibly steroid therapy. Heliox (helium-oxygen combination) can be used in an effort to prevent reintubation of the patient if some airway narrowing has occurred secondary to the bronchoscopy. When using Heliox, it is important that a maximum of 40% oxygen be used, otherwise the effect of the Heliox will be lost.

Complications related to the biopsy include bleeding and pneumothorax. If bleeding occurs, the patient should be placed with the head down and the bleeding side in a dependent position. This will protect the opposite lung from flooding. If possible, the bronchoscope should be used to occlude the bleeding segment, and local pressure should be applied in the hope of stopping the bleeding. If bleeding persists, an endotracheal tube may be required, and if bleeding is massive a double-lumen endotracheal tube can be placed to protect the opposite lung. Bleeding in most cases can be handled with local pressure, topical epinephrine, or direct cauterization. On occasion, an endobronchial blocker can be used on the side of the hemorrhage to protect the rest of the bronchial tree from being flooded with blood. If bleeding persists, a decision must be made by the surgeon about further treatment, which may include bronchial artery embolization or a thoracotomy to control the bleeding.

If a transbronchial biopsy is performed, the incidence of pneumothorax approaches 5%. Many small pneumothoraces can be managed with simple needle aspiration, but larger pneumothoraces or pneumothoraces that occur in a patient who is being ventilated should be treated with chest tube placement.

MEDIASTINOSCOPY

Cancer is the second most common cause of death in the United States today. Of all cancers, carcinoma of the lung is by far the leading cause of cancer deaths. Although the incidence of the majority of cancers has remained stable or declined over the past 50 years, carcinoma of the lung has had a linear increase as a cause of death, affecting 75 in 100,000 males and recently surpassing breast cancer to affect almost 28 in 100,000 females. The overall survival rate has remained unchanged at 8% to 13%.[15] Because of this, preoperative staging has become increasingly important to help determine which patients will most likely benefit from tumor resection.

Over the years, there has been continuing discussion concerning the indications for mediastinoscopy, as well as the use of noninvasive staging techniques, to help determine anatomic resectability. According to a survey on lung cancer management, 83% of nonsurgeons and 92% of surgeons do not recommend routine mediastinoscopy as a part of preoperative staging prior to attempted resection.[16] However, after a review of the literature concerning mediastinoscopy, we feel that there should be a move toward the routine use of preoperative mediastinoscopy rather than the currently accepted recommendation of selective mediastinoscopy. This is emphasized by the fact that a new staging system has been developed that distinguishes stage IIIA (which includes resectable N2 disease) from stage IIIB (which is surgically unresectable disease) (Table 36–1).[17]

In order to best determine the presence of surgically resectable disease, mediastinoscopy is necessary. Furthermore, it is difficult to justify the replacement of a relatively simple, accurate, low-cost procedure that is considered the "gold standard" with less accurate, although less invasive, techniques.

Table 36–1. LUNG CANCER STAGING

AJCC Stage		NIS Stage
Occult		*Occult*
I		0
I	T1, N0, M0	I
I	T1, N1, M0	II
II	T2, N1, M0	II
III	T3, N0, M0	IIIA
III	Any T, N3, M0	IIIB
III	Any T, Any N, M1	IV

AJCC = American Joint Committee on Cancer; NIS = New International System.

Rationale

Although some controversy exists about specific indications, mediastinoscopy remains an integral part of the prethoracotomy evaluation of bronchogenic carcinoma.

The original goal of mediastinoscopy was to obtain material for microscopic analysis in cases of bronchoscopically or radiographically suspected metastases or extension of cancer to the mediastinum. Vyas and coworkers feel that there are two major indications for mediastinal exploration. First, mediastinoscopy may be used for the diagnosis of pulmonary lesions, especially when there is evidence of hilar involvement. The second indication is in predicting resectability.[20]

Pearson found that 31% of patients presumably eligible for resection had mediastinal tumor spread detected by mediastinoscopy.[24, 42, 68, 76] This is somewhat greater than the 6.6% to 20% reported by Seydel and associates.[22] Anderson and coworkers found that if mediastinoscopy is carried out routinely in patients with bronchogenic carcinoma, tumor will be found in 30% to 40% of cases.[23] This seems to be in agreement with the finding of Luke and associates, who reported a 29.6% rate of abnormal mediastinoscopy results in a group of patients who did not have metastatic disease.[24] In further studies, Ashraf and colleagues and Fishman and Bronstein reported mediastinal node involvement in 27% and 28% of their patient groups, respectively.[25, 26] Maassen pulled statistical data on 8228 bronchogenic carcinomas that were investigated by mediastinoscopy. Mediastinal node involvement was detected in 35% of those cases.[27]

Once mediastinal lymph node metastases are detected, their relevance to survival must be considered. Several studies have addressed this point. Overall, 5-year survival rates based on lymph node status are reported as 25% to 40% for N0 disease, 15% to 20% for N1 disease, and less than 10% for N2 disease.[28–37] Naruke and associates reviewed their work to find that with complete mediastinal lymph node resection, the 5-year survival rate was improved to 59.9% for N0 disease, 39.1% for N1 disease, and 18.8% for N2 disease. This group found a significant difference in the presence or lack of metastases to the subcarinal nodes, with a decrease from a 29% survival rate with N2 metastases not involving the subcarinal nodes to a 9.1% survival rate if the subcarinal nodes were involved.[38] This seems to support the concept of high contralateral spread with subcarinal node involvement. In this study, no mention was made as to whether the decreased survival was due to contralateral disease.

In the study by Ashraf and coworkers, the operative mortality rate was three times higher when mediastinal lymph nodes were invaded— that is, 9%. When this fact is weighed against the 5-year survival rate of 3.7% for this particular group of patients, it may not seem appropriate to subject these patients to thoracotomy.[25]

In a different study, Bergh and Schersten showed that if there is only intranodal involvement of the mediastinal nodes, 43% of patients will be alive 2 to 10 years after resection for cure.[39]

Martini and colleagues did not perform mediastinoscopy as part of their staging procedure prior to thoracotomy; however, they did mediastinal lymph node dissections at the time of operation. In addition, the majority of these patients received intraoperative interstitial irradiation to treat residual tumor that could not be removed at the time of thoracotomy. These patients also received external beam radiotherapy. Even with all these modalities, there was still a recognized precipitous decrease in survival when either gross or microscopic disease was left behind.[40]

In the discussion of Martini's paper, Kirschner makes the observation that only 30% of N2 disease was totally resected, whereas there was an overall 17% unresectability rate.[41]

Pearson and associates reported a series of 141 patients over 17 years who underwent thoracotomy for presumably operable non–oat cell lung cancer with metastases to mediastinal nodes. The survival of those patients with N2 disease found at mediastinoscopy was 9%. If the N2 disease was found by thoracotomy after normal mediastinoscopy results, the overall survival rate was 24%, with a 41% survival rate for those who underwent a curative resection. Thus, mediastinoscopy appears instrumental in the selection of operable N2 disease (Table 36–2).[42]

Table 36–2. SURVIVAL RATES IN N2 DISEASE

Abnormal mediastinoscopy results	9%
Normal mediastinoscopy results with N2	24%
Disease detected at thoracotomy	(41% if curative resection is completed)

Although he did not use mediastinoscopy, Smith reported a 13.4% incidence of mediastinal lymph node invasion with a resectability rate of 97.4% and a hospital mortality rate of 2.8%.[43] Based on these results, he feels that mediastinoscopy is not necessary. However, he does report that no patient with paratracheal node involvement survived beyond 5 years. In addition, it is unclear how Smith staged his patients.

Sarin and Nohl-Oser observed that 40% to 50% of patients with lung cancers have abnormal mediastinoscopy results.[72] When cell type is considered, 76% of oat cell cancers have mediastinal spread at the time of presentation, whereas only 40% to 60% of adenocarcinomas and anaplastic cancers have abnormal results at mediastinoscopy. It appears that squamous cell carcinomas have the lowest rate of mediastinal spread, with about 35% of patients having abnormal findings at presentation.[44–47]

To illustrate the dismal prognosis for patients with only palliative operations, Shields has compiled some interesting data. In his group of patients, there was a 16.2% 30-day operative mortality rate. Thirty-eight percent of patients were dead within 3 months, 55% died within 6 months, and 74% died within 1 year. Only 4% of the patients in this series survived 5 years. All of the survivors had squamous cell carcinomas, with histologically detectable disease left behind and treated with adjuvant forms of therapy. When mediastinal disease was present, only 3.6% survived 2 years, and there were no 3-year survivors.[50]

Technique

Before beginning the procedure, it is very important that the surgeon review the computed tomography scan of the chest and mediastinum and that it be available for further review in the operating room. A general anesthetic is used and an endotracheal tube is placed. During the procedure, the patient is monitored in the usual fashion; however, the blood pressure monitor should be on the right arm because the brachiocephalic artery may be occluded by the medias-

tinoscope during some of the manipulations performed by the surgeon. Some anesthesiologists prefer to keep a hand on the right carotid artery so that if the carotid pulse disappears he or she can inform the surgeon that the brachiocephalic artery has been occluded.

The patient is prepared and draped for possible median sternotomy so that if surgical bleeding occurs during the mediastinoscopy, rapid entrance into the chest can be obtained without having to worry about preparing and draping the patient again. It is important not to hyperextend the neck, as this will decrease the space between the sternum and the trachea.

The standard mediastinoscopy is done through a suprasternal incision approximately one fingerbreadth above the sternal notch. Dissection is carried down to the pretracheal fascia, which is opened. If the right plane of dissection has been entered, it is very easy to place a finger along the trachea into the mediastinum. Care must be taken to go underneath the brachiocephalic artery during this finger dissection. At this time, the surgeon can palpate the nodal areas of interest in sampling. The brachiocephalic artery can be palpated, as can the arch of the aorta.

After the exploration with the finger has been completed, the mediastinoscope is brought onto the field and is hooked up to the light source. The mediastinoscope is placed directly down onto the trachea, and the tracheal rings are visualized as the scope is advanced into the mediastinum. By keeping the tracheal rings in view, the surgeon knows that he or she is going to be slipping underneath the brachiocephalic artery, keeping that vessel free from injury.

After the surgeon has placed the scope, sampling of the pertinent lymph node areas can begin. In general, for a patient with bronchogenic carcinoma, we make it a point to biopsy the region IV lymph nodes on both sides of the trachea underneath the brachiocephalic artery. We also make it a point to dissect the region VII area and biopsy lymph nodes from this area. On occasion, we can also find a region III and a region II lymph node for biopsy. For dissecting purposes, we have found a combined suction and coagulating device to help push the tissues aside while we try to find a suitable lymph node for biopsy. Before taking a biopsy specimen from any structure in the mediastinum, it is important to take a needle and aspirate the biopsy area. We do this with a long needle connected to a controlled-release syringe that contains approximately 1 to 2 ml of saline solution. If blood is withdrawn with the needle in position, biopsy of this region is not performed. If the biopsy proceeds, the biopsy forceps are then used to grab tissue in the area in question. At this point, the surgeon's tactile senses are very important because if the tissue does not come easily with the biopsy forceps, it is possible that a vascular structure has been grasped, and the surgeon should refrain from trying to tear it out of the mediastinum. If bleeding occurs after a biopsy, it is very important to leave the scope in place and put some packing over the area, leaving it there with some compression for approximately 15 to 20 minutes. If the bleeding persists after the packing is removed, we repack the area and prepare for a sternotomy. Bleeding may be coming from the pulmonary artery or the aorta or the brachiocephalic vessels. If these structures have been biopsied with the biopsy forceps, they most likely will need to be surgically repaired.

After the lymph node areas have been adequately sampled, hemostasis is obtained with the foot control cautery device, and the mediastinoscope is carefully removed. The wound is irrigated and the platysma muscle is approximated with three interrupted sutures of absorbable material. We close the skin with a subcuticular absorbable suture. A sterile dressing is placed.

In the recovery room, a chest x-ray film is obtained to make sure that the patient does not have a pneumothorax, which can occur if the pleura is injured during biopsy maneuvers (Figs. 36–1 through 36–9).

Chamberlain Procedure (Anterior Mediastinotomy)

When cervical mediastinoscopy cannot reach the nodal areas of interest, it may become

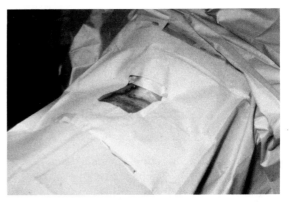

Figure 36–2. Final preparation and draping for mediastinoscopy.

necessary to perform an anterior mediastinotomy. This procedure allows biopsy of an anterior mediastinal mass, and it will allow sampling of region V and VI mediastinal nodes, which are areas where left upper lobe tumors are likely to spread.

To perform an anterior mediastinotomy, a transverse incision is made over the second or third costal cartilage on the side of interest. The costal cartilage is mobilized and excised in its subperichondrial plane. The posterior perichondrium is then incised. During this dissection, the internal mammary vessels may either be ligated individually or, if possible, retracted medially. Using the finger as a blunt dissector, the pleura is mobilized laterally and the mediastinum is then entered. The finger can be used to explore the node-bearing tissue in question. After the finger has done its blunt dissection, the mediastinoscope can be brought onto the field, and direct visualization of the nodal tissue to be biopsied can take place.

After hemostasis has been obtained, the scope is removed and the wound is closed. On occa-

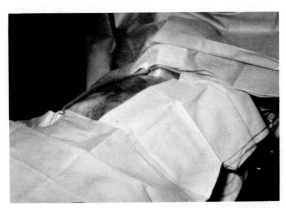

Figure 36–1. Patient is prepared and draped for possible median sternotomy.

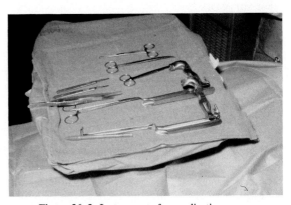

Figure 36–3. Instruments for mediastinoscopy.

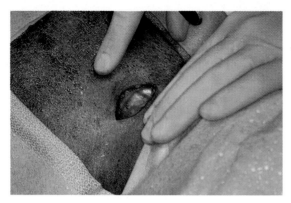

Figure 36–4. Skin incision for mediastinoscopy.

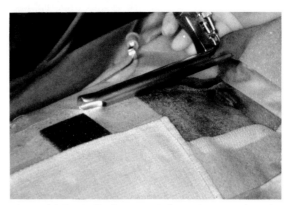

Figure 36–7. Mediastinoscope before placement into the mediastinum.

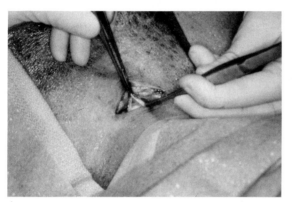

Figure 36–5. Pretracheal fascia incised before blunt dissection of the mediastinum.

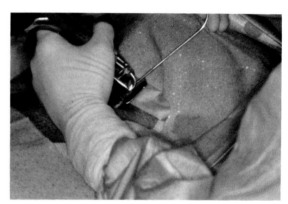

Figure 36–8. Scope in position. The right hand is used to manipulate various instruments.

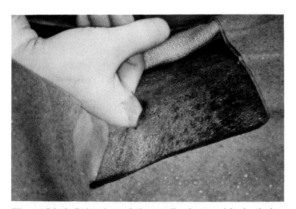

Figure 36–6. Palpation of the mediastinum with the index finger.

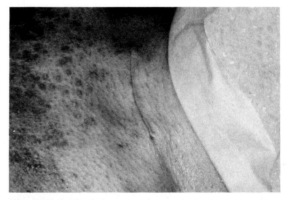

Figure 36–9. Final closure at the conclusion of mediastinoscopy.

sion it may be necessary to open the pleura to obtain adequate biopsy specimens. If this occurs, aspiration of air with a small red rubber catheter can be performed, with safe removal of the catheter after the wound is closed. On some occasions, it may be necessary to attach the catheter to a water seal drainage system.

Complications

Although Carlens reported no significant complications in his initial report of 100 cervical mediastinoscopies, other surgeons have not been as fortunate.[51] Reynders reported six complications, including pneumothorax, recurrent nerve paralysis, bleeding, subcutaneous emphysema, wound infection, and perforated traction diverticulum of the esophagus.[48, 52]

Bjork has stated that more than 2700 mediastinoscopies have been performed at his hospital (primarily by Carlens) with no mortality. He goes on to mention that Spect collected a series of 11,000 mediastinoscopies from 20 clinics and found an overall mortality rate of 0.17%.[53] Generally, mediastinoscopy is fairly safe, having a morbidity rate of 1.5% to 2.3% and a mortality rate of 0.09% to 0.10%.[21, 43, 54–57]

The most commonly reported complications of mediastinoscopy are hemorrhage (0.76%), pneumothorax (0.67%), recurrent laryngeal nerve injury (0.33%), and infection (0.18%). Tumor implantation has been reported in the mediastinoscopy scar in 0.12% of patients.[58] Other reported complications include chylothorax,[59, 60] pleural effusion, postoperative wheezing, unintentional removal of the endotracheal tube,[61] respiratory insufficiency,[57] cautery burn of the bronchus, avulsion of pulmonary artery branches,[62] cardiac arrhythmias (especially bradycardia), esophageal perforation, myocardial infarction, and hemiparesis[21] (Table 36–3).

Overall, the complication rate appears to be directly related to the experience of the surgeon,

Table 36–3. COMPLICATIONS OF MEDIASTINOSCOPY

Hemorrhage	Chylothorax
Pneumothorax	Wheezing
Recurrent nerve injury	Inadvertent extubation
Infection	Respiratory insufficiency
Tumor implantation	Bronchial burn
Pleural effusion	Esophageal perforation
Cardiac dysrhythmias	Myocardial infarction
Avulsion of pulmonary artery branch	

and Palva recommends that only in very select cases should mediastinoscopy be performed in hospitals without a thoracic surgeon present.[63, 64]

CONCLUSION

If the results of mediastinoscopy are normal, there is an overall 90% to 95% chance that an identified lung cancer will prove to be resectable at the time of thoracotomy. Mediastinoscopy has helped to identify that subgroup of patients who have resectable lesions and in whom surgery provides a 5-year survival rate that is significantly increased beyond that of the natural history of stage III disease.[22, 65]

The use of mediastinoscopy will decrease the frequency of backout thoracotomies while increasing the curative resection rate. Patients with squamous cell carcinoma of the right lung and ipsilateral low superior mediastinal nodes without extranodal disease may still benefit from resection.[42, 66–68]

Mediastinoscopy does not improve long-term survival, but it does increase the resectability rate to as high as 97% and decreases postoperative mortality without changing the patient's chance for a curative resection.[25]

Pearson and associates found an 8% false-negative rate with the use of mediastinoscopy. In most of these instances, the mediastinal nodes involved were found in locations not accessible to routine cervical mediastinoscopy. The rate of resectability in this particular series was 96%.[68]

Some authors consider mediastinal lymph node involvement to be a contraindication to operative intervention because of the dismal 5-year survival rate of less than 10%.[25, 39, 69–73] Conversely, some authors do not routinely perform mediastinoscopy based on the feeling that they would not withhold surgical treatment in any patient with a bronchogenic carcinoma involving the mediastinal lymph nodes.[25, 43, 74–76] However, since the 5-year survival rate of patients with mediastinal lymph nodes found preoperatively is 3.7%, it may be justified to withhold surgical treatment in such situations, since the 30-day postoperative mortality rate of 9% is high.[25]

When selecting patients for thoracotomy, Pearson recommends that only those with abnormal mediastinal biopsy results and ipsilateral nodal involvement below the level of the midtrachea without gross extranodal extension should undergo resection; postoperative adjuvant therapy is necessary in these cases. Patients with perinodal extension, high paratracheal involvement, contralateral spread, small cell carcinoma, or superior mediastinal nodes should not undergo thoracotomy.[68]

Mediastinoscopy merits an honored place among diagnostic and prognostic methods in thoracic disease. It assists in the diagnosis of malignant and benign disease and in prethoracotomy staging of bronchogenic carcinomas. Preferably, it should be performed by surgeons collaborating intimately with other chest specialists. The anesthesiologist must be experienced, and the facilities for median sternotomy must be available. Before the decision to perform mediastinoscopy is made, palpable lymph nodes in other sites should be studied histologically.[78, 79]

Based on our review, we feel that a more aggressive attitude toward the use of mediastinoscopy should be taken. Routine preoperative mediastinoscopy can assist in the staging and selection of patients who will benefit from thoracotomy while not denying any patient the opportunity for a curative resection.

References

1. Jackson C. The life of Chevalier Jackson, an autobiography. New York: Macmillian, 1938.
2. Ikeda S, Yawai N, Shikawa S. Flexible bronchofiberscope. Keio J Med 17:1, 1968.
3. Prakash UBS. The use of the pediatric fiberoptic bronchoscope in adults. Am Rev Respir Dis 132:715–718, 1985.
4. Zisholtz BM, Eisenberg H. Lung cancer cell type as a determinant of bronchoscopy yield. Chest 84:428–430, 1983.
5. Schenk DA, Bower JH, Bryan CL, et al. Transbronchial needle aspiration staging of bronchogenic carcinoma. Am Rev Respir Dis 134:146–148, 1986.
6. Shure D, Fedullo F. The role of transcarinal needle aspiration in the staging of bronchogenic carcinoma. Chest 86:5819–5823, 1984.
7. Williams D, Yungbluth M, Adams G, Glassroth J. The role of fiberoptic bronchoscopy in the evaluation of immunocompromised hosts with diffuse pulmonary infiltrates. Am Rev Respir Dis 131:880–885, 1985.
8. Meduri GU, Stover DE, Greeno RA, et al. Bilateral bronchoalveolar lavage in the diagnosis of opportunistic pulmonary infections. Chest 100:1272–1276, 1991.
9. Jackson C, Jackson CL. Bronchoesophagology. Philadelphia: WB Saunders, 1950.
10. Egbert LD, Batti GL, Turndorf H, Beecher HK. The value of a preoperative visit by the anesthetist. JAMA 185:553–555, 1963.
11. Zavala DC. Complications following fiberoptic bronchoscopy, the "good news" and the "bad news." Chest 73:783–785, 1978.
12. Dresin RB, Albert RK, Tally PA, et al. Flexible fiberoptic bronchoscopy in the teaching hospital. Chest 74:144–149, 1978.
13. Miller EJ. Hypoxemia during fiberoptic bronchoscopy. Chest 75:103, 1979.
14. Dajani AS, Bisno AL, Chung KJ, et al. Prevention of bacterial endocarditis: recommendations by the American Heart Association. JAMA 264:2919–2922, 1990.
15. Silverberg E, Lubera JA. Cancer statistics, 1988. CA 38:2–22, 1988.
16. Thurer RJ, Putman CE. Thoracic surgery survey on lung cancer management. Chest 91:913–916, 1987.
17. Moores DW. Staging of lung cancer. Ann Thorac Surg 44:225–226, 1987.
18. Bolton JWR, Weiman DS, Haynes JL, et al. Stair climbing as an indicator of pulmonary function. Chest 92:783–788, 1987.
19. Olsen GN, Weiman DS, Bolton JWR, et al. Invasive exercise testing in the assessment of risk of lung resection in patients with COPD. Unpublished data.
20. Vyas JJ, Desai PB, Rao ND. Relative accuracy of diagnostic method in bronchogenic carcinoma. J Surg Oncol 21:45–48, 1982.
21. Bone RC, Balk R. Staging of bronchogenic carcinoma. Chest 82:473–480, 1982.
22. Seydel HG, Chait A, Gmleich JJ. Cancer of the lung. New York: John Wiley & Sons, 1975.
23. Anderson RW, Arentzen CE. Carcinoma of the lung. Surg Clin North Am 60:793–814, 1980.
24. Luke WP, Pearson FG, Todd TRJ, et al. Prospective evaluation of mediastinoscopy for assessment of carcinoma of the lung. J Thorac Cardiovasc Surg 91:53–56, 1986.
25. Ashraf MH, Milsom PL, Walesby RK. Selection by mediastinoscopy and long term survival in bronchial carcinoma. Ann Thorac Surg 30:208–214, 1980.
26. Fishman NH, Bronstein MH. Is mediastinoscopy necessary in the evaluation of lung cancer? Ann Thorac Surg 20:678–686, 1975.
27. Maassen W. Accuracy of mediastinoscopy. In: Delarue NC, Eschapasse H, eds. International trends in general thoracic surgery, Vol I: lung cancer. Philadelphia, WB Saunders, 1985:42–53.
28. Higginson JF. Block dissection in pneumonectomy for carcinoma. J Thorac Surg 25:282–299, 1953.
29. Brock SR, Whytehead LL. Radical pneumonectomy for bronchial carcinoma. Br J Surg 43:8–24, 1955.
30. Nohl HC. The spread of carcinoma of the bronchus. London: Lloyd-Luke Medical Books, 1962.
31. Belcher JR, Anderson R. Treatment of carcinoma of the bronchus. Br Med J 1:948–954, 1965.
32. Boucot KR, Cooper DA, Weiss W. The role of surgery in the cure of lung cancer. Arch Intern Med 120:168–175, 1967.
33. Churchill ED, Sweet RH, Scannell JG, Wilkins EW Jr. Further studies in the surgical management of carcinoma of the lung. A further study of the cases treated at the Massachusetts General Hospital from 1950–1957. J Thorac Surg 36:301–308, 1958.
34. Clagett OT, Allen TH, Payne WS, Woolner LB. The surgical treatment of pulmonary neoplasms: a 10 year experience. J Thorac Cardiovasc Surg 48:391–400, 1964.
35. Gibbon JH Jr, Templeton JY III, Nealon TF Jr. Factors which influence the long term survival of patients with cancer of the lung. Ann Surg 145:637–643, 1957.
36. Cliffton EE. Criteria for operability and resectability in lung cancer. JAMA 195:1031–1032, 1966.
37. Paulson DL. Selection of patients for surgery for bronchogenic carcinoma. Am Surg 39:1–5, 1973.
38. Naruke T, Suemasu K, Ishikawa S. Lymph node mapping and curability at various levels of metastasis in resected lung cancer. J Thorac Cardiovasc Surg 76:832–839, 1978.
39. Bergh NP, Schersten J. Bronchogenic carcinoma: a follow-up study of a surgically treated series with special reference to the prognostic significance of lymph node metastases. Acta Chir Scand 347(Suppl):1–42, 1965.
40. Martini N, Flehinger BJ, Zaman MB, Beattie EJ. Prospective study of 445 lung carcinomas with media-

stinal lymph node metastases. J Thorac Cardiovasc Surg 80:390–399, 1980.

41. Kirschner PA. Discussion of Martini N, Flehinger BJ, Zaman MB, Beattie EJ. Prospective study of 445 lung carcinomas with mediastinal lymph node metastases. J Thorac Cardiovasc Surg 80:390–399, 1980.

42. Pearson FG, Delarue NC, Ilves R, et al. Significance of positive superior mediastinal nodes identified at mediastinoscopy in patients with resectable cancer of the lung. J Thorac Cardiovasc Surg 83:1–11, 1982.

43. Smith RA. The importance of mediastinal lymph node invasion by pulmonary carcinoma in selection of patients for resection. Ann Thorac Surg 25:5–11, 1978.

44. Shields TW, Fox RT. Surgical diagnostic procedures in general thoracic surgery. In: Shields TW, ed. General thoracic surgery. 2nd ed. Philadelphia: Lea & Febiger, 1983:220–223.

45. MacMahon H, Courtney JV, Little AG. Diagnostic methods in lung cancer. Semin Oncol 10:20–33, 1983.

46. Tucker JA. Mediastinoscopy: 300 cases reported and literature reviewed. Laryngoscope 82:2226–2248, 1972.

47. Goldberg EM, Shapiro CM, Glicksman AS. Mediastinoscopy for assessing mediastinal spread in clinical staging of lung carcinoma. Semin Oncol 3:205–214, 1974.

48. Reynders H. Mediastinoscopy in bronchogenic carcinoma. Dis Chest 45:606–611, 1964.

49. Baker RR. Mediastinoscopy. In: Siegelman SS, Stitik FP, Summer WR, eds. Pulmonary system: practical approaches to pulmonary diagnosis. New York: Grune & Stratton 1979:221–236.

50. Shields TW. The fate of patients after incomplete resection of bronchial carcinoma. Surg Gynecol Obstet 139:569–572, 1974.

51. Carlens E. Mediastinoscopy: a method for inspection and tissue biopsy in the superior mediastinum. Dis Chest 36:343–352, 1959.

52. Reynders H. Mediastinoscopy (thesis). 1963. In: Palva T. Mediastinoscopy. Chicago: Year Book Medical Publishers, 1964.

53. Bjork VO. Discussion of Fishman NH, Bronstein MH. Is mediastinoscopy necessary in the evaluation of lung cancer? Ann Thorac Surg 20:678–686, 1975.

54. Hashim SW, Baue AE, Geha AS. The role of mediastinoscopy and mediastinotomy in lung cancer. Clin Chest Med 3:353–359, 1982.

55. Schatzlein MH, McAuliffe S, Orringer MB, Kirsh MM. Scalene node biopsy in pulmonary carcinoma: when is it indicated? Ann Thorac Surg 31:322–324, 1986.

56. Cheung DK, Stibal D, Weinberg S, Poleksic S. Needle aspiration biopsy as an adjunct to mediastinoscopy. South Med J 79:1067–1069, 1986.

57. Foster ED, Munro DD, Dobell ARC. Mediastinoscopy: a review of anatomic relationships and complications. Ann Thorac Surg 13:273–386, 1972.

58. Sullivan WD, Passamonte PM. Mediastinoscopy incision site metastasis: response to radiation therapy. South Med J 75:1428, 1982.

59. Baggs KJ, Braun RA. An evaluation of mediastinoscopy as a guide to diagnosis and therapy. Arch Surg 111:703–706, 1976.

60. Kostiainen S, Meurala H, Mattila S, Appelqvist P. Chylothorax. Scand J Thorac Cardiovasc Surg 17:79–83, 1983.

61. Painter TD, Karpf M. Superior vena cava syndrome: diagnostic procedures. Am J Med Sci 285:2–6, 1983.

62. Coughlin M, Deslauriers J, Beaulieu M, et al. Role of mediastinoscopy in pretreatment staging of patients with primary lung cancer. Ann Thorac Surg 40:556–601, 1985.

63. Palva T. Mediastinoscopy. Year Book Medical Publishers, 1964.

64. Hashim SW, Baue AE, Geha AS. The role of mediastinoscopy and mediastinotomy in lung cancer. Clin Chest Med 3:353–359, 1982.

65. Tisi GM, Friedman PJ, Peters RM, et al. Clinical staging of primary lung cancer. Am Thorac Soc 659–664, 1981.

66. Spiro SC, Goldstraw P. The staging of lung cancer (editorial). Thorax 39:401–407, 1984.

67. Graves WG, Martinez MJ, Carter FL, et al. The value of computed tomography in staging bronchogenic carcinoma: a changing role for mediastinoscopy. Ann Thorac Surg 40:57–59, 1985.

68. Pearson FG, Nelems JM, Henderson RD, Delarue NC. The role of mediastinoscopy in the selection of treatment for bronchial carcinoma with involvement of superior mediastinal lymph nodes. J Thorac Cardiovasc Surg 64:382–390, 1972.

69. Fosberg RG, O'Sullivan MJ, Ah-Tye P, et al. Positive mediastinoscopy: an ominous finding. Ann Thorac Surg 18:346–356, 1974.

70. Paulson DL, Reisch JS. Long term survival after resection for bronchogenic carcinoma. Ann Surg 184:324–332, 1976.

71. Pearson FG. An evaluation of mediastinoscopy in the management of presumably operable bronchogenic carcinoma. J Thorac Cardiovasc Surg 55:617–625, 1968.

72. Sarin CL, Nohl-Oser HC. Mediastinoscopy: a clinical evaluation of 400 consecutive cases. Thorax 24:585–588, 1969.

73. Vincent RG, Takita H, Lane WW, et al. Surgical therapy of lung cancer. J Thorac Cardiovasc Surg 71:581–591, 1976.

74. Kirsch MM, Rotman H, Argenta L, et al. Carcinoma of the lung: results of treatment over ten years. Ann Thorac Surg 21:371–377, 1976.

75. Naruke T, Suemasu K, Ishikawa S. Surgical treatment for lung cancer with metastasis to mediastinal lymph nodes. J Thorac Cardiovasc Surg 71:279–285, 1976.

76. Rubenstein I, Baum GL, Kalter Y, et al. Resectional surgery in the treatment of primary carcinoma of the lung with mediastinal lymph node metastases. Thorax 34:33–35, 1979.

77. Jones DP. Diagnostic work-up of chest disease. Surg Clin North Am 60:743–755, 1980.

78. Bergh NP, Rydberg B, Schersten T. Mediastinal exploration by the technique of Carlens. Dis Chest 46:399–410, 1964.

79. Benfield JR, DeCaro ZF. When and how to invade for the diagnosis and staging of primary lung cancer. Am J Surg 143:670–674, 1982.

37

Diagnostic and Therapeutic Thoracoscopy

Carolyn E. Reed

Not infrequently in medicine, old ideas or tools combined with new technologies result in revived interest and excitement in techniques heretofore seldom used. Thoracoscopy, the visualization of the thorax through a tube containing an optical system and a light source, when married to the video camera, represented such a phenomenon in thoracic surgery. Because its application has depended on the development of technology (*i.e.*, imaging equipment) and the design of specialized instruments, the field is ever changing. The mechanics, instruments, indications, and procedures will continue to evolve. It should therefore be expected that much of the material presented in this chapter will require revision at the time of first reading.

HISTORY

The thoracoscope dates from 1910, and it actually is descended from the cystoscope, an instrument conceived in 1806. Jacobaeus in Sweden used a lighted cystoscope to explore the pleural cavity in patients with "idiopathic pleurisy," most of whom had tuberculosis.[1] He subsequently developed a technique for lysing pleural adhesions by introducing a galvanocautery device into the chest under the guidance of the thoracoscope to aid in "collapse" therapy of tuberculosis. Jacobaeus reported on 50 such cases in 1922[2] and further commented on the use of thoracoscopy to localize and diagnose pleural and pulmonary tumors.[3]

Thoracoscopy was widely used for the lysis of tuberculous adhesions until collapse therapy was abandoned in the late 1940s. Although some-what forgotten, especially in North America, European chest physicians continued to use thoracoscopy for the diagnosis of pleural diseases.

DIAGNOSTIC THORACOSCOPY

The most common and oldest indication for thoracoscopy is the diagnosis of pleural disease. Approximately 20% to 25% of patients with persistent pleural effusions will remain undiagnosed after thoracentesis, pleural biopsy, and bronchoscopy.[4, 5] Approximately 50% of these patients will ultimately be diagnosed as having malignancy. Closed needle biopsy for metastatic pleural malignancies is successful in only about 50% of cases.[5, 6] It is of little use when the tumor is very localized and is of no use when the tumor is confined to the visceral, mediastinal, or diaphragmatic pleura. On average, pleural cytologic studies are diagnostic in 50% to 60% of cases,[4, 7, 8] but results are dependent on the advanced state of the disease.

The results of a number of series that used thoracoscopy for the evaluation of pleural effusions and disease of unknown origin are summarized in Table 37–1. These series[5, 9–19] reveal that the diagnostic accuracy of thoracoscopy for malignancy ranges from 73% to 100%. A rigid instrument was used in all these reported cases. In the majority, a rigid thoracoscope (*i.e.*, the Storz endoscope) was used, but the mediastinoscope, laparoscope, and bronchoscope have also been employed. With the high-quality im-

Table 37–1. PLEURAL EFFUSION OR PLEURAL DISEASE OF UNKNOWN ORIGIN

| Series | No. of Patients | Findings | | | | | Sensitivity of Thoracoscopic Diagnosis of Malignancy (%) | Complication Rate (%)* | Deaths |
| | | Thoracoscopy | | | Follow-up | | | | |
		Not Diagnosed	Benign	Malignant	Benign	Malignant			
Hatch and DeCamp[9]	50	—	22	28	22	28	100	2/50(4)	0
Bergqvist and Nordenstam[10]	130	43	52	35	84	46	76	—	—
DeCamp et al[11]	121	3	71	47	71	50	94	7/126(5.6)	0
Lewis et al[12]	40	—	19	21	19	21	100	0	0
Canto et al[13]	204 (32 with mass)	2	73	129	67	137	94	7/208(3.4)	0
Oldenburg and Newhouse[14]	32	2	22	8	21	11	72.7	0	0
Weissberg et al[15]	80 (14 with mass)	4	8	68	—	—	—	1/80(1.2)	0
Baumgartner and Mark[16]	17	—	11	6	5	12	94	0	0
Boutin et al[5]	215	—	—	131	65	150	87.3	11/215(5.1)	0
Wu et al[17]	152	3	78	71	78	74	95.9	0	0
Menzies and Charbonneau[18]	102 (11 with mass)	7	57	38	53	42	90.5	10/104(9.6)	0
Hucker et al[19]	102	20	21	61	26	76	80.3	2/102(2.0)	0

*Minor and major complications/total thoracoscopies in reported series.

aging equipment now available, accuracy should approach 90% to 100%.

Thoracoscopy should be considered for patients with persistent or exudative pleural effusions that remain undiagnosed after routine studies. Thoracoscopy allows inspection of greater than 75% of the visceral pleural surface, as well as the parietal pleural surface. The endoscopic examination itself is often suggestive of the diagnosis,[20, 21] and biopsy can be visually directed to the location of the abnormality. Biopsy specimens can be obtained from multiple sites and are of greater size and depth, factors that lead to increased diagnostic yield. These advantages of thoracoscopy are especially useful in patients with a history of asbestos exposure and pleural effusion, as the diagnosis of malignant mesothelioma is difficult by cytologic examination and closed pleural biopsy procedures. Pleural effusion is present in 5% to 10% of cases of lung cancer at initial diagnosis. If cytologic findings are normal, thoracoscopy may identify those cases with pleural seeding (Fig. 37–1).

The employment of thoracoscopy for the evaluation of parenchymal disease, such as diffuse lung disease and peripheral localized opacities, has increased with the development of video imaging and stapling instruments. Boutin and associates studied the use of thoracoscopic biopsy as an alternative to open lung biopsy.[22] They achieved 100% sensitivity in diffuse lung disease and 70% sensitivity in peripheral localized lesions. Transthoracic needle aspiration is highly accurate for malignant nodules greater than 2 cm in diameter (80% to 95% true findings of malignancy) but decreases as the lesion becomes smaller.[23–25] A specific benign diagnosis is achieved in less than 20% of cases.[24] The diagnostic yield of transbronchial biopsy is about 50% to 80% in peripheral localized nodules, decreasing to less than 25% for lesions less than 2 cm,[25] and is about 40% to 70% in diffuse lung disease.[26] The ability to obtain an adequate portion of lung with preserved architecture for histopathologic analysis is an advantage of thoracoscopic biopsy in diffuse lung diseases. The limitation of thoracoscopy in the biopsy of peripheral nodules is one of visualization. Very small lesions that would be impossible to biopsy by needle are easily accessible with the thora-

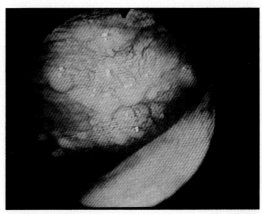

Figure 37–1. Metastatic adenocarcinoma "studding" parietal pleura.

coscope if they are pleural or just subpleural and pucker the visceral surface. Deeper nodules may be palpable by a probe. The use of the fluoroscope in the operating room and the development of techniques of needle localization similar to that used in breast biopsies will increase the diagnostic yield of deep lung lesions. A recent report describes the localization of nine deep pulmonary nodules using a hook wire placed percutaneously through the chest wall in the radiology suite under fluoroscopic or computed tomographic guidance. The patients were transported to the operating room suite and lung tissue was cored out around the wire imbedded in the nodule using the laser.[27]

Thoracoscopy has been a welcome alternative to open lung biopsy for patients with diffuse interstitial lung processes, and many of these patients are being referred earlier in the disease process. For patients at high risk for complications of thoracotomy, such as immunosuppressed transplant or human immunodeficiency virus–positive patients and patients with compromised pulmonary function, thoracoscopy represents a minimally invasive procedure that can supply sufficient tissue for histopathologic examination.[28]

Thoracoscopy for the staging of intrathoracic neoplasms, through either the demonstration of local invasion or lymph node involvement, has been infrequently reported.[29] The aortopulmonary window is often difficult to interpret by computed tomography and is easily accessible by thoracoscopy (Fig. 37–2). Tumors with questionable invasion of mediastinal pleura, and therefore properly staged as T4 lesions, can be viewed through the thoracoscope, thereby avoiding unnecessary thoracotomy. It is easy to visualize the aortic arch and great vessels on the left and the superior vena cava and azygos vein on the right, as well as peritracheal masses and suprahilar abnormalities. Mediastinoscopy and thoracoscopy should be viewed as complimentary procedures in the staging of lung cancer (see Chap. 36). The value of thoracoscopy in the staging of esophageal cancer needs further study.

THERAPEUTIC THORACOSCOPY

The therapeutic possibilities of thoracoscopy are just now being explored. With increased experience and better instrumentation, more complex thoracic procedures will become common. The indications, success rate, and complications of these procedures still need to be defined.

Like diagnostic thoracoscopy, early therapeutic applications of the thoracoscope involved pleural problems. Although most recurrent pleural effusions can be adequately managed by tube thoracostomy and chemical pleurodesis using agents such as tetracycline and its derivatives, bleomycin, or talc, approximately 20% of these effusions will be refractory to such management. Malignant pleural effusions can be especially distressing and costly to patients with limited life spans. Thoracoscopy can be diagnostic and therapeutic in many cases.[30, 31] Thoracoscopy can identify "trapped lung," which is a contraindication to chemical pleurodesis, and can evacuate loculations to increase the effectiveness of the pleurodesis. The use of talc poudrage pleurodesis has been highly successful in the control of malignant or chronic recurrent pleural effusions.[15, 32–37] There have been several trials illustrating the superiority of talc poudrage to other sclerosing agents,[36, 37] and the success rate is approximately 90%. In most cases, 2 to 5 g of talc is insufflated, and coating of the whole pleural cavity is confirmed under direct vision. The use of talc powder rather than a suspension has met with few complications.[33]

The role of the thoracoscope for debridement and drainage of empyema probably requires careful case selection. Early loculations can be broken up and gelatinous material removed. Adequate removal of a rind or peel on the lung may prove difficult. Thoracoscopic debridement of chronic empyema has a reported success rate of 60% to 80%.[38, 39]

Spontaneous pneumothorax requiring surgical intervention is easily treated with the thoracoscope. For the two groups at maximum risk— young males and the emphysematous patients— thoracoscopy offers less trauma with greater

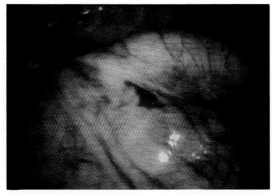

Figure 37–2. Cancerous lymph node in aortopulmonary window.

functional result for the first group and less operative risk for the second group. Pleural bullae can be ablated by electrocautery[40] or the CO_2 laser,[41] ligated with an Endoloop (Ethicon Endosurgery, Cincinnatti, OH),[42, 43] or stapled. Pleurodesis is usually performed. Mechanical pleurodesis is very easy to accomplish using a piece of gauze or mesh on a grasping forcep, or the laser can be used to scarify the parietal pleura. Talc poudrage by way of the thoracoscope has been highly successful for the treatment of pneumothoraces,[33, 34, 44] and the recurrence rate has been low (<10%).[44, 45]

Emergency thoracoscopy may be beneficial in cases of chest trauma in which ongoing hemorrhage from the pleural cavity requires a decision regarding the need for operative thoracotomy. Obviously, hemodynamic stability is a requirement. In a report of 36 patients who presented with hemothoraces, early thoracoscopy provided accurate assessment of the anatomic nature of injury in 35 patients and allowed determination of whether blood loss was continuing in all patients.[46] Management was altered as the result of thoracoscopy in 30.5% or 44.4% of patients, depending on the indication used for thoracotomy. For trauma patients in whom hemothorax is not evacuated by tube thoracostomy, thoracoscopy may be used to remove retained hematoma and avoid empyema.

The resection of peripheral lung lesions has become easier and more frequent with the advent of endoscopic stapling instruments[47] (Fig. 37–3), although the neodymium-doped yttrium-aluminum-garnet laser has also been useful.[48] Landreneau and associates[49] have reported on 85 pulmonary resections in 61 patients using the thoracoscope for nodules with a mean diameter of 1.3 cm. The majority of the nodules were benign (n = 46) or metastatic (n = 26). Thirteen peripheral lesions were primary lung carcinomas, and 5 of these patients then underwent formal resection. There was no mortality and minimal morbidity. The use of the thoracoscope for the resection of peripheral T1N0 lung cancers needs to be further defined. The ability to perform such an operation does not necessarily mean it is the best cancer procedure. For patients with compromised lung function, it may be the only option, but preoperative staging criteria, local recurrence rate, and disease-free and long-term survival need to be studied before it can be considered routine. Similarly, thoracoscopic lobectomy is possible, but the indications need to be defined.

The pericardium is easily approached through the thoracoscope and the creation of a window for drainage and resection for tissue biopsy performed using a grasping forcep and shears attached to an electrocautery device (Fig. 37–4). The superb imaging quality of the chest wall structures allows easy excision of the thoracic sympathetic chain.[50]

Esophageal surgery with the thoracoscope continues to develop. The resection of leiomyomas and cysts and vagotomy and myotomy will probably be routine. More complex procedures such as Collis-Nissen fundoplication and esophageal resection[51] require greater technical skill and more sophisticated instrumentation. The use of thoracoscopy in the preoperative staging of esophageal cancer needs further investigation.

At present, many surgeons use the thoracoscope as a "video assistant." Larger instruments and stapling devices are introduced through a small incision at the appropriate intercostal space to accomplish a procedure routinely requiring the separation of ribs. Pain following thoracotomy is therefore minimized.

The role of therapeutic thoracoscopy will continue to expand, and procedures formerly done

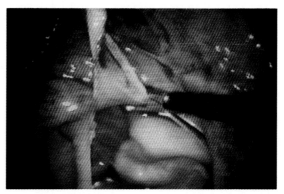

Figure 37–4. Creation of a pericardial window.

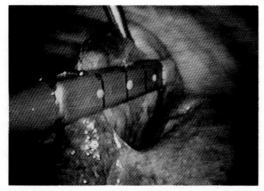

Figure 37–3. Resection of lung using the Endo-GIA (U.S. Surgical, Norwalk, CT).

by "open" technique will be accomplished routinely by means of the thoracoscope.[52] Because we are in the phase of "finding out what we can do," concerns such as cost-effectiveness, patient and procedure selectivity, and outcome variables await further investigation.

THORACOSCOPY TECHNIQUE

Although in the past, rigid thoracoscopy was frequently performed using local anesthesia, thoracoscopy today is done under general anesthesia. The use of a double-lumen endotracheal tube allows collapse of the lung, and frequently air insufflation is unnecessary. Most anesthesiologists insert a radial arterial line for constant blood pressure monitoring and follow O_2 saturation and end tidal CO_2 with respective monitors. The patient is routinely placed in the lateral decubitus position, although occasionally another approach may be useful. In the routine setup, the surgeon and first assistant stand on opposite sides of the table. The video monitor, light source, insufflator, and videocassette recorder are at the head of the table, and ideally, the surgeon and first assistant have separate viewing screens.

Unlike laparoscopic cholecystectomy, one must adapt the position of the incisions for the telescope and instrument ports to the pulmonary pathologic condition. Flexibility is key, and initial viewing of the pleural cavity often directs placement of subsequent instruments. In general, the telescope and attached camera are inserted in the middle to posterior axillary line in the fifth to seventh intercostal space. Working distance within the chest for the instruments usually requires ports placed anteriorly (midclavicular line) and posteriorly, often in "diamond fashion" around the camera.[53]

Thoracic surgeons initially had to adapt laparoscopic equipment to the thoracic cavity, but an array of trocars, entry ports, and instruments have been developed especially for thoracic use. Despite sheathed trocars, unless the lung is completely collapsed, damage to lung parenchyma is still possible. Entry into the pleural space is probably accomplished more safely using a Kelly clamp and blunt-tipped trocar. Modified trocar cannulas or "ports" are available in several sizes (5, 10.5, 11.5, 15 mm diameter) for instrument access. Some surgeons infrequently use air insufflation, although it may add to the visibility. For patients who will not tolerate single-lung anesthesia and need a diagnostic lung biopsy, use of air insufflation and careful cooperation with the anesthesiologist may still allow successful thoracoscopic biopsy. Air flow is usually 5 to 7 L at a pressure of 5 to 10 mm Hg.

Both disposable and nondisposable instruments are useful to the thoracic surgeon, and thoracoscopic instrumentation is a rapidly evolving field. The introduction of the endoscopic stapling device (Endo-GIA, U.S. Surgical, Norwalk, CT) quickly expanded the number of procedures that could be performed under thoracoscopic guidance. This device fires a 30 mm–long series of six rows of staples and cuts the tissue, leaving three rows of staples on each side of the blade. As longer stapling instruments become available, larger resections will become easier. The development of endoscopic lung clamps is of particular importance. Dissectors, biopsy forceps, shears, and suction cannulas are standard components of the thoracoscopy tray. For large resections of malignant lesions, various wrapping devices are available to prevent contact with the chest wall and possible seeding as the specimen is withdrawn through a separate incision.

For most procedures, a chest tube is inserted through a cannula site at the conclusion of the operation. As experience grows, simple procedures will require only evacuation of air by suction.

COMPLICATIONS OF THORACOSCOPY

Potential complications of thoracoscopy include intrapleural hemorrhage, air leak, pneumothorax, subcutaneous emphysema, empyema, cardiac complications (arrhythmia, hypotension, ischemia), respiratory distress, and thoracoscopy tract seeding. As seen in Table 37–1 and documented in two recent series,[49, 52] complications are rare. Tumor seeding at the thoracoscopy site is most common with malignant mesothelioma. Subcutaneous emphysema and "air leak" may be underreported.[34] Infection is very rare. Most deaths that have occurred within 30 days of thoracoscopy have been attributed to advanced malignant disease.[5, 34] The use of general anesthesia and its risks must be considered when selecting patients with terminal illness or marked cardiorespiratory reserve. The only absolute contraindication to thoracoscopy is an adherent pleural space.

THORACOSCOPY IN THE FUTURE

As experience and instrumentation develop, the full potential of thoracoscopy will become defined. There are thoracic surgeons who believe that nearly all procedures will eventually be performed through or with the assistance of the thoracoscope. Thoracoscopy represents a powerful diagnostic and therapeutic tool. The thoracic surgeon must devote the time to learn how to use this tool skillfully and develop the judgment to use it when it results in maximum benefit to the patient.

References

1. Bloomberg AE. Thoracoscopy in perspective. Surg Gynecol Obstet 147:433–443, 1978.
2. Jacobaeus HC. The cauterization of adhesions in artificial pneumothorax treatment of pulmonary tuberculosis. Am Rev Tb 6:871–897, 1922.
3. Jacobaeus HC. The practical importance of thoracoscopy in surgery of the chest. Surg Gynecol Obstet 34:289–296, 1922.
4. Salyer WR, Eggleston JC, Erozan YS. Efficacy of pleural needle biopsy and pleural fluid cytopathology in the diagnosis of malignant neoplasm involving the pleura. Chest 67:536–539.
5. Boutin C, Viallat JR, Cargnino P, Farisse P. Thoracoscopy in malignant pleural effusions. Am Rev Respir Dis 124:588–592, 1981.
6. Poe RH, Israel RH, Utell MJ, et al. Sensitivity, specificity, and predictive values of closed pleural biopsy. Arch Intern Med 144:325–328, 1984.
7. Graham GG, McDonald JR, Clagett OT, Schmidt HW. Examination of pleural fluid for carcinoma cells. J Thorac Surg 25:366–370, 1953.
8. Dines DE, Pierre RV, Franzen SJ. The value of cells in the pleural fluid in the differential diagnosis. Mayo Clin Proc 50:571–572, 1975.
9. Hatch HB, DeCamp PT. Diagnostic thoracoscopy. Surg Clin North Am 46:1405–1410, 1966.
10. Bergqvist S, Nordenstam H. Thoracoscopy and pleural biopsy in the diagnosis of pleurisy. Scand J Respir Dis 47:64–74, 1966.
11. DeCamp PT, Moseley PW, Scott ML, Hatch HB. Diagnostic thoracoscopy. Ann Thorac Surg 16:79–84, 1973.
12. Lewis RJ, Kunderman PJ, Sisler GE, MacKenzie JW. Direct diagnostic thoracoscopy. Ann Thorac Surg 21:536–539, 1976.
13. Canto A, Blasco E, Casillas M, et al. Thoracoscopy in the diagnosis of pleural effusion. Thorax 32:550–554, 1977.
14. Oldenburg FA, Newhouse MT. Thoracoscopy. Chest 75:45–50, 1979.
15. Weissberg D, Kaufman M, Zurkowski Z. Pleuroscopy in patients with pleural effusion and pleural masses. Ann Thorac Surg 29:205–208, 1980.
16. Baumgartner WA, Mark JB. The use of thoracoscopy in the diagnosis of pleural disease. Arch Surg 115:420–421, 1980.
17. Wu M-H, Hsiue R-H, Tseng K-H. Thoracoscopy in the diagnosis of pleural effusions. Jpn J Clin Oncol 19:116–119, 1989.
18. Menzies R, Charbonneau M. Thoracoscopy for the diagnosis of pleural disease. Ann Intern Med 114:271–276, 1991.
19. Hucker J, Bhatnagar NK, Al-Jilaihawi AN, Forrester-Wood CP. Thoracoscopy in the diagnosis and management of recurrent pleural effusions. Ann Thorac Surg 52:1145–1147, 1991.
20. Boutin C, Astoul Ph, Seitz B. The role of thoracoscopy in the evaluation and management of pleural effusions. Lung (Suppl)168:1113–1121, 1990.
21. Sattler A. Pleural biopsy—results obtained and their practical significance. Ciba Found Symp 9:109–121, 1961.
22. Boutin C, Viallat JR, Cargnino P, Rey F. Thoracoscopic lung biopsy. Chest 82:44–48, 1982.
23. Zavala DC, Schoell JE. Ultrathin needle aspiration of the lung in infectious and malignant disease. Am Rev Respir Dis 123:125–131, 1981.
24. Perketh AR, Robinson AA, Barker V, Flower CD. Use of percutaneous needle biopsy in the investigation of solitary pulmonary nodules. Thorax 42:967–971, 1987.
25. Wallace JM, Deutsch AL. Flexible fiberoptic bronchoscopy and percutaneous needle aspiration for evaluating the solitary pulmonary nodule. Chest 81:665–671, 1982.
26. Wall CP, Gaensler EA, Carrington CB, Hayes JA. Comparison of transbronchial and open biopsies in chronic infiltrative lung diseases. Am Rev Respir Dis 123:280–285, 1981.
27. Mack MJ, Gordon MJ, Postma TW, et al. Percutaneous localization of pulmonary nodules for thoracoscopic lung resection. Ann Thorac Surg 53:1123–1124, 1992.
28. Krasna M, Flowers JL. Diagnostic thoracoscopy in a patient with a pleural mass. Surg Laparosc Endosc 1:94–97, 1991.
29. Rodgers BM, Ryckman FC, Moazam F, Talbert JL. Thoracoscopy for intrathoracic tumors. Ann Thorac Surg 31:414–420, 1981.
30. Oakes DD, Sherck JP, Brodsky JB, Mark JBD. Therapeutic thoracoscopy. J Thorac Cardiovasc Surg 87:269–273, 1984.
31. Rusch VW, Mountain C. Thoracoscopy under regional anesthesia for the diagnosis and management of pleural disease. Am J Surg 154:274–278, 1987.
32. Weissberg D, Kaufman M. Diagnostic and therapeutic pleuroscopy. Chest 78:732–735, 1980.
33. Daniel TM, Tribble CG, Rodgers BM. Thoracoscopy and talc poudrage for pneumothoraces and effusions. Ann Thorac Surg 50:186–189, 1990.
34. Ohri SK, Oswal SK, Townsend ER, Fountain SW. Early and late outcome after diagnostic thoracoscopy and talc pleurodesis. Ann Thorac Surg 53:1038–1041, 1992.
35. Aelony Y, King R, Boutin C. Thoracoscopic talc poudrage pleurodesis for chronic recurrent pleural effusions. Ann Intern Med 115:778–782, 1991.
36. Fentiman IS, Rubens RD, Hayward JL. A comparison of intracavitary talc and tetracycline for the control of pleural effusions secondary to breast cancer. Eur J Cancer Clin Oncol 22:1079–1081, 1986.
37. Hamed H, Fentiman IS, Chaudary MA, Rubens RD. Comparison of intracavitary bleomycin and talc for control of pleural effusions secondary to carcinoma of the breast. Br J Surg 76:1266–1267, 1989.
38. Ridley PD, Braimbridge MV. Thoracoscopic debridement and pleural irrigation in the management of empyema thoracis. Ann Thorac Surg 51:461–464, 1991.

39. Wakabayashi A. Expanded applications of diagnostic and therapeutic thoracoscopy. J Thorac Cardiovasc Surg 102:721–723, 1991.

40. Wakabayashi A. Thoracoscopic ablation of blebs in the treatment of recurrent or persistent spontaneous pneumothorax. Ann Thorac Surg 48:651–653, 1989.

41. Wakabayashi A, Brenner M, Wilson AF, et al. Thoracoscopic treatment of spontaneous pneumothorax using carbon dioxide laser. Ann Thorac Surg 50:786–790, 1990.

42. Nathanson LK, Shimi SM, Wood RAB, Cuschieri A. Videothoracoscopic ligation of bulla and pleurectomy for spontaneous pneumothorax. Ann Thorac Surg 52:316–319, 1991.

43. McLaughlin MJ, McLaughlin BH. Thoracoscopic ablation of blebs using PDS-Endoloop in recurrent spontaneous pneumothorax. Surg Laparosc Endosc 1:263–264, 1991.

44. Vanderschueren RGJRA. The role of thoracoscopy in the evaluation and management of pneumothorax. Lung (Suppl)168:1122–1125, 1990.

45. Almind M, Lange P, Viskum K. Spontaneous pneumothorax: comparison of simple drainage, talc pleurodesis, and tetracycline pleurodesis. Thorax 44:627–630, 1989.

46. Jones JW, Kitahama A, Webb WR, McSwain N. Emergency thoracoscopy: a logical approach to chest trauma management. J Trauma 21:280–284, 1981.

47. Krasna M, Nazem A. Thoracoscopic lung resection: use of a new endoscopic linear stapler. Surg Laparosc Endosc 1:248–250, 1991.

48. Landreneau RJ, Herlan DB, Johnson JA, et al. Thoracoscopic neodymium:yttrium-aluminum garnet laser-assisted pulmonary resection. Ann Thorac Surg 52:1176–1178, 1991.

49. Landreneau RJ, Hazelrigg SR, Ferson PF, et al. Thoracoscopic resection of 85 pulmonary lesions. Ann Thorac Surg 54:415–420, 1992.

50. Lin C-C. A new method of thoracoscopic sympathectomy in hyperhidrosis palmaris. Surg Endosc 4:224–226, 1990.

51. Leahy PF, Pennino RP, Hinshaw JR, et al. Minimally invasive esophagogastrectomy: an approach to esophagogastrectomy of the left thorax. J Laparoendosc Surg 1:59–62, 1990.

52. Mack M, Aronoff R, Acuff T, et al. The present role of thoracoscopy in the diagnosis and treatment of diseases of the chest. Ann Thorac Surg 54:403–409, 1992.

53. Landreneau RJ, Mack MJ, Hazelrigg SR, et al. Video-assisted thoracic surgery: basic technical concepts and intercostal approach strategies. Ann Thorac Surg 54:800–807, 1992.

38

Endoscopic Training for the General Surgeon

Richard M. Satava and Irwin B. Simon

HISTORICAL PERSPECTIVE

The education of a surgeon continues to evolve. The initial organization of a training program by Billroth focused around individual mentoring. Halsted pioneered the formal approach to resident education using a very rigid, disciplined system consisting of many residents under the watchful eye of the chief of surgery. Within these systems, the quality and content of the educational experience varied greatly and was dependent solely on the stature and dedication of the individual surgeon. The American Board of Surgery (ABS) established the Residency Review Committee (RRC) with the intent of providing a uniform set of guidelines to assist the individual chiefs of residency programs in ensuring the highest caliber of surgical training. The focus was a broad-based education in all the diverse facets of surgery, with the implication that as new technologic advances occurred, they would be incorporated into the fundamental core of surgical knowledge.

Despite the pioneering efforts of surgeons such as Overholt, Way, Shinya, and Berci,[1] the true potential of the endoscope was overlooked by most surgeons in clinical practice. In fact, few surgeons were trained in flexible endoscopy from its conception in 1958 until 1985, when the ABS first mandated that all surgical training programs include exposure to the principles and applications of fiberoptic flexible endoscopy.[2]

This mandate was not widely heeded, and as recently as 1989, only 76% of general surgery residency programs had a rotation in gastrointestinal endoscopy, and only 44% of these programs had designated a surgeon as director of endoscopy training.[3]

The majority of surgical training programs relegated the surgical resident's "exposure" to a 1- or 2-month rotation on the gastroenterology service. At the Society of American Gastrointestinal Endoscopic Surgeons (SAGES) Program Directors' Workshop in 1988 entitled The Incorporation of Endoscopic Training into a Surgical Residency, two key tenets were proposed.[4]

1. A separate surgical endoscopic service provides the most effective vehicle for this training. It is difficult to achieve endoscopic training by a rotation on the gastroenterology endoscopy service, for the surgical resident is often relegated to a position as second-class citizen. Medical gastroenterology instructors are often unfamiliar with the surgical considerations pertinent to some endoscopic examinations, such as the margin of resection or adherence to adjacent organs.

2. A surgeon designated as the surgical endoscopy director is unequivocally the most important factor for an effective endoscopic teaching program. This individual should assume full responsibility for the program and coordinate the efforts of all surgeons as endoscopy instructors.

Beginning in 1989, the laparoscope was rediscovered by the general surgical community as a diagnostic and therapeutic instrument. Dubois

The opinions or assertions contained herein are the private views of the authors and are not to be construed as official, or as reflecting the views of the Department of the Army or the Department of Defense.

and Perrissat in France and Reddick in the United States brought laparoscopic surgery to the forefront of general surgical practice.

Unlike flexible endoscopy, laparoscopic surgery was immediately embraced, and training was rapidly incorporated into the body of surgical education. Although there may be some experienced surgeons still seeking training in laparoscopic procedures, residency training programs have regarded laparoscopic surgery as a variation of open operative surgery, not as a separate discipline like flexible endoscopy. Therefore, all the standard established mechanisms for training in open operative surgery have been applied to laparoscopic surgery.

The goal of this chapter is to provide insight into the incorporation of flexible endoscopic training into a surgical residency program. These same principles apply to any training acquired by a staff surgeon who has already completed a surgical residency. A surgical endoscopy training program must be based on a structured educational foundation and be supported by a dedicated physical facility, personnel, and adequate equipment and resources.

STRUCTURED STANDARD TRAINING PROGRAM

The goals of a surgical training program must incorporate the philosophies of education, clinical practice, and research. In accordance with the 1985 mandate of the ABS, the RRC offered a broad generalization of the requirements for endoscopy. Subsequent guidelines have been recommended by SAGES,[5] which are conceptually in accord with previous position statements released by the American Society of Gastrointestinal Endoscopy, the American Gastroenterological Association, the American College of Gastroenterology,[6] and the Society for Surgery of the Alimentary Tract.

Introduction to endoscopic principles should be accomplished through a series of didactic lectures, which will most often be concurrent with assisting at endoscopic procedures. Additional educational aids include 35-mm slides, videotapes, and atlases, as well as textbooks.

As with any procedure, the ultimate skill level of the surgeon as endoscopy trainee will vary, as will the interest and competence in performing these procedures in later clinical practice. Individual programs will certainly experience difficulties in accomplishing all three philosophic goals. Research experience is commonly the most difficult to provide. The program director

should attempt to provide such opportunity to any resident and surgeon who demonstrates an interest or aptitude for endoscopy. As with any surgical skill, endoscopic training must be maintained within the guidelines of sound, compassionate patient care and never at the expense of the patient. Video endoscopy is not an interactive video game that must be "won" by the trainee at any cost.

Goal 1: Education

It is advised that each surgical residency program have one surgical staff member designated as the director of surgical endoscopy. This individual will be responsible for establishing the appropriate endoscopy unit and bringing the resident endoscopy training program to fruition. It is not anticipated that this individual will be the only surgeon-endoscopist within the training program. His or her responsibility will be to assume the role of coordinator for didactic, as well as hands-on, clinical training to be provided by numerous staff surgeons.

The education of the surgical resident is often conceptualized as being divided into three categories: clinical teaching, didactic teaching, and research. These categories are often inseparable but will be discussed individually for the sake of practicality. These educational concepts represent a common theme that will be seen to repeat in the other philosophic goals of the training program.

Clinical Teaching

Clinical teaching in endoscopic training is simply a subset of resident education as a whole. It incorporates patient evaluation and determination of the indications for an endoscopic procedure. As with the performance of any surgical procedure, the trainee is expected to perform or participate in the care of the patient both before and after the procedure. The concepts of informed consent hold true. The trainee must be knowledgeable in the indications, contraindications, risks, and benefits of each procedure for a given patient. The staff member is expected to provide direct supervision of all training.

Teaching should begin on inert models. If an animal facility is available, the early stages of technical proficiency should be attained on an appropriate animal model. Direct supervision on patients follows. Video endoscopy should be universally employed in training programs, as it inherently adds to both patient safety and efficiency in attaining proficiency.[7] The final stage is to allow the trainee to work independently while still under the watchful eye of the experienced instructor.

Although the postgraduate level at which hands-on endoscopic training should begin may vary, exposure to the principles and practice of endoscopic surgery should begin in the first year of postgraduate study. In fact, the earliest exposure will be made in some fashion while the individual is still an undergraduate medical student. Dent and associates[8] have recommended that the resident have a 1- or 2-month rotation on the endoscopy service in the third postgraduate year. Patient care duties as outlined previously may be combined with the presentation of a monthly endoscopic conference (Table 38–1). An often overlooked but absolutely critical aspect of the resident's education is learning the mechanics and maintenance of the endoscopic equipment. When mechanical problems occur during a procedure, the surgeon must be knowledgeable enough about the equipment to determine the cause.

In lieu of a specific rotation in endoscopy, training may be incorporated into the general surgery rotations of the early postgraduate years. Mastering the basic concepts and skills during the early years allows experience and maturity to be gained in more senior years.

For teaching to be effective, the director of surgical endoscopy must be not only an accomplished technical endoscopist but also a competent administrator. To facilitate resident research, a comprehensive, computerized database should be maintained under the director's guidance. Record keeping, quality assurance, and assessment and incorporation of expanding technologies are paramount to any surgical educational program. The issue of quality assurance includes morbidity and mortality and it is felt that surgical endoscopic morbidity and mortality should be presented within the framework of the existing general surgery quality assurance conference, rather than as a separate quality improvement issue.

Didactic Teaching

Didactic teaching requires a regularly scheduled endoscopy conference. Although this may include case reviews and a parallel subject review by the residents, there is a definite place for a core series of lectures to be presented by the attending staff. The Resident Education Committee of SAGES has available an example of teaching guidelines.[9]

To assist in the preparation of conferences, there is also a plethora of well-made educational slide and video series (including interactive video presentations). They allow the resident an excellent opportunity to learn to recognize the endoscopic appearance of varying pathologic states in a rapid fashion, facilitating the interpretation of findings during clinical procedures.

Histopathologic correlation of slides from previous cases should be accomplished within the didactic series. This is best done in a joint conference between the surgical endoscopy service and the pathology service and should include appropriate histopathologic and cytopathologic specimens.

Research

Basic science research laboratories may not be readily available to the surgical resident. However, there are a multitude of ways that the resident may participate in clinical research. Specific aspects of a procedure can be evaluated or a new procedural technique may be developed in an animal research facility.

Table 38–1. GENERIC MONTHLY ENDOSCOPIC CONFERENCE SCHEDULE

January: *Basic principles of endoscopy*
   Principles of mechanics, fiberoptics, and video
	July: *Lower endoscopy*
	   Malignant diseases

February: *Basic principles of endoscopy*
   Therapeutic modalities and accessories
	August: *Lower endoscopy*
	   Therapeutic modalities

March: *Upper endoscopy*
   Benign disease
	September: *Intraoperative endoscopy*
	   Choledochoscopy
	   Enteroscopy
	   Colonoscopy

April: *Upper endoscopy*
   Malignant diseases
	October: *ERCP*
	   Diagnostic

May: *Upper endoscopy*
   Therapeutic modalities
	November: *ERCP*
	   Therapeutic

June: *Lower endoscopy* Benign diseases	December: *New technology in endoscopy*

ERCP = endoscopic retrograde cholangiopancreatography.

The maintenance of a thorough endoscopy patient database is a key element to both prospective and retrospective studies of a clinical nature.[10] The sheer number of procedures performed over a 6- to 12-month period in a moderately busy surgical endoscopy unit provides an adequate sampling for meaningful clinical research.

Submission of a resident's research to appropriate medical journals is to be encouraged: this is one measure of commitment to complete resident training and reflects favorably on the academic quality of an entire program. These articles may be submitted to any medical, surgical, or pathology journal for publication. It should be noted that there is now a sizable list of journals devoted to the topic of flexible endoscopy.

Goal 2: Clinical Practice

As with any surgical skill, training in endoscopy requires the acquisition and integration of both cognitive and technical abilities. Satava[11] has delineated four skills: deductive, technical, interpretive, and therapeutic.

The deductive skills involve acquisition of the individual patient's clinical information. This begins with a proper history and physical examination and is supplemented by appropriate laboratory and radiologic testing. Based on this information, the indications or contraindications for an endoscopic procedure are delineated. Preprocedural requirements and informed consent are obtained and counseling is performed, if necessary.

Prior to video endoscopy, the acquisition of technical skills in endoscopic training was almost entirely dependent on a system of one-on-one instruction between instructor and trainee. This required a cumbersome teaching head attached to the endoscope. Video opens a new dimension to teaching, permitting greater teacher-student interaction and involvement of all members of the team. Even though an individual resident may not actually be performing the "hands-on" procedure, significant instruction may be imparted to any number of "viewing" trainees.

There is a basic armamentarium of endoscopic technical skills that has been identified as essential. These skills must be mastered by the trainee in a stepwise gradation from instructed to independent performance (Table 38–2).[11, 12] The conduct of endoscopy from patient sedation to recovery following the procedure must be mas-

Table 38–2. BASIC ENDOSCOPIC TECHNICAL SKILLS

Administrative skills
    Care, maintenance, and cleaning of endoscopic equipment
    Preparation of pathologic specimen
    Creation of photographic and video documentation
    Computerized database management
Global skills
    Preparation and monitoring for endoscopy
    Administration of intravenous sedation
    Endoscopic intubation for EGD
    Intubation of the rectum for colonoscopy
Diagnostic skills

Biopsy	Standard forceps technique
	Electrocoagulating (hot biopsy) forceps technique
Cytologic	Brush technique
	Aspiration technique
Radiologic	Introductory familiarization with ERCP images

Therapeutic skills

Polypectomy	With standard snare types
	Electrocoagulating
	Monopolar
	Bipolar
Electrocoagulation	For hemorrhage
	For palliation of malignancy
Foreign body	Retrieval by forceps
	Retrieval by snare
	Use of oventube
Sclerotherapy	For hemorrhage
	Variceal
	Nonvariceal

EGD = esophagogastroduodenoscopy; ERCP = endoscopic retrograde cholangiopancreatography.

tered. The techniques of passing the endoscope, as well as the execution of diagnostic maneuvers (biopsy, brush cytology) and therapeutic maneuvers (polypectomy, foreign body removal, sclerotherapy) proceeds from the "watching stage of the endoscopic neophyte" through increasing levels of independence. Thus the trainee is ultimately performing the procedure in both elective and emergent procedures.

The interpretive aspects of endoscopy may be acquired only through experience. Once again this visual-cognitive experience may be obtained in a much more rapid fashion because of the video technology currently available. Identification of pathologic lesions is the emphasis, and this "experience" may be gained from clinical practice as well as from the previously mentioned libraries of both still photographs and video presentations currently available. The interpretive skill cannot be separated completely from the technical aspects, as the resident must learn to anticipate where to search and what to search for, as well as what diagnostic or therapeutic adjunct is appropriate to the situation.

Therapeutic skills must be considered within the basic armamentarium of the surgeon as endoscopist. It is inappropriate to expect all endoscopists to be proficient in all skills, particularly those requiring advanced training such as endoscopic retrograde cholangiopancreatography (ERCP) with sphincterotomy or laser ablation of tumors. It is equally inappropriate to perform a diagnostic procedure and find a colon polyp or bleeding ulcer and then be forced to withdraw and refer the patient to another endoscopist, subjecting the patient to another session of sedation and the inherent procedural risk. Basic therapeutic skills are listed in Table 38–2. Appropriate follow-up is mandatory to evaluate the adequacy of therapy.

Goal 3: Research

Research is the "wellhead" for future generations. Its value is recognized and highly recommended in many academic programs, resulting in the residency experience expanding to 6 and 7 years of postgraduate training to include time for research. The individual, as well as the entire training program, can only benefit from experience in research, and this certainly applies to the endoscopic training program carried out within the auspices of a surgical residency.

Research may be conveniently divided into three areas: training, clinical investigation, and basic science research. Although the latter two are aimed at acquisition of academic skills,

training research may be used to effectively facilitate the trainee's acquisition of technical skills. Laboratory animals as live training models can be used to teach the essentials of endoscopy and normal anatomy at an entry level. Despite recent advances such as an interactive video endoscopy simulator,[13] no inert model currently available can substitute for the training afforded by such live models. Resident feedback indicates that this laboratory experience shortens the learning curve and rapidly builds confidence by providing endoscopic experience prior to actual patient experience. This model has been essential in recent years for training surgeons in procedures such as laparoscopic surgery.

Clinical investigation, as noted earlier, is readily available in any program in which a proper database is maintained. A wide variety of topics may be included—for example, the efficacy of intravenous sedation, the aspects of monitoring during procedures,[14] and the relative benefits of one diagnostic-therapeutic modality versus another. Retrospective studies are easily researched through a proper database, and prospective studies may also be entertained. The trainee may easily be the principal investigator in a retrospective project that may be completed within the time constraints of a 1- to 3-month rotation.

Basic science research is difficult to perform over a short time. However, this can be accomplished over the period of a full surgical residency. This investigation is directed toward the understanding of normal or pathologic physiologic disease processes or techniques, without orientation to a specific disease entity. Examples might include the rate of mucosal regeneration after biopsy or the number of antral G-cells present in the normal versus H_2-blocked animal.

DOCUMENTATION

Modern surgical practice requires responsible documentation to fulfill numerous federal and local regulations. The ability to educate, by definition, mandates a method to document that education has occurred. The care of any patient must be documented in the patient's medical record. Quality assurance, as well as clinical research, is best served by the ability to retrieve and interpret data on large numbers of patients. Numeric documentation of the individual trainee's experience must be maintained. With all these various requirements for data collection and documentation, a computer-compiled database is strongly recommended as the most efficient means of maintaining a consolidated information management system.

Computerized databases may be maintained on a local personal computer in the endoscopy suite. If possible, the endoscopy database should be integrated into the overall surgical residency database. This allows rapid cross-referencing and data searches and analysis, and results may be compiled and printed with a modicum of effort.

The two areas of documentation include the medical record (for individual patient and individual procedure) and the trainee education record (for the training program and ABS requirements).

Medical Record Documentation

As with any medical procedure, appropriate documentation in the patient record is mandatory and generally takes the form of a dictated report. Although such reports may be completed in myriad ways, they must include the following fundamental information at a minimum: indications, procedure, findings, specimens taken, final diagnosis, complications, and recommendations for further medical or surgical therapy. Photographic or video documentation, or both, of any pathologic condition should be included whenever possible.

Documentation of Trainee Education

At the completion of each procedure, it is recommended that the trainee complete a worksheet with information regarding the procedure (Fig. 38–1). The data obtained from this worksheet are entered into the training program's computer database. At any time, a compilation of an individual trainee's experience may be culled from the database.

In addition, the preceptor must document the evaluation of the trainee. Such forms may be locally generated or a standardized form may be obtained from the ASGE.[15] The frequency of such reporting is at the discretion of each endoscopy program director. These evaluation reports allow ongoing evaluation of the trainee and overall evaluation for certification of competence. This same information can serve for ABS recommendations and review by regulatory organizations such as the RRC and the Joint Commission on Accreditation of Healthcare Organizations.

Although documentation of experience is important, there is no universally accepted numeric quota of cases beyond which competence is implied. In this context, the determination of competency is that ". . . the training director's opinion and recommendation should be considered as prima facie evidence for the trainee's acceptance as an individual qualified in gastrointestinal endoscopy."[16]

Documentation for Quality Improvement

Assessment of quality improvement is necessary for endoscopic procedures, as for any other surgical procedure. The RRC and the Joint Commission on Accreditation of Healthcare Organizations rely heavily on such data for their ongoing evaluation of hospitals and their surgical training programs.

If findings in all endoscopic procedures are documented as suggested earlier, little effort should be required to retrieve information for quality improvement. Such documentation includes pathologic and cytologic evaluation of specimens obtained. Photographic and videotape documentation offers significant advantages. All endoscopic complications, including those of sedation, must be recorded and presented at regularly held quality assurance meetings. Endoscopy performed by surgeons is a skill that makes up only one portion of the surgeon's armamentarium; therefore, endoscopic procedural complications should not be isolated but rather presented at surgical morbidity and mortality conferences and integrated into general surgery quality assurance.

LOGISTIC SUPPORT

Logistic support must not be taken for granted or compromised; to accept a less than adequate level of support will jeopardize the entire training process and afford poor patient care. Since there is never enough hospital space, personnel, or finances for capital equipment, the temptation to accept a converted closet, a part-time technician, and borrowed or used fiberoptic equipment just to be able to begin endoscopy must be avoided at all costs. Surgical endoscopy is a high revenue generator; the administration must be made aware of the necessity of "up front" commitment to reap the substantial monetary rewards. Even if there is a complete medical gastroenterology endoscopy unit, there

Endoscopy Worksheet   Date_____

Name_____   SSN_____   Age_____   Sex_____

Procedure: <u>Colonoscopy</u>   Premed   Demerol_____   Versed_____

Indication:

Complications:

Findings:

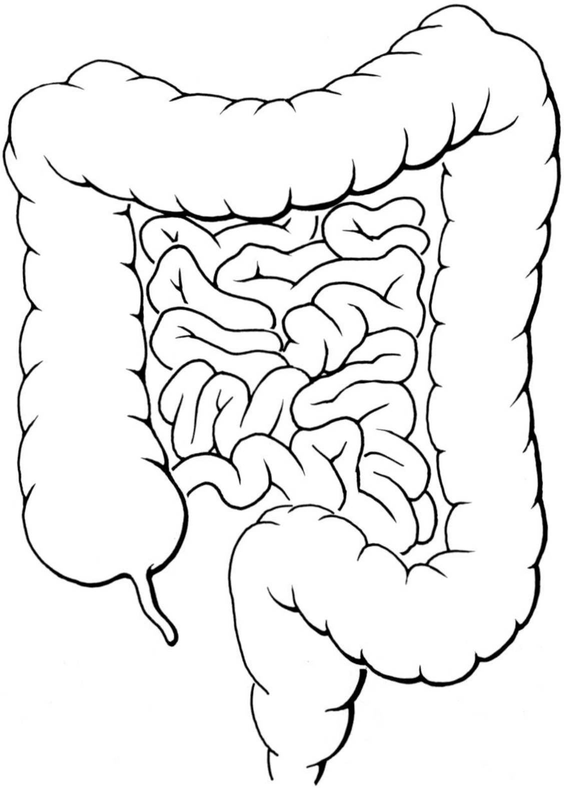

Additional Procedures:

    Specimens:

    Pathology Report:

Photographs:
    Video:

Final Diagnosis:

Recommendations:

Signature_____   Attending_____

Figure 38–1. Basic endoscopy worksheet for the database.

is ample evidence that an independent surgical endoscopy suite will not detract from the former unit and will actually increase the institution's total revenues.[11, 17]

Personnel

At the very least, all endoscopy units require a registered nurse (RN). The RN may function as the gastrointestinal assistant (GIA) or may be aided by a trained GIA who is not necessarily an RN. It is estimated that one GIA is required for each 600 to 800 procedures/year.[11, 18] This breaks down to four to five procedures/day/assistant. The presence of only one assistant mandates that sedated patients complete their recovery in an ambulatory surgery area or recovery room.

Additionally, when a surgical endoscopy unit approaches the level of 600 procedures/year, a full-time secretary is essential. In these days of cost containment, one may expect that the secretary will also serve the role of clerk and receptionist.

Facilities

A dedicated endoscopy suite is to be used for all elective procedures; most emergency procedures are performed at the patient's bedside in the intensive care unit with a mobile endoscopy unit. It is difficult to justify an expensive fluoroscopic unit in the typical endoscopy suite unless a high volume of ERCP or balloon dilation procedures is expected. For this reason, most of these procedures are performed in a radiology suite with portable endoscopy equipment. The presence of a radiologist is at the discretion of the surgeon-endoscopist and the political encumbrances of the hospital.

There have been several treatises written on the design and setup of endoscopic units.[11, 18–20] As the volume of patients increases, the number of rooms and assistants, as well as floor space must grow accordingly. Estimates for space-room requirements have been compiled and range from 600 to 1200 procedures/year/endoscopic procedure room.

The requirements for equipment and space necessary to perform and teach endoscopy go well beyond the scope of this chapter. Larson and Ott,[18] Sivak and Senick,[19] Green,[20] and Satava[11] have written extensively on this subject.

A surgical program initiating an educational endeavor today may, of necessity, begin by coexisting with medical gastroenterologists in an established unit. This is not only a matter of economics and space allocations but also appropriate use of expensive capital equipment without the need to duplicate.

If the director of surgical endoscopy education finds that there is no suitable existing endoscopy unit, a basic endoscopy unit must be established. The previously mentioned authors should be consulted by anyone contemplating the design of a new endoscopy unit.

The minimum of endoscopy equipment includes the endoscope system and the accessories (Table 38–3). It is essential to initiate training with video endoscopy equipment at the outset. This ensures safer procedures and enhances the educational efforts of all involved. The basic system consists of gastroscope and colonoscope, video processor and light source, and one video monitor. A flexible sigmoidoscope could be included; however, it is readily apparent that the colonoscope can serve equally well in cases in which flexible sigmoidoscopy is planned. It is the recommendation of the authors that all endoscopy units have a minimum of two gastroscopes and two colonoscopes. Multiple scopes allow rapid turnover time, increasing the use of the endoscopy room or rooms and personnel. The high-technology nature of video endoscopes is such that they are subject to mechanical or electrical breakdown on occasion, or both. These occasions may be more frequent within the context of training programs. Although most manufacturers will readily oblige with overnight shipment of loaned endoscopes, the availability of only one colonoscope that malfunctions on the first patient of the day precludes the per-

Table 38–3. ESSENTIAL EQUIPMENT TO INITIATE SURGICAL ENDOSCOPY TRAINING

Processor—light source
Upper endoscopes (2)
Lower endoscopes (2)
Video monitors (2)
Electrocautery unit
Mobile endoscopy cart
Endoscope cleaning unit
    Manual or automatic
Patient monitoring
    EKG
    BP and pulse
    Pulse oximeter
High-speed (wall) suction
Oxygen supply (wall)
Video still photograph recorder
Video cassette recorder
Database management system (PC-based)

EKG = electrocardiogram; BP = blood pressure, PC = personal computer.

Table 38–4. ENDOSCOPIC ACCESSORIES

Basic	Advanced	ERCP
Biopsy forceps	Oventube	Diagnostic cannulas
Hot biopsy forceps	Endoscopic ultrasound	Sphincterotomes
Retrieval forceps	Heater probe	Biliary balloons-Fogarty balloons
Coagulating snares	Bicap electrocautery unit	Stents
Cytology brushes	Variceal ligator	Stone baskets and crushers
Sclerotherapy needles	Balloon dilators	
	Esophageal stents	
	Lasers	

ERCP = endoscopic retrograde cholangiopancreatography.

formance of the remainder of the day's procedures on already prepared patients. Furthermore, once an endoscopy unit is established, the numeric growth of procedures often exceeds expectations. The availability of two gastroscopes and two colonoscopes provides a built-in capacity to accommodate the rapid increase in procedural volume.

The minimal essential accessories include biopsy forceps, retrieval forceps, injection needles, electrocautery snares, a monopolar electrocautery unit, and cleaning accessories. Depending on the level of endoscopic volume and available expertise, additional accessories may be required (Table 38–4) such as pediatric endoscopes, dual-channel endoscopes for intervention in rapidly bleeding lesions, and side-viewing duodenoscopes for ERCP and sphincterotomy. Increased volume may justify the addition of an automatic endoscope washer. To supplement the video systems, information management systems are now available and may include computers, video cassette recorders (VCRs), photographic accessories, and image management systems, such as the Sony Promavica and Mavigraph.

There are additional requirements and procedures to take into account when teaching endoscopy to trainees, including the availability of a VCR, creation of teaching files with x-ray studies performed before the procedure, and still and video recordings of findings. Although a computer database is essential within a teaching program, for a modest investment, image storage and manipulation capabilities can also be acquired. Since research and publication is to be encouraged, editorial and audiovisual support, which is usually available through the hospital's existing programs, should be used.

Advanced therapeutic techniques may later require the purchase of additional equipment such as bipolar electrocautery, heater probe units, lasers, PEG sets, balloon dilators, and even a fluoroscopic unit (fixed or C-arm). Ul-

trasound probes and processing units are available to those investigating endolumenal ultrasound. A commitment to ERCP adds the need for a diagnostic duodenoscope and a larger therapeutic duodenoscope, along with various cannulas, stents, sphincterotomes, and biliary balloons.

TRAINING IN ADVANCED ENDOSCOPIC TECHNIQUES

This chapter has focused on the deliverance of comprehensive education and acquisition of skills considered to be basic to all endoscopists. Now there is a greater interest in adding advanced therapeutic endoscopic training for surgeons. It is unrealistic to expect that every surgical program should offer advanced endoscopic training to all surgical residents. In fact, it has been advocated that an additional year of fellowship (the "third tier") be available in medical gastroenterology training. It is within this third tier that advanced techniques are taught, including therapeutic ERCP (sphincterotomy, stenting, stone extraction), peroral cholangioscopy (mother and baby scopes), endoscopic ultrasonography, laser ablation of gastrointestinal neoplasms, and use of the laser in gastrointestinal bleeding.

Recently Cameron[21] advocated that fellowship training in specific areas of alimentary tract surgery be made available to interested and talented graduates of general surgery residencies. One such area would include fellowship training in advanced therapeutic endoscopy. There is a small cadre of surgeons in the United States and worldwide with expertise in these advanced techniques. These surgeons work mainly at tertiary referral centers, performing the volume of procedures necessary to maintain a level of proficiency within the areas of specialization; many offer fellowship training within their areas of expertise. The fundamental premise is that the completely trained surgeon can offer all the options for a specific medical problem—from diagnostic and therapeutic endoscopy to open surgery. Within the surgical residency program, the director of surgical endoscopy training should advise all interested surgeons as to the availability of advanced fellowships after completion of residency. These fellowships currently require 3 months to 2 years, depending on the training desired and the caseload volume required to acquire adequate experience. It may be anticipated that the graduates of these fellowships will slowly promote training of their own residents and fellows over the course of the next several decades.

ENDOSCOPY IN THE OPERATING ROOM

Standard flexible endoscopic procedures may be performed in the confines of the operating room whenever and wherever circumstances make this an attractive alternative; however, as a routine, it is not recommended. It is an inefficient use of operating room time, space, and personnel. Furthermore, the performance of such procedures in the operating room generally requires the participation of anesthesia personnel, increasing the cost of the procedure. Regardless of the cost, the addition of anesthesia personnel detracts from the trainee's experience. As part of endoscopic training, the endoscopist is expected to become proficient in the safe and efficacious administration of intravenous sedation.[14]

Nonetheless, there are occasions when the performance of endoscopy is most appropriate within the operating room. One should not hesitate to enlist the operating room and anesthesia personnel in such circumstances. The experienced gastrointestinal assistant can mobilize a video endoscope and bring it to the operating room on short notice. In addition, a few programs may have planned intraoperative enteroscopy as a means to evaluate obscure sources of small bowel bleeding.

Perhaps the most common flexible endoscopic procedure the general surgeon should be performing in the operating room is operative choledochoscopy. Until recently, this generally would be an open procedure. The advent of laparoscopic surgery has added a new dimension. The most common procedure now is likely to be translaparoscopic choledochoscopy. Whenever a common duct exploration is performed in the course of residency training, we

would recommend that some form of video endoscopic visualization be employed.

The most common endoscopic procedures performed in the operating room today are those that employ the rigid laparoscope. The venue of this chapter is not a detailed discussion of training in laparoscopic surgery; this subject has been addressed in many chapters elsewhere within this text. Resident training in laparoscopic surgery should be incorporated into the basic structure of general surgery and not considered a separate discipline.[22]

FUTURE SPECULATION

There are two main areas in resident education that will continue to show significant changes: the regulatory requirements for documentation and the simulated teaching experience. The former demands vigilance with the highest moral integrity, and the latter provides the exhilaration of a limitless future.

The era of overregulation is upon us, and every aspect of surgery, including endoscopy, requires voluminous documentation. The vast majority of record keeping does not significantly improve patient care, rather it serves to provide an audit trail for one oversight body or another to monitor the administrative process. The usual response to a request for new documentation is to devise another form to fulfill the new regulation. Medical records are already overflowing with superfluous data. Rather than creating new forms, we must view all new regulations with an analytic eye, perceive the essential information required, be certain that it truly enhances patient care, and provide a legitimate response, either with existing forms or by replacing previous forms. We must ensure that the medical profession continues to protect the moral high ground and that the future demands for data are not merely a paper screen that buries the question rather than answers it.

The exciting innovations in the field of endoscopy will continue to become more complex by adding three-dimensional stereoscopic images, changing the shape and function of the endoscope and accessories, devising new procedures, and adding new technologies. All these changes will require further education in basic principles and training in technical skills. To respond to these needs, a new generation of simulators is being developed, such as the endoscopic and ERCP simulator of Noar,[13] which will permit a fully interactive training experience. The technologies of telepresence and virtual reality offer the promise of a simulator so realistic that it may actually substitute for actual patient training in the same manner that sophisticated flight simulators provide "flight time" for commercial and military pilots. We must not only conduct our own medical research but must also look to the leaders in industry, business, and academia to see where the technologies of the future might direct us.

CONCLUSION

The purpose of endoscopic training in general surgery is to reflect and complement the entire surgical residency experience. This is best achieved by selecting a member of the surgical staff to be the designated director of surgical endoscopy with full authority and responsibility for incorporating endoscopic training as an integral portion of the residents' education. The ideal method would be to provide a specific rotation in surgical endoscopy, preferably in the second or third postgraduate year, under the tutelage of the surgical endoscopy staff. This experience must encompass both didactic and clinical education; if possible, the opportunity for endoscopic research should be provided. In some centers, advanced endoscopic training, such as ERCP, could allow certain residents to pursue these advanced techniques. These surgeons could then offer the complete spectrum of medical care to the patient, from diagnostic and therapeutic endoscopy to open surgery. Under all circumstances, accurate documentation of the trainee's progress and of the training program is essential to meet regulatory requirements; this is best accomplished with a computerized consolidated database.

A productive program cannot be achieved without adequate resources in equipment, personnel, and facilities. Since surgical endoscopy greatly enhances patient care at a favorable cost–benefit ratio while at the same time providing a significant source of revenue, initiation and maintenance of a surgical endoscopy program must be undertaken with the understanding that advance investment is necessary and will be rapidly recouped.

The future holds a mixed promise. Although the increasing demands of documentation and review agencies portend a suffocating influence on the ability to provide quality education, the recent explosion of innovative technology, in particular educational simulation, points to an ambitious future for endoscopy and surgical education.

References

1. Haubrich WS. History of endoscopy. In: Sivak MV, ed. Gastroenterologic endoscopy. Philadelphia: WB Saunders, 1986:2–19.
2. American Board of Surgery. Booklet of information. Philadelphia: American Board of Surgery, 1986.
3. Satava RM, Unger SW. Resident education in surgical endoscopy: the 1990 SAGES survey. Presented at the 6th annual scientific session of SAGES, Monterey, CA, April 1991.
4. Ponsky JL. The incorporation of endoscopic training into a surgical residency. Newsletter of the Society of American Gastrointestinal Endoscopic Surgeons, Spring 1988:2.
5. Society of American Gastrointestinal Endoscopic Surgeons. Guidelines for general surgery residency education in gastrointestinal endoscopy. Los Angeles: Society of American Gastrointestinal Endoscopic Surgeons, 1992.
6. American Society of Gastrointestinal Endoscopy. Statement on endoscopic training. Manchester, MA: American Society of Gastrointestinal Endoscopy, 1986.
7. Satava RM. The impact of video endoscopy on surgical training. Am Surg 54:263–266, 1989.
8. Dent TL, Kukora JS, Leibrandt TJ. Teaching surgical endoscopy of the gastrointestinal tract. World J Surg 13:202–205, 1989.
9. Society of American Gastrointestinal Endoscopic Surgeons. Curriculum guide for resident education in GI surgical endoscopy. Los Angeles, CA: Society of American Gastrointestinal Endoscopic Surgeons, 1991.
10. Cunningham ER, Satava RM. Development of a surgical endoscopy database for quality assurance. Am Surg 57:271–273, 1991.
11. Satava RM. Establishing an endoscopy unit for surgical training. Surg Clin North Am 69:1129–1145, 1989.
12. Dent TL, Leibrandt TJ. Teaching surgical endoscopy of the gastrointestinal tract. In: Dent TL, Strodel WE, Turcotte G, eds. Surgical endoscopy. Chicago: Year Book Medical Publishers, 1985:487–492.
13. Noar MD. Endoscopy in simulation: a brave new world? Endoscopy 23:147–149, 1991.
14. Simon IB, Lewis RJ, Satava RM. A safe method for sedating and monitoring patients for upper and lower gastrointestinal endoscopy. Am Surg 57:219–221, 1991.
15. American Society for Gastrointestinal Endoscopy. Training evaluation form. Manchester, MA: American Society for Gastrointestinal Endoscopy. 1982.
16. Society of American Gastrointestinal Endoscopic Surgeons. Granting of privileges for gastrointestinal endoscopy by surgeons. Los Angeles: Society of American Gastrointestinal Endoscopic Surgeons, 1991.
17. Smale BF, Reber HA, Terry BE, et al. The creation of a surgical endoscopy program: is there sufficient material? Surgery 94:180–185, 1983.
18. Larson DE, Ott BJ. The structure and function of the outpatient endoscopy unit. Gastrointest Endosc 32:10–14, 1986.
19. Sivak MV, Senick JM. The endoscopy unit. In: Sivak MV, ed. Gastroenterologic endoscopy. Philadelphia: WB Saunders, 1987:42–66.
20. Green ML. Physical structure of the endoscopy unit. In: Endoscopic training director's manual. Manchester, MA: American Society for Gastrointestinal Endoscopy, 1984.
21. Cameron JL. Fellowship training in alimentary tract surgery: is it necessary? Society for Surgery of the Alimentary Tract Presidential Address, San Francisco, May 1992.
22. Society of American Gastrointestinal Endoscopic Surgeons. Position statement. Arch Surg 127:82–83, 1992.

39

Credentialing and Privileging for Endoscopic and Laparoscopic Surgery

Thomas L. Dent

Clinical privileges are those functions and procedures that a physician is permitted to perform in the course of caring for patients in a given hospital. In the recent past, the granting of clinical privileges was less complicated than it is today: all a physician had to show was that training had been obtained in a clinical discipline, and he or she was granted privileges for all clinical tasks common to that discipline. Nonsurgeons performed few, if any, invasive procedures, and the chief of surgery controlled operating room privileges. If surgeons felt comfortable performing any of the procedures that fell within their specialty, their right to do so was unquestioned. There were no lists of privileges. Everyone "knew" what each surgical specialty did, and the chief of surgery resolved any disagreements by fiat. Today, the performance of invasive procedures by nonsurgeons, the "turf" battles among surgical specialists over the exclusive right to perform certain procedures, and the greater scrutiny of the privileging process by regulatory agencies, the news media, patients, legislators, attorneys, and courts have all contributed to the development of a more rigorous and complex mechanism for granting clinical privileges.

THE INITIAL PRIVILEGING PROCESS

The privileging process is intended to ensure that patients receive skillful care by competent practitioners. The granting of clinical privileges is, ultimately, the responsibility of the hospital governing board.[1] Each hospital is responsible for developing its own mechanism for granting all clinical privileges; frequently, "national" criteria developed by specialty boards or specialty societies are adopted.[2] The hospital usually asks a credentials committee or the chief of a clinical service to evaluate each request for clinical privileges by reviewing the following criteria: the requesting physician's credentials, including board certification; general and specific training and experience in the privileges requested; and certification of competence by the residency program director, instructors, and peers. Competence is defined as a safe and acceptable level of skill and can refer either to a physician's general ability within a specialty to care for patients or to the ability of the physician to perform a specific technical procedure or operation. Based on the evaluation by the credentials committee or clinical service chief, each physician's clinical privileges are granted by the hospital governing board. Some hospitals initially grant privileges provisionally or require that physicians be proctored for a period before full privileges are granted, or both, whereas others do not. Individual hospitals and department chairmen are charged by the Joint Commission on Accreditation of Healthcare Organizations with assuring the competence of each member of the medical staff. Clinical privileges must be reevaluated and regranted at least every 2 years.[1]

PRIVILEGE LISTS

Basically, there are three methods of deciding which procedures should be included in a physician's privilege list. With a *categorical* approach, privileges are granted in all procedures common to a physician's specialty, as defined by that specialty's accrediting board. Two disadvantages to this approach are (1) that not every surgical specialist has received adequate training and experience in every procedure claimed by that specialty during his or her residency and (2) that significantly new procedures will be developed after the applicant's residency training. Board certification, or even recertification, cannot guarantee competence in procedures not taught during residency training.

A second approach is to grant each surgeon privileges from a constantly updated, exhaustive *list* of every possible procedure and variation within his or her specialty. Such lists would include thousands of procedures and are difficult to develop and even more difficult to maintain. Also, performance of any procedure or variation inadvertently not included in such a list would automatically mean that the surgeon has exceeded his or her clinical privileges, creating unnecessary administrative and medicolegal difficulties.

In my experience, the best approach to the granting of privileges is to combine the *categorical* and *list* approaches. Categories, such as gastric operations or colon operations, group similar surgical procedures; additional listings are then developed only for those procedures that require separate privileges (see further on). Periodic review is necessary to add newly developed procedures and to move previously separate procedures into a standard privilege category after they have been incorporated into the residency curriculum for that specialty.

ADDITIONAL PRIVILEGES

Residency education in the United States is rigorous and is regulated by the Accreditation Council for Graduate Medical Education through residency review committees for each of the 24 major surgical specialties and an additional 56 medical and surgical subspecialties. Each specialty and subspecialty has specific requirements regarding the amount and content of educational exposure to the specialty and the type and number of procedures that must be performed before a resident is eligible to sit for board examination in that specialty. Therefore, when a physician receives board certification, there is reasonable assurance that he or she is competent to perform the procedures included in that specialty's procedure list at the time of certification.

If a staff physician applies for clinical privileges to perform a procedure not previously included in his or her residency training, most hospitals will require documentation of additional training, experience, competence and, possibly, proctoring in the additional procedure before privileges are granted.[2]

Most problems in the privileging process are associated with such new privileges, because it is difficult for a physician or surgeon to obtain adequate hands-on training once residency training is completed. New *cognitive* information can be learned at a seminar or postgraduate course in the traditional manner of continuing medical education. Learning a new *technical* procedure, however, is not as easy. Many "new" procedures are only minor variations of existing procedures and can be learned simply and quickly by reading about the technique, observing the procedure, or taking a short postgraduate course. For example, highly selective vagotomy is a minor variation for a surgeon already privileged to perform truncal vagotomy. Such minor variations in procedures do not require the granting of additional privileges, and their performance and outcomes can then be monitored through traditional peer review mechanisms.

Other procedures, such as endoscopy and laparoscopy, require more extensive training and experience than can be obtained from a postgraduate seminar because they are sufficiently different or complicated; therefore, clinical privileges should not be granted in these cases before such training and experience are obtained.[3–8] Unfortunately, there are no formally established and regulated postresidency training programs that provide the necessary technical training in such new procedures, and already established residency programs are not organized to provide additional hands-on training to surgeons in practice.

There are two steps that must be taken by chiefs of clinical services or credentials committees, or both, to identify which new procedures require additional privileges. The first and most important is to decide if the proposed new procedure is safe and efficacious, (*i.e.,* not experimental). If the new procedure has not been demonstrated to be safe and efficacious, privileges should not even be considered unless the procedure is being performed as part of an experimental trial under the supervision of the hospital's institutional review board.

Once the procedure has been shown to be reasonably safe and efficacious, the second step is to determine if the proposed new procedure is "sufficiently different" from other similar procedures. A good test of this is to decide whether the new procedure requires additional formal training in an animal laboratory. If so, the credentialing committee should advise the hospital that additional privileging is required for this procedure. Additional privileging should also be considered for new procedures that are controversial, risky, or of high visibility, as well as for those procedures that will be performed by more than one clinical specialty.[2, 3] It is also important that the requested privilege be in a clinical area in which the requesting physician is already knowledgeable. For example, it would be illogical to grant privileges in diagnostic and therapeutic gastroscopy to an otolaryngologist simply because he or she is privileged to perform a similar procedure (esophagoscopy) with a similar instrument. A specific knowledge base of the clinical anatomy and pathophysiology of the organ or organs involved should be required.

After it has been decided that a new procedure requires a separate application for clinical privileges, and before any physician in the hospital is allowed to perform it, the criteria for the granting of such privileges should be formulated.[2, 3] The criteria should include the certification and credentials required, the method of assessing competence in the procedure, and whether or not proctoring will be required. Lists of criteria and guidelines for the granting of clinical privileges in new procedures are often available from national specialty organizations, but these criteria and guidelines must be reviewed carefully for bias and protectionism. The criteria must specify the training and credentials required, the necessary didactic and laboratory experience, the method of documenting competence in the procedure, and whether or not proctoring is required prior to the granting of full privileges.

GASTROINTESTINAL ENDOSCOPY

Gastrointestinal endoscopy is an example of a group of procedures for which the privileging process has been complicated because many specialties have incorporated endoscopy into their procedural armamentaria.[6, 8–16] Selected gastrointestinal endoscopic procedures are now performed by gastroenterologists, internists, family practitioners, general surgeons, thoracic surgeons, otolaryngologists, pediatric surgeons, and colon and rectal surgeons.[17]

Prior to 1970, endoscopy of the gastrointestinal tract consisted of only rigid proctoscopy and rigid esophagoscopy. These procedures were primarily diagnostic, uncomfortable for the patient, and not particularly remunerative for the physician. The development of flexible fiberoptic endoscopes has revolutionized the diagnosis and treatment of diseases of the gastrointestinal tract by allowing the endoscopist to accurately visualize the entire esophagus, stomach, duodenum, and colon with excellent patient comfort and safety, and to perform surgical procedures, such as gastrostomy, polypectomy, ablation of esophageal varices, and biliary sphincterotomy, that could not be accomplished previously except through laparotomy. Not surprisingly, the ease of performance, accuracy of diagnosis, simplified surgical techniques, and increased income stimulated the imagination and enthusiasm of all physicians whose practice included either the medical or surgical treatment of gastrointestinal diseases. Since many of these specialists were not trained in gastrointestinal endoscopy during their residencies, since the procedures are sufficiently different and technically demanding as to require additional formal training, and since more than one specialty performs them, separate privileging for each major procedure (flexible sigmoidoscopy, esophagogastroduodenoscopy [EGD], colonoscopy, and endoscopic retrograde cholangiopancreatography [ERCP]) is appropriate.

There is an adequate volume of cases in teaching hospitals for all general surgery residents to become trained in flexible sigmoidoscopy, colonoscopy, and EGD.[7, 16–18] At present, most surgeons, and some gastroenterologists, are not being trained in ERCP because of the small number of available cases. Potential solutions to this problem include initial training on a model to develop the manual skills needed in ERCP prior to performing the procedure in humans[19] and on endoscopic simulators, which are still in development.[20]

Both the American Society of Gastrointestinal Endoscopy (ASGE) and the Society of American Gastrointestinal Endoscopic Surgeons (SAGES) have published guidelines advising hospitals how to privilege physicians to perform these procedures (Table 39–1). Both of these "competing" specialty organizations agree that to be competent in the performance of endoscopic procedures, the physician must be trained in a formal fellowship in a specialty that cares for patients with gastrointestinal dis-

Table 39–1. COMPARISON OF THE AMERICAN SOCIETY OF GASTROINTESTINAL ENDOSCOPY'S (ASGE) AND THE SOCIETY OF AMERICAN GASTROINTESTINAL ENDOSCOPIC SURGEONS' (SAGES) GUIDELINES FOR GRANTING HOSPITAL PRIVILEGES IN GASTROINTESTINAL ENDOSCOPY

	ASGE[15]		SAGES[12]	
Uniformity of standards	Should apply equally to all hospital staff		Should apply equally to all hospital staff	
Specificity of credentialing	For each major category of endoscopy		For each major category of endoscopy	
Training	Fellowship or residency in gastroenterology or surgery		Residency in surgery	
Competence	Must be demonstrated and documented		Must be demonstrated and documented	
Minimum number of supervised cases	EGD	50–75	EGD	25
	Colonoscopy	50	Colonoscopy	50
	Polypectomy	15	Flexible sigmoidoscopy	15
	ERCP	35–50		
Proctoring	Recommended if any question of competence		Recommended if any question of competence	
Certification	Endoscopic training directors should confirm in writing the training, experience, and actual observed level of competence		Endoscopic training directors should confirm in writing the training, experience, and actual observed level of competence	
Short courses	Not acceptable as substitute for supervised hands-on training		Not acceptable as substitute for supervised hands-on training	
New procedures	Individualize		Individualize	
Quality assurance monitoring	Multidisciplinary endoscopy committee		Existing mechanisms or multidisciplinary endoscopy committee	
Continuing education	Required as part of periodic renewal of endoscopic privileges		Required as part of periodic renewal of endoscopic privileges	
Responsibility for credentialing	Hospital; multidisciplinary endoscopic procedure committee desirable		Hospital; chief of surgery for surgeons	

EGD = esophagogastroduodenoscopy; ERCP = endoscopic retrograde cholangiopancreatography.

eases. They also agree that since individual trainees may differ significantly in technical ability and that some may require more training than others in these procedures, the trainee's endoscopic instructor should be the primary judge of competence. Although the suggested minimum number of completed cases for each procedure was similar in both guidelines when first published (Table 39–1), the ASGE has recently published a new document increasing the minimum number of supervised cases significantly (100 EGDs, 100 colonoscopies, 20 polypectomies, and 75 ERCPs).[6] Since these procedures have not become any harder to perform since 1988, one possible explanation of the motive for these increased numbers is to make it harder for nongastroenterologists to become trained and privileged in flexible endoscopy. Surgeons actually may require fewer supervised procedures than nonsurgeons because "by virtue of completing a residency program in surgery, the surgeon endoscopist will have acquired at least 5 years of cognitive experience in anatomy, physiology, and disease processes, combined with the progressive development of visual and psychomotor skills and experience necessary for the performance of diagnostic and therapeutic procedures in the gastrointestinal tract."[12] Both organizations believe, however, that competence, rather than a specific number of procedures performed, should be the deciding factor in the granting of privileges. Both societies also agree that when competence cannot be verified by submitted written material or by the endoscopy instructor, proctoring of applicants by an unbiased endoscopist, preferably from the same clinical discipline, should be considered.[11]

Despite these published guidelines, "turf" battles between gastroenterologists and surgeons continue at many hospitals,[5, 8–10, 13, 14] usually over the exact number of procedures necessary for endoscopic privileges. In most instances, these battles could be resolved simply by following the published guidelines for each discipline (Table 39–1). At Abington Memorial Hospital (Abington, PA), the chief of surgery evaluates the credentials of surgeons applying for endoscopic privileges, and the chief of gastroenterology evaluates the credentials of nonsurgeons, each using the guidelines of their respective societies and requiring proctoring as necessary. Each then makes privileging recommendations to the executive committee of the medical staff, which, in turn, makes a recommendation to the board of trustees. Endoscopic procedures are performed by both surgeons and gastroenterologists (and in the case of flexible sigmoidoscopy, family practitioners and internists as well) in a shared gastrointestinal procedures unit. This cooperation, in the author's experience, is unusual but works quite well for us and should be considered by other hospitals.

LAPAROSCOPIC CHOLECYSTECTOMY

Laparoscopic general surgery has created privileging difficulties of a different sort. Since it is generally agreed that surgeons already privileged to perform open abdominal procedures should be the ones to learn and perform therapeutic laparoscopic procedures, there are no significant "turf" battles among different specialties. However, since most surgeons currently in practice did not learn laparoscopic techniques during their residencies, the content of what constitutes adequate additional training before performing laparoscopic surgery has become a subject of debate.[3, 4, 21–26] Laparoscopic surgical procedures are new to general surgeons, are significantly different from other general surgical techniques, are technically demanding and, like any major surgical procedure, are associated with morbidity and mortality. In addition, laparoscopic surgery is both controversial and of high visibility.[24, 27] Until these procedures are taught in adequate numbers in all surgical residency programs, separate privileges are necessary and appropriate.

SAGES developed and published privileging guidelines for laparoscopic surgery as soon as it became evident that laparoscopy was about to radically change the way surgeons treat diseases of the biliary and gastrointestinal tracts (Table 39–2). Abington Memorial Hospital modified SAGES' guidelines to develop criteria for the granting of privileges in laparoscopic cholecystectomy (Table 39–3). We agreed that only those surgeons privileged to perform open biliary tract surgical procedures should be permitted to seek privileges in laparoscopic general surgery[29] and that "surgeons who are experienced in operating upon abdominal organs are familiar with anatomy, tissue tolerance, organ compliance, and pathological processes and should readily develop laparoscopic proficiency . . . and [also that the] criteria [should not be] . . . unreasonably stringent."[28]

We first included a requirement and a mechanism for obtaining privileges in diagnostic laparoscopy. Some have recommended more ex-

Table 39–2. THE SOCIETY OF AMERICAN GASTROINTESTINAL ENDOSCOPIC SURGEONS' GUIDELINES FOR GRANTING OF PRIVILEGES FOR LAPAROSCOPIC GENERAL SURGERY[28]

1. Completion of a surgical residency/fellowship program that incorporates structured experience in laparoscopic surgery. Competence should be documented by the instructor or instructors.
2. Proficiency in laparoscopic surgical procedures and clinical judgment equivalent to that obtained in a residency/fellowship program. Documentation and demonstration of competence is necessary.
3. For those without residency training or fellowship that included laparoscopic surgery or without documented prior experience in laparoscopic surgery, the basic minimum requirements for training should be:
   a. completion of approved residency training in general surgery.
   b. credentialing in diagnostic laparoscopy.
   c. training in laparoscopic general surgery by a surgeon experienced in laparoscopic surgery or completion of a university-sponsored or academic society–recognized didactic course with clinical experience and hands-on laboratory practice.
   d. observation of laparoscopic surgical procedures performed by a surgeon (or surgeons) experienced in the performance of such procedures.
4. Attendance at short courses that do not provide supervised hands-on training is not an acceptable substitute for the development of competency.

tensive training and experience in diagnostic laparoscopy prior to learning laparoscopic cholecystectomy,[30] but surgeons at our institution have learned diagnostic laparoscopy readily during a short preceptorship with either a gynecologist or another surgeon experienced in laparoscopy.

A training course in laparoscopic surgery, including both didactic instruction and hands-on experience in live animals, is important for surgeons whose training did not include laparoscopic techniques. A comprehensive curriculum, an experienced faculty, and an extensive animal laboratory experience are the essential elements of a good postgraduate training course.[4]

Although SAGES recommends only observation of the procedure in humans, I feel that assisting during laparoscopic operations is an important component of learning the procedure. SAGES' guidelines also include proctoring only as a recommendation, but recommend it as an important patient safeguard. The proctor must certify the applicant's competence in the performance of the procedure before full privileges are granted.

As laparoscopic cholecystectomy is incorporated into the general surgery residency training curriculum, residents will be trained as they are trained in other surgical procedures: by assisting

Table 39–3. ABINGTON MEMORIAL HOSPITAL'S CRITERIA FOR BEING GRANTED CLINICAL PRIVILEGES IN LAPAROSCOPIC CHOLECYSTECTOMY

For a surgeon to be granted privileges to perform laparoscopic cholecystectomy, the following requirements must be met:

1. The surgeon must be privileged to perform biliary tract operations through an accredited residency program in General Surgery.
2. The surgeon must be privileged in diagnostic laparoscopy. For those not privileged, privileging requires all of the following:
   a. tutoring by someone already privileged in laparoscopy (*e.g.,* gynecologist) in the indications, contraindications, technique, risks, complications, and results of diagnostic laparoscopy,
   b. participating (performing or first-assisting) in a sufficient number of procedures (minimum number: five) to become proficient in laparoscopy,
   c. having the tutor certify in writing that the surgeon is competent in both the understanding and techniques of diagnostic laparoscopy.
3. The surgeon must have taken a formal course in laparoscopic cholecystectomy that includes both didactic instruction and hands-on experience in live animals.
4. The surgeon must have assisted in at least five laparoscopic cholecystectomies in humans.
5. The surgeon must be proctored by a surgeon with privileges in biliary tract surgery and/or laparoscopic cholecystectomy in at least three laparoscopic cholecystectomies. The proctor must certify in writing that the surgeon is competent to perform the procedure.
6. Provisional privileges in laparoscopic cholecystectomy may be granted by the Division Chief of General Surgery after the completion of requirement No. 4, but full privileges will not be recommended to the Executive Committee of the Medical Staff and the Board of Trustees until completion of requirement No. 5.

From Dent TL. Training, credentialling, and granting of clinical privileges for laparoscopic general surgery. Am J Surg 161:402, 1991.

an experienced surgeon and then performing the procedure under gradually decreasing supervision.[3, 21, 22, 25, 31, 32] In just a few years, when laparoscopic cholecystectomy is taught in all residency programs and animal laboratory experience will be unnecessary, laparoscopic cholecystectomy will then become a part of the biliary tract category of general surgical privileges for all newly trained general surgeons and will no longer require a separate privileging mechanism.

OTHER ENDOSCOPIC AND LAPAROSCOPIC PROCEDURES

New surgical variations and procedures using laparoscopes and endoscopes are being developed constantly. Additional training for surgeons to perform these procedures once they are already trained in basic general, endoscopic, and laparoscopic surgery will probably consist of learning by lecture, videotape, or "scrubbing in" with a colleague, or a combination of these techniques. Learning by using an endoscopic or laparoscopic simulator, similar to those used by pilots learning to fly, is an exciting possibility.[20, 33] However, as with other clinical privileges and in keeping with traditional medical ethics, the surgeon, monitored by the clinical service chief or the credentials committee, or both, should recognize when and how much additional training in each new variation is necessary, and when the "variation" is actually a new procedure that requires additional formal training and additional privileges.

Since the development of biliary sphincterotomy and endoscopic polypectomy in the 1970s, most recent advances in flexible gastrointestinal endoscopy, such as rubber band ligation of esophageal varices and biliary stent placement, have been minor variations in technique that do not require additional formal training or separate privileges.

Laparoscopic surgery, in contrast, is being used to perform many truly new procedures in this rapidly expanding field. Some would like to see laparoscopic surgery restricted to academic centers that "participate in current or planned prospective studies designed to optimize the technique and carefully refine its indications"[30] prior to allowing the procedure to be performed by all surgeons. As imperfect as the system is, the author believes that progress would be severely impeded if every logical surgical innovation, such as laparoscopic cholecystectomy, had to undergo extensive prospective randomized trials prior to clinical use. There are many examples of logical procedures that have been performed before their efficacy was scientifically proved. Once performed safely, the procedures were so obviously superior to prior treatments that they were never scientifically validated by randomized trials. Aortic resection for aneurysm and open appendectomy for acute appendicitis are just two examples.

There is an important difference between performing a procedure that is a logical amalgamation of proven surgical techniques with known outcomes and one that is completely new and unproved, amounting to uncontrolled human experimentation. Laparoscopic cholecystectomy is a logical combination of the accepted surgical techniques of laparoscopy and open cholecystectomy. Removal of the gallbladder by any method obviously removes the diseased organ, and the laparoscopic method has been shown in large series to be reasonably safe.[34–41] Laparoscopic cholecystectomy is currently the only laparoscopic general surgical procedure that can be considered "standard."[3, 41, 42] However, even for laparoscopic cholecystectomy, some authors[27, 30, 43] are not yet willing to agree to its unrestricted acceptance, citing the increased incidence of common bile duct injuries and other complications when compared with open cholecystectomy. In the author's opinion, as long as the local and national surgical results of laparoscopic cholecystectomy are continually monitored by the hospital, it is appropriate to grant privileges now in this procedure to appropriately trained surgeons.

Some laparoscopic procedures currently in development are also a logical combination of open and laparoscopic techniques. Laparoscopic appendectomy, pelvic lymphadenectomy, common bile duct exploration, and highly selective vagotomy, for example, are virtually identical to open procedures and can be learned with minimal additional training once basic laparoscopic surgical techniques are mastered. Therefore, they would not require additional privileges for general surgeons already privileged in laparoscopic cholecystectomy. However, since these procedures have not yet been shown to have any advantage over their open surgery counterparts and their comparative safety is still unknown, they should be used cautiously, if at all, until more information on outcome is available.

Other laparoscopic procedures are still experimental. Despite initial enthusiastic reports of "successful" laparoscopic inguinal hernia repair,[44] gastric antireflux operations,[45] and intestinal resection,[46, 47] in the author's opinion, these procedures and certain others performed laparoscopically differ significantly from open techniques and warrant more scientific study and standardization before their widespread clinical use is appropriate. These procedures are still in the developmental phase and their short- and long-term efficacy and safety are unknown.[48–50] Privileges to perform these procedures should be withheld by hospitals (unless their surgeons are participating in an experimental study or a clinical trial) until more information on outcome is available. Abington Memorial Hospital's institutional review committee requires that each patient undergoing a laparoscopic herniorrhaphy sign a consent form that explains the experimental nature of the procedure and the lack of scientific data regarding its safety, efficacy, and outcome.

MONITORING OF QUALITY

The quality of a surgeon's performance in endoscopic[51] and laparoscopic[3] procedures, as in all other surgical procedures, should be monitored through the hospital's quality improvement programs. Proctoring, additional training, or even restriction of privileges may be required if individual poor outcomes or high complication rates are identified. Continuing education in endoscopic and laparoscopic surgery is important because new variations in technique and equipment are inevitable in these rapidly evolving fields.

CONCLUSION

Hospitals in the United States are charged by the Joint Commission on Accreditation of Healthcare Organizations to evaluate the credentials of and grant specific clinical privileges to their staff physicians, as well as assure the quality of the care rendered. Each hospital must determine: (1) if a new procedure is safe and efficacious, (2) whether the procedure is sufficiently different from other procedures to require additional privileges, (3) what the privileging criteria should be, and (4) how the quality of the performance of these procedures should be monitored and assured.

Since most surgeons currently in practice were not taught endoscopic and laparoscopic surgical techniques during their residency training, additional formal training should be necessary before they are permitted to perform these procedures. SAGES has published guidelines addressing the granting of privileges in endoscopy and laparoscopy for surgeons, which have been adapted for successful use in the author's hospital.

Once privileges have been granted in the "standard" *endoscopic* categories of flexible sigmoidoscopy, EGD, colonoscopy, and ERCP, current variations within these categories are minor and should not require separate privileges.

Conversely, laparoscopic cholecystectomy is the only general surgical *laparoscopic* procedure that can be considered "standard," in the author's opinion. Some laparoscopic procedures such as appendectomy, common bile duct exploration, and highly selective vagotomy are, except for the laparoscopic approach, identical to their open surgery counterparts, and once they are deemed safe and efficacious might be added to a laparoscopic surgeon's privileges with minimal additional training. Other procedures, especially laparoscopic inguinal herniorrhaphy, are markedly different from traditional operations and their performance should not be permitted, except as part of an experimental study, until outcome data are available.

References

1. Joint Commission on Accreditation of Healthcare Organizations. The 1992 joint commission accreditation manual for hospitals. Oakbrook Terrace IL: Joint Commission on Accreditation of Healthcare Organizations, 1991.
2. The Credentialling Institute. Delineating clinical privileges: laparoscopic cholecystectomies. Pittsburgh: The Credentialling Institute.
3. Dent TL. Training, credentialling, and granting of clinical privileges for laparoscopic cholecystectomy. Am J Surg 161:399–403, 1991.
4. Greene FL. Training, credentialing, and privileging for minimally invasive surgery. Probl Gen Surg 8:502–506, 1991.
5. Myers JO, Ragland JJ, Candelaria LA. Fiberoptic endoscopy of the gastrointestinal tract in surgical training. Surg Gynecol Obstet 170:283–286, 1990.
6. American Society for Gastrointestinal Endoscopy. Principles of training in gastrointestinal endoscopy. Manchester MA: American Society for Gastrointestinal Endoscopy, 1992.
7. Cullado MJ, Porter JA, Slezak FA. The evolution of surgical endoscopic training. Meeting the American Board of Surgery requirements. Am Surg 57:250–253, 1991.
8. Kukora JS, Clericuzio CP, Dent TL. The case *for* surgical training in gastrointestinal endoscopy (letter). Am J Gastroenterol 79:907–909, 1984.
9. Dent TL. Surgeons, gastroenterologists, endoscopists. Surg Gynecol Obstet 153:733, 1981.
10. Dent TL. The surgeon and fiberoptic endoscopy. Surg Gynecol Obstet 137:278, 1973.
11. American Society for Gastrointestinal Endoscopy. Proctoring and hospital endoscopic privileges. Gastrointest Endosc 37:666–667, 1991.
12. Society of American Gastrointestinal Endoscopic Surgeons. Granting of privileges for gastrointestinal endoscopy by surgeons. Los Angeles: Society of American Gastrointestinal Endoscopic Surgeons, 1989.
13. Achord JL. The credentialing process: rational decisions of hospital committees for granting of privileges in gastrointestinal endoscopic procedures (editorial). Am J Gastroenterol 82:1064–1065, 1987.
14. Gandolfi L, Orlandi F. Problems of gastrointestinal endoscopy in Italy. Ital J Gastroenterol 22:218–221, 1990.
15. American Society for Gastrointestinal Endoscopy. Methods of granting hospital privileges to perform gastrointestinal endoscopy. Gastrointest Endosc 34(Suppl):28S–29S, 1988.
16. Pearl RK, Nelson RL, Abcarian H, et al. Establishing a flexible sigmoidoscopy/colonoscopy program for surgical residents. The University of Illinois experience. Am Surg 52:577–580, 1986.
17. Dent TL, Kukora JS, Leibrandt TJ. Teaching surgical endoscopy of the gastrointestinal tract. World J Surg 13:202–205, 1989.
18. Dasmahapatra KS, Najem AZ, Cheung NK. Surgical endoscopy training in a university program. Am Surg 52:287–290, 1986.
19. Leung JW, Chung RS. Training in ERCP (editorial). Gastrointest Endosc 38:517–518, 1992.
20. Noar MD, Soehendra N. Endoscopy simulation training devices. Endoscopy 24:159–166, 1992.
21. Bailey RW, Imbembo AL, Zucker KA. Establishment of a laparoscopic cholecystectomy training program. Am Surg 57:231–236, 1991.
22. Laws HL. Credentialling residents for laparoscopic surgery: a matter of opinion. Curr Surg 48:684–685, 1991.
23. Asbun HJ, Reddick EJ. Credentialing in laparoscopic surgery: a survey of physicians. J Laparoendosc Surg 2:27–32, 1992.
24. Altman LK. Surgical injuries lead to new rule. The New York Times 1992: June 14, p 1, column 1; p 47, column 1.
25. Sigman HH, Fried GM, Hinchey EJ, et al. Role of the teaching hospital in the development of a laparoscopic cholecystectomy program. Can J Surg 35:49–54, 1992.
26. Tompkins RK. Laparoscopic cholecystectomy: threat or opportunity? Arch Surg 125:1245, 1990.
27. Braasch JW. Laparoscopic cholecystectomy and other procedures. Arch Surg 127:887, 1992.
28. Society of American Gastrointestinal Endoscopic Surgeons. Granting of privileges for laparoscopic (peritoneoscopic) general surgery. Los Angeles; Society of American Gastrointestinal Endoscopic Surgeons, 1992.
29. American College of Surgeons. Statement on laparoscopic cholecystectomy. Bull Am Coll Surg 75(6):22, 1990.
30. Cuschieri A, Berci G, McSherry CK. Laparoscopic cholecystectomy. Am J Surg 159:273, 1990.
31. Cohen MM. Initial experience with laparoscopic cholecystectomy in a teaching hospital. Can J Surg 35:59–63, 1992.
32. Schirmer BD, Edge SB, Dix J, et al. Incorporation of laparoscopy into a surgical endoscopy training program. Am J Surg 163:46–52, 1992.
33. Baillie J, Jowell P, Evangelou H, et al. Use of computer graphics simulation for teaching of flexible sigmoidoscopy. Endoscopy 23:126–129, 1991.
34. Graves HA Jr, Ballinger JF, Anderson WJ. Appraisal of laparoscopic cholecystectomy. Ann Surg 213:655–664, 1991.
35. Neugebauer E, Troidl H, Spangenberger W, et al. Conventional versus laparoscopic cholecystectomy and the randomized controlled trial. Br J Surg 78:150–154, 1991.
36. Reddick EJ, Olsen DO. Laparoscopic laser cholecystectomy: a comparison with mini-lap cholecystectomy. Surg Endosc 3:131–133, 1989.
37. The Southern Surgeons Club. A prospective analysis of 1518 laparoscopic cholecystectomies. N Engl J Med 324:1073–1078, 1991.
38. Airan M, Appel M, Berci G, et al. Retrospective and prospective multi-institutional laparoscopic cholecystectomy study organized by the Society of American Gastrointestinal Endoscopic Surgeons. Surg Endosc 6:169–176, 1992.
39. Bailey RW, Zucker KA, Flowers JL, et al. Laparoscopic cholecystectomy: experience with 375 consecutive patients. Ann Surg 214:531–541, 1991.
40. Cushieri A, Dubois F, Mouiel J, et al. The European experience with laparoscopic cholecystectomy. Am J Surg 161:385–387, 1991.
41. Larson GM, Vitale GC, Casey J, et al. Multipractice analysis of laparoscopic cholecystectomy in 1,983 patients. Am J Surg 163:221–226, 1992.
42. Ebert PA. As I see it. Bull Am Coll Surg 75:2–3, 1990.

43. Keith RG. Laparoscopic cholecystectomy: let us control the virus. Can J Surg 33:435–436, 1990.

44. Dion YM, Morin J. Laparoscopic inguinal herniorrhaphy. Can J Surg 35:209–212, 1992.

45. Geagea T. Laparoscopic Nissen's fundoplication: preliminary report on ten cases. Surg Endosc 5:170–173, 1991.

46. Wexner SD, Johansen OB, Nogueras JJ, et al. Laparoscopic total abdominal colectomy: a prospective trial. Dis Colon Rectum 35:651–655, 1992.

47. Schlinkert RT. Laparoscopic-assisted right hemicolectomy. Dis Colon Rectum 34:1030–1031, 1991.

48. American Society of Colon and Rectal Surgeons. Colon and rectal surgeons adopt position on laparoscopic cholecystectomy. Dis Colon Rectum 34:8A, 1991.

49. Nyhus LM. Laparoscopic hernia repair. Arch Surg 127:137, 1992.

50. Lichtenstein IL, Shulman AG, Amid PK. Laparoscopic hernioplasty. Arch Surg 126:1449, 1991.

51. Fleischer DE, AL-Kawas F, Benjamin S, et al. Prospective evaluation of complications in an endoscopy unit: use of the A/S/G/E quality care guidelines. Gastrointest Endosc 38:411–414, 1992.

40

Cleaning and Disinfecting Endoscopic Equipment

Anna D. Miller and Robert E. Schmieg, Jr.

Endoscopic procedures are widely performed in the United States for both diagnostic and therapeutic purposes. The safety of these procedures depends on both the technical competence of the operator and properly cleaned and disinfected endoscopic equipment. Infectious complications are an infrequent but acknowledged risk of endoscopic procedures. The incidence of nosocomial infections can be estimated at approximately 8 in 1 million upper gastrointestinal endoscopies.[1] The number of endoscopic procedures being performed is growing; at the University of Virginia, the number of flexible gastrointestinal endoscopic procedures increased 175% from 1989 to 1992. The subset of therapeutic endoscopic procedures is also increasing. A relatively greater number of reports of nosocomial infections is associated with these more invasive procedures, implying a greater risk of infection. The pool of patients at risk for nosocomial infections from endoscopic procedures thus continues to expand. The potential for endoscopy-related infections cannot be completely eliminated but can be minimized with proper attention to the disinfection of equipment.

INFECTION CONTROL

Infectious pathogens can be transmitted between patients via the endoscopic equipment or to a patient from opportunistic colonization of the endoscope during cleaning, disinfection, and storage. This chapter considers the epidemiology and prevention of these two mechanisms. The additional infectious route of autologous infection—for example, aspiration pneumonia or endocarditis from bacteremia—will not be considered here.

The probability of infection is proportional to the amount of inoculum and the virulence of the pathogen and is inversely proportional to host resistance. Patients who present for an endoscopic procedure often have malnutrition, liver disease, cancer, or other debilitating disorders. These difficulties can cause significant immunosuppression and increase the risk of nosocomial infection. Immunocompromised patients are more likely to become seriously ill from infectious insults, with potentially fatal results. A heightened awareness of such disorders is part of the preprocedural evaluation of the patient but only occasionally allows prophylactic measures to be taken.

Virulent pathogens are increasingly common in the general population and thus also in the patient population undergoing endoscopy. More than 230,179 cases of acquired immunodeficiency syndrome (AIDS) were reported in the United States from 1982 through June 1, 1992;[2] the number of patients infected with the human immunodeficiency virus (HIV) but not yet diagnosed with AIDS is even larger. Other viruses, such as hepatitis B, are also prevalent in the endoscopic patient population. Outbreaks of highly resistant tuberculosis are now being reported.[3–6] Patients are often asymptomatic with such disorders for a time. Contagious diseases may thus be entirely undiagnosed and unsuspected at the time of an endoscopic procedure.

The step of the infectious process that offers the greatest opportunity for preventive interven-

508

tion is that involving the inoculating amount of viable pathogen. The goal of cleaning and disinfecting endoscopic equipment is to eliminate infectious hazards to the patient from the procedural equipment by reducing the amount of inoculum of any viable pathogen to near-zero levels. Guidelines for these processes were historically based on the risks of bacterial and mycobacterial infection and have evolved as other pathogens have been identified. Many physician and nursing societies involved in endoscopic procedures, along with individual practitioners, have published guidelines in an attempt to develop standard procedures.[7-13] Instrument manufacturers have made additional recommendations specific to their equipment.[14] Advances in technology have produced more complex instruments that pose new and unique challenges to the traditional cleaning and disinfection processes. The rarity of infectious complications from endoscopic procedures demonstrates the excellent results achievable by current cleaning and disinfection procedures. The final responsibility for protecting patients from nosocomial infections transmitted by contaminated instruments must ultimately be borne by the practitioners and personnel of the modern endoscopy unit.

INFECTIONS DUE TO CONTAMINATED EQUIPMENT

Nosocomial infections associated with endoscopy typically occur in an epidemic fashion. The origin of pathogens has been traced to a variety of deficiencies in the decontamination process, including use of ineffective or contaminated chemical disinfectants, poor mechanical cleaning, and contamination of automatic washers and storage cases. Gram-negative bacilli are isolated most frequently. *Pseudomonas aeruginosa* is the most commonly reported organism in outbreaks of endoscopy-related infections;[15-20] other gram-negative pathogens have included *Salmonella newport* and *S. typhi*,[21-27] *Proteus* species,[28] and *Serratia marcescens*.[29] Serotyping of *Pseudomonas* isolates frequently identifies serotype 10, which may possess characteristics that enable it to survive nonrigorous decontamination methods.[30] Transmission of the hepatitis B virus by endoscopy has been reported,[31] but the risk of viral transmission appears to be relatively small. Epidemic outbreaks of *Mycobacterium tuberculosis* and *M. chelonae* infection have been isolated to contamination of the rinse

water of automatic washers.[32] Endoscopy-related infectious outbreaks have usually been terminated by identification of the probable sources and modification of infection control practices.

HISTORICAL INFECTION CONTROL MEASURES

In the past, certain instruments have been designated as "contaminated" and were to be used only for patients with a known potentially contagious infection, such as hepatitis B. Accessory equipment (biopsy forceps, snares, water bottles, and so on) was also segregated from the total inventory and was used only for "contaminated" cases. These "contaminated endoscopes" were then cleaned, disinfected, and often, but not always, sterilized after each procedure. The risk of cross-contamination with other infectious pathogens between patients within such groups, as well as the inability to clearly identify all patients for the designated group, illustrates the deficiencies of this approach in protecting patients in either the "contaminated" group or the "uncontaminated" group from nosocomial infections. Modern cleaning and disinfection techniques have outdated this approach and it should be abandoned.[13]

Another approach for handling endoscopic equipment used in known contagious cases has been modification and supplementation of decontamination procedures, such as increasing the exposure time to glutaraldehyde or sterilization using ethylene oxide gas. If deficiencies in the standard procedures exist, the patients not in the known contagious group are at risk for cross-contamination from those patients whose contagious diseases are not yet identified, and a false sense of security is generated. If the endoscopy unit's standard procedures are adequate and sufficient to prevent cross-contamination, added measures are redundantly wasteful of resources and provide no additional protection. However, actual practices continue to lag behind current recommendations. In one 1991 survey, 58% of respondents still altered the cleaning and disinfection process for endoscopes used in patients with confirmed cases of bloodborne pathogens and *M. tuberculosis*.[33] In addition, the lifetime of delicate endoscopic equipment may be shortened by any added measures.

Primarily driven by the HIV epidemic, the Centers for Disease Control and Prevention (CDC) published new guidelines in 1988 on infection control to be used in all hospital settings.[34] "Universal precautions," as these guidelines became known, extend the use of blood and body precautions to all patients and consider all patients to be potentially infected with blood-borne pathogens. In the endoscopy setting, the practice of universal precautions protects personnel working with patients and decreases the chance of spreading pathogens from patient to patient.

Modern endoscopy units should now employ these universal precautions for *all* endoscopic procedures. Similarly, only those cleaning and disinfection procedures that eliminate the potential spread of all possible pathogens should be used. Both hepatitis B and HIV transfer can be prevented by proper cleaning and disinfection of endoscopes and endoscopic instruments.[7, 13, 35–37] With incorporation of the principles of the universal precautions in the routine protocols of an endoscopy unit, the decontamination process for endoscopic equipment used for patients diagnosed with HIV or other infectious diseases need not be altered from standard procedures.

DEFINITIONS

Sterilization is the complete inactivation of reproductive capacity with ensuing permanent loss of infectivity for all forms of life, including bacteria, viruses, mycobacteria, and spores. Because evidence of microbial life is usually determined by microbiologic culture techniques, "sterilization" commonly means complete destruction of all microbial life. The destruction of viable organisms does not ensure destruction of their toxic metabolic products. After sterilization, pyrogenic bacterial products can still produce a febrile response when no viable bacteria are present. Sterilization is an absolute term; an item cannot be partially sterilized.

Disinfection is removal of the infective potential of any microbial life, except bacterial spores. The CDC has drawn further distinctions of the level of disinfection based on the destruction of viruses, bacterial spores, and mycobacteria.[38] *High-level disinfection* is defined as any disinfection process that inactivates all microbial life, except for high levels of bacterial spores. High-level disinfectants destroy both lipophilic and hydrophilic viruses and kill 100% of *M. tuberculosis*. *Intermediate-level disinfection* destroys vegetative bacteria, most viruses and fungi, and tubercle bacilli but does not ensure destruction of bacterial spores. *Low-level disinfection* inactivates some viruses and fungi and kills most

bacteria but does not destroy resistant pathogens such as bacterial spores or tubercle bacilli.

Cleaning is the removal of all foreign material from an item, including blood, mucus, and other proteinaceous matter. This step must precede disinfection and sterilization. Rinsing with water, detergents, and mechanical action are common methods of cleaning.

Deciding which treatment of reusable instruments is appropriate can be difficult. Sterilization of all equipment is both unnecessary and impractical. The choice of sterilization versus disinfection has traditionally been based on the nature and planned use of the instrument, host factors, and the nature and amount of possible contaminating organisms. Suspicion of contamination is not an appropriate criterion, as asymptomatic, infected patients may cause unsuspected contamination of the equipment. Spaulding proposed a rational categorization of surgical equipment more than 25 years ago that is still relevant.[39] This approach bases the infective risk of equipment on the complexity of the item and the degree to which it will invade a patient's body.

Noncritical items are those that will come into contact only with intact skin surfaces and include items such as blood pressure cuffs and patient linens. Noncritical items can be appropriately handled by intermediate or low-level disinfection, such as hospital detergents and less potent disinfectants.

Semicritical items are instruments that will come into contact with mucous membranes or broken skin surfaces. Flexible endoscopes and bronchoscopes are in this category. Both the CDC and the Association for Practitioners in Infection Control (APIC) recommend that all semicritical items receive high-level disinfection.[7]

Critical items are those that will come into contact with sterile tissues, body cavities, or the vascular system—for example, items such as needles, scalpels, and most surgical instruments. These instruments call for the highest level of scrutiny, with sterilization following a rigorous cleaning and disinfection procedure. Endoscopic procedures that invade the mucous membranes, such as endoscopic retrograde cholangiopancreatography (ERCP), endoscopic biopsies, and polypectomies, can result in transient bacteremia in a healthy patient. These invasive procedures can initiate life-threatening episodes of sepsis in immunocompromised patients.[18] Preparation of instruments to be used in an immunosuppressed patient may include treating the equipment as critical rather than semicritical.

Minimally invasive surgery has expanded rapidly since the initial performance of laparoscopic cholecystectomy in the United States in 1987. Rigid endoscopes such as arthroscopes and laparoscopes, endoscopic and bronchoscopic biopsy forceps, and nondisposable ERCP cannulas and polypectomy snares are ideally classified as critical items but are frequently treated as semicritical items. High-level disinfection is a minimal standard for treating these instruments. The necessity of sterilization in these cases remains under debate without definitive data. The history of gynecologic laparoscopic procedures has revealed few reported cases of transmission on the basis of contaminated equipment[33] when high-level disinfection alone is used; the majority of nosocomial infections in these cases were due to common skin microorganisms such as *Staphylococcus epidermidis*. Until this debate is resolved, sterilization of these items should be performed according to the recommendations of the CDC and the APIC. When sterilization is not feasible, the minimally acceptable standard is high-level disinfection.

CLEANING AND INSPECTION

Mechanical cleansing is an essential but often underestimated step in the proper care of endoscopic equipment. Cleaning alone can reduce the number of viral particles and bacteria by several orders of magnitude.[35–37] The presence of organic material markedly reduces the efficacy of many disinfectants. Foreign proteins can create a mechanical barrier preventing the disinfecting agent from reaching viable pathogens and can inactivate the disinfecting agent by chemical bonding or surface adsorption. In order for high-level disinfection or sterilization to be consistently effective, all contaminated endoscopes and accessory equipment must first be thoroughly cleaned, a step often requiring some dismantling of the instruments. This can be problematic with more complex equipment, such as endoscopes used for ERCP with a blind channel for the elevator cable.

Enzymatic detergents are recommended for cleaning prior to disinfecting. When properly used, these detergents start breaking down organic debris, thus decreasing the chance for such matter to be retained in the inner channels of the endoscopes. Soaking instruments in the detergent for 10 minutes assists in dissolving blood and other organic debris. Thorough brushing of all endoscopic channels is an essential step (Fig. 40–1). Careful inspection of the equipment follows cleaning, and the cleaning process should be repeated until all gross contamination is eliminated. Inspection should also reveal equipment problems and failures such as cracked or split seals. Details of improper functioning of the equipment and potentially damaging events during the endoscopic procedure should be conveyed to those responsible for cleaning and inspecting the instruments. Prompt repair of disabled equipment will reduce the exposure of patients and endoscopy personnel to infectious and other hazards. Surveillance and maintenance of endoscopic equipment are thus readily incorporated into these routine procedures.

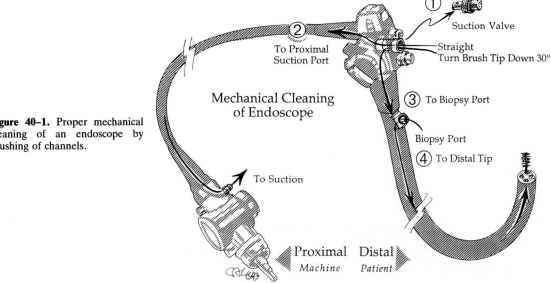

Figure 40–1. Proper mechanical cleaning of an endoscope by brushing of channels.

DISINFECTION AND STERILIZATION

It is recommended that endoscopes and accessory equipment, including cleaning brushes, receive at least high-level disinfection between each use. After the decision of sterilization versus disinfection has been made, the choice of an agent or method for practical use is governed by several criteria. The specific agent must possess activity against potential infective agents. The efficacy of several chemical disinfectants against a variety of pathogens is shown in Table 40–1. Other criteria include patient safety from exposure to the processed equipment, prevention of excessive damage to or degradation of the quality of the equipment, minimal side effects of the disinfection process to endoscopy unit personnel, ease and economy of use, time required for completion of the full process, economic constraints, availability and accessibility of the process, and environmental issues of waste disposal. Historically, the slow acceptance in the late nineteenth century of carbolic acid disinfection, as proposed by Lister, illustrates how failure to meet these criteria can impede the acceptance of an agent for routine use even after its efficacy has been proved. Environmental factors such as the concentration of the agent, length of time of exposure, presence of extraneous organic matter, pH, and temperature often significantly affect the potency of an agent in actual use.

Although heat is the most reliable and easily implemented method of sterilization, most endoscopic instruments are heat-sensitive and are unacceptably damaged by this process. Likewise, sodium hypochlorite solutions corrode the metallic parts of the endoscope, and ionizing radiation degrades plastic and rubber parts, making them more brittle. These agents are thus not acceptable for decontamination of endoscopy equipment because of their damaging effects.

Quaternary ammonium compounds such as benzalkonium chloride are easily inactivated by organic material and other environmental factors. They are not sporicidal or tuberculocidal and do not inactivate hydrophilic viruses. For these reasons, the quaternary ammonium compounds are not recommended for high-level disinfection.

Alcohols act by disorganizing the lipid structure of cell membranes and denaturing cellular proteins. These agents are not sporicidal at room temperature. Their efficacy is markedly reduced by the presence of organic material and is thus dependent on a compulsively thorough cleaning step. They pose a potential fire hazard and may damage the flexible portion of the endoscope after repeated and prolonged exposure. As single agents or when mixed with detergents, the alcohol solutions do not provide high-level disinfection.

Since the introduction of carbolic acid by Lister, chemical modifications of the phenol molecule have enhanced the antimicrobial properties of this group of agents and have decreased their toxicity and caustic nature. Commonly used phenol derivatives include *o*-phenylphenol, *o*-benzyl-*p*-chlorophenol, and hexachlorophene. These agents act by cell wall disruption and irreversible inactivation of certain membrane-bound enzymes. Although the phenols can provide bactericidal, fungicidal, and tuberculocidal activity, they are not sporicidal. Data on the viricidal activity of phenols are sparse and often conflicting. Even with the less toxic derivatives, residual disinfectant can cause irritation. Absorption through skin or mucous membranes can cause neurotoxicity, especially in infants. For these reasons, the phenolic compounds are not recommended for high-level disinfection in the endoscopy setting.

Table 40–1. EFFICACY OF VARIOUS DISINFECTANTS AND STERILIZING AGENTS

	Bactericidal	Viricidal	Sporicidal	Mycobacterium	HIV
Ethylene oxide	High	High	High	High	Yes
2% glutaraldehyde	High	High	High*	High	Yes
0.13% glutaraldehyde-0.44% phenol-0.08% sodium phenate	Moderate†	Moderate	No	Moderate‡	Yes
70% isopropyl or 70% ethyl alcohol	Moderate	Low‖	Low	Low	Yes
Iodophors	High	Moderate	Moderate§	Moderate	No data
Guaternary ammonium compounds	Moderate**	No	No	No	No data

*Exposure time of at least 20 minutes required.
†Loses bactericidal activity in presence of organic matter.
‡Only 90% kill ratio.
‖Limited activity against picornaviruses; ineffective against hepatitis B.
§Requires fairly long exposure times.
**Activity low against gram-negative bacilli.

Iodine disinfects by combining irreversibly with proteins. The active form is the elemental I_2 and not the ion; maximal bactericidal action is at a pH less than 6. Solutions of iodine mixed with surface-active agents or carriers such as neutral polymers are available as iodophors. Unlike solutions of iodine alone, iodophor products are relatively nontoxic and nonirritating. Iodophor solutions are available as both antiseptic solutions and disinfectant solutions; however, the antiseptic iodophor solutions contain significantly lower levels of elemental iodine and are not appropriate for equipment disinfection purposes. The bactericidal effects of iodophors are dependent on proper dilution, and bacterial contamination of full-strength iodophor solutions has been documented. Sporicidal effects are attainable but require prolonged contact times. Although iodophor solutions can provide high-level disinfection, the preceding disadvantages hinder the practical application of this agent in routine disinfection procedures.

Alkylating agents include ethylene oxide, formaldehyde, and glutaraldehyde; they achieve their biocidal activity by the alkylation of sulfhydryl, hydroxyl, phenolic, carboxyl, and amino groups of proteins. This alkylation, in turn, alters the synthesis of RNA, DNA, and protein.

Ethylene oxide is a water-soluble gaseous epoxy compound that, in addition to normal alkylation, also reacts with DNA and RNA. This agent is appropriate for true sterilization of endoscopic equipment, and it is noncorrosive. Theoretic human toxicities include mutagenicity and carcinogenicity. Fairly long exposure times (3 to 6 hours) for sterilization, as well as airing times to remove residual gas, are required. Sterilization by ethylene oxide is usually available in hospital settings and typically is performed by nonendoscopy personnel. Overall, this sterilization process is more time-consuming and costly than proper high-level disinfection. The necessity of sending delicate endoscopic equipment to a central sterilization department also increases the risk of damage to the equipment. Sterilization of endoscopic equipment by ethylene oxide is appropriate only for critical items, such as endoscopes to be used in severely immunocompromised patients.

Formaldehyde is an effective high-level disinfectant, being sporicidal at high concentrations. Relative disadvantages of formaldehyde versus glutaraldehyde have caused glutaraldehyde to be used more frequently. The drawbacks of formaldehyde include a 10-fold lesser bactericidal potency and formation of the polymer paraformaldehyde on surfaces, with later reversal of the polymerization process, resulting in an irritating residue.

The most commonly used high-level disinfectant at this time is glutaraldehyde, a saturated five-carbon dialdehyde. In 88% of endoscopy units surveyed in 1988 in the United States, glutaraldehyde was the disinfectant of choice.[15] This agent is relatively noncorrosive to flexible endoscopes. Commercially available as a 20% weight/volume solution, this liquid chemical becomes sporicidal only after "activation" by alkalating agents to a pH of 7.5 to 8.5.[7] A 2% solution of glutaraldehyde at a pH of 7.5 to 8.5 is effective in killing vegetative bacteria in less than 2 minutes, as well as killing M. tuberculosis, fungi, and viruses in less than 10 minutes.[7, 40] The CDC recommends endoscopic equipment be exposed to the chemical disinfectant for at least 20 minutes to kill M. tuberculosis and at least 3 hours for inactivation of spores of Bacillus and Clostridium spp. To achieve high-level disinfection, the minimum effective concentration of glutaraldehyde is a 1% solution.

When used correctly, glutaraldehyde provides rapid, high-level germicidal activity even in the presence of organic material. For maximal effectiveness and safety, the number of times a solution of glutaraldehyde can be reused must be limited. The Environmental Protection Agency defines a "reuse day" as three immersion loads of clean, dry instruments into the same glutaraldehyde solution over a day. If the instruments are wet, contaminated with organic debris, or make up one of many instrument loads placed in the solution, biocidal efficiency and reuse life may be decreased markedly. The use of reagent strips (test strips) are recommended for determining the efficacy of reused glutaraldehyde solutions.

Both the liquid and vapor forms of glutaraldehyde pose irritant hazards to endoscopy unit personnel. Glutaraldehyde vapors at 0.2 ppm concentration are irritating to the eyes and exposed mucous membranes; repeated exposures to the liquid form can cause skin irritation. Adequate ventilation of the cleaning area and the use of gloves when handling this agent may reduce these problems. The use of automated washers can limit the exposure of endoscopy unit personnel to both forms of glutaraldehyde during the disinfection process. Mucous membranes exposed to glutaraldehyde can develop marked inflammation and, therefore, residual disinfectant must be rinsed from both the outer surface and channels of the endoscope.

A 1:16 dilution of a 2% solution of glutaraldehyde combined with phenate is available commercially. The bactericidal efficacy of this diluted solution of two agents is markedly reduced in the presence of organic material, and fungicidal and tuberculocidal activities are limited even with 30- to 60-minute exposure times. This combination solution does not provide high-level disinfection and is not recommended for use in the endoscopy setting.[7]

Peracetic acid is a combination of hydrogen peroxide and acetic acid. It is fungicidal, bactericidal, and sporicidal at relatively low temperatures and retains activity even in the presence of some organic material. Although peracetic acid itself is quite corrosive, one manufacturer (STERIS Corporation, Mentor, OH) recently developed a sterilization process involving a combination of peracetic acid and anticorrosive agents.[41] The available system, consisting of a tabletop sterilizing unit and sealed containers of sterilant, can provide true sterilization for precleaned endoscopic equipment with a 20- to 30-minute processing time. Approval of this process as a sterilization procedure by the Food and Drug Administration has been based on available data demonstrating impressive laboratory results even with large quantities of spores (10^7) placed inside endoscopic channels. The advantages of an automated system, a single-use process, protection of cleaning personnel from corrosive solutions, reasonable effective processing times, and nonhazardous waste end products make this an attractive process for endoscopy units. Although additional reports of the effectiveness of this method in the clinical endoscopy setting are needed, this process can be recommended for at least high-level disinfection based on current data.

In summary, precleaned endoscopic equipment can be appropriately sterilized with either ethylene oxide or peracetic acid processes, and high-level disinfection can be attained by exposure to 2% glutaraldehyde solution for 30 minutes at room temperature. As previously stated, thorough cleaning is essential prior to any of these recommended methods of disinfection or sterilization for these methods to be effective.

RINSING AND DRYING AGENTS

Rinsing and drying endoscopic equipment after disinfection removes any residual disinfectant and eliminates any residual water pockets that would provide a fertile site for colonization of pathogens during storage, especially *Pseudomonas* species. Linkage of *P. aeruginosa*

transmission to contaminated automatic endoscope washers has resulted in a manufacturer's recall of that specific model.[30, 42] The addition of a drying step in the decontamination process has eliminated contamination of endoscopic equipment despite continued contamination of these automatic washers.[30, 32] In one outbreak, the duration between cleaning and use was highly significant.[19] These cases illustrate the ability of microorganisms to colonize residual water pockets after equipment rinsing; proper forced-air drying is effective in eliminating these residual shelters for pathogens. Rinsing with sterile water, followed by a 70% isopropyl alcohol rinse and forced-air drying, is recommended after disinfection. This step is not necessary between immediately consecutive cases but is essential prior to storage of the endoscope for any length of time.

STORAGE

Endoscopic equipment should be stored after disinfection and drying in a setting that provides both physical and microbial protection. Equipment should be stored only when dry, never when wet. Endoscopes should be hung straight after drying in a well-ventilated dedicated cabinet. The carrying case is solely for transportation purposes and is not appropriate for storage prior to use. If an endoscope has been stored in the carrying case, high-level disinfection is recommended prior to use in a patient.

QUALITY CONTROL, COMPLIANCE, AND EDUCATION

The most important factor for the success of any decontamination process is the human behavioral component. Compliance with infection control practices is variable[12, 15] but appears to be most laudable in the area of instrument cleaning procedures. One report identified the primary factor impairing appropriate infection control as lack of administrative support; other factors included insufficient equipment and a lack of clearly defined institutional procedures.[15] Each endoscopy unit should establish written protocols for cleaning and disinfection based on the scientific data available. A sample protocol for cleaning and disinfection procedures is given in Table 40–2.

Cleaning and disinfection procedures should be evaluated on a periodic basis by culturing

Table 40–2. EXAMPLE PROTOCOL FOR CLEANING AND DISINFECTING FLEXIBLE
ENDOSCOPIC EQUIPMENT

Stage I: Cleaning and Inspection
To be completed before leaving the examination room:
1. Immediately following all endoscopic procedures, wipe down the insertion tube with a 4 in × 4 in gauze wet with either detergent, water, or enzymatic detergent.
2. Suction approximately 200 ml of enzymatic detergent through the endoscope.
3. For video endoscopes, attach the water-resistant cap.

In designated cleaning area:
1. For video and fiberoptic endoscopes, remove the air-water valve, the suction valve, and the biopsy valve. If the distal end has a removable tip, unscrew the tip and place it with the other valves for cleaning.
2. Pass the cleaning brush repeatedly down the biopsy channel and the suction channel. Alternate the brushing with (1) suctioning detergent through the channels to help loosen debris and (2) rinsing with tap water. *Repeat this step until all organic debris is rinsed from the channels.*
3. After brushing the channels, brush all valves and removable tips, making sure that all tiny crevices are cleaned.
4. The biopsy valve should be cleaned and inspected for any defects. If cracks in the rubber are found, discard it and replace with a new rubber biopsy valve.
5. Once the brushing is completed, suction water through the channels and finish by aspirating air for approximately 10 seconds.

Stage II: Leakage Test
The leakage test should be performed after each endoscopic procedure to identify damaged endoscopes. In reality, it is impossible for a busy endoscopy unit to accomplish this task after each procedure. A more realistic expectation would be for all endoscopes to be tested for leaks at the end of the day or the week. Those endoscopes that do not pass the leakage test are then sent for repairs.

Communication between the endoscopist and the individual responsible for cleaning and disinfection of all equipment is vital. If the endoscopy was a difficult one (*e.g.,* the patient may have bitten the endoscope) and damage to the endoscope is suspected, that particular endoscope should be tagged and not used until it has been thoroughly examined and tested for leaks. Early detection of leaks and other damage will help lower repair costs. The leakage tester accompanies all endoscopes and can be found in the case. Only after complete cleaning should the leakage test be performed.
1. Attach the leakage tester to the venting connector of the endoscope.
2. Immerse the entire scope in water and observe carefully for 30 seconds. If tiny bubbles appear in the water, the endoscope has a leak and should not be used again prior to repair. If there is no noticeable bubbling, continue following the other stages of the cleaning and disinfection process.

Stage III: Disinfection
This step can be performed manually or with an automatic washer specifically designed for endoscopes. Familiarity with the specific equipment at hand is essential. These machines are not capable of adequately brushing out organic debris and do *not* provide complete mechanical cleansing of the instruments.

Manual disinfection
1. Attach the all-channel irrigator to the endoscope.
2. Immerse the endoscope and all-channel irrigator in a 2% activated glutaraldehyde solution and pump the disinfectant through all channels.
3. After all channels have been saturated with disinfectant, disconnect the all-channel irrigator from the endoscope and allow the endoscope to soak in the glutaraldehyde for 20 minutes. Place all valves and caps in the glutaraldehyde solution for soaking.
4. After 20 minutes, remove the endoscope from the disinfectant solution and reattach the all-channel irrigator to the endoscope. Irrigate sterile water through all channels to ensure complete rinsing of all the glutaraldehyde from them. This will require approximately 500 ml of sterile water. Wipe down the external insertion tube and the umbilical tube with sterile water.

Automatic washer disinfection
1. Attach channel irrigator to the endoscope and place the endoscope in the washer.
2. The automatic washers available today have many different capabilities. Follow the manufacturer's instructions for the specific model used.
3. After the cycle has finished, remove the endoscope from the washer. Never leave the endoscopes in the machine overnight.

Drying procedure
1. Flush 30 ml of 70% alcohol down all channels. Force air down the channels after the alcohol.
2. Reattach the valves and tip.
3. Hang the endoscope in a well-ventilated designated cabinet until the next use. Do *not* store in the carrying case except for transportation.

the patient-ready equipment and by testing the potential efficacy of any reusable disinfectant solutions. Any reusable agents must be tested periodically for potency, and records of the days and volume of use should be readily available. Identification of an index case of nosocomial infection should initiate prompt investigation using modern epidemiologic methods.

Adequate preparation of endoscopic equipment requires specific training of all personnel involved in handling the equipment. An active education program with periodic in-service reviews is essential to the modern endoscopy unit. Open communication between the endoscopist and the cleaning personnel is essential for both infection control and equipment maintenance. Practitioners of endoscopy should be acquainted with all stages of equipment care and familiar with protocols of the endoscopy unit.

CONCLUSION

Transmission of infectious pathogens is a limited but real risk of endoscopic procedures. Strict adherence to stringent guidelines for cleaning and disinfection must be followed to minimize the risk of these nosocomial infections. All patients undergoing gastrointestinal endoscopy must be considered at risk for bacterial, viral, and mycobacterial infections. Endoscopy should be performed only with equipment that has been properly cleaned and has undergone high-level disinfection between each use; this includes both the endoscopes and all reusable accessory equipment. Explicit institutional guidelines and protocols assist in the uniform and consistent application of basic infection control principles. The endoscopy unit should establish a continuing education program covering both the basic principles of infection control and the specific institutional guidelines and protocols. The efficacy of the steps in the decontamination process must be continually reassessed. Infection control personnel can be a valuable resource in developing and implementing the cleaning and disinfection procedures of the endoscopy unit. With these measures, the infectious hazards of endoscopy can be minimized.

References

1. Silvis SE, Nebel OT, Rogers G, et al. Endoscopic complications. JAMA 9:928, 1976.
2. Stroube RB. Surveillance report for acquired immunodeficiency syndrome (AIDS) and human immunodeficiency virus (HIV) infection. Commonwealth of Virginia, Richmond, VA, 1993.
3. Abrutyn E. Multidrug-resistant nosocomial TB: newest facet of the HIV epidemic. Hosp Pract 27:11, 15, 1992.
4. Anonymous. Management of persons exposed to multidrug-resistant tuberculosis. MMWR 41:61, 1992.
5. Anonymous. National action plan to combat multidrug-resistant tuberculosis. MMWR 41:5, 1992.
6. Anonymous. Transmission of multidrug-resistant tuberculosis among immunocompromised persons in a correctional system—New York, 1991. MMWR 41:507, 1992.
7. Rutala WA. APIC guideline for selection and use of disinfectants. Am J Infect Control 18:99, 1990.
8. Anonymous. Guidelines for establishment of gastrointestinal endoscopy areas. Gastrointest Endosc 37:661, 1991.
9. McGregor P, Connell P. Society of Gastrointestinal Assistants, Inc: Recommended guidelines for infection control in gastrointestinal endoscopy settings. SGA J 10:265, 1988.
10. Axon ATR. Disinfection and endoscopy: summary and recommendations. J Gastroenterol Hepatol 6:23, 1991.
11. Axon AT. Disinfection of endoscopic equipment. Baillieres Clin Gastroenterol 5:61, 1991.
12. Axon AT, Cotton PB. Endoscopy and infection. Gut 24:1064, 1983.
13. Weller IVD, Williams CB, Jeffries DJ. Cleaning and disinfection of equipment for gastrointestinal flexible endoscopy: interim recommendations of a Working Party of the British Society of Gastroenterology. Gut 29:1134, 1988.
14. Anonymous. Instructions, Olympus GIF type 100 Evis Gastrointestinal Videoscope. Olympus Corporation, 1993.
15. Gorse GJ, Messner RL. Infection control practices in gastrointestinal endoscopy in the United States: a national survey. Infect Control Hosp Epidemiol 12:289, 1991.
16. Cryan EMJ, Falkiner FR, Mulvihill TE, et al. *Pseudomonas aeruginosa* cross-infection following endoscopic retrograde cholangiopancreatography. J Hosp Infect 5:371, 1984.
17. Earnshaw JJ, Clark AW, Thom BT. Outbreak of *Pseudomonas aeruginosa* following endoscopic retrograde cholangiopancreatography. J Hosp Infect 6:95, 1985.
18. Greene WH, Moody M, Hartley R, et al. Esophagoscopy as a source of *Pseudomonas aeruginosa* sepsis in patients with acute leukemia: the need for sterilization of endoscopes. Gastroenterology 67:912, 1974.
19. Classen M, Jacobson JA, Burke JP, et al. Serious Pseudomonas infections associated with endoscopic retrograde cholangiography. Am J Med 84:590, 1988.
20. Allen JI, Allen MO, Olson MM. *Pseudomonas* infection of the biliary system resulting from use of a contaminated endoscope. Gastroenterology 92:759, 1987.
21. Dean AG. Transmission of *Salmonella typhi* by fiberoptic endoscopy. Lancet 2:134, 1977.
22. Hawkey PM, Davies AJ, Viant AC, et al. Contamination of endoscopes by *Salmonella* species. J Hosp Infect 2:373, 1981.
23. Beecham HJ, Cohen ML, Parkin WE. *Salmonella typhimurium*: transmission by fiberoptic upper gastrointestinal endoscopy. JAMA 241:1013, 1979.
24. Chmel H, Armstrong D. *Salmonella oslo*: a focal outbreak in a hospital. Am J Med 60:203, 1976.
25. Dwyer DM, Klein EG, Istre GR, et al. *Salmonella newport* infections transmitted by fiberoptic colonoscopy. Gastrointest Endosc 33:84, 1987.
26. O'Connor BH, Bennett JR, Alexander JG, et al. Sal-

monellosis infection transmitted by fibreoptic endo-scopes. Lancet 2:864, 1982.

27. Schliessler KH, Rozendaal B, Taal C, Meawissen SGM. Outbreak of *Salmonella agona* infection after upper intestinal fibreoptic endoscopy. Lancet 2:1246, 1980.

28. Weinstein HJ, Bone RC, Ruth WE. Contamination of a fiberoptic bronchoscope with a *Proteus* species. Am Rev Respir Dis 116:541, 1977.

29. Webb SF, Vall-Spinosa A. Outbreak of *Serratia marcescens* associated with the flexible fiberbronchoscope. Chest 68:703, 1975.

30. Alvarado CJ, Stolz SM, Maki DG. Nosocomial infections from contaminated endoscopes: a flawed automated endoscope washer. An investigation using molecular epidemiology. Am J Med 91:272S, 1991.

31. Birnie GG, Quigley EM, Clements GB, et al. Endoscopic transmission of hepatitis B virus. Gut 24:171, 1983.

32. Anonymous. Nosocomial infection and pseudoinfection from contaminated endoscopes and bronchoscopes—Wisconsin and Missouri. MMWR 40:675, 1991.

33. Rutala WA, Clontz EP, Weber DJ, Hoffmann KK. Disinfection practices for endoscopes and other semi-critical items. Infect Control Hosp Epidemiol 12:282, 1991.

34. Anonymous. Update: Universal precautions for prevention of transmission of human immunodeficiency virus, hepatitis B virus, and other bloodborne pathogens in health-care settings. MMWR 37:377, 1988.

35. Hanson PJV, Gor D, Clarke JR. Contamination of endoscopes used in AIDS patients. Lancet 2:86, 1989.

36. Hanson PJV, Gor D, Jeffries DJ, Collins JV. Elimination of high titre HIV from fibreoptic endoscopes. Gut 31:657, 1990.

37. Hanson PJV, Gor D, Clark JR. Recovery of the human immunodeficiency virus from fibreoptic bronchoscopes. Thorax 46:410, 1991.

38. Garner JS, Favero MS. CDC guidelines for the prevention and control of nosocomial infections. Guideline for handwashing and hospital environmental control, 1985. Am J Infect Control 14:110, 1986.

39. Spaulding EH. Chemical disinfection of medical and surgical materials. In: Lawrence CA, Block SS, eds. Disinfection, sterilization and preservation. Philadelphia: Lea & Febiger, 1968:517.

40. Scott EM, Gorman SP. Sterilization with glutaraldehyde. In: Block SS, ed. Disinfection, sterilization and preservation. 3rd ed. Philadelphia: Lea & Febiger, 1983:65.

41. Crow S. Peracetic acid sterilization: a timely development for a busy healthcare industry. Infect Control Hosp Epidemiol 13:111, 1992.

42. Daschner FD. Nosocomial infection and pseudoinfection from contaminated endoscopes could have been avoided. Infect Control Hosp Epidemiol 13:254, 1992.

41

New Technologies and Future Developments for Endoscopic Surgery

Michael R. Treat

We are privileged to be living in an era in which surgery is undergoing a profound change. Despite occasional misgivings and misadventures, the craft of surgery has taken an epochal step forward. In the past, the *surgical interface* has been the surgeon's gloved hands acting on the patient's tissues, guided by the surgeon's physical senses. This traditional surgical interface uses "low" technology, is reliable, and is universally available. However, this interface imposes a high physiologic price on the patient because it requires access through large incisions. The rapid acceptance of video laparoscopic surgery is due to the benefits of using a more technologically complex interface that can minimize the traumatic impact of surgery. As patients and surgeons have realized, the video laparoscopic surgical interface enables us to avoid the trauma associated with surgical access with the old interface, which is based on the unaided eye and hand of the surgeon.

Although our present video laparoscopic interface offers advantages to the patient, it imposes major handicaps on the surgeon. This interface is awkward and limited in capability, compared with what might be possible from a truly advanced technologic standpoint. Consequently, there is much interest worldwide in extending and improving the video laparoscopic approach by using technologies that are currently outside the traditional surgical domain.[1, 2] The purpose of this chapter is to review the technologies that will have an impact on endoscopic surgery in the near and far future. In-

cluded in this review are the following areas: imaging and sensing, mechanized instruments, computer-assisted instruments, autonomous instruments, alternative methods of tissue closure, new laser-tissue interactions, teleoperating, telerobotics, telepresence, and virtual reality.

All of these technologies already exist, and many are in use in the aerospace and military environments. Because of the geopolitical situation of the past 40 years, the military-industrial complex has enjoyed access to far greater resources and consequently more sophisticated technologies than has the medical sector. Now, however, the resolution of the Cold War provides a great impetus for the peaceful use of these technologies. A real cornucopia of technologies and human scientific talent from the military-industrial complex is now available and indeed is in search of a market. Consideration of the issues will reveal that there are parallels between the military and surgical missions: both are concerned with the destruction or removal of undesirable targets while minimizing collateral damage. Because of the anticipated adaptability of military and aerospace technologies to the surgical arena, we may see the rise of a "medical-industrial complex," which hopefully will be regarded as a more benign entity than its military predecessor.

The ideal surgical interface would be one that is just as natural to use as the old interface but that provides the benefits of technologic enhancement. There will not be an imminent introduction of a full-blown, full-featured advanced surgical interface because there are too many problems that would have to be overcome simultaneously, including issues of patient safety, surgeon training, governmental regulation, product liability, cost, and reimbursement. However, it should be possible to implement the new interface in an incremental fashion, gradually introducing individual components of what might eventually be a totally new way of doing surgery.

In the following sections, specific components that will contribute to the evolution of our surgical interface will be reviewed. In the final sections, some concepts for unifying these components into a completely new surgical interface will be discussed.

REBUILDING THE SURGICAL INTERFACE

"Intelligent" Scopes

The video endoscopic interface improves some aspects of the visual capabilities of the surgeon but takes away from others. The aspect that is most improved is the size (magnification) of the image presented to the surgeon. With an excellent video system it is possible to see anatomic details that are very difficult if not impossible to appreciate with the naked eye. The advantages of magnification have long been appreciated by the microsurgeon, and general laparoscopic surgeons have recently caught on to this fact.

On the negative side, what is lost is chiefly depth perception and the ease of varying the point of perspective. The reason for these losses is the reliance on traditional rigid telescope technology. Current imaging techniques are really a hybrid of conventional lensed endoscopes (telescopes) with video cameras added. In this adaption of the monocular telescope, the video camera is almost an afterthought that was certainly not engineered into the visual system from the beginning. One consequence of this oversight is the limited ability to vary perspective. At present, the rigid telescope is constrained to move in arcs of a sphere whose center is the port through which the scope enters the abdomen. To obtain a very different perspective on the laparoscopic field requires replacement of the telescope into another port, a step that, although feasible, is time-consuming and awkward. Placing the video chip into the distal end of the laparoscope is an obvious next step that is already beginning to appear in the marketplace. This evolutionary step will even-

tually lead to visual instruments that might, for example, be positioned on a rotating, extensible mount on the undersurface of the abdominal wall. The flexible laparoscope embodies this concept, but using the flexible laparoscope is not as easy or intuitive as the use of the traditional rigid scope. What would help in this situation (and this is a general theme) is the use of a computer to relieve the human operator of the burden of having to work out the detailed control movements needed to position the flexible laparoscope to obtain the desired view.[3] Ideally, the human surgeon could instruct the scope as to what sort of view was wanted, and the scope would be "intelligent" enough to assume the proper configuration to provide the desired view.

Stereoscopic Vision

Another deficiency of the conventional telescope is being addressed with the arrival of early versions of stereoscopic endoscopes. Most current systems are based on a scope with separate distal optical apertures. The two spatially different views of the operative field are conveyed to the video camera or cameras mounted proximally on the scope. A computer system presents the left and right views alternatively on the video monitor. An infrared beacon driven by the computer is used to trigger polarized goggles or glasses to alternately allow the right and left eyes to accept an image from the video screen. Current systems have limitations in terms of image quality (resolution and color), as well as a noticeable flickering sensation. Qualitative and semiquantitative evaluation of these systems for the performance of complex laparoscopic tasks (e.g., suturing) indicate that there probably is a real advantage compared with monocular systems. Although in their infancy, stereoscopic visual systems will no doubt assume a leadership role in video technology as they are refined. Interestingly, these systems employ essentially no new technology or concepts but are based on "off-the-shelf" components and methods.

In the more distant future, virtual reality and holography may be part of the surgical interface. Such developments hinge on the availability of computing power at levels of cost-effectiveness that are not possible today.

Laser-Induced Fluorescence

Although lasers have been used as therapeutic devices in endoscopic surgery and other areas,

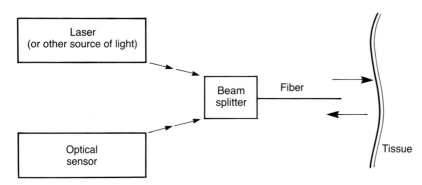

Figure 41–1. Information about tissue can be derived by analyzing light reflected back after the tissue is illuminated by a diagnostic light source (laser). Pulsing the laser allows the same fiber to be used for transmitting the outgoing (fluorescent) light and for collecting the reflected light.

including cardiovascular interventions and dermatology, we are just beginning to explore the possibilities of using lasers as information-producing devices, that is, as a way of "seeing" tissue better than we can with the naked eye.

A promising example of this approach is laser-induced tissue fluorescence (Fig. 41–1). In this technique, tissue is exposed to a very low power laser (a few milliwatts), and the tissue then fluoresces. Fluorescence is the phenomenon by which absorbed light is reradiated at a different, usually longer wavelength. What happens in the fluorescing substance is that the absorbed light energy is used to move electrons up into higher energy levels. The electrons occupy these higher energy states for only a short time and then fall back to their initial state. When they fall, the electrons give up the energy, and some of that energy is transformed back into light. The outgoing light is the fluorescent light. This fluorescence is not necessarily just one wavelength and in fact is usually a spectrum of wavelengths. The details of the chemical and physical nature of the illuminated target determine the spectral distribution of the fluorescent emissions. The central hypothesis of tissue fluorescence–based diagnostics is that there is enough uniqueness in this spectral "signature" to differentiate different histologic types of tissue. This approach has been used in early clinical trials to differentiate adenomatous tissue of the colon from normal or hyperplastic tissue.[4] An ultraviolet laser system (337-nm pulsed N_2 laser, with a pulse width of 3 nsec) was fiber-optically delivered through a colonoscope and used to illuminate colonic polyps. The resulting fluorescence from the polyp was collected through the same fiber, amplified, and sent to a multichannel analyzer that resolved the fluorescence into its spectral components. Mathematical analysis of the spectrum was then used to differentiate the spectra from adenomatous tissue and the spectra from hyperplastic tissue. The polyp was also sampled by standard biopsy forceps for routine pathologic analysis. A diag-

nostic accuracy rate of 86% was achieved by the laser-induced fluorescence method, which was similar to the diagnostic rate achieved by the concordance of two senior pathologists using standard light microscopy to classify the samples as either adenomatous or hyperplastic. In addition, the same technique has been used in transcatheter laser angioplasty[5, 6] to provide real-time guidance in the removal of atherosclerotic tissue with minimal collateral injury to normal arterial wall.

An obvious logical extension of this concept is the use of monoclonal antibodies that would be specific for tumor metastases and would fluoresce when selectively illuminated.

Ultrasound

Ultrasound is a modality that needs to be exploited further by the laparoscopic surgeon. It can restore the surgeon's sense of touch and extend this sense below the surface of organs. Clinically, endoscopic or transcatheter ultrasound is finding application in cardiovascular and gastrointestinal (GI) areas, including laparoscopy.

Intraluminal GI endosonography[7, 8] was initially accomplished with blind, rigid probes introduced transrectally. Because of the lack of optics and the rigidity of these devices, their range of action was limited to the rectum. More recently, a flexible endoscope with oblique viewing optics and a distally mounted ultrasonic transducer has been used to stage cancers of the upper GI tract and has also been used for rectal cancers. A further refinement has been the development of a colonoscopic instrument that incorporates end-viewing optics, biopsy capability, and a radial scanning ultrasound transducer.

Endosonography is performed after filling the intestinal lumen with water or by filling a balloon that covers the end of the transducer. Preliminary experience suggests that this technique is of value in staging the depth of invasion of malignancies.

For intravascular applications,[9] size constraints are more severe than for GI applications, and a flexible device must be used. Applications in the vascular systems include delineation of an anatomic pathologic condition, monitoring of valvular therapies, and steering of radiofrequency ablation devices in arrhythmia therapy. These flexible No. 7 to No. 10 French ultrasonic imaging devices may also be used for intraluminal evaluation of the bile duct by way of a transpapillary approach using a side-viewing duodenoscope.

Both phased-array and rotating scan methods may be employed. The phased-array approach consists of 32 to 64 tiny ultrasound elements circumferentially located at the tip of the catheter. The elements are sequentially activated and then a computer algorithm is used to reconstruct the cross-sectional image. In the rotating scan method, a single ultrasonic crystal is rapidly rotated axially at the end of the device, which radially scans the surrounding tissues. An alternative to rotating the crystal consists of an ultrasonic reflector that may be rotated around an axially placed crystal. This modification is said to reduce image artifact. The phased-array catheters are more flexible and rugged than the mechanical scanners, since no moving parts are involved at the catheter tip. The mechanical scanners may currently offer superior image quality. Ultrasonic frequencies from 3.5 MHz to 40 MHz have been used. The higher frequencies are better suited to detailed resolution of structures close to the transducer.

Ultrasound will likely be clinically useful in the detection of liver metastases; localization of pancreatic, renal, and adrenal neoplasms; and evaluation of mesenteric and retroperitoneal adenopathy. It will also be used in evaluating intraductal biliary pathologic conditions, including stones. Although clinically useful endoscopic ultrasound systems are now available, additional refinements are needed in terms of probe size and flexibility and acoustic coupling requirements (i.e., underwater versus direct contact). Rapid improvements in this technology are expected. In addition to improvements in the technology, surgeons will have to learn yet another skill in order to be able to interpret these two-dimensional images.

Three-Dimensional Imaging

Computer integration of the two-dimensional scan "slices" into a three-dimensional representation is now possible in real time. The underlying imaging modality may be ultrasound, computed tomography, or magnetic resonance imaging. With sufficient computing power, the three-dimensional image may be colorized, rotated, and sliced to provide in-depth three-dimensional views that would be impossible to achieve with the unaided eye or with two-dimensional scanning alone. Computer manipulation of three-dimensional images can provide the surgeon with a powerful and intuitive way of examining complex body structures.

Magnetic Resonance Imaging in Real Time

Real-time magnetic resonance imaging is already possible. What is required is its integration into the operating room routine. As discussed further on, there are opportunities to combine magnetic resonance imaging with other sensing modalities to enhance the surgeon's view.

Integrated Data Displays

The basic premise in integrated data displays is that we want to be able to add or overlay data to the basic video visual image. These data will come from sensors or imaging modes such as ultrasound, real-time magnetic resonance imaging, spectroscopy, and thermal sensing. Many other forms of data (e.g., immunochemical or immunofluorescent labeling) can be combined with the basic image. The integration of these data acquisition technologies into the conventional video data display will result in an "image" that goes far beyond the video picture, since the surgeon would be able to "see" below the surface features that are visible to the unaided eye. For example, using real-time magnetic resonance imaging or ultrasound, a surgeon would be able to instruct the computer to superimpose onto the video image a colored diagram of ductal or vascular structures that are below the surface and hidden from view during the course of a difficult dissection. The possibilities for integrating different data streams are endless. The capability of taking the data from one sort of imaging modality and blending it in real time with the data from one or several other modalities requires a great deal of computing power. With greater availability of computing power, we would like to have blending and reconstruction of all the data channels into a unified, informative, and intuitive display. This display will give the surgeon the ability to "see" further, deeper, and with more knowledge of the tissues than ever before.

Mechanized Instruments

Current laparoscopic instruments are not user-friendly. Conventional laparoscopic instruments are too long to be handled with the same degree of ease that is possible with the tools used in open surgery. In addition, there is a "fulcrum effect" working against the surgeon because the shaft of the instrument is constrained to move in spherical arcs determined by the site of entry through the abdominal wall. Being constrained to move in an arc is far from ideal and is a great drawback when complex three-dimensional tasks such as suturing are attempted. Another deficit of the fulcrum effect is that instrument tip motion is not related to the motion of the operator's handle in a constant way. As the instrument is advanced into the abdominal cavity, the point of the fulcrum changes, and small movements of the handle produce larger swings of the tip of the instrument. As with other user-unfriendly aspects of our current video laparoscopic interface, a skilled operator can overcome these problems. However, there should be a better way.

The concept of the servomechanism ("servo") is relevant here. A servo will faithfully follow the motions of the controlling device (proportional control). A servo incorporates some kind of mechanical actuator (such as an electrical motor) and some kind of feedback device to measure how far the actuator has moved. A simple example of a servo system is a radio-controlled model airplane. The rudder of the model airplane is actuated by a servomechanism whose motion is directly proportional to the amount of deflection of a joystick on the controlling radiotransmitter. There is no intelligence or computer control implied here, merely a faithful replication of the master unit's range of motion. If this concept were incorporated into a surgical instrument, we would have a device that has several joints and a rotatable base. The joints would be servomotorized and would be controlled by a joystick, trackball, or foot pedal. The new line of articulated and "roticulating" instruments that we are seeing are simple embodiments of this concept. Although not mechanized, the additional degree of freedom allowed by these instruments is of value in approaching situations in which the simple straight-stick instruments would not work well.

Computer-Assisted Instruments

A more ambitious solution to the problem of user-unfriendly instruments is the use of computer-assisted positioning of these more complicated surgical devices. The idea is to use a computer to take over some of the functions of the surgeon's cerebellum in coordinating eye-hand movements. The "many degrees of freedom" instruments already mentioned would be difficult for a surgeon to control if each joint of the device had to be "micromanaged." This is a good job for a computer to assist the surgeon in performing (Fig. 41-2). The general concept is similar to the use of on-board computers that allow human pilots to handle certain very maneuverable jet fighters. These airplanes employ an aerodynamic design that allows great maneuverability, but the tradeoff is that the plane is inherently unstable and requires so many millisecond by millisecond adjustments of the control surfaces that no human could fly it. The computer is, in this case, an extension and augmentation of the human pilot's cerebellum. It accepts high-level commands from the pilot (*e.g.,* "bank left") and translates the command into the multitude of millisecond by millisecond microadjustments required to control the highly unstable aircraft. In an analogous way, a computer "cerebellum" might allow the human surgeon to control instruments with multiple joints operating at "unnatural" angles or around corners in ways that would normally be very difficult. In this scenario, the surgeon would operate wearing gloves and perhaps a shoulder harness that would be wired into the computer, which would translate the upper extremity movements into motions of the mechanized instrument. The computer would free the surgeon of having to micromanage the motion of the various joints of the arm and would allow the mechanized instrument to mimic the surgeon's movements in a natural and intuitive way. This sort of device

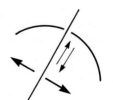 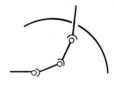

"Stick" instrument with 2 degrees of freedom   Complex instrument with 4 degrees of freedom

Figure 41-2. Computer assistance is needed to allow the surgeon to intuitively use complex instruments that have several joints or "degrees of freedom."

already exists in certain military-industrial applications.

Another step in the development of computer-assisted instruments is the incorporation of sensors into the instrument itself. A major deficiency of conventional laparoscopic instruments is the lack of operator awareness about how much force is being applied to the tissues. The length of the instruments and their narrow diameter means that leverage has to be used to generate enough force at the jaws of the instrument. However, with a leverage system, it is very easy to produce traumatic levels of tissue force and not be aware that this is occurring. In the same way that our hands have pressure-force sensors built into the working surfaces (*i.e.*, fingertips), intelligent instruments should measure the force being exerted at the tissue interface and convey this information back to the surgeon or to the computer that is responsible for positioning the instrument. Silicon chip technology (microelectromechanical systems) exists such that microscopic strain gauges and force sensors could be integrated into the working surfaces of instruments.

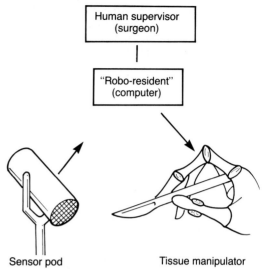

Figure 41-3. The "roboresident" is a semiautonomous machine assistant to the human surgeon. It incorporates sensing elements and mechanized tissue manipulators. Its central computer provides enough on-board intelligence to execute complex "surgical macros" such as suture placement and knot tying for wound closure or constructing an anastomosis, but the *judgment* of what macros to invoke and when to invoke them resides with the surgeon.

Autonomous Instruments

A further extension of the computer-assisted instrument concept is the autonomous instrument. Ideally, the surgeon should not completely give up control to the instrument, but rather should interact with the instrument as though it were a capable, reliable, and highly accurate assistant ("robo-resident") (Fig. 41-3). A useful concept in this regard is the "surgical macro." In computer parlance, a "macro" is a small program or series of steps that the computer will execute upon receipt of a single command. Macros are useful in spread sheets and word processing programs to simplify the execution of repetitive multistep instruction sequences. A surgical macro would be a well-defined series of tissue manipulation movements. An example of a surgical macro might be as follows:

Make an incision 3 cm long and 0.5 mm deep
Grasp edges and lift tissue
Place suture 1 cm from left edge
Place suture 1 cm from right edge
Cross sutures and tie knot
Repeat preceding steps six times and then stop

An autonomous instrument could be programmed to execute a surgical macro on tissue that is designated by the supervising human surgeon. The autonomous instrument would offer the advantage of greater speed, precision, and reproducibility of the execution of the surgical macro, whereas the human surgeon would retain overall control of the process, especially the decision of where and when to invoke the process. In current practice, the analogous situation would be a senior surgeon (maybe with slightly shaky hands) supervising a very capable surgical resident in the performance of a vascular anastomosis. The senior surgeon is the judgment and supervisory element of the team; the surgical resident is the steady hands.

An autonomous instrument does not have to be directly held or positioned by the human surgeon. The instrument might be capable of moving itself into position and setting itself up to perform the surgical macro.

Shifting our focus away from laparoscopic surgery for a moment, an ideal situation for an autonomous instrument would be in intraluminal endoscopic surgery. A miniature self-contained robotic "video bug" would be introduced into the rectum and could then walk or crawl along the lumen, executing a preprogrammed search pattern, perhaps using reflectance spectroscopy (by means of a tiny on-board diode laser) to sense abnormal tissue. Such a video bug could make semiautomated mass screening of the entire GI tract a possibility, eliminating the discomfort associated with pushing a long, flexible shaft into the bowel. In conjunction with a supervisory endoscopic surgeon, the video bug could also perform the usual biopsies or polypectomies using its micromanipulators to obtain tissue samples for histopathologic analysis.

Alternative Methods of Tissue Closure

There is continued interest in alternative means of tissue closure besides mechanical methods such as sutures or staples. Although endoscopic stapling technology has made remarkable progress in the past few years, the technical problems imposed by the limited access may be pushing existing mechanical tissue closure technologies to their limits. Also, mechanical stapling devices, whether for open or laparoscopic surgery, have a generic failing, which is that they cannot completely adapt to tissues of different thicknesses and strengths (or lack of strength) and an irregular or nonstandard geometry of the closure. In fact, for completely customized and versatile tissue closure, handsewn sutures are unmatched, but it is well known that laparoscopic suturing is fairly difficult.

Tissue "welding" by a laser or other controllable heat source may be a way of transcending these limitations. A related concept is tissue "gluing" or "soldering" using both laser- and nonlaser–activated tissue adhesives. Situations in which these alternative tissue closure methods might be useful are those in which it is awkward or difficult (e.g., because of size constraints) to place sutures or staples, and when high mechanical strength is not required but watertightness is desired.

The mechanism of tissue welding is not known, but it probably involves the heat denaturation of collagen or other tissue structural proteins, with subsequent formation of noncovalent bonds (eletrostatic or hydrogen bonds) between the edges of the tissues being joined. There appears to be a fairly narrow range of tissue heating that results in maximum bond formation without thermally induced, irreversible damage. Also, tissue edge apposition during the welding process must be precise. Currently, tissue welding is somewhat of an art but will become more reliable and predictable by means of automated control of the welding process based on tables of optimum laser parameters or

by means of real-time monitoring of tissue temperature. Recently, protein tissue solders and light-absorbing dyes have been employed to improve the quality and reliability of laser welds.[10–12] Protein solders that have been used consist of plasma cryoprecipitate (fibrinogen) or albumin–hyaluronic acid. Other proteins are being investigated. The solder is applied prior to laser energy and bonds with the tissue edges during the welding process. The solder helps because it absorbs most of the applied heat energy, thereby protecting the substrate tissues from thermal damage. The solder also greatly increases the adhesive area of the weld, which greatly contributes to increased strength. By mixing an energy-absorbing dye with the protein solder prior to laser exposure, the amount of laser power that is required to effect the weld is reduced by a factor of 10. The ability to use lower power lasers, such as the solid state diode lasers, to achieve welding is an important step forward in the art of tissue welding, since these lower powered lasers are less likely to cause collateral thermal damage and are also cheaper and logistically more convenient than high-power lasers. The lowered cost of these solid state diode lasers is of major importance in making tissue welding an economically viable alternative to mechanical tissue closure methods.

It is not necessary to use a laser as the source of the welding heat energy. Electrical energy (as in electrosurgical use) or microwave energy could be used. The advantages of the laser are that it is a noncontact method of delivering the energy, which is important in not disturbing the tissues or solder during the act of producing the weld. Also, lasers are uniquely suited to taking advantage of selective absorption by using exogenous dyes or endogenous tissue chromophores. In addition, the level of control of the energy delivery parameters is much greater with a laser than with other methods of energy delivery, since the laser output can be pulsed and modulated in virtually any way desired.

Experimentally, tissue welding has proved to be useable in blood vessels, intestine, and biliary tissues. A relevant recent experiment[13] is one in which fibrinogen solder and the 810-nm diode laser were used to close longitudinal choledochotomies in a canine model. In this model, immediate bursting pressures were obtained that were well in excess of pathologic biliary pressures. Excellent healing was observed when the animals were sacrificed at 1 week.

Clinical application of this technique has been limited. The chief concern is that the initial weld strength may be insufficient. Although under optimal experimental conditions, excellent weld strengths are routinely achieved, it is not clear whether this could be routinely and reliably accomplished in a clinical setting.

Probably the most successful and appropriate example of clinical tissue welding is in the urologic area. Another area of the possible appropriate use of tissue soldering is to reinforce anastomoses that are at high risk for postoperative leakage. In this application, the anastomosis would be sutured in the usual way and then the laser-activated glue would be used to additionally strengthen and seal the suture line. Experimental work has shown that this approach is of value.[14] Limited early clinical results with the use of laser-activated tissue glues to reinforce high-risk gastrointestinal anastomoses (esophagogastric and pancreatojejunal anastomoses) have been good.

New Laser-Tissue Therapeutic Interactions

There is much interest in basic science laboratories and from clinically oriented groups in exploring therapeutic low-energy laser-tissue phenomena, including photodynamic therapy ("laser-activated photosensitizers") and photobiomodulation ("switching on") of subcellular processes. In short, we are learning that there is much more to therapeutic lasers than the high-energy, photothermal, ablative approach that is essentially all we have seen in surgical lasers to date.

Photodynamic therapy (PTD) is the use of light-activated exogenous agent to kill cells.[15] The light-activated agent is known as a photosensitizer. The mechanism by which cells are affected is different from the purely physical process of laser energy altering tissue by heating it. The photosensitizer is taken up relatively selectively by the target cells. When appropriately activated, it releases a cytotoxic substance that produces cell death. The classic example is the use of hematoporphyrin derivative to kill tumor cells. When activated by light, hematoporphyrin derivative releases singlet oxygen in the tumor cells, which have absorbed it in greater concentration than normal cells. Because of the concentration difference, normal tissue is relatively unharmed. PDT can be improved by finding photosensitizers that have a greater selectivity for target tissue than do current photosensitizers. Another method of improvement is to link light-activated cytotoxic agents to monoclonal antibodies against tumor cells. PDT will become a more useful modality as it is coupled to immunodiagnostic and therapeutic techniques. Since the delivery of PDT is simply accomplished by means of fiberoptics, and since it is technically easy to perform, it should be amenable to endoscopic delivery in many situations.

Photobiomodulation refers to the use of very low energy light to produce biologic effects on tissue. The light energy does not directly produce a physical change on the tissue, as is the case with high-energy interactions. Unlike PDT, an exogenous photosensitizer is not required, and the laser energies involved are about 100 times less. Photobiomodulation does not involve production of a cytotoxic intermediary. Rather, the light energy is thought to trigger or modulate normal intracellular biochemical processes through some indigenous photoacceptor molecule that can absorb the incoming photon of light. After absorbing the light energy, the photoacceptor molecule undergoes a change in energy state, reactivity, or molecular conformation. Changes in the photoacceptor molecule will eventually be reflected in the metabolic processes of the cell. A typical system that has been studied extensively is the response of fibroblasts in vitro to 632-nm helium-neon laser operating at powers of a few milliwatts. Favorable experimental studies have shown increases in collagen production and proliferation rates.

Despite an extensive literature, photobiomodulation remains poorly understood, and there is abundant skepticism that the phenomenon even exists. The implication of the positive in vitro studies is that wound healing rates could be enhanced in the clinical setting, but this claim remains unproved. The clinical studies on wound healing rates that have been done to date are not convincing owing to lack of adequate controls and standardization of experimental parameters. Indeed, even the in vitro studies done to date are far from unanimous in defining the parameters for achieving positive effects. The central issue in photobiomodulation is the identification of the photoacceptor molecule and subsequently working out the detailed mechanism for the cellular response. However, there is a fairly widespread, if unofficial, consensus among photobiologists that the general assumptions underlying the concept of photobiostimulation are valid and that there is great potential if the process could be understood. The potential importance to surgeons of photobiomodulation is obvious, and better scientific work needs to be done to resolve the controversies.

Alternative Methods of Tissue Ablation

In the far term, we see the need to explore completely noninvasive methods of tissue ablation such as focused energy beams that will eliminate the need for any access incision. Although extracorporeal shock wave lithotripsy has been disappointing for eliminating biliary stones, the general concept is valid and may have application in selective destruction of soft tissue targets. It should be possible to use several converging energy beams (ultrasonic or laser) and to monitor (temperature or magnetic resonance imaging) the response of the target area to ensure that the desired effect is obtained while minimizing collateral damage. Ideally, this technique should be combined with real-time three-dimensional imaging of target and surrounding structures.

Teleoperating, Telerobotics, Telepresence, and Virtual Reality

The following concepts and definitions are taken from Thomas Sheridan's outstanding new book *Telerobotics, Automation, and Human Supervisory Control.*[16] Owing to the clarity and generally nontechnical nature of the explanations, this book is extremely useful to a person with a nonengineering background.

Teleoperating is defined as the direct and continuous human control of a teleoperator, which is a machine that extends a person's sensing and manipulation capabilities to a location remote from that person. For the purposes of this discussion, the term will be limited to imply a master-slave relationship between the human operator and the teleoperator, without any intelligence on the part of the teleoperator. The next step upward is telerobotics, which refers to an advanced form of teleoperating in which the human operator supervises through a computer intermediary. The operator communicates intermittently with the computer intelligence of the telerobot and defines the goals, constraints, and contingencies relative to the remote task. The telerobot executes the task on the basis of input from the human operator plus its own artificial sensing and intelligence. In surgical parlance, the telerobot is like a resident acting under the supervision of an attending surgeon.

Telepresence and virtual reality are related terms. Telepresence means that the operator receives sufficient information from the teleoperator about the task environment, displayed in a sufficiently natural way that the operator feels physically present at the remote site. Virtual presence or virtual reality is experienced by a person when sensory information generated only by and within a computer compels a feeling of being present in an environment other than the one the person is actually in. Stated in other words, virtual reality refers to the creation of a complete illusion or impression on the part of the operator that he or she is actually a part of or inside a scenario that is totally computer-generated. Besides the reliance on computer-generated images instead of direct video camera input, the difference between telepresence and virtual reality is one of degree.

The first modern master-slave teleoperators were developed in 1945 for manipulation of radioactive materials. Subsequent developments included force reflection (feedback) and stereo vision by two remote cameras whose positioning was controlled by a head-mounted display. Application of teleoperator concepts to space exploration revealed problems in direct master-slave control of the teleoperator because of the transmission time delay. This led to the development of supervisory control, in which the human operator provides intermittent guidance to the teleoperator, which has a certain level of innate artificial intelligence. For undersea exploration for oil and other purposes, the high cost associated with human divers and the risk to life was a major impetus to the development of remotely operated vehicles. In addition to undersea and space use, teleoperators have also been useful in nuclear power plant operation, toxic waste cleanup, construction, agriculture, mining, warehousing, fire fighting, policing, and military operations.[17, 18]

Telepresence has its roots in the work of Goertz[19] and Chatten[20] who showed in the 1960s and early 1970s that when a video display is fixed relative to the operator's head, and the remote video camera's motion is linked to that of the operator's head, the operator feels as if he or she were physically present at the camera location.

An important series of experiments in telepresence was carried out by Tachi et al. in 1985,[21] in which he defined some of the basic components of telepresence systems. These components are a head-mounted binocular display, a six degree of freedom position input device, and an anthropomorphic slave robot (the teleoperator).

When a computer-generated picture of the

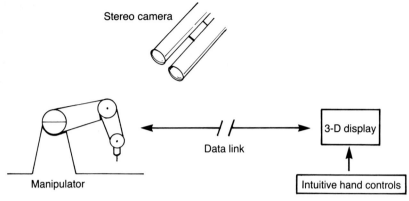

Figure 41–4. Schematic diagram of a generic teleoperating system. Teleoperating allows the surgeon to perform actions as if physically present. This concept may have tremendous implications for battlefield surgery. In civilian life, it will enable surgical "teleconsulting" to remote areas.

world is substituted for direct video images, and the view is referenced to the position of the operator's head, the operator can be made to feel present in an artificial world.[22] Virtual reality is certainly not a new idea, but the attainment of a realistic substitute for the real world is a fairly recent development. In the 1940s, Link developed a crude mechanical ancestor of today's flight simulators. Truly compelling virtual reality systems have been made possible owing to the availability of computer graphic systems having sufficient power. Another crucial piece of technology is the multiple degree of freedom (*i.e.,* six axis) position sensors ("super joysticks") that are necessary to translate head and free limb movements into corresponding movements of the computer-generated display.

Probably the most influential demonstrations of virtual reality were the efforts at the NASA Ames Research Center and at the Wright-Patterson Air Force Base Aerospace Medical Research Laboratory.

A recent effort to create a practical surgical teleoperating system is under way at the Stanford Research Institute.[23] This system employs a powered teleoperator station that mimics the surgeon's hand movements in a natural and intuitive way (Fig. 41–4).

Teleoperating and virtual reality will have an important long-term impact on the nature of surgical education and practice. We envision the development of a "medical center without walls" in which the diagnostic and therapeutic (*i.e.,* surgical) skills of a surgical or medical specialist will be available to patients in remote locations. In the short term, fairly conventional teleoperating technology can make this possible. In the long term, virtual reality technology will be the underpinning of telesurgery. We have not quite attained sufficient computing power to create a virtual reality display with sufficient detail for surgical requirements, but this will eventually happen. As truly "real" virtual reality becomes possible, we should see fundamental changes in the way in which medical students and residents are taught the elements of surgical practice (*i.e.,* anatomy, pathology, physiology, and psychomotor skills).

CONCLUSION

Tremendous opportunities exist for developing an enhanced *surgical interface* (Fig. 41–5) using the technology that is available to us from military, aerospace, and industrial sources. The development of this interface is part of the continuing evolution of surgery and is something in which we all can participate.

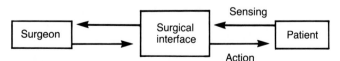

Figure 41–5. The surgical interface is the means by which the surgeon accomplishes a physical intervention for the benefit of the patient. This concept is a generalization of the teleoperating scenario. In addition to video, the evolving surgical interface of the near future will include other sensory modalities (*e.g.,* CT, MRI, ultrasound) that will be registered onto the basic video data display. This computer-assisted synthesizing of different sensory data sets will allow the surgeon to "see" the tissues in an enhanced, multimedia way. The action of the interface component will be versatile and dexterous computer-assisted manipulator mechanisms capable of great speed, precision, and consistency.

References

1. Treat MR, Oz MC, Bass LS. New technologies and future applications of surgical lasers—the right tool for the right job. Surg Clin North Am 72(3):705–742, 1992.
2. Reports and Surveys: "An ant-like robot." Robotica 10:5–10, 1991.
3. Taylor R, Funda J, LaRose D, Treat MR. A telerobotic system for augmentation of endoscopic surgery. Proc of the Fourteenth Annual International Conference of the IEEE Engineering in Medicine and Biology Society, Paris, France, Oct 29–Nov 1, 1992:1054–1056.
4. Schomacker KT, Frisoli JK, Compton CC, et al. Ultraviolet laser-induced fluorescence of colonic polyps. Gastroenterology 102:1155–1160, 1992.
5. Deckelbaum LI, Lam JK, Cabin HS, et al. Discrimination of normal and atherosclerotic aorta by laser-induced fluorescence. Laser Surg Med 7:330–335, 1987.
6. Gaffney EJ, Clarke RH, Lucas AR, et al. Correlation of fluorescence emission with the plaque content and intimal thickness of atherosclerotic coronary arteries. Laser Surg Med 9:215–228, 1989.
7. Kimmey MB, Martin RW, Silverstein FE. Endoscopic ultrasound probes. Gastrointest Endosc 36:S41–S46, 1990.
8. Boyce GA, Sivak MV Jr. New approaches to the diagnosis of malignant and premalignant lesions: colonoscopic endosonography and laser-induced fluorescence spectroscopy. Semin Colon Rectal Surg 2(1):17–21, 1991.
9. Coy KM, Maurer G, Siegel RJ. Intravascular ultrasound imaging: a current perspective. J Am Coll Cardiol 18:1811–1823, 1991.
10. Oz MC, Johnson JP, Parangi S, et al. Tissue soldering using indocyanine green dye enhanced fibrinogen with the near infrared diode laser. J Vasc Surg 11:718–725, 1990.
11. Grubbs PE, Wang S, Marini C, et al. Enhancement of CO_2 laser microvascular anastomoses by fibrin glue. J Surg Res 45:112–119, 1988.
12. Poppas DP, Schlossberg SM, Richmond IL, et al. Laser welding in urethral surgery: improved results with a protein solder. J Urol 139:415–417, 1989.
13. Bass LS, Libutti SK, Oz MC, Rosen J, Williams MR, Nowygrod R, Treat MR. Canine choledochotomy closure using diode laser activated fibrinogen solder. Surgery, 1993 (in press).
14. Moazami N, Oz MC, Bass LS, et al. Reinforcement of colonic anastomoses with a laser and dye-enhanced fibrinogen. Arch Surg 125:1452–1454, 1990.
15. Herrera L, Madrid-Franco R, Petrelli NJ, et al. Photodynamic therapy in colorectal cancer. In: Schrock TR, ed. Perspectives in colon and rectal surgery. St. Louis: Quality Medical Publishing Inc., 3:256–273, 1990.
16. Sheridan TB. Telerobotics, automation, and human supervisory control. Cambridge, MA: MIT Press, 1992.
17. Fogle RF, Heckendorn FM. Teleoperated equipment for emergency response applications at the Savannah river site. J Robotic Systems 9(2):169–185, 1992.
18. Smith FM, Backman DK, Jacobsen SC. Telerobotic manipulator for hazardous environments. J Robotic Systems 9(2):251–260, 1992.
19. Goertz RC. An experimental head-controlled television system to provide viewing for a manipulator operator. Proc Thirteenth RSTD Conference, 1965:57.
20. Chatten JB. Foveal hat: a head-aimed television system with foveal-peripheral image format. Proc Symp Visually Coupled Systems: Developments and Applications. Aerospace Medical Division, Brooks AFB, Texas, 1972.
21. Tachi S, Arai H, Maeda T. Development of anthropomorphic tele-existence slave robot. Proc International Conference on Advanced Mechatronics, Tokyo, Japan, May 21–24, 1989:385–390.
22. Stone R. Virtual reality and telepresence. Robotica 10:461–467, 1992.
23. Satava RM. High tech surgery: speculation on future directions. In: Hunter JG, Sackier JM, eds. Minimally invasive surgery. New York: McGraw-Hill Inc., 1993:339–347.

42

Transanal Microsurgical Techniques

Samir Said and Gerhard Buess

CONSERVATIVE APPROACHES TO TREATMENT

Pedunculated polyps present few problems in treatment. The use of a diathermy snare permits complete removal of these lesions anywhere in the colon, as healthy mucosa forms the stalk of these polyps. However, large, sessile polyps (defined by Christie[1] as lesions 2 cm or larger), particularly in the middle (8 cm or more from the anal verge) and upper thirds of the rectum, create difficulties when the goal is to remove the tumor as a "total biopsy" specimen.[2]

Transanal Electrofulguration, Transanal Electrocoagulation, and Endocavitary Irradiation

Taking conservative procedures into consideration, there is general agreement that local recurrence is less following complete surgical excision of a rectal tumor than following transanal fulguration,[3, 4] electrocoagulation,[5, 6] or endocavitary irradiation as described by Papillon and Berard[7] and Sischy and associates.[8]

Transanal electrofulguration differs from electrocoagulation in that the tissue is destroyed by electric current at about 300°C and disappears because of fast dehydration and carbonization, instead of remaining in situ to become sequestrated.[3, 4] The penetration of heat from electrofulguration is thought to be greater than that from electrocoagulation; however, experience with electrofulguration is limited. Generally, its primary objective is to dilate tumor-related stenoses.

Transanal electrocoagulation is performed through a proctoscope with an outside diameter of 40 mm and a length of 15 cm. A bipolar coagulating current is used without cutting current. The charred tumor is then sharply removed with angulated biopsy forceps or sharp uterine curettes. The tumor is burned repeatedly until it is completely destroyed.[6]

Endocavitary irradiation includes contact x-ray therapy with the 50-kV machine and Curie therapy with ^{192}Ir. Contact x-ray therapy is an ambulatory treatment and requires four endorectal applications within 6 weeks. It destroys the tumor layer by layer. ^{192}Ir, a supplementary modality, delivers a booster dose of 20 to 30 Gy to the tumor bed in 24 hours.[7]

Laser Photoablation

Recently, the neodymium-doped:yttrium-aluminum-garnet (Nd:YAG) laser has been used as an alternative method for the treatment of colorectal tumors.[9–11] The endoscopic equipment consists of either a flexible colonoscope or a rectoscope. The tumor is vaporized and, if possible, the underlying region is coagulated. The total laser energy applied during one session ranges from 2500 to 9000 J (mean of 4000 J). The wavelength of the Nd:YAG laser beam is 1064 nm, with an energy range of 10 to 100 W.

Cryosurgery

The basic principles of cryosurgery, which is used mainly as a palliative measure, include rapid freezing (−170°C to −190°C) of the tumor and its tissue, slow thawing to enhance the destructive effect of recrystallization, and immediate repetition of the freeze-thaw cycle.[12]

THE TRANSANAL APPROACH VERSUS EXTENSIVE SURGERY

The principal criticism of the conservative approaches already discussed is that tumor destruction is imprecise, no specimen is obtained to evaluate the level of invasion of the rectal wall, and multiple sessions are needed to eliminate the tumor.

To date, exposure of tumors in the lower rectum has been managed mainly by means of retractors such as the type used by Parks.[13] However, this transanal surgical approach can be more difficult than extensive surgical techniques when the tumor is not adjacent to the anus (>8 cm from the anal verge) or when the surgeon encounters large (>3 cm) polyps. Considerable experience is needed with the Parks retractor to manage broad-based polyps situated high in the rectum. Using the transanal approach, Parks found a recurrence rate of 10%,[14] which was probably due to the inherent limitations of dissection.

The precision of the transanal techniques and the increased rate of complications seen in the extensive surgery techniques (anterior rectal resection, abdominoperineal resection, the posterior approach according to Kraske,[15] or Mason's transsphincteric posterior approach[16]) led to the development of an endoscopic surgical system. The endoscopic method allows the performance of all the conventional surgical techniques within the whole rectal cavity. This minimally invasive surgical system has been developed at the Surgical Department of the University of Cologne by Buess and coworkers and has been in clinical use since 1983.[17, 18]

INDICATIONS FOR ENDORECTAL MICROSURGERY

The main indication for endorectal surgery is the removal of *sessile adenomas* (Table 42–1).

According to a study at the Mayo Clinic, the common tubular adenoma is usually small and rarely contains invasive cancer (just 1.3% of polyps less than 1 cm in diameter are malignant). As it grows, however, the malignant potential increases, and about a third of polyps

Table 42–1. INDICATIONS FOR ENDORECTAL SURGERY

1. Local excision of sessile adenomas and early rectal carcinomas in "low-risk" cases
2. Palliative treatment of local excisions of nonstenosing rectal carcinomas
3. Correction of stenosis
4. Rectopexy

larger than 2 cm in diameter are malignant. The incidences of tubulovillous and villous adenomas, which constitute the majority of large sessile polyps, are 15% and 10%, respectively. The incidence of malignant transformation of tubulovillous adenomas is 22%. This figure can rise to 41% for villous adenomas.

Not infrequently, gastroenterologists remove broad-based tumors located high in the rectum using the piecemeal colonoscopic technique.[19] Proper histologic evaluation cannot be achieved with this technique, and it is associated with high recurrence rates of up to 24% as reported in the literature.[20, 21] Using the transanal endoscopic technique, however, clinically benign lesions that are confined to the mucosal layer are removed by mucosectomy with a wide margin of clearance.

Local excision of early stage rectal carcinomas, defined as a carcinoma that has penetrated to the submucosa only, has been widely accepted.[22–24] Early rectal carcinomas with favorable histologic features, as well as moderately or well-differentiated carcinomas (grades 1 and 2) of the "low-risk" type that do not reveal mucinous adenocarcinoma, signet cell carcinoma, pleomorphic undifferentiated carcinoma, or invasion of lymphatic vessels[22, 25] (in which the probability of regional lymph node metastasis is low—approximately 3%), are managed endoscopically by full-thickness excision of lesions located within the extraperitoneal portion of the rectum. Criteria for a definitive local approach also include histologically proven disease-free excisional margins.[26, 27] According to the literature, there is no significant difference in survival rates when local excision of early rectal cancer is compared with radical surgery (80% and 90%, respectively). Thus, we tentatively suggest that in these cases, adjuvant therapy such as irradiation is overtreatment because one can hardly justify potentially harmful pelvic radiotherapy to treat lymph nodes that have only an approximate 3% chance of harboring lymph node metastases.

A clear distinction has to be made between "malignant polyps," which are adenomas having a focal carcinoma, and tumors that appear as clinical cancer from the outset of treatment so that accurate comparisons can be made to results of other series.

Like many other surgeons, we initially lacked confidence in the results of local excision for rectal cancer. Therefore, most of our patients with rectal cancer, who underwent curative local excision, had large sessile adenomas of the rectum with a final postoperative histologic appearance showing a focus of invasive carcinoma (malignant polyps).

With increasing experience, our selection criteria for the use of endorectal surgery also included bioptically proven *carcinomas* under the following circumstances: In accordance with the selection criteria of other authors,[28-30] we perform local excision of carcinomas that have invaded the muscular layer (pT2 or greater) only in cases in which there is a medical contraindication to radical surgery or in cases in which the patient is unwilling to undergo extensive surgery. These patients undergo full-thickness disc excision.

Our other selection criteria for local excision of rectal cancer include the following:

- A tumor diameter of less than 4 cm with a margin of clearance of 1 cm
- A tumor confined to the rectal wall, mainly early rectal carcinomas (pT1 carcinomas), and in very selected cases pT2 carcinomas when the patient is at increased operative risk because of advanced age (>70 years) or medical reasons; these cancers, which have invaded the muscularis propria, may require adjuvant therapy
- A low-grade malignancy (moderate or well-differentiated)
- The margins of the locally excised specimen must be histologically tumor-free

One should always keep in mind that the avoidance of a permanent stoma or extensive surgery is an advantage to the patient only if the cure of cancer is not jeopardized by local resection.

Our experience with *palliatively treated cases* suggests that patients need not undergo several tumor-reducing interventions. The tumor is resected in one session. There is no peranal discharge of detritus following the procedure, and the duration of hospitalization averages less than 1 week.

A further indication for endorectal surgery is the correction of benign rectal strictures by creating vertical incisions or the circular resection of stricture-inducing tissue. Our experience with this technique is limited as yet, as is our experience with transanal endoscopic rectopexy,

which has been performed several times in the surgical department of the University of Tübingen.

THE ROLE OF ADJUVANT THERAPY IN LOCALLY EXCISED RECTAL CANCER

In spite of advances in surgical technique and supportive care of patients with rectal cancer, the overall 5-year survival rate remains at approximately 50%. Unfortunately, roughly half of the patients presenting with colorectal cancer are not cured. Therefore, to expand the chance of local control, adjuvant therapy has become more appropriate.

Investigations by the Gastrointestinal Tumor Study Group[31-33] and the Mayo/North Central Cancer Treatment Group[34] have shown that the combined-modality regimen of sequential single-agent 5-fluorouracil (5-FU) and high-dose (4500 to 5040 cGy) multiple-field pelvic irradiation combined with 5-FU as a radiation sensitizer is more effective at decreasing local failure rates and improving survival (reduction of the local tumor recurrence by 46% and cancer-related death rate by 36%) than radiation therapy alone. Both trials have independently determined that methyl-CCNU (*N*-[2-chloroethyl]-*N*-cyclohexal-*N*-nitrosurea]; lomustine) does not produce additive benefits over irradiation plus 5-FU. Chemotherapy as a single modality has also been shown to be ineffective with regard to local tumor control, disease-free survival, or overall survival.

As far as surgical adjuvant therapy for rectal cancer is concerned, a clinical trial in the United States is now evaluating a combination of postoperative radiation and chemotherapy, consisting of 5-FU plus levamisol, which has significantly decreased the overall tumor relapse rate by 41% in patients with Dukes' C colon cancer.[33]

Several authors[35, 36] suggest that the combined therapy of radiation plus chemotherapy is standard adjuvant therapy for patients with Dukes' stages B and stage C cancer. Concerning advanced metastatic colorectal cancer, controlled clinical trials[37, 38] have demonstrated improved response rates with 5-FU plus low-dose leucovorin (folinic acid). In addition, the use of adjuvant therapy for local excision of rectal cancer is now becoming more widespread.[7, 8, 39, 40] Two approaches are now being used: endocavitary irradiation as proposed by Papillon and Berard[7] and Sischy and associates[8] and the combination of local excision with external beam radiation therapy.[41, 42] A major advantage of the latter approach is the possibility of accurate patient selection. The true extent of the tumor is determined by local excision, so that patients at high risk for lymphatic involvement (pT2 or greater) can be referred for radical surgery immediately, whereas patients with low-risk early stage rectal cancers can be considered to have been treated sufficiently by full-thickness local excision only.

Pelvic irradiation eventually combined with intracavitary radiotherapy has been proposed as an attractive treatment modality after local excision of rectal cancers, especially for elderly, poor-risk patients with T2 or T3 tumors of the lower rectum.[43, 44] In 67 patients, Papillon and Berard[7] reported a 59.7% 5-year disease-free survival rate. Their report also included a 5-year disease-free survival rate of 74% in 312 patients who have been treated with endocavitary irradiation with or without ^{192}Ir for T1 and T2 adenocarcinoma. Radiotherapy cannot be performed at every hospital, which restricts adjuvant therapy to a few centers. More experience in adjuvant therapy after local excision of rectal lesions is necessary to clarify its exact role. Neither radiotherapy nor chemotherapy was routinely given perioperatively in our series of transanal endoscopic surgical procedures.

PREOPERATIVE ASSESSMENT

It is important to bear in mind that successful local treatment of rectal lesions is based primarily on appropriate patient selection. Hence, a thorough knowledge of preoperative assessment is mandatory. To avoid severe complications, such as intraperitoneal perforations with possible subsequent peritonitis, rectovaginal fistulas, or injury to the bladder, sphincter muscles, or other adjacent structures, it is of utmost importance to be acquainted with the anatomy of the rectum.

Rectal Digital Examination

After obtaining the medical history—especially in regard to bowel habits, bleeding, peranal (mucoid) discharge, difficulty in defecation, incontinence, and weight loss—a careful rectal digital examination should be carried out, palpating the rectal mucosa, the rectal wall, and extrarectal structures. Mason[45] has demonstrated that the digital assessment of local spread of palpable tumor can be performed quite accurately; he based his findings not only on the mobility but also on the configuration of the tumor, its consistency, and its histologic grade.

Although some authors[45, 46] claim up to 80% accuracy in clinically identifying rectal cancers confined to the wall of the rectum and up to 50% accuracy in identifying clinically apparent lymph nodes, we tentatively suggest that such accuracy can hardly be duplicated by most clinicians.

A further limiting factor of rectal digital examination is that the average index finger can examine the rectum only up to 8 to 10 cm from the anal verge, and clinical examination cannot differentiate between fixation due to malignant spread and fixation due to an inflammatory reaction next to the tumor, which can be found in as many as 50% of patients in some series.[47]

Rigid Rectoscopy

All of our patients in whom endorectal surgery was performed had rigid rectoscopy preoperatively. The goal of this examination is to record the site of the tumor, its size, its distance from the anal verge, and its morphologic appearance. Usually, patients with polypoid (exophytic) or plateau-like tumors are considered to be good candidates for local excision, even when there is a superficial ulceration above the mucosal level.

Deeply ulcerated carcinomas are associated with a high incidence of regional node metastases in up to 57% of patients,[60, 61] and thus ulceration should at least be taken into account when making the decision to perform local excision of rectal cancer.

Although a review of the literature indicates that the size of the tumor cannot be regarded as an independent variable when estimating the probability of lymph node metastasis or local recurrence,[62] several studies have demonstrated a lower local recurrence rate when local excision is limited to rectal lesions less than 4 cm in diameter.[5, 26, 63] Not infrequently, lesions that are less than 3 cm in diameter are considered suitable for local transanal resection, mainly from a technical point of view. The size of the tumor is recorded by specifying the number and clock position of the quadrants of the rectal circumference involved.

Determining the correct site and circumferential involvement of the tumor is an important factor in determining the correct position of the patient on the operating table (Fig. 42–1). For the tumor to always be situated below the

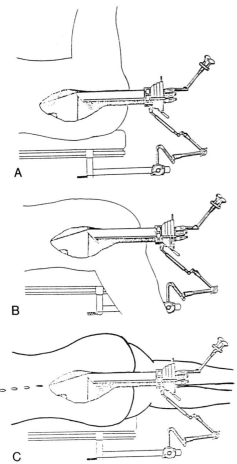

Figure 42–1. Positioning of the patient on the operating table. The tumor should always be located below the optical system. **(A)** Lithotomy position. **(B)** Prone position. **(C)** Lateral position.

endoscope, the prone position with legs spread is used for anterior tumors, the lithotomy position is used for posterior tumors, and the lateral (left or right) position is used for lateral lesions.

To determine the feasibility of transanal endoscopic resection, the distance from the anal verge is determined in centimeters. The precise location of rectal tumors can also be difficult to assess with rigid rectoscopy because of hidden lesions just above the valves of Houston or occult prolapses in which the sigmoid colon containing tumor falls into the rectal cavity and appears to be a tumor lying within the rectum and providing optimal access. Hence, to be on the safe side in determining the accurate distance of the tumor from the anal verge, a double–air contrast barium enema is recommended. In addition, flexible colonoscopy or barium enema examination should be carried

out preoperatively to exclude synchronous lesions.

Endorectal Sonography

Currently, endoluminal ultrasound is the most reliable technique for measuring the depth of tumor infiltration within the rectal cavity. It is of particular value in assessing lesions confined to the rectal wall (adenomas and T1 and T2 carcinomas).

In a large number of studies that have included more than 700 patients,[48–51] the mean accuracy of endorectal sonography in the staging of local excision of rectal carcinoma has been reported to be between 80% and 85%. Although some authors report an overall accuracy in predicting nodal involvement of up to 80%,[52, 53] it is generally acknowledged that the accuracy of endoluminal ultrasound in detecting lymph nodes is limited because most lymph nodes metastases are smaller than 5 mm[54] and because metastases may be present in lymph nodes that are not enlarged.[55]

Because experienced endoluminal sonographers are generally uncommon, not all patients who underwent endorectal surgery at the University of Cologne were preoperatively examined by endoluminal ultrasound. Conversely, Buess and coworkers have had good experience regarding endoluminal sonography within the past few years and have also developed a new endoluminal scanning probe.[56, 57]

Computerized Tomography and Magnetic Resonance Imaging

Although computed tomography (CT) of the pelvis is less accurate than endoluminal ultrasound in defining the depth of invasion within the rectal wall, it can accurately stage extrarectal spread of carcinoma of the rectum. The reported accuracy of pelvic CT in assessing local spread of rectal tumors is up to 93%.[53, 58]

Although at present magnetic resonance imaging (MRI) is generally reported to be less accurate than CT, both CT and MRI can correctly identify lymph node metastases in slightly more than 50% of patients.[59]

These findings indicate that neither endoluminal sonography nor MRI or pelvic CT can reliably identify lymph node metastases, and at present their use for selecting patients to undergo local excision of rectal lesions is limited. Neither pelvic CT nor MRI has been used routinely as a preoperative assessment for endorectal surgery.

Histologic Assessment

It is acknowledged that a preoperative biopsy specimen may not be representative of the main tumor because rectal tumors are mostly heterogeneous. There is wide subjective variation among pathologists in the assessment of biopsy specimens.

Because the accurate grading of tumors belongs to the "fine tuning" of a patient's assessment, the authors believe, in agreement with others, that a preoperative biopsy should not be performed routinely in lesions suitable for local excision (<4 cm in diameter, mobile tumors, no deep ulceration) because it may lead to an erroneous therapeutic decision. In these cases, total disc excision with a margin of clearance (>1 cm) should be carried out as a "total biopsy" for complete histologic analysis. In the case of favorable histologic features and tumor extension, local excision can then mean a definitive local approach. Undoubtedly, poor access has hitherto usually meant poor exposure of rectal lesions, which has led to incomplete local resections, as well as disruption of the excised specimen. It is the authors' belief that endorectal surgery, as described further on, is a technique that allows more precise surgery in an operative field difficult to reach with other local measures.

Interview With the Patient

After preoperative assessment has led to the conclusion that transanal endoscopic resection should be performed, all possible complications (bleeding, rectal stenosis, intraperitoneal perforation, and septic complications, with the possible necessity of extensive surgery) should be thoroughly discussed with the patient, as should the advantages of the procedure. It is the clinician's duty to make the patient understand that regular follow-up examinations are mandatory to detect a possible recurrent tumor at an early stage. The authors suggest follow-up examination at the following intervals: every 3 months in the first year, every 6 months in the second year, and yearly thereafter.

PERIOPERATIVE COURSE OF ENDORECTAL SURGERY

Preoperative patient preparation consists of orthograde intestinal lavage with, on average,

10 L of saline solution. Perioperative antibiotics (metronidazole and one of the second-generation cephalosporins) are routinely administered. The operation is usually carried out with the patient under general anesthesia, but regional anesthesia is also feasible in the case of endorectal surgery conducted in a lithotomy position. The operation averages 90 minutes. Parenteral nutrition is usually carried out only on the first postoperative day, and patients generally walk on the evening of the operation. Pain necessitating oral analgesics for an average of 3 days occurs if the tumor resection was adjacent to the anus. The postoperative hospitalization is 6 days on average.

SYSTEM FOR TRANSANAL ENDOSCOPIC OPERATION

A rectoscope (Fig. 42–2) with an outside diameter of 40 mm keeps the anal orifice open. Depending on the site of the lesion in the rectum, either the 120-mm or the 200-mm rectoscope tube, together with its obturator (atraumatic introducer), is used. The tip of the tubes are slanted 45° so that the upper part of the rectoscope offers protection for the telescope, and underneath the operative field is simultaneously kept open mechanically. The rear end of the rectoscope's main element can be equipped with either an adapter with a viewing window and illumination insert for the initial survey of the rectal cavity or a working insert for the telescope and auxiliary instruments. Loss of gas is prevented by rubber-sealing sleeves and caps with different diameters for auxiliary instruments.

In addition to the wide-lumen rectoscope, automatic pressure-controlled gas insufflation is applied for constant exposure of the operating area. The combined endosurgical unit (Fig. 42–3) includes three functions: (1) preselectable, pressure-controlled insufflation of carbon dioxide gas at a constant pressure of about 10 to 15 mm Hg, (2) rinsing of the optic lens with distilled water through the use of a foot switch, and (3) suctioning of blood, secretions, and coagulating fumes.

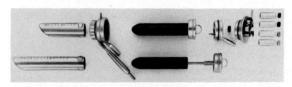

Figure 42–2. Wide-lumen endosurgical rectoscope and accessories.

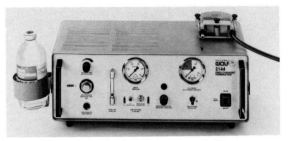

Figure 42–3. Combination endosurgical unit.

The stereoscopic telescope (Fig. 42–4) that is provided with up to a sixfold magnification transmits a three-dimensional image to the surgeon. The assistant sitting on the left side of the surgeon can aid in the operation with a semirigid (monocular) telescope (Fig. 42–4), which is inserted in the probe channel of the stereo telescope or, if available, a video system can be used. Automatic gas insufflation to the tip of the optical system prevents clouding over, and the optic lens can be rinsed by water injection.

Most of the auxiliary instruments (Fig. 42–5) are angulated at the tip to enlarge the operating area. They include a coagulation-suction tube with a monopolar high-frequency connection to perform electrocoagulation of minor bleeding as well as suction, an almost fully insulated high-frequency knife for the excision of the bowel wall, a retractable needle for eventual injection of saline solution beneath the tumor, a needle holder with jaws shaped so that the needle automatically clings when grasped, high-frequency combination forceps for grasping tissue or holding the needle, scissors for cutting the thread, and stapling forceps for securing the thread that is used in a continuous suture technique with special silver clips.

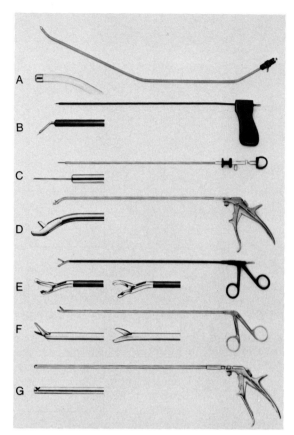

Figure 42–5. Auxilliary instruments for transanal endoscopic microsurgery. **(A)** Coagulation-aspiration tube. **(B)** High-frequency knife. **(C)** Injection needle. **(D)** Needle holder. **(E)** Forceps. **(F)** Scissors. **(G)** Suture clip forceps.

TECHNIQUE OF TRANSANAL ENDOSCOPIC MICROSURGERY

After placing the patient on the operating table in such a way that the tumor is located below the viewing range of the optical system (in a prone, lithotomy, or lateral position), the perianal skin is disinfected without previous local skin shaving. The region around the anus is then covered with sterile drapes.

A gradual digital dilation of the anal sphincter up to four fingerbreadths follows so that the appropriate rectoscope tube (120 or 200 mm), together with the lubricated atraumatic obturator (Fig. 42–6), can be introduced smoothly. Care must be taken not to injure the rectal wall because the sphincter region is passed blindly. After equipping the outer orifice of the proctoscope with the adapter and viewing window, the rectoscope is advanced to the tumor-bearing area under visual control by manual insufflation. The rectoscope is then stabilized in its ideal

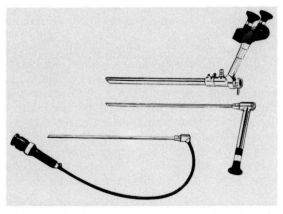

Figure 42–4. Stereoscopic telescope, documentation telescope, and semirigid telescope.

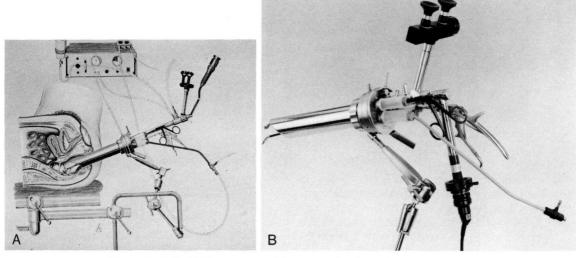

Figure 42–6. (A, B) The system used for transanal endoscopic microsurgery.

position throughout the operation with the help of a supporting arm with a clamping device (Martin arm) that is attached to the operating table. Not infrequently during the operation, the position of the rectoscope must be changed by activating a central adjusting screw on the clamping mechanism.

After the adapter with viewing window is removed, the working insert with the sealing sleeves and caps is fitted into the rectoscope's main element. Next, the stereo telescope, together with the documentation telescope for the video camera or the semirigid telescope, is introduced halfway into the rectoscope tube to avoid soiling the optic lens. Only at this point are the endoscopic instruments inserted into three of the four sealing sleeves. The usual equipment that goes into the sealing caps includes the high-frequency knife, which goes into the right upper cap; the forceps, which goes into the left upper cap; and the coagulation-suction device, which goes into the left lower cap. The right lower sealing sleeve is usually armed with a cap and is not opened.

Finally, the tube systems are connected, and when pneumatic distention of the rectum is achieved in a gas-tight environment, the telescope is pushed forward to attain optimal exposure of the operative field. Occasionally, the position of the rectoscope needs fine adjustment so that the procedure can commence.

The microsurgical operation can be divided into three steps as illustrated in Figure 42–7. Initially, a margin of clearance of 5 mm in the case of benign lesions and at least 10 mm in the case of carcinomas is outlined using the high-frequency knife (coagulation current). The reason for this is to ensure sufficient margins around the tumor, which could be difficult when intraoperative hemorrhage obscures the local anatomy. The next step consists of preparing the tumor using either mucosectomy, partial wall excision, or full-thickness disc excision. The technique depends on the localization of the lesion and the outcome of the clinical assessment. Adenomatous tissue does not extend further than the muscularis propria, so in these cases *mucosectomy* is sufficient treatment. After excising the mucosa, the aboral margin is grasped with the forceps, and the polyp is gradually removed from its base with cutting current from the monopolar-frequency knife as a total biopsy specimen, thus finally exposing the circular layer of the muscularis propria. Slight bleeding that occurs during preparation can be managed easily with the coagulation-aspiration tube. The mucosectomy technique can be applied within the entire rectum and lower sigmoid colon.

In the case of huge polyps and those polyps located in the intraperitoneal region, very careful preparation is compulsory so that the adjacent organs are not injured accidentally and intraperitoneal perforation does not occur. When there is an adhesion at the submucosa–muscularis propria border caused by either scarring following previous polypectomies or uncertain infiltrative growth, partial wall excision (resection of the circular layer) can be carried out. The resection line would then be between the longitudinal and circular layers of the muscularis propria.

Microsurgical procedure of endorectal operation:

- **circumcision of the sessile growth**
- **excision of the tumor**
- **closure of the defect by a continous transverse suture**

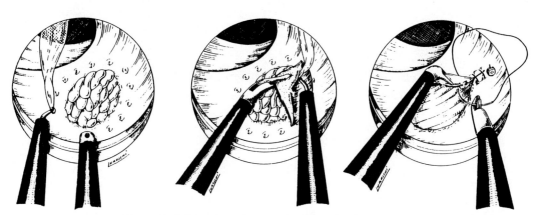

Figure 42–7. Procedure of transanal endoscopic microsurgery.

The magnification (up to sixfold) of the muscularis propria fibers with the stereo telescope allows microsurgical techniques to be performed under three-dimensional endoscopic control. This means that whenever possible, *full-thickness excision* with resection of perirectal fat should be carried out within the extraperitoneal region of the rectum and away from the sphincter region. The reason for giving preference to full-thickness excision is that this technique ensures the most reliable safety margin adjacent to the tumor. In addition, this technique makes it more likely that the pathologist can carry out an exact assessment of the histologic specimen. Especially if carcinoma is to be locally excised for cure, full-thickness removal of the tumor has to be considered mandatory. Caution must be exercised by removing just a small rim of perirectal tissue if the tumor is located anteriorly or laterally to avoid injury to the urethra, vagina, or the urinary bladder.

Not infrequently during full-thickness excision, arteries spurt and need to be compressed with forceps and coagulated. This is carried out by removing the high-frequency knife and inserting a second high-frequency combination forceps, since the other forceps is needed to expose the site of bleeding. Meanwhile the coagulation-suction tube is advanced to the spurting blood vessel, and suction and intermittent coagulation are activated. If coagulation does not control the hemorrhage, arterial he-

morrhage can be managed by a stitch suture under endoscopic control. Bear in mind that excessive coagulation can also create injuries to the peritoneum or adjacent structures. Inevitably, full-thickness excision should be reserved for more experienced endorectal surgeons.

After ensuring complete hemostasis and irrigating the wound, the defect is closed in transverse fashion with continuous absorbable sutures to avert strictures and bleeding. Continuous suturing is done by clamping silver clips onto both ends of the thread. In the case of large wall defects, further precautions can be taken to avoid rectal stenosis and reduce tension on the sutures by placing several continuous sutures, one behind the other. The stitches should be placed at least 5 mm away from the margin of the rectal wall defect so that tears do not occur at the edges of the excision, which can lead to dehiscence of the suture line. Prior to concluding the operation, one has to make sure that the suture has not created any marked stenoses. Finally, the rectoscope is withdrawn from the anal canal under visual control.

POSTOPERATIVE HISTOLOGIC EXAMINATION

The locally resected specimen is pinned on a piece of cork and fixed in formaldehyde solution (Fig. 42–8). The specimen must be handled very

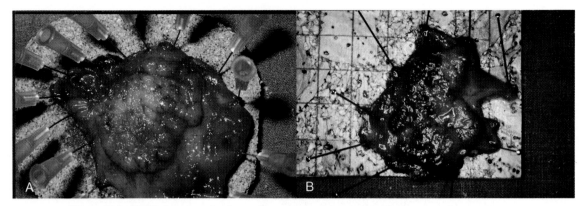

Figure 42–8. (A, B) Samples of endorectally excised specimens that have been pinned to cork.

cautiously so that the pathologist's analysis is not jeopardized. A precise pathology report is of extreme importance in deciding whether the local excision can be considered adequate or further therapy is needed. Therefore, histologic type, grade of malignancy, depth of invasion in the rectal wall, and lack of neoplastic infiltration in the specimen margins have to evaluated.

TEACHING PROGRAMS

It is the authors' belief that by striving for optimal access to the entire rectum with minimal invasiveness and superior overall results, the introduction of the sophisticated microsurgical technique is justified. As in all endoscopic techniques, professional handling of the system is mandatory. Besides special talent, this requires continuous training to avoid severe complications during the clinical learning phase. Regular video-supported intensive training courses in

Table 42–2. ENDORECTAL SURGERY AT THE UNIVERSITY OF COLOGNE DEPARTMENT OF SURGERY
July 1983–December 1990

	No. Patients	%
Total	233	100
Average age of 65.6 yr (29–99 yr)		
Male	105	45.1
Female	128	54.9
	No. Operations	%
Total	251	100
Therapeutic local excision	211	84
Radical surgery subsequent to local excision of cancer	19	7.6
Palliative excision	17	6.8
Correction of benign stenosis	4	1.6

transanal endoscopic microsurgery, of 5 days' duration and using phantom models, are offered in the surgical department at the University of Tübingen, Germany. A videotape regarding the technique of transanal endoscopic microsurgery can be obtained from Richard Wolf Medical Instrument Corp. (Vernon Hills, IL).

The short postoperative hospital stay after this minimally invasive procedure, as well as the reduced cost of postoperative patient rehabilitation, makes up for the expense of the sophisticated transanal endoscopic equipment within a short period.

RESULTS OF ENDOSCOPIC TRANSANAL MICROSURGICAL PROCEDURES

During the period from July 1983 to December 1990, the transanal endoscopic operation system was carried out in 233 patients (Table 42–2) in the surgical department of the University of Cologne, where the system has been introduced primarily into clinical use. The age of the patients at the time of operation ranged from 29 to 99 years, with an average age of 65.6 years. One hundred five were men (46.8%), and 128 patients were women (53.2%). The total number of operations rose to 251 because of recurrences and metachronous tumors within the rectum.

In 211 patients, therapeutic local excision of the tumor was achieved endoscopically, as confirmed by histologic evaluation (84%). Nineteen patients did not fulfill the criteria for local excision (7 high-risk early cancer, 12 more infiltrative cancers) and therefore went on to extensive surgery immediately (7.6%). In 17 cases in which infiltrative carcinoma had been verified

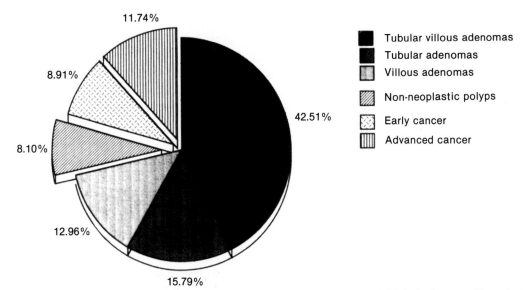

11.74%

8.91%

42.51%

8.10%

12.96%

15.79%

Tubular villous adenomas

Tubular adenomas

Villous adenomas

Non-neoplastic polyps

Early cancer

Advanced cancer

Figure 42–9. Histologic findings of endoscopically excised specimens. Of 247 patients, 79.5% had adenoma without dysplasia, 6.3% had adenoma with moderate dysplasia, and 14.2% had adenoma with severe dysplasia.

preoperatively, local excision remained the final treatment because of medical reasons or because of the will of the patients (6.8%). Four benign rectal stenoses that occurred from previous polypectomies or anterior rectal resections were managed by vertical incision of the mucosa (1.6%).

Postoperative Histologic Results

One hundred seventy-six (71.3%) of the locally excised tumors were adenomas. Thirty-nine of these adenomas were tubular, 32 were villous, and 105 were tubulovillous; 14.2% of the adenomas contained severe dysplasia, 6.3% contained moderate dysplasia, and 79.5% did not reveal any dysplasia (Fig. 42–9). Twenty (8.1%) of the excised polyps proved to be

nonneoplastic. Twenty-two (8.9%) of the resected tumors contained focal carcinoma with only submucosal spread, indicating early rectal cancer (pT1) or a "malignant polyp." All 5 patients with "high-risk early carcinoma" underwent further radical operation immediately, with an uneventful postoperative course. Twenty-nine (11.7%) of the locally treated tumors were microscopic cancers that had already invaded the muscularis propria (pT2 or greater).

Localization and Extent of Tumor Circumference

The tumors operated on were located along the entire course of the rectum and lower sigmoid colon (Fig. 42–10). Localization of the lesions ranged from 6 to 22 cm from the ano-

Figure 42–10. Tumor distance from the anocutaneous line.

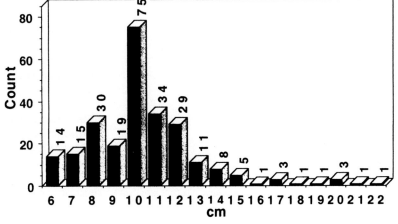

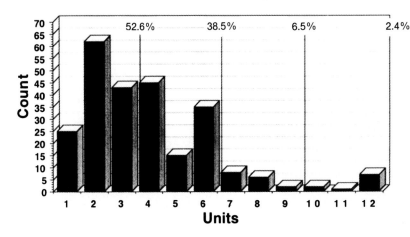

Figure 42–11. Circumferential involvement of endoscopically excised rectal tumors.

cutaneous line. Most of the locally excised tumors were situated 8 to 10 cm from the anal verge, and their longitudinal extension was up to 8 cm.

Of the 247 tumors located in the rectum (Fig. 42–11) or lower sigmoid colon, 2.4% extended over three quarters of the rectal circumference. Seven tumors encompassed the entire circumference of the rectum, demanding segmental resection. In 38.5% of the tumors, from one quarter to one half of the circumference was involved, and approximately 52.6% of the tumors involved one quarter of the circumference or less.

Major sessile polyps occasionally had to be removed in piecemeal fashion in one session to shorten the operative time.

Complications

Early postoperative complications occurred as outlined in (Table 42–3). Five patients suffered

Table 42–3. RESULTS OF ENDORECTAL SURGERY AT THE UNIVERSITY OF COLOGNE

Early Postoperative Complications (N = 251)

Complication	No. of Patients	%
Intraperitoneal perforation	5	2
Bleeding	4	1.6
Peritonitis	—	—
Fistula	4	1.6
Ileus	—	—
Incontinence	—	—
Lethality (cardiac failure)	2	0.8
TOTAL	15	6

intraperitoneal perforations, which were treated by laparotomy with an uneventful postoperative course. Hemorrhages were recorded four times and were controlled using the transanal route. Four rectovaginal fistulas occurred. Two of the patients had advanced cancers and underwent extensive surgery. The other 2 patients with minimal lesions were treated conservatively. There were two postoperative deaths in elderly patients because of cardiopulmonary failure. This figure corresponds to clinical mortality rates after conventional transanal local excision. All the complications occurred within the first 3 years of our transanal endoscopic experience.

Long-term Results

Long-term follow-up information has been obtained in 215 of 233 cases (Table 42–4). Hence, the overall follow-up rate is 92.3%. (The range of follow-up was from 1 month to 6.6 years, with a mean follow-up period of 29 months.)

In patients who had adenomas and nonneoplastic polyps removed by the transanal endoscopic route, 8 patients had recurrences. Thus, the recurrence rate was 4.9%. After full-thickness excision of an early cancer with moderate differentiation, we found one local recurrence of an adenoma that was managed by the transanal endoscopic route. Among the patients treated palliatively, 1 patient underwent a sigmoidostomy 5 months postoperatively because of tumor progression. There were four slight strictures that did not need any further therapy. Two elderly patients mentioned incontinence for gas, and 9 patients with advanced cancer died of cancer-related causes.

Table 42–4. LONG-TERM RESULTS OF TRANSANAL ENDOSCOPIC MICROSURGERY IN 215 OUT OF 233 PATIENTS (FOLLOW-UP RANGE 1 MO TO 6.6 YR; FOLLOW-UP RATE 92.3%)

	Adenoma and Benign Polyps (N = 163)	Early Rectal Cancer (N = 22)	Advanced Cancer (N = 27)	Benign Stenosis (N = 3)
Local recurrence	8	1 (adenoma)	—	1
Tumor progression	—	—	1	—
Stenosis	3	0	1	—
Incontinence	0	0	2	—
Fistula	0	0	0	—
Mortality due to rectal cancer	0	0	9	—

CONCLUSION

Transanal endoscopic operations permit curative local excision of large adenomas and "low-risk early cancers" with minimal morbidity and excellent presentation of specimens for complete histologic analysis.

Local excision of T2 carcinomas should be done only in elderly and high-risk patients or when the patient is not willing to undergo radical surgery. In these cases, adjuvant therapy might become an increasingly encouraging modality.

Thorough training is mandatory to become acquainted with the technique of transanal endoscopic microsurgery.

References

1. Christie JP. Colonoscopic excision of large sessile polyps. Am J Gastroenterol 67:430–438, 1977.
2. Morson BC. Histological criteria for local excision. Br J Surg 72(Suppl):S53–S54, 1985.
3. De Graaf PW, Roussel JG, Gortzak E, et al. Early-stage rectal cancer: electrofulguration in comparison to abdomino-perineal extirpation or low-anterior resection. J Surg Oncol 29:123–128, 1985.
4. Hoekstra HJ, Verschueren RCJ, Oldhoff J, van der Ploeg E. Palliative and curative electrocoagulation for rectal cancer. Cancer 55:210–213, 1985.
5. Salvati EP, Rubin RJ, Eisenstat TE, et al. Electrocoagulation of selected carcinoma of the rectum. Surg Gynecol Obstet 166:393–396, 1988.
6. Eisenstat TE, Oliver GC. Electrocoagulation for adenocarcinoma of the low rectum. World J Surg 16:458–462, 1992.
7. Papillon J, Berard PH. Endocavitary irradiation in the conservative treatment of adenocarcinoma of the low rectum. World J Surg 16:452–457, 1992.
8. Sischy B, Remington JH, Sobel SH. Treatment of rectal carcinomas by means of endocavitary irradiation: a progress report. Cancer 46:1957–1961, 1980.
9. Joffe SN. Contact neodymium-YAG laser surgery in gastroenterology. Surg Endosc 1:25–27, 1987.
10. Kiefhaber P, Huber F, Kiefhaber K. Palliative and preoperative endoscopic Nd-YAG laser treatment of colorectal carcinoma. Endoscopy 19(Suppl):43–46, 1987.
11. Mathus-Vliegen EMH, Tytgat GNJ. Nd-YAG laser photocoagulation in gastroenterology: its role in palliation of colorectal cancer. Arch Surg 37:17–19, 1987.
12. Gage AA. Cryosurgery in the treatment of cancer. Surg Gynecol Obstet 174:73–92, 1992.
13. Parks AG. A technique for excising extensive villous papillomatous change in the lower rectum. Proc R Soc Med 61:441–442, 1968.
14. Parks AG, Stuart AE. The management of villous tumours of the large bowel. Br J Surg 60:688–695, 1973.
15. Christiansen J. Excision of the mid-rectal lesions by Kraske sacral approach. Br J Surg 67:651–652, 1980.
16. Mason AY. Trans-sphincteric surgery of the rectum. Prog Surg 13:66–97, 1974.
17. Buess G, Hutterer F, Theiss R, et al. Das system für die transanale endoskopische rektumoperation. Chirurg 55:677–680, 1984.
18. Buess G, Theiss R, Günther M, et al. Endoscopic surgery in the rectum. Endoscopy 17:31–35, 1985.
19. Shinya H, Wolff WI. Morphology, anatomic distribution and cancer potential of colonic polyps. Ann Surg 190:679–683, 1979.
20. Nivatvongs S, Snover DC, Fang DT. Piecemeal snare excision of large sessile colon and rectal polyps: is it adequate? Gastrointest Endosc 30:18–20, 1984.
21. Thomson JPS. Treatment of sessile villous and tubulovillous adenomas of the rectum: experience of St. Mark's Hospital, 1963–1972. Dis Colon Rectum 20:467–472, 1977.
22. Hermanek P, Gall FP. Early (microinvasive) colorectal carcinoma. Pathology, diagnosis, surgical treatment. Int J Colorectal Dis 1:79–84, 1986.
23. Curley StA, Roh MS, Rich TA. Surgical therapy of early rectal carcinoma. Hematol Oncol Clin North Am 3:87–102, 1989.
24. Bailey HR, Huval WV, Max E, et al. Local excision of carcinoma of the rectum for cure. Surgery 111:555–561, 1992.
25. Gall FP. Cancer of the rectum—local excision. Int J Colorectal Dis 6:84–85, 1991.
26. Hager Th, Gall FP, Hermanek P. Local excision of cancer of the rectum. Dis Colon Rectum 26:149–151, 1983.
27. Stearns MW, Sternberg StS, DeCosse JJ. Treatment alternatives. Localized rectal cancer. Cancer 54:2691–2694, 1984.
28. Cooper HS. Surgical pathology of endoscopically removed malignant polyps of the colon and rectum. Am J Surg Pathol 7:613–623, 1983.
29. Wolff WL, Shinya H, Cwern M, Hsu M. Cancerous colonic polyps. "Hands on" or "hands off"? Am Surg 56:148–152, 1990.
30. Nivatvongs S, Wolff BG. Technique of per anal excision for carcinoma of the low rectum. World J Surg 16:447–450, 1992.

31. The Gastrointestinal Tumor Study Group: Prolongation of the disease-free interval in surgically treated rectal carcinoma. N Engl J Med 312:1465–1472, 1985.
32. The Gastrointestinal Tumor Study Group: Survival after postoperative combination treatment of rectal cancer. N Engl J Med 315:1294–1295, 1986.
33. Moertel CG, Childs DS, Reitemeier RI, et al. Combined 5-fluorouracil and supervoltage radiation therapy of locally unresectable gastrointestinal cancer. Lancet 2:865–867, 1969.
34. Krook J, Moertel CG, Gunderson LL, et al. Effective surgical adjuvant therapy for high risk rectal carcinoma. N Engl J Med 324:709–715, 1991.
35. Tepper JE. Role of radiation therapy in the treatment of carcinoma of the rectum. J Surg Oncol 2(Suppl):51–53, 1991.
36. O'Connell MJ, Gunderson LL. Adjuvant therapy for adenocarcinoma of the rectum. World J Surg 16:510–515, 1992.
37. Poon M, O'Connell M, Wieand H, et al—Mayo Clinic and North Central Cancer Treatment Group: Biochemical modulation of fluorouracil with leucovorin: confirmatory evidence of improved therapeutic efficacy in advanced colorectal cancer. J Clin Oncol 9:1967–1972, 1991.
38. Gunderson LL, O'Connell MJ, Dozios RR. The role of intra-operative irradiation in locally advanced primary and recurrent rectal adenocarcinoma. World J Surg 16:495–501, 1992.
39. Despretz J, Otmezguine Y, Grimard L, et al. Conservative management of tumors of the rectum by radiotherapy and local excision. Dis Colon Rectum 33:113–116, 1990.
40. Marks G, Mohiuddin MM, Masoni L, Pecchioli L. High-dose preoperative radiation and full-thickness local excision. Dis Colon Rectum 33:735–739, 1990.
41. Rich TA, Weiss DR, Mies C, et al. Sphincter preservation in patients with low rectal cancer treated with radiation therapy with or without local excision or fulguration. Radiology 156:527–531, 1985.
42. Willett CG, Tepper JE, Donnelly S, et al. Patterns of failure following local excision and local excision and postoperative radiation therapy for invasive rectal adenocarcinoma. J Clin Oncol 7:1003–1008, 1989.
43. DeCosse JJ, Wong R, Quan SH, et al. Conservative treatment of distal rectal cancer by local excision. Cancer 63:219–223, 1989.
44. Minsky B, Rich TA, Recht A, et al. Selection criteria for local excision with or without adjuvant radiation therapy for rectal cancer. Cancer 63:1421–1429, 1989.
45. Mason AY. Rectal cancer: the spectrum of selective surgery. Proc R Soc Med 69:237–244, 1976.
46. Nicholls RJ, Mason AY, Morson BC, et al. The clinical staging of rectal cancer. Br J Surg 69:404–409, 1982.
47. Durdey P, Williams NS. Pre-operative evaluation of patients with low rectal carcinoma. World J Surg 16:430–436, 1992.
48. Feifel G, Hildebrandt U, Dhom G. Assessment of depth of invasion in rectal cancer by endosonography. Endoscopy 19:64–69, 1987.
49. Dragsted J, Milton P, Jorgensen T, et al. Endoluminal rectal ultrasound scanning of patients with rectal carcinomas (Abstract). Endoscopy 20(Suppl):94, 1988.
50. Yamashita Y, Machi J, Shirouzu K, et al. Evaluation of endorectal ultrasound for the assessment of wall invasion of rectal cancer: report of a case. Dis Colon Rectum 31:617–623, 1988.
51. Jochem RJ, Reading CC, Dozios RR, et al. Endorectal sonographic staging of rectal carcinoma. Mayo Clin Proc 65:1571–1577, 1990.
52. Hildebbrandt U, Feifel G. Preoperative staging of rectal cancer by intrarectal ultrasound. Dis Colon Rectum 28:42–46, 1985.
53. Beynon J. An evaluation of the role of rectal endosonography in rectal cancer. Ann R Coll Surg Engl 71:131–139, 1989.
54. Gall FP, Hermanek P. Cancer of the rectum—local excision. Surg Clin North Am 68:1353–1365, 1988.
55. Killingback M. Local excision of carcinoma of the rectum: indications. World J Surg 16:437–446, 1992.
56. Buess G, Heintz A, Frank K, et al. Endoluminale sonographie des rektums. In: Buess G, ed. Endoskopie. Von der diagnostik bis zur neuen chirurgie. Köln: Deutscher Ärzte-Verlag, 1990:76–82.
57. Buess G. Endoskopie. Von der diagnostik bis zur neuen chirurgie. Köln: Deutscher Ärzte-Verlag, 1990.
58. Williams NS, Durdey P, Quirke P, et al. Preoperative staging of rectal neoplasm and its impact on clinical management. Br J Surg 72:868–874, 1985.
59. Holdsworth PJ, Johnston D, Chalmers AG, et al. Endoluminal ultrasound and computed tomography in the staging of rectal cancer. Br J Surg 75:1019–1022, 1988.
60. Abrams JS. Clinical staging of rectal cancer. Am J Surg 139:539–543, 1980.
61. Cohen AM, Wood WC, Gunderson LL, Shinnar M. Pathological studies in rectal cancer. Cancer 45:2965–2968, 1980.
62. Whiteway J, Nicholls RJ, Morson BC. The role of surgical local excision in the treatment of rectal cancer. Br J Surg 72:694–697, 1985.

43

Endoscopic Surgery in Children

David E. Wesson, Vito Forte, and Thom E Lobe

Gans[1] and Rogers[2] introduced diagnostic laparoscopy and thoracoscopy to pediatric surgery during the 1960s and 1970s shortly after the Hopkins rod-lens system was developed and endoscopes were miniaturized. Until very recently, however, endoscopic surgery played only a small role in the surgical care of children. In a few short years, beginning in the late 1980s, endoscopic surgery has revolutionized the practice of general surgery; the same is now happening in pediatric surgery.

Endoscopy has many advantages over "open" surgery. Often it allows an operation to be done more effectively or more easily than with conventional methods; in the not too distant future, endoscopy will almost certainly make it possible to perform operations that could not be performed by conventional techniques. The advantages of endoscopic surgery include (1) better visualization of the operative field because of improved exposure, illumination, and magnification; (2) less tissue trauma because of smaller incisions and elimination of vigorous retraction of the body wall; (3) less postoperative pain; and (4) shorter hospitalization and a quicker return to normal health.

Originally, endoscopic surgery was performed through a natural opening in the body such as the mouth, anus, or urethra. Now it is most often done through an incision in a body cavity, as in thoracoscopy and laparoscopy.

Three main technologic advances have contributed to the development of endoscopic surgery in children: (1) the Hopkins rod-lens system and fiberoptic light carriers, (2) miniature endoinstruments, and (3) miniature video cameras and high-resolution monitors. The basic principles, equipment, and techniques of endoscopic surgery apply to patients of all ages. The guiding principle is that the operator must have the training and experience to convert the procedure to open surgery if necessary.

Since the explosion of operative laparoscopy and thoracoscopy in the late 1980s and early 1990s, we have learned that the techniques and instrumentation used in adult practice are also suitable for children. Endoscopic surgical techniques can be applied to a wide variety of conditions commonly seen in infants and children. Now the most pressing question is: Which endoscopic procedures actually benefit children? This is very difficult to answer because of the lack of controlled trials and the dearth of information concerning morbidity and long-term effects. It is obvious that no operation should be performed just because it is technically possible.

Endoscopic surgery in adults is justified by the reduction in postoperative pain and a shortened hospital stay. For many adults this means less time lost from work and lost income. Although shorter hospitalization may decrease the total hospital cost, this is partly offset by the increased cost of disposable instruments. There is no question that endoscopic procedures are better tolerated by most adult patients and are being performed with increasing frequency.

In older children and adolescents, the techniques of endoscopic surgery are essentially the same as in adults. In neonates and preschool-aged children, the working distances are considerably reduced, and the optics are poorer when small telescopes are used.

Endoscopic procedures should be assisted by video whenever possible to allow the assistants,

543

nurses, and anesthesiologists the same view as that of the operator so that they can provide optimal assistance. In addition to the lenses and carriers, the setup should include bipolar cautery, a suction-irrigation device, a selection of instruments that can be placed through the instrument channel of the scope or a separate trocar, and clips and sutures as required. Laser equipment, which should be used only by those with special training and experience, is not essential.

The purpose of this chapter is to describe the endoscopic procedures that a pediatric surgeon might find useful in the care of children. We will emphasize therapeutic procedures over diagnostic procedures. The reader should bear in mind that this field is changing very rapidly. New procedures are reported almost weekly. Therefore, anyone practicing endoscopic surgery must make a special effort to keep up to date through the literature and continuing education.

LARYNGOTRACHEAL ENDOSCOPIC SURGERY

Technical Considerations

Many laryngotracheal problems that previously required open procedures can now be corrected endoscopically. It is preferable to perform procedures on the trachea and larynx with the patient breathing spontaneously and, for the larynx, without endotracheal intubation. This gives a better view and a larger field in which to carry out the procedure.

Endoscopic surgery of the child's airway has been greatly facilitated by the miniaturization of bronchoscopic equipment, the development of microsurgical instruments that can be used through the bronchoscope, and the advanced optical instruments that give excellent visualization without compromising ventilation. The ability of children to breathe spontaneously and of the anesthesiologist (who is armed with highly advanced monitoring equipment) to warn the surgeon of impending problems adds greatly to the safety of these procedures.

Although both rigid and flexible instruments have undergone technologic advances, the flexible systems are limited to diagnostic procedures in neonates and infants. The main problem with these smaller instruments is in maintaining adequate ventilation. For all practical purposes, rigid systems must be used for endoscopic airway surgery in children.

The development of the modern miniaturized bronchoscopic system is the main factor that makes endoscopic surgery of the child's airway possible. Storz bronchoscopes and telescopes allow treatment of even the most premature babies.

Optic foreign body forceps of several different varieties are now available to allow the surgeon to visualize and treat a variety of endobronchial lesions. This has revolutionized the removal of foreign bodies; video makes it possible to teach these techniques far more effectively. CO_2, yttrium-aluminum-garnet, argon, and tunable dye laser systems for both flexible and rigid bronchoscopes allow treatment of lesions even in the most distal airway. Electrodessicators and instruments for fulguration are also available for resecting endobronchial lesions. Endoscopic treatment of short strictures of the trachea and esophagus using radiographically controlled balloon dilation and stenting came from interventional cardiology. Although currently experimental, these methods will no doubt soon be routine.

Papillomas of the Larynx

Papillomas are the most common benign laryngeal tumor of childhood, presenting with hoarseness or airway obstruction (Fig. 43–1). A viral cause has been postulated but not proved. Despite the occasional response to interferon, the mainstay of treatment of papillomas of the larynx is CO_2 laser excision with preservation of normal vocal cord structures. The pediatric laryngoscope is introduced and suspended, and the microscope is used to inspect the larynx. Large lesions can be removed with cup forceps; remaining tissue is removed with the CO_2 laser. Papillomas in the anterior commissure should be removed in a serial fashion at repeated sessions to avoid web scar formation. An atraumatic telescopic examination of the trachea should be carried out at the same time, without introducing the bronchoscope if possible to avoid mucosal injury and minimize "seeding."

Vocal Cord Cysts and Nodules

Vocal cord nodules must be distinguished from inclusion cysts of the vocal cord because the former may respond to voice rest and voice therapy, whereas the latter ultimately require endoscopic surgery. Either type of lesion can be easily excised microsurgically or vaporized with the CO_2 laser, taking care to minimize damage to the free edge of the vocal cord.

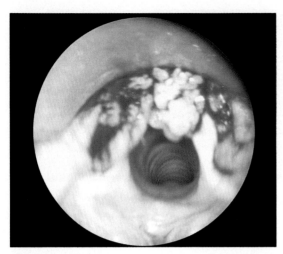

Figure 43–1. Papilloma of the larynx, including anterior commissure.

Epiglottic and Laryngeal Cysts

Mucus retention cysts that cause either hoarseness or obstruction can also be removed by either microsurgical dissection or CO_2 laser excision and vaporization (Fig. 43–2). If the lining is completely removed or vaporized, recurrence is uncommon.

Hemangiomas

Large isolated subglottic hemangiomas can be excised by microlaryngoscopy and laser treatment (Fig. 43–3). If the lesion is extremely large it may obstruct the airway. In such cases, intra-

operative tracheotomy will allow aggressive laser excision. The tracheotomy tube can be removed at the end of the procedure and replaced with a nasotracheal tube, which is left in place for 5 to 7 days. In this way, it may be possible to remove large lesions at one sitting without the need for even short-term tracheotomy. For more diffuse hemangiomas, repeated CO_2 laser treatment supplemented by oral steroid administration is recommended.

Subglottic Stenosis and Webs

Isolated soft stenoses, subglottic cysts, or subglottic webs may be vaporized with the CO_2 laser or excised with microsurgical techniques (Fig. 43–4). With judicious use in selected patients, open laryngeal surgery, including the cricoid split procedure, may often be avoided.

Tracheal Webs, Granulomas, and Cysts

The CO_2 laser readily treats tracheal webs, granulomas, and cysts (Fig. 43–5).

Foreign Bodies

Optic forceps are used to remove foreign bodies under direct visualization, with extreme

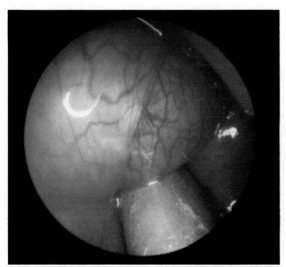

Figure 43–2. Large obstructing left ventricular cyst (false cord tensed over lesion—bronchoscope seen posteriorly).

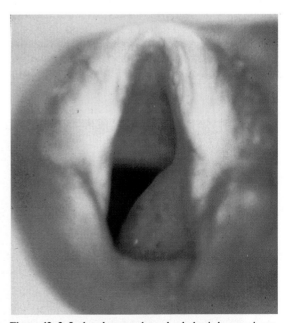

Figure 43–3. Isolated posterolateral subglottic hemangioma, which is easily treated with CO_2 laser.

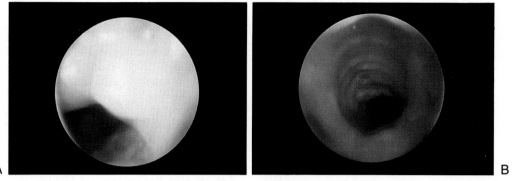

Figure 43–4. (A) Intubation-induced subglottic cyst in neonate in whom extubation failed. **(B)** Two weeks following laser excision.

safety and accuracy. They can be pulled back from the distal airway with an embolectomy catheter and removed from the trachea (Fig. 43–6). Alternatively, intraoperative postural chest physiotherapy may dislodge distal foreign material into larger airways, facilitating its removal. A sharp foreign body should be shielded with the tip of the bronchoscope at all times if possible.

Tracheal Stenosis

Short segments of tracheal stenosis can be managed with radiographically controlled balloon dilation or laser therapy. Some success has been achieved in very premature infants with balloon dilation and splitting of the posterior trachea, followed by 1 week of endotracheal stenting. Longer stenoses have been managed by open surgery, even though this often requires repeated endoscopic dilation and removal of granulation tissue to achieve success. Long-term

stenting of the trachea and bronchi has recently been performed using balloon-expandable intravascular stents placed under radiographic control (Fig. 43–7).

Telangiectasia

Obliteration of telangiectasias may be accomplished with applications of argon or tunable dye laser through a flexible channel.

Massive Hemoptysis

Endoscopic measures may be necessary in preparation for embolization or open surgery in children with massive hemoptysis. Balloon occlusion of the involved bronchus with ventilation of the remaining lung under bronchoscopic control may provide temporary relief while other measures are being carried out.

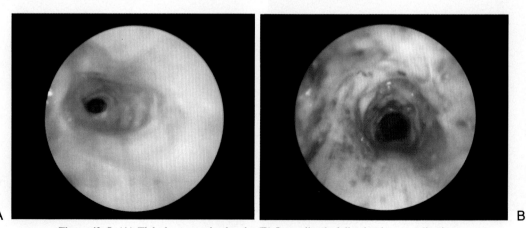

Figure 43–5. (A) Tight lower tracheal web. **(B)** Immediately following laser application.

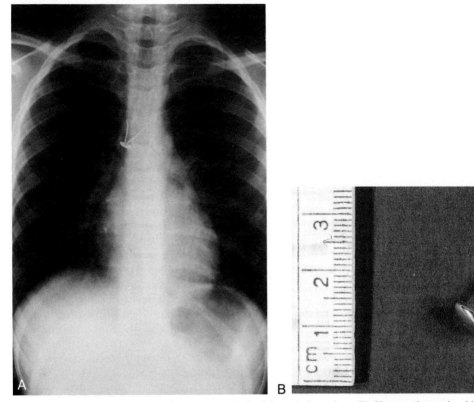

Figure 43–6. (A) Radiograph showing paper staple in right main bronchus. **(B)** Sharp end must be shielded in bronchoscope during removal.

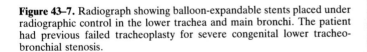

Figure 43–7. Radiograph showing balloon-expandable stents placed under radiographic control in the lower trachea and main bronchi. The patient had previous failed tracheoplasty for severe congenital lower tracheobronchial stenosis.

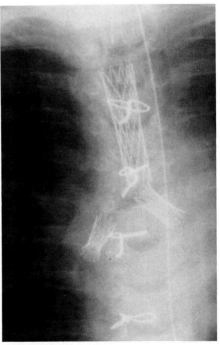

Tracheoesophageal Fistula

In rare cases, it may be necessary to occlude a tracheoesophageal fistula with an embolectomy catheter to achieve adequate ventilation and to prevent aspiration prior to definitive surgical correction.

Granulomas of the Bronchus

Granulomas are not uncommon in the neonate following long-term intubation and are likely related to deep suctioning. Long, flexible forceps may be used under telescopic guidance or laser to remove granulation tissue from the distal airway.

THORACIC ENDOSCOPIC SURGERY

Technical Considerations

Endoscopic thoracic surgery has major advantages over conventional open thoracotomy. The most obvious is the avoidance of a painful incision. Thoracoscopy is useful for treatment of pulmonary blebs, nodules and tumors, and mediastinal cysts and tumors. (See Chap. 37)

Thoracoscopy is best performed under general anesthesia with positive pressure breathing. Patients are monitored by pulse oximetry. We do not use arterial lines routinely. The patient should be placed in the lateral decubitus position and prepared as for a standard thoracotomy. The incision line and the chest tube site should be marked and used as a guide for placement of the trocars. A diamond-shaped configuration of trocar sites is used to surround the lesion. The telescope can be placed through the planned chest tube site, if one is required, and the operating instruments through one or more trocars in the incision line. To establish an adequate pneumothorax, the lung must be completely collapsed. In older children and teenagers, a double-lumen tube can be used. For smaller children and infants, contralateral intubation with a cuffed endotracheal tube is necessary. In these smaller infants, inflating the endotracheal tube cuff can push the tube out of the bronchus and result in some air leakage. This results in inflation of the lung on the side of the thoracoscopy. When this occurs, it is helpful to insert a Fogarty balloon catheter to occlude the bronchus. A flexible bronchoscope passed through the endotracheal tube can facil-itate balloon catheter placement. In spite of these maneuvers, it may be necessary to use CO_2 insufflation of the chest to 6 to 8 mm Hg to collapse the lung. This generally does not cause any significant hemodynamic instability or respiratory embarrassment.

The patient's position can be adjusted according to the location of the lesion. We use gravity to facilitate dependent retraction of the lung. Thus, for a superior lesion, we place the patient in the reverse Trendelenburg position. For a posterior lesion, we rotate the patient anteriorly so that the lung will fall forward.

For biopsy of mediastinal masses, evacuation of loculated pleural effusions or empyema, pleurodesis, and other routine procedures, a two-trocar technique is usually performed. The first cannula is for the telescope. The second cannula is placed in an appropriate position to allow access for the biopsy forceps (in the case of the mediastinal mass) or for the cannula (to evacuate an empyema or to perform pleurodesis).

For simple biopsies (when there is no significant hemorrhage and the pleura is not violated), a chest tube is not necessary. For evacuation of fluid, decortication, or pleurodesis, a chest tube is inserted through a trocar site at the end of the procedure.

Wounds are closed with absorbable sutures and dressed with adhesive strips and a moisture/vapor–permeable occlusive dressing. Patients are allowed a full diet and activity as tolerated without restriction as soon as they are comfortable. This is usually within 36 to 48 hours.

Esophageal Foreign Bodies

Retained esophageal foreign bodies are common in children 1 to 5 years of age. Many of these objects will pass spontaneously, but those that do not should be removed. There are several options: (1) balloon extraction under radiologic guidance (blunt objects only), (2) endoscopic removal using a rigid esophagoscope (for sharp or blunt objects), and (3) endoscopic removal with a flexible esophagoscope. The latter two techniques usually require general anesthesia. The choice depends on the exact nature of the patient's problem and the experience of the operator. Rigid endoscopy is the standard method and is both safe and reliable.[3, 4] Occasionally, in a patient who is well known to the surgeon and has a stricture or motility disorder, a food bolus may be safely pushed down into the stomach with a Maloney bougie. This is quick and safe.

Esophageal Varices

Bleeding from esophageal varices usually ceases, at least temporarily, with supportive measures only. Direct injections of a sclerosant solution, such as ethanolamine oleate, reduce the chance of rebleeding episodes and may eventually obliterate the varices after a course of repeated injections.

Esophageal Strictures

Repair of esophageal atresia is occasionally complicated by esophageal strictures, especially if there is excessive tension on the anastomosis or an anastomotic leak. Acid reflux causes esophagitis, which can, in turn, lead to a peptic stricture. Acid reflux may also contribute to stricture formation after esophageal atresia repair. A less common cause of esophageal stricture is candidal esophagitis.

Simple dilation with a Maloney bougie often provides temporary relief, but most cases in which reflux is a factor are best managed by a combination of dilation and surgical correction of the reflux. Very tight or recalcitrant strictures can sometimes be overcome with coaxial pneumatic balloon dilation over a guidewire under fluoroscopic guidance.

Spontaneous Pneumothorax

Spontaneous pneumothorax is common, especially in healthy adolescents and young adults. Failure to resolve spontaneously, continued air leakage after intercostal drainage, or recurrence after successful nonoperative treatment are generally considered to be indications for surgery, which can be performed thoracoscopically, as described previously. The bullous lung, usually the apex of the upper lobe, can be removed using an endoscopic linear stapling and cutting device such as the Endo-GIA stapler (U.S. Surgical Corp., Norwalk, CT). Alternatively, the argon beam coagulator can be used to "shrink" the blebs and seal the air leak.

Pulmonary Nodules and Metastases and Lung Biopsy

Thoracoscopic lung biopsy is best performed using a linear stapler. In small children, the 12-mm cannula that is required for the stapler is best placed in the sulcus between the chest wall and the diaphragm as inferiorly as possible. At least 5 cm of the stapler must be inserted into the chest for the instrument to function properly. This means that children younger than 3 or 4 years of age cannot have thoracoscopic lung biopsies using the linear stapler because there is not sufficient room in the chest to use the stapler.

For a biopsy using the stapler, one cannula is initially placed for inspection. Another 5-mm cannula is placed for insertion of a grasper to secure the lung, and a 12-mm cannula is placed for insertion of the linear stapler. A gauge is used to determine the appropriate staple length, and the stapler is applied to the lung tissue. After the desired segment is resected, it is withdrawn through the largest cannula. We have not used tube thoracostomy routinely for patients not on mechanical ventilation. Patients on positive pressure ventilation or those with respiratory stress that is sufficient to require mechanical ventilation undergo tube thoracostomy to prevent postoperative tension pneumothorax.

Isolated pulmonary nodules and metastatic lesions can be removed by thoracoscopy, as described for lung biopsy, provided that they can be seen on the lung surface. If not, a small incision can be made and the lung palpated to localize the lesion or lesions, which can then be removed endoscopically with the aid of the thoracoscope and the Endo-GIA stapler, or they can be wedged out through the limited incision—a type of video-assisted open surgery.

Major Pulmonary Resections

Formal lobectomy and pneumonectomy have been accomplished in adults. One of us (TEL) has performed video-assisted lobectomy in a child, but the exact role of this procedure is not yet established.

Mediastinal Cysts and Tumors

Simple bronchogenic cysts are excised thoracoscopically in toto or in part. Laser or electrosurgical techniques are used to excise the presenting wall of the cyst. We prefer to use the KTP/532 Laser (Laserscope, San Jose, CA) to ablate the lining of the cyst. A chest tube is not routinely used unless the cyst is adherent to the airway and an air leak is likely to persist.

Complications

The complications of thoracoscopic surgery are listed in Table 43–1. In addition to those listed, we have had several other isolated complications. In one patient, a needle and syringe were used to establish a pneumothorax before trocar placement. Selective intubation of the left lung had been accomplished, and the needle was introduced through the right fourth intercostal space. Upon injection of air, the patient experienced hemodynamic instability consistent with an air embolism. She recovered and thoracoscopy was continued. It was apparent from this event that when selective intubation is performed and a pneumothorax has not yet been established, the diaphragm will rise as the lung deflates and the subdiaphragmatic viscera may lie directly under the fourth or fifth intercostal space. When this approach is used, air should be injected into the second or third intercostal space.

In one teenager who had received chemotherapy and thoracic radiation, thoracoscopy was undertaken to evaluate a thickening of the diaphragm. This patient had nearly complete pleural symphysis and it was difficult to gain access. A tear was made in the diaphragm and a formal thoracotomy was performed. There was no subdiaphragmatic injury.

ABDOMINAL ENDOSCOPIC SURGERY

Technical Considerations

Laparoscopy is useful for the diagnosis of jaundice, chronic ascites, abdominal pain (acute and chronic), abdominal masses (endoscopically guided biopsy), intersex, cryptorchidism, and trauma. It can be used even in neonates.[5] It can also be used therapeutically in cases of peritoneal adhesions, abdominal cysts and tumors, gonadectomy, staged orchidopexy, appendectomy, and cholecystectomy. Other less common procedures have also been reported, including laser coagulation of liver hemangiomas, pullthrough procedures for Hirschsprung's disease, and irrigation of the biliary system in the inspissated bile syndrome. Waldschmidt and Schier reported their experience with 136 abdominal operations performed laparoscopically in neonates and infants.[6]

Preoperative preparation for most patients includes prophylactic antibiotic administration. Depending on the procedure, some patients undergo bowel preparation with either a sodium biophosphate and sodium phosphate enema or an osmotic cathartic bowel preparation to empty the colon of gas and feces.

Wounds are closed with absorbable sutures and dressed with adhesive strips and a moisture/vapor–permeable occlusive dressing. Patients are given metoclopramide postoperatively to combat nausea. Patients 10 years of age or older are also treated with a scopolomine skin patch applied behind the ear to combat nausea. Patients are allowed a full diet and activity as tolerated without restriction as soon as they are comfortable. This is usually within 36 to 48 hours.

Laparoscopy is best performed with the patient under general anesthesia and lying in the supine position. General anesthesia allows full relaxation and control of ventilation, which may be compromised by the pneumoperitoneum. Nitrous oxide may be used, at least for procedures lasting less than 75 minutes, without causing excessive bowel distention.[7] Laparoscopic procedures can be done on an outpatient basis; the need for admission depends on the nature of the procedure and the patient's condition. The patient must be strapped securely to the table to allow safe repositioning during the procedure. In most cases, a nasogastric tube and a Foley catheter should be inserted, although for short operations the bladder may be emptied by the Credé maneuver. The patient should be prepared and draped as for laparotomy, and the necessary instruments for laparotomy should be immediately available. Standard surgical skin preparation and draping are used in all cases. A closed technique using a Veress needle for CO_2 insufflation is usually performed. When there has been previous surgery or when peritonitis or adhesions are suspected, an open technique using a blunt Hasson trocar for atraumatic access is used. In this method, the first incision is placed in the inferior margin of the umbilicus and is carried down through the linea alba so that the peritoneum can be entered under direct vision. This allows placement of the Hasson trocar and creation of the pneumo-

Table 43–1. COMPLICATIONS OF THORACOSCOPIC SURGERY

Bleeding
Air leak
Pneumothorax
Air embolus
Diaphragmatic injury

peritoneum. Two absorbable sutures are placed in the fascia to hold the trocar in place and to close the abdominal wall at the end of the procedure. Because of the frequent presence of an umbilical hernia and the smaller size of the abdominal cavity in infants, it is safer to use the Hasson trocar than the Verres needle for laparoscopy in very young children. In infants, care must be taken to avoid the bladder, which rises to a point near the umbilicus. For this reason, a supraumbilical incision may be used. The telescope with attached video camera is placed through the umbilical trocar for inspection of the peritoneal cavity. The pressure of the pneumoperitoneum should be carefully controlled at 8 to 10 mm Hg in infants and 10 to 15 mm Hg in older children. Secondary trocars are placed, as required, under direct vision. Trocars must be placed far enough apart to avoid "duelling" instruments during the procedure. Standard 0° Storz laparoscopes are satisfactory for most cases, but a 30° lens is very useful in certain applications.

Contraindications to laparoscopy include multiple previous laparotomies, peritonitis, active abdominal wall infection, and coagulopathy.

Gastrostomy

The technique of percutaneous gastrostomy (PEG) described by Ponsky is a useful alternative to the conventional open method and works well in children weighing as little as 5 kg.[8] In small children, a No. 15 French catheter should be used. A recent controlled study showed that when compared to nasogastric tube feeding, PEG is safe and effective and offers important advantages, the most significant being that it is more reliable.[9, 10] Another recent controlled trial comparing percutaneous gastrostomy to Stamm gastrostomy did not reveal any clinically important differences between the two techniques; however, the percutaneous method proved to be less expensive.[11] Laparoscopy may be added to the standard PEG procedure to avoid bowel injury.

Gastroesophageal Reflux

Surgery for gastroesophageal reflux is one of the most common abdominal procedures in pediatric surgery. Nissen fundoplication is the operation most commonly performed. This operation may be done endoscopically.[12]

The bowel is prepared to keep colonic contents from interfering with visualization. The procedure is essentially the same as an open fundoplication. It may be helpful to place the patient in the lithotomy position to allow the surgeon to stand between the patient's legs and to elevate the head of the operating table 20 to 30°.[12] An upper midline 5-mm cannula is used as a retractor to elevate the left lobe of the liver and expose the esophageal hiatus. At least three other cannulas are necessary. A useful arrangement is to place one 5-mm cannula in the right midclavicular line, one 10-mm cannula in the left midclavicular line below the costal margin, and one 5-mm cannula in the left anterior axillary line above the iliac crest. The patient's stomach is emptied, and an esophageal dilator as large as the lumen of the esophagus will accommodate is passed by way of the mouth to facilitate dissection.

Initially, the esophagus is dissected free at the hiatus, and an umbilical tape is passed around the gastroesophageal junction for retraction. With the hiatus exposed, the diaphragmatic crura are reapproximated with interrupted sutures. The cardia of the stomach is passed behind the esophagus from left to right, and the wrap is completed with interrupted sutures tied extracorporeally.

In our first few cases, we divided several short gastric vessels between clips to mobilize the fundus. However, because the laparoscopic wrap leaves the suture line facing the patient's right side rather than anteriorly, and much of the wrap is formed by bringing the stomach anterior to the esophagus, it is unnecessary to divide the short gastric vessels routinely.

For concurrent gastrostomy, we bring part of the anterior gastric wall through the left midclavicular line trocar site and suture a Stamm gastrostomy under direct vision.

Hypertrophic Pyloric Stenosis

Endoscopic treatment of hypertrophic pyloric stenosis is possible; however, the conventional open operation is so quick and reliable that the wisdom of doing it endoscopically is questionable.

Cholelithiasis

Although gallstones are less common in children than in adults, they do occur, especially in children with hemolytic anemias, such as sickle cell anemia and hereditary spherocytosis. The indications for operation are essentially the same in children as in adults.

The standard four-trocar technique for cholecystectomy can be used even in young children.[13-16] The main difference between adults and children undergoing biliary surgery is the size of the bile ducts, especially the cystic duct, which makes it more difficult to perform cholangiograms and common duct explorations in children. For cholecystectomy, initial trocar placement is determined by the patient's age. In teenagers and larger children, trocar placement is the same as in adults. In smaller patients, a 10-mm or 12-mm cannula is placed to the left of the midline about 2 cm below the costal margin. By placing this cannula to the left of the falciform ligament, the trajectory of the dissecting instruments is better suited to the small abdomen. Similarly, the cannula to be placed in the right side should be situated as inferiorly as possible, usually just above the iliac crest in the anterior axillary line. By placing it inferiorly, instruments inserted through this cannula do not interfere with the other instruments.

We prefer a percutaneous cholangiogram technique. A needle catheter is passed through the anterior abdominal wall and inserted in the cystic duct. We either clip the catheter in place or use a balloon catheter to occlude the duct for the cholangiogram.

Many children referred for cholecystectomy have sickle cell anemia and have been evaluated for recurring episodes of abdominal pain. In these patients, we routinely perform an appendectomy using the linear stapler passed through one of the cholecystectomy cannulas.

Splenic Diseases

Patients are prepared for a splenectomy with a bowel preparation and preoperative antibiotic administration. Two cannulas are placed in the left midclavicular line: one 12-mm cannula above and one 5-mm cannula below the umbilicus. Two more 5-mm cannulas are placed in the left anterior axillary line: one below the costal margin and one just above the iliac crest. With the patient in an exaggerated reverse Trendelenburg position, the greater curvature of the stomach is retracted to the patient's right and the short gastric vessels are divided between surgical clips. The patient is then turned to a right lateral decubitus position. Through the two anterior axillary line cannulas, grasping or dissecting instruments elevate the spleen to ex-

pose the splenic hilum. Smaller vessels are dissected from the splenic hilum using surgical clips or electrosurgical technique until the splenic artery and vein are identified. We divide the hilar vessels using a linear stapler. The ligaments to the body wall and diaphragm are then taken down using endoscopic shears. A retrieval bag (Tissue Sac, Cook Urological, Spencer, IN) is inserted through the 12-mm cannula. Using grasping forceps on the tabs at the opening of the sac, the spleen is gently maneuvered into the sac. The drawstring is used to cinch up the neck of the sac and the sac is withdrawn into the 12-mm cannula; the tissue morcellator is then inserted through the neck of the sac and the spleen is morcellated inside the retrieval bag until it is small enough to allow the bag to be withdrawn from the abdomen.

Acute Appendicitis

Although most general surgeons consider appendicitis to be a relatively innocuous disease, it may be complicated by wound infection, intraabdominal and pelvic abscess, intestinal obstruction, and incisional hernia. Laparoscopic appendectomy for acute appendicitis is still controversial because there is no proof that it is better than conventional appendectomy. However, early experience suggests that laparoscopic appendectomy may result in a cosmetically better scar, less postoperative pain, and a shorter convalescence, at least in adults.[17]

We use a 30-mm linear stapler to remove the appendix. When there is a preoperative diagnosis of ruptured appendix, we prefer the conventional open approach. When laparoscopy is undertaken and the patient is found to have a ruptured appendix, we continue laparoscopically, if feasible, using the stapler.

Many authors have reported performing appendectomy during laparoscopy for chronic pelvic pain. In acute cases, laparoscopy can be used for diagnostic purposes and, if the diagnosis of appendicitis is confirmed, appendectomy can be performed endoscopically.

With the patient in the Trendelenburg position, three cannulas are inserted: a 5-mm or 10-mm 0° telescope is passed through an umbilical cannula; a 5-mm cannula is placed in the right lower quadrant below the "bikini line," and a 12-mm cannula for introduction of the stapler is placed in the left lower quadrant. A dissector is passed through the cannula on the left side to make an opening between the base of the appendix and its mesentery. The Endo-GIA stapler of appropriate staple length is used to divide the appendix, its base, and the mesentery. The appendix is placed in a retrieval bag that is withdrawn through the 12-mm cannula to avoid wound contamination. Any blood or fluid is aspirated. Cultures are performed if the fluid is cloudy or there is gross pus.

Inguinal Hernia

There is no indication for endoscopic repair of inguinal hernias in children because they can be repaired very easily on an outpatient basis by conventional methods. The inguinal canal may be inspected laparoscopically in patients with undescended testes. Even in these cases, however, it is preferable to perform the orchidopexy and concomitant hernia repair by the usual open technique.

Cryptorchidism

Cryptorchidism occurs in 0.5% to 1% of boys. Ten to 20% of these patients have nonpalpable testes.[18] Twenty to 50% of nonpalpable testes are not present.[19] Undescended testes that are not palpable have an increased risk of malignancy and infertility. When the testis is not palpable, and this is confirmed by examination under general anesthesia, laparoscopy may help to locate it or to prove that it is not present as in the vanishing testes syndrome, thus obviating laparotomy. Therefore, laparoscopy is indicated in all cases of nonpalpable testes. It is more accurate than other techniques used to localize the testes, including ultrasonography, nuclear scanning, computed tomography, arteriography, and venography.

The procedure is performed with the patient under general anesthesia; exploration can be done under the same anesthetic, if indicated. The bladder is drained and the abdomen insufflated with a Veress needle. A 5-mm trocar is then inserted and a pediatric cystoscope lens is passed through it.[19] For small infants, we use a 3-mm port through which a 2-mm 0° telescope passes easily. The patient is placed in a 15° to 20° Trendelenburg position. On the normal side, the spermatic vessels and the vas deferens can be seen in their retroperitoneal position. The vas deferens courses laterally from the pelvis over the external iliac vessels; the spermatic vessels run caudally lateral to the external iliacs to meet the vas deferens at the internal ring. One may see a veil-like process covering a patent processus vaginalis, a small hernia sac, or a funnel with no apparent bottom, indicating the presence of an indirect hernia.

There are several possible findings at laparoscopy for nonpalpable testes:

1. The gonad may be found at the internal ring or more proximally, within the peritoneal cavity.
2. The cord structures may end blindly, indicating previous torsion.
3. The cord structures may enter the inguinal canal normally, indicating either a missed ectopic or undescended testis or an atrophic inguinal testis.

A blind-ending vas deferens and testicular vessels are proof that there is no testis. In fact, blind-ending vessels alone are considered adequate evidence of anorchia. A blind-ending vas deferens without an obvious testis or vessels may still be associated with a high intraabdominal testis. Adequate visualization of the entire retroperitoneum may require an additional instrument introduced through a second trocar. We prefer to insert a cannula from the contralateral lower quadrant and to pass an instrument to deflect the intestines medially. When no testicular vessels can be seen by laparoscopy, a laparotomy is indicated. In cases of high intraabdominal testes, preliminary endoscopic clipping of the testicular vessels may allow later orchidopexy based on the collateral blood supply from the gubernaculum testis and along the vas deferens.[19] When the vas deferens and vessels are seen to enter the inguinal canal, exploration of the groin usually confirms testicular atrophy. The testicle may be seen at or just inside the internal inguinal ring. If so, immediate orchidopexy can usually be accomplished.

Published reports of laparoscopy in cases of nonpalpable testes indicate that one third to two thirds of testes are not present.[19] In one series, approximately one third of patients had a testis that was not present, one third of patients had a canalicular testis that was easily placed in the scrotum, and one third of patients required a staged procedure.[20]

It is also important to note that an intraabdominal testis is found in a significant minority of patients with previous negative groin explorations.

A high intraabdominal testis that is considered nonsalvageable can be removed endoscopically. Alternatively, the testicular vessels may be clipped for a staged Fowler-Stephens orchidopexy based on the collateral blood supply to the testis. Finally, if normal anatomy is observed at the internal ring, inguinal exploration is indicated.

Colonoscopy and Polypectomy

Colonoscopy is indicated for diagnosis in selected cases of rectal bleeding, diarrhea, and abdominal pain in children. The technique is similar to that recommended for adults[21] and can almost always be accomplished under analgesia-sedation with meperidine and midazolam. Polypectomy using a snare cautery is indicated for diagnosis and treatment of juvenile polyps, which are the most common type of polyps in young children. Low rectal polyps can often be intussuscepted out the anus so that the base can be suture ligated before excision.

Abdominal Trauma and Other Miscellaneous Conditions

Laparoscopy has great potential for diagnosis in abdominal trauma, but this application has not been well studied. For victims of trauma in whom there remains a question of intraabdominal injury or even of penetration through the abdominal wall into the peritoneal cavity, laparoscopy is used to inspect the peritoneal and visceral surfaces. In rare instances, a bleeding vessel can be clipped or ligated, or a hole in the bowel can be repaired. A single umbilical cannula may suffice. More often, an additional instrument is necessary to move and inspect the viscera.

Laparoscopic inspection to evaluate biliary

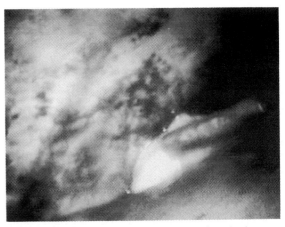

Figure 43–9. Suction cannula *(right center)* aspirating pus from suprahepatic intraabdominal abscess.

tract anatomy in infants with jaundice is easy to perform. When a gallbladder is identified and the presence of ducts remains in doubt, a cholangiogram is performed by passing a needle through the anterior abdominal wall directly into the gallbladder. When the cholangiogram is completed, the hole in the gallbladder is either sutured or clipped to avoid a bile leak. Under inspection, liver biopsy should be performed using a percutaneously passed core biopsy needle or a standard biopsy forceps (Fig. 43–8).

In patients with multiple abdominal abscesses secondary to trauma or a ruptured appendix, laparoscopy may be performed to drain persistent abscesses. In these cases, open access with the Hasson trocar is used to avoid injuring bowel loops that may be adherent to the undersurface of the abdominal wall. CO_2 insufflation dissects loose adhesions. The insertion of a second or third cannula facilitates further blunt dissection. Computed tomographic guidance pinpoints the location of the abscesses so that they can be approached directly. Abscesses are aspirated and specimens are sent to be cultured (Fig. 43–9).

Patients with intestinal lesions such as Meckel's diverticulum can be diagnosed laparoscopically. Meckel's diverticulum containing gastric or other aberrant mucosa toward its tip is resected by placing a linear stapler transversely across the base of the diverticulum at its junction with the small bowel (Fig. 43–10). Alternatively, if the diverticulum is thickened down to its base, a laparoscopic resection is performed using techniques that have been described elsewhere.[22]

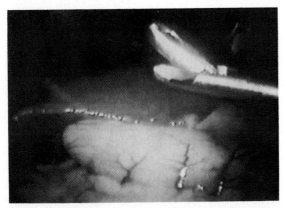

Figure 43–8. Cup biopsy forceps poised to obtain specimen of white lesion in liver edge below.

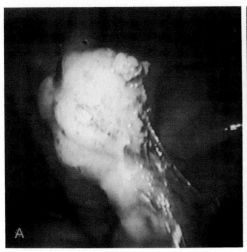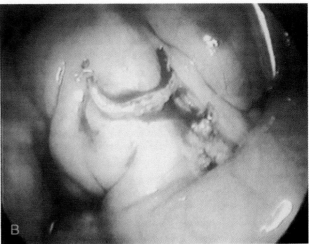

Figure 43–10. (A) Meckel's diverticulum being held in grasper. **(B)** Staple line from resection of Meckel's diverticulum.

Complications

The potential complications of laparoscopic surgery are listed in Table 43–2. In general, the complications are the same as those described for adults except that there is a greater risk of bladder injury in infants. Preliminary drainage of the bladder should prevent this complication. If a bladder injury occurs, catheter drainage of several days' duration usually allows satisfactory healing.

There has been no death, major hemorrhage, or major visceral injury from endoscopic surgical procedures in our experience.

DISCUSSION

Endoscopic surgery has earned a prominent place in pediatric surgery. Its use will almost certainly increase if for no other reason than the fact that patients prefer it to open surgery. One issue of concern is the possible increased frequency of complications, particularly in the hands of less experienced endoscopic surgeons. This has been addressed recently in the lay media. National standards have not yet been set

Table 43–2. POTENTIAL COMPLICATIONS OF LAPAROSCOPIC SURGERY

Bleeding
Bowel injury
Abscess
Adhesive bowel obstruction
Respiratory distress/hypercarbia

for training and credentialing for endoscopic surgery, although many national surgical organizations have established guidelines or approved course curricula that may well become standard prerequisites for credentialing.

We will review the possible advantages of endoscopic surgery in children in light of our own experience. The procedures that can be performed fall into four major categories: (1) operations for which the endoscopic approach may lengthen the procedure and subject the patient to unnecessary risks without offering any obvious advantages, (2) diagnostic procedures that could be performed operatively but do not in all likelihood alter the patient's course of management, (3) therapeutic or diagnostic procedures that have an operative alternative but that tend to decrease morbidity and hospitalization, and (4) reconstructive procedures that shorten hospitalization and decrease operative morbidity. Table 43–3 lists the average operating times for various endoscopic procedures, and Table 43–4 presents the average postoperative hospital stay for these same procedures.

In the first category are procedures such as pyloromyotomy, which can be performed endoscopically but for which this approach appears to offer no obvious benefits. The standard open operation for pyloric stenosis is performed through a small incision, has few complications, and is followed by a brief hospitalization. Laparoscopic pyloromyotomy has no obvious advantage because patients do not resume feeding any sooner. Thus, we cannot recommend laparoscopy for this procedure.

Table 43–3. AVERAGE OPERATING TIME FOR ENDOSCOPIC PROCEDURES (INCLUDES ANESTHESIA TIME)

Operation	First Procedure	With Experience
Laparoscopic		
Acute appendicitis	45 min–1 h 30 min	30 min–1 h
Ruptured appendicitis	1 h 30 min–3 h	45 min–1 h 30 min
Cholecystectomy	2 h 30 min–4 h	1 h–2 h 30 min
Exploration for undescended testis or inguinal hernia	30 min–45 min	5 min–15 min
Splenectomy	2 h 30 min–4 h	2 h 30 min–3 h
Nissen fundoplication with gastrostomy	4 h 30 min–5 h	1 h 30 min–2 h
Thoracoscopic		
Biopsy of mass	1 h–1 h 30 min	20 min–45 min
Lung biopsy	1 h 30 min–2 h	30 min–45 min
Evacuation empyema	1 h 30 min–2 h	30 min–1 h
Bronchogenic cyst	2 h 30 min–4 h	1 h 30 min–3 h

In the second of these categories are diagnostic procedures that may not alter the patient's management. Laparoscopy for the evaluation of undescended testes is an example. These procedures are useful to locate intraabdominal testes and guide the surgeon's decision to perform inguinal exploration. When the vas deferens and spermatic vessels end blindly before they traverse the inguinal canal, and no testicle is found, the diagnosis of previous testicular torsion with atrophy can be made. Inguinal exploration is not necessary unless an inguinal hernia is apparent. In this instance, one can avoid an exploration and thus potentially decrease morbidity. The "down side" of the procedure is the risk of potential visceral injury at the time of Veress needle or trocar insertion. Although the risk exists, our experience supports the findings of others that this risk is minimal.

The third category is more complex to assess. In this category are procedures such as cholecystectomy, appendectomy, splenectomy, and others. One must consider the risks and added expense of endoscopy and weigh them against the benefits. The alleged benefits may not be as great in pediatrics as in adults. The average patient who undergoes a routine appendectomy usually goes home on the second or third postoperative day. The patient may return to unrestricted activities within a couple of weeks of the operation. In contrast to this, the average patient who undergoes a laparoscopic appendectomy for acute appendicitis leaves the hospital within 1 to 2 days and can return to

unrestricted activity within 2 or 3 days. Although this may be better for the patient and will allow him or her to participate in competitive sports and so on, there is little economic advantage except that if the child returns to school sooner, the parents may not have to stay home from work. However, there are inevitably some added expenses to the endoscopic operation if one uses disposable instruments, varying from a few hundred to approximately a thousand dollars. Although these costs are not necessary if one uses nondisposable instruments, there is at least some additional cost over an open appendectomy when the linear stapler is used.

A similar situation exists for cholecystectomy. Routine operative cholecystectomy in pediatrics is a relatively simple procedure performed through a small incision. Patients rarely spend more than 2 to 3 days in the hospital. Laparoscopic cholecystectomy is also easily performed, and patients usually spend 1 or 2 days in the hospital. Thus, the decreased time spent in the hospital is minimal with this procedure. Patients can return to unrestricted activities within 2 to 3 days after a laparoscopic procedure, whereas after an incision is made, the surgeon usually restricts the child's activities for several weeks. The real advantage of the laparoscopic procedure is evident in the decreased pulmonary complications associated with the lack of an abdominal incision. This is particularly true of patients with sickle cell anemia in whom pulmonary complications are common after abdominal surgery.

The advantages of endoscopic surgery are more clear in patients who undergo lung biopsy,

Table 43–4. AVERAGE POSTOPERATIVE HOSPITAL STAY FOR ENDOSCOPIC PROCEDURES

Procedure	Postoperative Hospital Stay
Laparoscopic	
Acute appendicitis	12 h–24 h
Ruptured appendicitis	36 h–5 d
Cholecystectomy	24 h–36 h
Exploration of undescended testis or inguinal hernia	2 h–6 h
Splenectomy	48 h
Nissen fundoplication with ≤ gastrostomy	36 h
Thoracoscopic	
Biopsy of mass	2 h–24 h
Lung biopsy	12 h–34 h
Empyema	2 d–5 d
Bronchogenic cyst	2 d–3 d

splenectomy, or Meckel's diverticulectomy. In these patients, an operation may mean 2 to 4 days in the hospital and some period of restriction after the procedure to allow resolution of the postoperative ileus. In contrast, although there may be some additional costs because of the disposable instrumentation, the endoscopic procedure allows the patient a significantly more rapid recovery and earlier return to unrestricted activities.

We believe that the advantages are best illustrated in the case of reconstructive procedures such as Nissen fundoplication. In this instance, the abdominal procedure requires an abdominal incision and several days of hospitalization before feeding is reestablished. In our experience with the laparoscopic approach, patients tolerate full feedings within 36 to 48 hours and can be discharged to unrestricted activities at that time. Although this may be an advantage in the normal child, many children undergoing Nissen fundoplication are mentally impaired or in some other way debilitated so that a return to unrestricted activities may be of little concern. An advantage in this latter group, however, is the decreased risk of pulmonary complications that occur because of an incision. To date, we have seen no pulmonary complications after the laparoscopic procedure, whereas these complications are common after an abdominal incision has been performed.

We are still assessing the value of endoscopic surgical procedures in children. It will likely take several years to gain enough experience with some of the procedures to properly compare them to their operative counterparts. Prospective studies will be required before we know their true value and their proper place in the armamentarium of the pediatric surgeon.

A similar assessment can be made of thoracoscopic procedures. There is no question that thoracoscopic lung biopsy is better tolerated than an open lung biopsy by means of a thoracotomy. In children younger than 2 to 3 years of age, however, a lung biopsy performed by way of a thoracotomy using a small incision may be as well tolerated as thoracoscopy. There are some procedures, such as early thoracoscopy with evacuation of loculated pleural effusion or empyema, that appear to have some value but for which controlled studies are necessary to properly compare the results of this approach with the standard therapy.

Whether or not more extensive procedures, such as bronchogenic cystectomy and so on, are of value is difficult to judge at this time. It could be argued that any time a large incision is required for thoracotomy, it is better to perform the procedure thoracoscopically if it can be accomplished safely and effectively. Patients often do not require a tube thoracostomy after thoracoscopy, and many can be discharged the day after surgery. When it is likely because of the patient's condition that the child will require prolonged perioperative hospitalization regardless of how the surgery is performed, thoracoscopy may not offer any advantage other than greater patient comfort.

Whether a more extensive procedure such as lobectomy should be performed thoracoscopically should be determined by considering the patient's potential for early discharge and return to unrestricted activity. A possible advantage in oncology patients relates to concern over the healing of incisions, which often delays radiation therapy. Radiotherapy can be initiated immediately after thoracoscopy without regard to incisional complications.

There are some procedures that can be performed best thoracoscopically. An example is an esophagomyotomy for achalasia. Although this is not often performed in children, the techniques have been well described and are successful in adult patients. Even advocates of bag dilation for achalasia admit that patients treated in this manner require a general anesthetic and run the risk of esophageal perforation at the time of forceful dilation. Thoracoscopy converts a Heller esophagomyotomy to a procedure requiring short hospitalization and eliminates the major objections to the postoperative discomfort of thoracotomy. Because the procedure is performed under direct vision and the risks of perforation are minimal, we believe that this is a better alternative than dilation under general anesthesia. Similarly, if a procedure such as thymectomy can be performed adequately, and all of the thymus can be removed thoracoscopically, this is a better alternative than a median sternotomy with its associated complications. Thus far, in the limited adult experience, this appears to be a reasonable option. It is still too early in the assessment of these procedures in children to say definitively what percentage of procedures should be performed endoscopically. Currently, most pediatric surgeons are well versed in standard operative techniques but have not yet been trained in endoscopic surgery. This is rapidly changing as surgeons now entering pediatric surgical training programs have had a substantial endoscopic surgical experience during their general surgery training. The next generation of pediatric surgeons will be as well versed in endoscopic surgery as the current generation is in open surgery.

We are convinced that endoscopic surgery

offers many advantages. In our practice, we have to ask ourselves the question: Is it better for the patient to perform open surgery or will it be best to perform the procedure endoscopically? We are comfortable with the low complication rate we have encountered. With the obvious patient satisfaction after thoracoscopy and laparoscopy in children, particularly as it relates to earlier discharge from the hospital and early return to unrestricted activities, we have adopted the use of these techniques as a major part of our practice.

References

1. Gans SL, Berci G. Advances in endoscopy of infants and children. J Pediatr Surg 6:199–233, 1971.
2. Rodgers BM, Talbert JL: Thoracoscopy for diagnosis of intrathoracic lesions in children. J Pediatr Surg 11:703–708, 1976.
3. Hawkins DB. Removal of blunt foreign bodies from the esophagus. Ann Otol Rhinol Laryngol 99:935–940, 1990.
4. Myer CM. Potential hazards of esophageal foreign body extraction. Pediatr Radiol 21:97–98, 1991.
5. Schier F, Waldschmidt J. Experience with laparoscopy for the evaluation of cholestasis in newborns. Surg Endosc 4:13–14, 1990.
6. Waldschmidt J, Schier F. Laparoscopical surgery in neonates and infants. Eur J Pediatr Surg 1:145–150, 1991.
7. Taylor E, Feinstein R, White PF, Soper N. Anesthesia for laparoscopic cholecystectomy: is nitrous oxide contraindicated? Anesthesiology 76(4):541–543, 1992.
8. Ponsky JL, Gauderer MWL: Percutaneous endoscopic gastrostomy: a non-operative technique for feeding gastrostomy. Gastrointest Endosc 27:9–11, 1981.
9. Park RHR, Allison MC, Lang J, et al. Randomised comparison of percutaneous endoscopic gastrostomy and nasogastric tube feeding in patients with persisting neurological dysphagia. BMJ 304:1406–1409, 1992.
10. Forgacs I, MacPherson A, Tibbs C. Percutaneous gastrostomy: the end of the line for nasogastric feeding? BMJ 304:1395–1396, 1992.
11. Stiegmann GV, Goff JS, Silas D, et al. Endoscopic versus operative gastrostomy: final results of a prospective randomized trial. Gastrointest Endosc 36(1):1–5, 1990.
12. Dallemagne B, Weerts JM, Jehaes C, et al. Laparoscopic Nissen fundoplication: preliminary report. Surg Laparosc Endosc 1(3):138–143, 1991.
13. Holcomb GW III, Olsen DO, Sharp KW. Laparoscopic cholecystectomy in the pediatric patient. J Pediatr Surg 26(10):1186–1190, 1991.
14. Newman KD, Marmon LM, Attorri R, Evans E. Laparoscopic cholecystectomy in pediatric patients. J Pediatr Surg 26(10):1184–1185, 1991.
15. Sackier JM. Laparoscopy in pediatric surgery. J Pediatr Surg 26(10):1145–1147, 1991.
16. Sigman HH, Laberge J-M, Croitoru D, et al. Laparoscopic cholecystectomy: a treatment option for gallbladder disease in children. J Pediatr Surg 26(10):1181–1183, 1991.
17. Loh A, Taylor RS. Laparoscopic appendicectomy. Br J Surg 79(4):289–290, 1992.
18. Winfield HN, Donovan JF, See WA, et al. Urologic laparoscopic surgery. J Urol 146(4):941–948, 1991.
19. Elder JS. Laparoscopy and Fowler-Stephens orchiopexy in the management of the impalpable testis. Urol Clin North Am 16(2):399–411, 1989.
20. Guiney EJ, Corbally M, Malone PS. Laparoscopy and the management of the impalpable testis. Br J Urol 63:313–316, 1989.
21. Steffen RM, Wyllie R, Sivak MV Jr, et al. Colonoscopy in the pediatric patient. J Pediatr 115(4):507–514, 1989.
22. Lobe TE, Schropp KP. Pediatric laparoscopy and thoracoscopy. Philadelphia: WB Saunders, 1993.

Index

Note: Page numbers in *italics* refer to illustrations;
page numbers followed by t refer to tables.